KU-609-171

Anaesthesia Science

Anaesthesia Science

EDITED BY

Nigel R. Webster

AND

Helen F. Galley

Academic Unit of Anaesthesia and Intensive Care
School of Medicine
University of Aberdeen
Aberdeen, UK

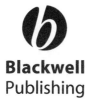

Blackwell
Publishing

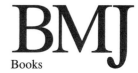

Books

© 2006 by Blackwell Publishing Ltd
BMJ Books is an imprint of the BMJ Publishing Group Limited, used under licence

Blackwell Publishing, Inc., 350 Main Street, Malden, Massachusetts 02148-5020, USA
Blackwell Publishing Ltd, 9600 Garsington Road, Oxford OX4 2DQ, UK
Blackwell Publishing Asia Pty Ltd, 550 Swanston Street, Carlton, Victoria 3053, Australia

The right of the Author to be identified as the Author of this Work has been asserted in accordance with the Copyright, Designs and Patents Act 1988.

All rights reserved. No part of this publication may be reproduced, stored in a retrieval system, or transmitted, in any form or by any means, electronic, mechanical, photocopying, recording or otherwise, except as permitted by the UK Copyright, Designs and Patents Act 1988, without the prior permission of the publisher.

First published 2006

1   2006

ISBN-13: 978-0-7279-1773-7
ISBN-10: 0-7279-1773-0

A catalogue record for this title is available from the British Library and the Library of Congress

Set in 10/12 pt Galliard by SNP Best-set Typesetter Ltd., Hong Kong
Printed and bound in Singapore by C.O.S. Printers PTE Ltd

Commissioning Editor: Mary Banks
Development Editor: Helen Harvey
Production Controller: Debbie Wyer

For further information on Blackwell Publishing, visit our website:
http://www.blackwellpublishing.com

The publisher's policy is to use permanent paper from mills that operate a sustainable forestry policy, and which has been manufactured from pulp processed using acid-free and elementary chlorine-free practices. Furthermore, the publisher ensures that the text paper and cover board used have met acceptable environmental accreditation standards.

Blackwell Publishing makes no representation, express or implied, that the drug dosages in this book are correct. Readers must therefore always check that any product mentioned in this publication is used in accordance with the prescribing information prepared by the manufacturers. The author and the publishers do not accept responsibility or legal liability for any errors in the text or for the misuse or misapplication of material in this book.

Contents

List of Contributors

Peter Andrews MD, MBChB, FRCA
Consultant and Reader in Anaesthesia and Intensive Care
University of Edinburgh Department of Anaesthesia, Critical Care and Pain Medicine
Intensive Care Unit
Western General Hospital
Crewe Road
Edinburgh EH4 2XU
Scotland, UK

Peter Århem PhD
Professor, Nobel Institute for Neurophysiology
Department of Neuroscience
Karolinska Institute
SE-171 77 Stockholm
Sweden

Andrew D. Axon MBChB, FRCA
Department of Anaesthesia
University of Liverpool
Duncan Building
Daulby Street
Liverpool L69 3GA
UK

Stephen Ball PhD, FRCP
Professor of Cardiology
Institute for Cardiovascular Research
Yorkshire Heart Centre
Leeds General Infirmary
Great George Street
Leeds LS1 3EX
UK

Roxanna Bloomfield MBChB, FRCA
Specialist Registrar in Intensive Care Medicine
Hon. Clinical Tutor, University of Aberdeen
Intensive Care Unit
Aberdeen Royal Infirmary
Foresterhill
Aberdeen AB25 2ZN
Scotland, UK

Daniel Burke MBChB, FRCA
Department of Anaesthesia
St John's Hospital
Livingston EH54 6PP
Scotland, UK

Jeremy Cohen MBBS, BSc, MRCP, FRCA, FJFICM
Department of Intensive Care Medicine
3rd Floor Ned Hanlon Building
Royal Brisbane and Women's Hospital
Butterfield Street
Herston 4029
Queensland, Australia

Lesley Colvin MBChB, FRCA, PhD
Department of Anaesthesia, Critical Care and Pain Medicine
Western General Hospital
Crewe Road
Edinburgh EH4 2XU
Scotland, UK

Leanne Coyne
Thomas J Long School of Pharmacy & Health Sciences
University of the Pacific
Stockton
California 95211
USA

Peter De Paepe MD, PhD
Professor in Clinical Pharmacology
Department of Pharmacology and Department of Emergency Medicine
Ghent University Hospital
De Pintelaan 185
900 Ghent
Belgium

Thomas Engelhardt MD, FRCA
Institute Medical Sciences
Anaesthesia and Intensive Care
Foresterhill
Aberdeen AB25 9ZD
Scotland, UK

Professor Malcolm Fisher AO, MBChB, MD, FANZCA, FRCA, FJFICM
Clinical Professor, Intensive Therapy Unit
University of Sydney at Royal North Shore Hospital
St Leonards NSW 2065
Australia

Helen F. Galley PhD, FIMLF
Senior Lecturer in Anaesthesia and
  Intensive Care
Academic Unit of Anaesthesia and
  Intensive Care
School of Medicine
University of Aberdeen
Aberdeen AB25 2ZD
Scotland, UK

**Fiona J. Gilbert MBChB, FRCR,
FRCP**
Professor of Radiology, Department of
  Radiology
University of Aberdeen
Lilian Sutton Building
Foresterhill
Aberdeen AB25 2ZD
Scotland, UK

George M. Hall
Professor of Anaesthesia
Department of Anaesthesia and
  Intensive Care Medicine
St George's Hospital, University of
  London
London SW17 0RE
UK

Susan Hill MA, PhD, FRCA
Consultant Neuroanaesthetist
Shackleton Department of Anaesthesia
Southampton General Hospital
Tremona Road
Southampton SO16 6YD
UK

**Anita Holdcroft MBChB, MD,
FRCA**
Reader in Anaesthesia and Honorary
  Consultant Anaesthetist
Department of Anaesthetics, Pain
  Medicine and Intensive Care
Division of Surgery, Oncology,
  Reproductive biology and
  Anaesthetics (SORA)
Faculty of Medicine
Imperial College London
Chelsea and Westminster Hospital
369 Fulham Road
London SW10 9NH
UK

**Jennifer M. Hunter MBChB, PhD,
FRCA**
Department of Anaesthesia
University of Liverpool
Duncan Building
Daulby Street
Liverpool L69 3GA
UK

Praveen Kalia FRCA, DA, MD
Consultant in Anaesthesia
North Tees and Hartlepool NHS Trust
Holdforth Road
Hartlepool TS24 9AH
UK

Alain Kalmar MD
Research Fellow
Department of Anaesthesia
Ghent University Hospital
De Pintelaan 185
900 Ghent
Belgium

**John A. Kellum MD, FACP, FCCP,
FCCM**
The CRISMA Laboratory
Department of Critical Care Medicine
University of Pittsburgh School of
  Medicine
608 Scaife Hall
Pittsburgh, PA 15213 2582
USA

Anand Kumar MD
Associate Professor of Medicine
Health Sciences Centre/St. Boniface
  Hospital
Department of Medicine
University of Manitoba
710 Park Blvd South
Winnipeg, MB
Canada R3P-0X1

Martin Kuper BM, BCh
SPR Anaesthesia
Royal Brompton Hospital
Sydney Street
London SW3 6NP
UK

George Lees PhD, FRPharmS
Professor of Neurophysiology and
  Neuropharmacology
Chair Department of Pharmacology &
  Toxicology
School of Medical Sciences
Otago University
PO Box 913
Dunedin
New Zealand

**Jeffrey Lipman MBBCh, DA (SA),
FFA (Crit Care), FJFICM**
Professor and Head
Anaesthesiology and Critical Care
University of Queensland
Department of Intensive Care Medicine
3rd Floor Ned Hanlon Building
Royal Brisbane and Women's Hospital
Butterfield Street
Herston 4029
Queensland, Australia

Andrew Lumb MB, BS, FRCA
Consultant Anaesthetist
Department of Anaesthetics
St James's Univesity Hospital
Leeds LS9 7TF
UK

Karen M. Maddison MRPharmS
University of Sunderland Pharmacy
  School
Sunderland SR1 3SD
UK

Amr Mahdy MBChB, MD, FRCA
Lecturer in Anaesthesia
Academic Unit of Anaesthesia and
  Intensive Care
School of Medicine
University of Aberdeen
Aberdeen AB 25 2ZD
Scotland, UK

**Stuart Murdoch MBChB,
MMedSc, FRCA**
Consultant in Intensive Care
  Medicine/Anaesthesia
St James's University Hospital
Beckett Street
Leeds LS9 7TF
UK

Nanotechnology Study Group
K. Al-Tarrah, L. Balchin, T. Gilbertson, Y. Gourtsoyannis, F. Khiard, J. Partridge, R. Sidhu, N.R. Webster, J. Weir-McCall
University of Aberdeen
Scotland, UK

Grainne Nicholson
Senior Lecturer in Anaesthesia
Department of Anaesthesia and Intensive Care Medicine
St George's Hospital, Universty of London
London SW17 0RE
UK

Johanna Nilsson
Nobel Institute for Neurophysiology
Department of Neuroscience
Karolinska Institute
SE-171 77 Stockholm
Sweden

David Noble BMedBiol, MBChB, FRCA
Consultant in Anaesthesia and Intensive Care Medicine
Hon. Clinical Senior Lecturer, University of Aberdeen
Intensive Care Unit
Aberdeen Royal Infirmary
Foresterhill
Aberdeen AB25 2ZN
Scotland, UK

Sze-Yuan Michael Ooi MD, MBBS
Research Registrar in Cardiology
Institute for Cardiovascular Research
Yorkshire Heart Centre
Leeds General Infirmary
Great George Street
Leeds LS1 3EX
UK

Christopher Pepper MD, MRCP
Consultant Cardiologist
Yorkshire Heart Centre
Leeds General Infirmary
Great George Street
Leeds LS1 3EX
UK

Bryce Randalls
Consultant and Hon. Senior Lecturer in Intensive Care Medicine
Intensive Care Unit
Aberdeen Royal Infirmary
Foresterhill
Aberdeen AB25 2ZN
Scotland, UK

Thomas W. Redpath BSc, MSc, PhD
Professor, Department of Radiology
University of Aberdeen
Lilian Sutton Building
Foresterhill
Aberdeen AB25 2ZD
Scotland, UK

Charles S. Reilly
Professor, Academic Anaesthesia Unit
Floor K
Royal Hallamshire Hospital
Glossop Road
Sheffield S10 2JF
UK

Jonathan Rhodes MBChB, FRCA
Clinical Lecturer
University of Edinburgh Department of Anaesthesia, Critical Care and Pain Medicine
Intensive Care Unit
Western General Hospital
Crewe Road
Edinburgh EH4 2XU
Scotland, UK

Michael Rose MBBS, BSc(Med), FANZCA
Staff Specialist
Department of Anaesthesia and Pain Management
University of Sydney at Royal North Shore Hospital
St Leonards NSW 2065
Australia

Kristoffer Sahlholm
Nobel Institute for Neurophysiology
Department of Neuroscience
Karolinska Institute
SE-171 77 Stockholm
Sweden

John Robert Sneyd MD, FRCA
Associate Dean and Professor of Anaesthesia
Peninsula Medical School, C304
Portland Square
University of Plymouth
Drake Circus
Plymouth PL4 8AA
UK

Neil Soni
Consultant, Intensive Care and Anaesthetics
Magill Department of Anaesthetics and Critical Care
Chelsea and Westminster Hospital
London SW10 9NH
UK

Michel M.R.F. Struys MD, PhD
Professor in Anaesthesia and Research Coordinator
Department of Anaesthesia
Ghent University Hospital
De Pintelaan 185
9000 Ghent
Belgium

Susan Walwyn MBChB, FRCA
Specialist Registrar in Anaesthetics
Department of Anaesthetics
St James's Univesity Hospital
Leeds LS9 7TF
UK

Nigel R. Webster BSc, MBChB, PhD, FRCA, FRCP, FRCS
Professor, Anaesthesia and Intensive Care
School of Medicine
University of Aberdeen
Aberdeen AB25 2ZD
Scotland, UK

Preface

Basic science underlies the practice of anaesthesia. *Anaesthesia Science* aims to present the scientific foundations upon which the clinical practice of anaesthesia and care of the critically ill are based. Other volumes provide more comprehensive texts and it was not our intention to replace these well known and valuable textbooks, but rather to complement areas given less emphasis elsewhere. This book aims to give the reader detailed coverage on less well appreciated aspects of the subject. Each up-to-date chapter encompasses salient features of the scientific foundations of anaesthesia not found elsewhere in a single volume. We aimed to integrate anaesthesia with basic sciences with no artificial boundaries separating the two.

The basic medical sciences are all represented in the discipline of anaesthesia and technological advances have contributed to the development of modern safe anaesthetic practice. We hope that we have presented basic science in a readable and fascinating way to enthuse those practising anaesthesia and its sub-specialities.

Helen F. Galley
Nigel R. Webster
Aberdeen, 2006

PART 1
Pharmacology

CHAPTER 1
Pharmacokinetic principles

Michel M.R.F. Struys, Alain Kalmar and Peter De Paepe

Introduction

Pharmacokinetics can be defined as the characterization and prediction of the time course of the concentration of a drug in the body. This includes the characteristics of drug absorption, distribution, metabolism and elimination. Pharmacokinetic models can be used to predict the time course of this drug concentration. Variations in body composition or organ function — for example, in children, in pregnant women and fetuses *in utero*, in elderly populations and in patients with organ dysfunction — may affect anaesthetic drug distribution and elimination and therefore drug responses. In this chapter, we first briefly describe some of the basic concepts governing pharmacokinetics. Secondly, we focus on the concepts of pharmacokinetic modelling and, thirdly, the influence of various physiological changes on the pharmacokinetics of drugs is described.

Drug absorption

Transfer of drugs across membranes

To reach a therapeutic concentration at their site of action, drugs need to pass through the cell membranes that separate different compartments in the body [1]. These membranes are 5–10 nm wide and are arranged in a lipid bilayer structure. This bilayer is present in a fluid state embedding a mosaic of dispersed proteins that can penetrate both outer or inner leaflet of the lipid sheet [1,2]. The structure of the lipids in cell membranes varies widely, although all of them are amphipatic. The membrane lipids comprise phospholipids, sphingolipids and cholesterol, and most membrane proteins are glycoproteins carrying carbohydrates on their outer surface. In the same way, some phospholipids are glycolipids. The molecules in cell membranes are orientated in such a way that non-polar elements are confined to the core and polar elements are exposed on either side. The hydrophobic core favours the crossing of lipid-soluble molecules and hampers the movement of water-soluble ones across the cell membranes [2]. The nature of the compartmentalization by membranes strongly depends on the specific structure of the barrier in different tissues. In some tissues, such as the gastrointestinal tract, the lining cells are closely connected. In other tissues, such as the glomerulus of the kidney, there are gaps between cells allowing filtration [1]. The permeability of vascular endothelium throughout the body also varies. There are gaps between endothelial cells of the capillary wall, but in some tissues, such as the central nervous system (CNS), there are tight junctions between the endothelial cells of the capillaries forming the blood–brain barrier [1,3].

Theoretically, drugs can move across cell membranes by passive mechanisms or by active processes [4]. Lipophylic drugs cross cell membranes very easily by simple diffusion. The rate of diffusion across the membrane depends on the concentration gradient, the size of the molecules (smaller molecules diffuse more easily than large ones), the lipid solubility, membrane properties such as the membrane area and thickness, and the diffusion coefficient. Drugs in a charged, ionized form cannot pass through membranes by simple diffusion; only the uncharged fraction can [1]. The Henderson–Hasselbalch equation makes it possible to calculate the uncharged fraction of a drug, given its pKa and the ambient pH. From:

$$pH = pKa + \log base/acid \qquad (1)$$

For acidic drugs, this results in:

$$pH = pKa + \frac{\text{log ionized concentration/}}{\text{unionized concentration}} \quad (2)$$

For basic drugs, this results in:

$$pH = pKa + \frac{\text{log unionized concentration/}}{\text{ionized concentration}} \quad (3)$$

Ionization is not only important in determining the rate of which a compound can move across a membrane, it is also important in determining the partition of a drug between compartments with a different ambient pH. Diffusion of water-soluble drugs is restricted by passage through aqueous pores that span the cell membrane. However, these channels are too small to let most drugs pass through them. Endothelial membranes in the capillaries can have larger pores allowing bulky molecules to pass through [4]. Diffusion can also be facilitated by carrier-mediated mechanisms that operate along a concentration gradient without making use of an energy source. This is called 'facilitated diffusion' [1].

Active transfer mechanisms require energy. The energy can be supplied by the hydrolysis of adenosine triphosphate (ATP) directly, as for instance in the case of Na^+/K^+ ATPase, or indirectly by the coupling of the passive transfer of one compound along its ionic gradient with the movement of another molecule against its concentration gradient [3]. An example of such a transport system is the absorption of amino acids from the small bowel lumen into intestinal cells [1]. This transfer is achieved by a coupling with Na^+ diffusion that occurs down its electrochemical gradient. Maintenance of the latter requires energy and ultimately depends on the Na^+/K^+ ATPase system [3].

Pinocytosis transports large molecules [3]. In this process a part of the cell membrane is invaginated to form a vesicle, which engulfs extracellular material, and is removed via exocytotic mechanisms.

Drug administration techniques in anaesthesia

There are many ways in which a drug can be given. Although most drugs are given orally, in anaesthesia many drugs are administered intravenously. Because absorption is bypassed, drug action is very fast by this route. However, for all other routes of drug administration, the drug must be absorbed from the site of application before being carried in the circulation to its site of action.

Intramuscular or subcutaneous administration

Many factors affect the rate of absorption after intramuscular or subcutaneous injection. The molecular weight of the compound, the vehicle in which the drug is dissolved, the volume that is given and, last but not least, the local perfusion of the muscle and fat tissue are important [5]. Some drugs are absorbed very easily, but for others the absorption is poor or unpredictable (e.g. diazepam) [6]. After the injection of water-soluble drugs, the plasma level can increase rapidly, because these compounds enter the circulation very fast. This is especially true for drugs with low molecular weight, which can reach the systemic circulation by entering the capillaries directly [5]. The use of vasoconstrictors or vasodilators, as well as individual patient haemodynamics, can also markedly influence the rate of absorption.

Inhalation

Depending on the particle size, inhaled drugs will mainly reach airway mucosa from the larynx to the bronchioles, creating local effects, or reach the alveolus, allowing largely systemic effects. However, systemic absorption may still occur in both cases [5]. Volatile molecules readily reach the alveolar space and can enter the systemic circulation within seconds. The rate of absorption of volatile anaesthetics is determined by adequacy of pulmonary ventilation, cardiac output, inspired concentration and anaesthetic solubility [7].

Epidural, intrathecal and perineural administration

Epidural, intrathecal or perineural administration of drugs is used for providing regional analgesia and anaesthesia. The onset time depends on the concentration of unionized local anaesthetic around the axon. Because local anaesthetics are bases, adding sodium bicarbonate reduces onset time in epidural solutions. Addition of a vasoconstrictor increases the duration of the block [1].

Oral administration

Multiple factors are involved in the absorption of the drug from the gastrointestinal tract to the systemic circulation. First-pass metabolism, unpredictable pharmacokinetics and a latent period before maximal concentration in plasma make this route unsuitable for many anaesthetics [8].

Rectal administration

The rectal blood flow partly drains directly into the systemic circulation, avoiding first-pass metabolism, although absorption is unpredictable [1].

Sublingual, buccal and nasal administration

While permitting very fast absorption of certain drugs, these routes directly drain into the systemic circulation, avoiding first-pass effect [5].

Bioavailability

Bioavailability is generally defined as the fraction of an extravascularly administered dose that reaches the systemic circulation [5]. An orally administered dose is only partially absorbed from the gut and partially metabolized in the gut wall and liver before reaching the systemic circulation.

Drug absorption and first-pass effect

Before the drug can cross the mucosal membranes after oral intake, the tablets must disintegrate and dissolve. Pharmaceutical factors such as chemical formulation, particle size, coatings or the inclusion of inert filters influence this dissolution process [8]. Because most drugs only pass the lipid membranes in their unionized form, the regional pH greatly influences absorption. Consequently, acidic drugs would mainly be absorbed in the stomach, but the large surface area and anatomical properties of the small intestine make this the main absorption site for all drugs [4]. The speed of gastric emptying, simultaneous intake of other drugs or food and pathological conditions also influence the speed and degree of drug absorption [1]. Before reaching the systemic circulation, the drugs need to pass through the intestinal mucosa and the liver [8]. Metabolism of the drug may occur in the gut wall or by the liver,

further reducing the amount that reaches the target organ.

Drug distribution

The basic pharmacokinetic parameter to describe drug distribution is the apparent volume of distribution (V_d), calculated as:

$$V_d = \text{amount of drug/concentration} \tag{4}$$

It must be noted, however, that this has been simplified by assuming that the drug is administered into a single, well-mixed compartment. If the drug remains unbound in the plasma and does not distribute into other tissues, the V_d would be the same as the plasma volume. However, most drugs leave the plasma and distribute into and bind to other tissues. Drug distribution throughout the body depends largely on organ blood flow and physicochemical properties of the drug, such as lipid solubility and protein binding.

Blood flow

Shortly after a drug enters the systemic circulation, tissue concentrations rise in the more highly perfused organs, such as the brain and liver. Organs with lower blood flow will take longer to equilibrate, and, in some cases, this may take several hours or even days [4].

Lipid solubility

After passing into the extravascular space, water-soluble drugs are mostly limited to the extracellular fluid, while lipid-soluble drugs easily cross cell membranes and can accumulate in certain tissues. For instance, lipophilic drugs such as thiopental may accumulate in fat, and be redistributed to other organs afterwards, prolonging the duration of drug action [4]. This indicates that drug distribution throughout the body depends largely on physicochemical properties.

Protein binding

In plasma, many drugs are bound to a variable degree to plasma proteins and, because only free unbound drug is able to move across capillary membranes, this protein-bound fraction cannot be regarded as pharmacologically active [4,9]. The plasma proteins have multiple binding sites and the amount of drug bound depends on its total concentration, the competition for binding by other compounds for the same binding sites, the concentration of protein and the affinity between drug and protein [10]. As a rule, neutral and acidic drugs bind to albumin and basic drugs bind also to α_1-acid glycoprotein and lipoproteins [1]. Plasma protein binding is particularly important for drugs that occupy a large portion of the available binding sites at therapeutic concentrations. With these drugs, a small increase in the bound fraction can increase the unbound fraction out of proportion [1,6].

Special membranes

Blood–brain barrier
Contrary to most tissues, where capillary membranes are freely permeable, cerebral capillaries form tight junctions, restricting free diffusion of drugs into the cerebral extracellular fluid. Besides this structural barrier, astrocytes form a metabolic or enzymatic blood–brain barrier that neutralize certain agents before they reach the CNS. Penetration of drugs into the brain depends on ionization, molecular weight, lipid solubility and protein-binding [5]. However, peptides such as bradykinin and enkephalins and certain conditions such as inflammation can increase the blood–brain barrier permeability, allowing normally impermeable substances to enter the brain [6].

Placental barrier
Most low molecular weight, lipid-soluble drugs can easily cross the placental barrier while large molecular weight or polar molecules cannot [8]. Differences in fetal blood pH, placental blood flow, protein binding and fetal metabolism influence fetal free drug levels [1]. As a rule, drugs that affect the CNS — and consequently pass the blood–brain barrier — can also cross the placenta [8].

Drug metabolism

After administration, most drugs (certainly if they are lipid-soluble) have to be metabolized before they can leave the body. In most cases metabolism reduces the activity of a drug, but in some cases metabolic conversion of a drug may increase or only partially decrease its activity. Generally, metabolism results in a more water-soluble molecule that can be excreted more easily. The main organ for drug metabolism is the liver [8], but processes also take place in the gut, plasma, gastric mucosa, lung or other organs [1]. Metabolism consists of two phases.

Phase I
In phase I, molecules are chemically activated to prepare for possible phase II reaction [5]. Three types of enzymatic reactions may occur: oxidation, reduction and hydrolysis.

Oxidation
Many oxidative reactions take place in the endoplasmatic reticulum of the liver, the microsomes, and are catalysed by the cytochrome P450 system. The P450 superfamily comprises more than 30 different isoenzymes in humans. However, the majority of P450s involved in drug metabolism belong to three distinct families: CYP1, CYP2 and CYP3. These are essential in the elimination of drugs as well as in the synthesis or metabolism of endogenous compounds. Monoamines are metabolized by monoamine oxidase in the mitochondria. Alcohol dehydrogenase is localized in the cytoplasm.

Reduction
These reactions typically take place in the hepatic endoplasmic reticulum and cell cytoplasm. As in oxidation, the cytochrome P450 system is responsible for many reduction reactions [8].

Hydrolysis
Esterases are active in plasma as well as in the liver. They are able to hydrolyse an ester to the alcohols and the carboxylic acid.

Phase II
Conjugation or synthesis
These reactions include glucuronidation, sulphation, acetylation, methylation or glycination. This generally increases the water solubility, favouring renal or biliary excretion, and most of these reactions

take place in the liver microsomes, but the lung is also involved [1].

Drug excretion

Either directly or after biotransformation, drugs are eliminated out of the body in urine or bile. Small amounts are also excreted in saliva, sweat and milk, but this is usually of little quantitative significance [5]. Small molecules are mainly excreted in urine; high molecular weight molecules (>400–500 Da) are preferentially eliminated in bile.

Renal excretion

Three processes account for renal drug excretion: filtration, secretion and diffusion.

Glomerular filtration

Glomerular filtration is a passive process involving filtration of mainly unbound fraction of water-soluble molecules. Large or highly protein-bound molecules will not cross the glomerular membrane [8].

Tubular secretion

Tubular secretion is an active carrier-mediated secretion that may take place against a concentration gradient. For some drugs, complete clearance may be achieved in a single renal circulation [8].

Tubular diffusion

In the distal renal tube, depending on urine pH, important passive diffusion may take place between the urine and the plasma. This mechanism is restricted to substances capable of crossing tubular cell membranes and can result in marked reabsorption of excreted drugs. In addition, the elimination of certain drugs can be increased by alterations in urine pH; after diffusion of the non-ionized fraction of certain basic drugs from the relatively alkaline plasma to the acid urine, they are trapped as cations and excreted [8].

Biliary excretion

Hepatocytes actively transport high molecular weight molecules, such as the steroid-based muscle relaxants, to the bile. This is a saturable process which can be inhibited by other drugs. Active transport may result in significant concentration of certain drugs, up to 100 times the plasma level [5]. Some drugs require conjugation, but others are excreted unchanged in bile. Conjugated drugs excreted in the bile may be subsequently hydrolysed by bacteria in the gut and reabsorbed, increasing their biological half-life [1], a process called enterohepatic recirculation.

Drug clearance

The two main organs responsible for drug excretion are the liver and kidneys. Clearance is defined as the volume of plasma from which a drug is completely removed per time unit. Many drugs are metabolized by the liver and although their metabolites may stay in the blood for some time before actual excretion, they often have no or little residual pharmacological effect. On the other hand, a drug may be removed from the body both by urinary excretion of unchanged drug and by hepatic metabolism.

Clearance values can be considered as the sum of the clearances by the various organs involved for a certain drug:

$$Cl = Cl_R + Cl_H + CL_X \tag{5}$$

whereby Cl_R is renal clearance, Cl_H is hepatic clearance and CL_X is clearance by other routes. The clearance of most drugs is mainly dependent on the liver, either by hepatic metabolism and/or biliary excretion [8].

The pharmacokinetic concept of hepatic clearance takes into consideration that the drug is transported to the liver by the portal vein and the hepatic artery and leaves the organ by the hepatic vein [11]. It diffuses from plasma water to reach the metabolic enzymes. There are at least three major parameters to consider in quantifying drug elimination by the liver: blood flow through the organ (Q), which reflects transport to the liver; free fraction of drug in blood (f_u), which affects access of drug to the enzymes; and intrinsic ability of the hepatic enzymes to metabolize the drug, expressed as intrinsic clearance (Cl_{int}). Intrinsic clearance is the ability of the liver to remove drug in the absence of flow limitations and blood binding. Taking into account these three parameters, the hepatic clearance can be expressed by:

$$Cl = \frac{Q \cdot f_u \cdot Cl_{int}}{Q + f_u \cdot Cl_{int}} \qquad (6)$$

It is obvious that the hepatic clearance cannot be larger than the total volume of blood reaching the liver per unit time (i.e. the liver blood flow Q). The ratio of the hepatic clearance of a drug to the hepatic blood flow is called the extraction ratio of the drug (E), which can be expressed as:

$$E = \frac{C_a - C_v}{C_a} = \frac{f_u \cdot Cl_{int}}{Q + f_u \cdot Cl_{int}} \qquad (7)$$

where C_a is the concentration in the mixed portal venous and hepatic arterial blood and C_v is the hepatic venous blood concentration. The value of the extraction ratio can vary between 0 and 1. It is 0 when $f_u \cdot Cl_{int}$ is zero (i.e. when the drug is not metabolized in the liver); it is 1 when the hepatic clearance equals hepatic blood flow (approximately 1.5 L/min in humans).

The extraction ratio can be generally classified as high (>0.7), intermediate (0.3–0.7) or low (<0.3) according to the fraction of drug removed during one pass through the liver. The effect of critical illness on hepatic clearance depends on these extraction characteristics of the drug as explained below (see p. 18). Table 1.1 lists the hepatic extraction ratio in humans for some sedative and analgesic drugs.

Table 1.1 Some example drugs with various hepatic extraction ratios (ER).

Low ER (ER < 0.3)	Intermediate ER (ER 0.3–0.7)	High ER (ER > 0.7)
Diazepam	Alfentanil	Fentanyl
Lorazepam	Chlorpromazine	Flumazenil
Methadone	Diphenhydramine	Ketamine
Pentobarbital	Droperidol	Morphine
Chlordiazepoxide	Etomidate	Nalmefene
	Haloperidol	Naloxone
	Hydromorphone	Propofol
	Midazolam	Sufentanil
	Pethidine	

High extraction drugs

Drugs with a high hepatic extraction have a high intrinsic hepatic metabolizing capacity ($f_u \cdot Cl_{int} \gg Q$) and are rapidly and extensively cleared by the liver from the blood. Their clearance depends primarily on hepatic blood flow, and binding to blood components is not an obstacle for extraction; the extraction is said to be non-restrictive or blood flow dependent. This results in a simplification of equation 6:

$$Cl \approx Q \qquad (8)$$

Changes in protein binding will have no influence on the clearance of high extraction drugs. The importance of changes in protein binding must also be assessed by evaluating the influence on the drug concentrations, particularly on the free drug concentrations as they determine the drug effect. This is made clear by the following equations, which illustrate the relationship between total (C_{SS}) and unbound ($C_{SS,u}$) drug concentrations at steady state, and Cl following intravenous drug administration:

$$C_{SS} = \frac{R_0}{Cl} \qquad (9)$$

and

$$C_{SS,u} = \frac{f_u \cdot R_0}{Cl} \qquad (10)$$

where R_0 represents the rate of drug input. Because $Cl \approx Q$ (equation 8) for high extraction drugs, one can substitute Q for Cl in equations 9 and 10. It is apparent that C_{SS} is not affected by changes in protein binding, whereas $C_{SS,u}$ changes directly with f_u. The latter implies that for high extraction drugs, changes in free drug fraction may result in alterations in drug effect.

Low extraction drugs

Drugs with a low hepatic extraction have a low intrinsic hepatic metabolizing capacity ($f_u \cdot Cl_{int} \ll Q$) and are extracted less avidly and incompletely from hepatic blood. Their clearance is relatively independent of hepatic blood flow, and is primarily determined by the intrinsic metabolizing capacity of the liver and by the free drug fraction; the extraction is said to be restrictive or capacity limited. This results in a simplification of equation 6:

$$Cl \approx f_u \cdot Cl_{int} \tag{11}$$

Changes in free fraction may occur during critical illness and will result in alterations of clearance of low extraction drugs. When substituting equation 11 into equations 9 and 10, it is clear that for low extraction drugs changes in protein binding are inversely related to C_{SS}, but have no effect on $C_{SS,u}$.

Intermediate extraction drugs

The clearance of drugs with intermediate extraction is dependent on hepatic blood flow, the intrinsic metabolizing capacity of the liver and free drug fraction.

Pharmacokinetic analysis of the time course of the drug concentration

Pharmacokinetic analysis in the individual patient

The study of the time course of drug concentrations in plasma, urine and other sampled sites has been helped by the development of sensitive analytic techniques such as high performance liquid chromatography (HPLC), mass spectrometry and radioimmunoassay. Changes in measured drug concentration in relation to time are used to derive pharmacokinetic constants that describe the behaviour of drugs in the body. The two most important pharmacokinetic constants to describe the characteristics of a drug are the volume of distribution (V_d) and clearance (Cl). The volume of distribution represents the apparent volume available in the body from the distribution of the drug. The clearance represents the body's ability to remove drug from the blood or plasma. Both V_d and Cl can be determined from a decline in their plasma concentration after drug administration.

Two methods to determine V_d and Cl are discussed in this chapter. Although model-independent analysis still represents the gold standard by which the estimates of other techniques should be compared, this approach does not offer sufficient information to facilitate the development of rational drug dosing guidelines. Therefore, compartmental or physiological model-dependent analysis is mandatory.

Model-independent pharmacokinetic analysis

Model-independent pharmacokinetics represents a straightforward approach based purely on mathematical descriptions of blood or plasma profiles of drugs or metabolites without invoking a particular model. In many situations, such as during drug development, it is sufficient to characterize plasma profiles in terms of maximum plasma concentration levels, C_{max}, time of maximum level, t_{max}, and area under the plasma curve, AUC. These parameters can be obtained by simple inspection of the plasma or blood concentration of the drug versus time, as seen in Fig. 1.1. From AUC, one can determine the clearance and volume of distribution [12].

The AUC, representing the change in concentration (C) during time (t) (starting at the moment of drug administration) can be calculated by using the integral:

$$AUC = \int_0^\infty C(t) \cdot dt \tag{12}$$

In practice, the AUC can be estimated using the 'trapezoidal rule'. Because the total amount of drug eliminated between the moment of drug administration and infinity must be equal to the dose, we can rewrite equation 12 as follows:

$$Dose = CL \cdot AUC \tag{13}$$

From equation 13, we can calculate the drug clearance (CL) as:

$$CL = Dose / AUC \tag{14}$$

The second basic pharmacokinetic parameter, volume of distribution (V_d), can also be determined as:

$$V_d = CL \cdot MRT \tag{15}$$

Whereby MRT stands for the 'mean residence time', calculated as the ratio between the total area under the first moment of the plasma concentration–time curve (i.e. the area under the plasma concentration $\times$ time versus time curve, extrapolated to infinity) or AUMC and the AUC:

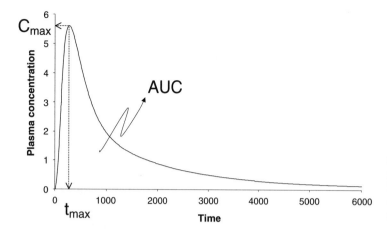

Figure 1.1 Time course of the plasma concentration of a drug after bolus injection. AUC, area under the curve; C_{max}, maximum plasma concentration; t_{max}, time at C_{max}.

$$MRT = AUMC/AUC \qquad (16)$$

It has to be stated that the V_d calculated here is the apparent volume of distribution. If the drug remains unbound in the plasma and does not distribute into other tissues, the V_d would be equal to the plasma volume. As most drugs distribute through extravascular sites in the body and bind to other tissues, the apparent V_d might be much larger than the whole body volume. In contrast, the initial volume is usually reported, which, for an intravenous bolus dose, is determined using equation 16:

$$V_d = Amount/Concentration = dose/C_0 \qquad (17)$$

whereby the drug concentration is 'back-extrapolated' to time zero (C_0).

Model-dependent pharmacokinetic analysis

Two approaches towards model dependent pharmacokinetic analysis are discussed: *compartmental* and *physiological models*. In the *compartmental* model, the body is assumed to be made up of one or more compartments. These compartments might be special or chemical in nature but, in most cases, the compartment is used to represent a body volume or group of similar tissues or fluids into which a drug is distributed. In the physiological model approach, pharmacokinetic modelling is based on known anatomical or physiological values and the modelling of drug movement is based on the flow rates through partic-

ular organs or tissues and experimentally determined blood-tissue concentration ratios. Although compartmental models are dramatically simplifying the 'pharmacokinetic reality' and physiological models might be a more realistic approximation, compartmental models are often used clinically in anaesthesia to predict the plasma concentration of various drugs (e.g. propofol, opioids). Since the introduction of computer-controlled drug delivery systems into clinical practice (so-called target controlled infusion devices), it is crucial to understand the underlying theoretical concepts of compartmental models. Therefore, the development of these models is explained in more detail below.

Compartmental models

The simplest pharmacokinetic model is the 'one-compartment model' with a single volume (V) and clearance (CL), as shown in Fig. 1.2. Clearance is calculated as $k_{10} \cdot V$, whereby k_{10} is the rate constant for drug elimination. Although almost none of the drugs used in anaesthesia can be accurately characterized by the one-compartment model, it allows the introduction of some mathematical concepts. There are two forms of processes: zero-order and first-order. A zero-order process is one that happens at a constant rate. The mathematics of the rate of change (dx/dt) is simple:

$$Constant\ rate\ of\ change = k = dx/dt \qquad (18)$$

where x is the amount of drug and t is time.

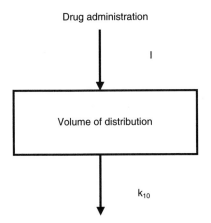

Drug administration

I

Volume of distribution

k_{10}

Figure 1.2 The one-compartment pharmacokinetic model.

If the value of x at time t is needed, $x(t)$, it is found as the integral of the equation 18 from time 0 to time t:

$$x(t) = x_0 + k \cdot t \qquad (19)$$

where x_0 is the value of x at $t = t_0$. This is a straight line with a slope of k and an intercept of x_0.

A first-order process is much more complex. The rate of change for a first-order process is:

$$dx/dt = k \cdot x \qquad (20)$$

where the units of k are simply 1/time. If a value of x at time t is needed, $x(t)$, it can be found as the integral of the equation 20 from time 0 to time t:

$$x(t) = x_0 \cdot e^{-kt} \qquad (21)$$

By using the equation $C_0 = x_0/V$, where C_0 is the concentration at time 0, x_0 is the initial dose of drug and V is the volume of the compartment, the plasma concentrations over time after an IV bolus of drug are then described by:

$$C(t) = C_0 \cdot e^{-kt} \qquad (22)$$

This is the commonly used expression relating concentration to time and initial plasma concentration and the rate constants. It defines the 'concentration over time' curve for the one-compartment model and has a log-linear shape. The one-compartment model is frequently used in pharmacology to describe the pharmacokinetics of drugs. It demonstrates the

concepts of volumes, clearances and rate constants. In this model, no distribution phenomenon occurs. Unfortunately, none of the intravenous hypnotic anaesthetic drugs used in clinical anaesthesia can be characterized accurately by a one-compartment model because of their distribution into and out of the peripheral tissues. Therefore, it is necessary to extend this one-compartment model to a multicompartmental one.

Several multicompartment models are described in the literature [13,14]. Although a two-compartmental model is used commonly in general drug research, the most popular one in anaesthesia is the three-compartment mammalian model, as shown in Fig. 1.3. In anaesthesia, all clinically used, target controlled, infusion techniques and pharmacokinetic computer simulations are based on this model.

The fundamental variables of the compartment model are the volume of distribution (central, rapidly and slowly equilibrating peripheral volumes) and the clearances (systemic, rapid and slow intercompartmental). As shown in Fig. 1.3, the drug is injected into and eliminated either by metabolism or renal excretion from this central compartment (compartment 1). The drug is quickly distributed into a rapidly equilibrating peripheral compartment (compartment 2) and this compartment quickly reaches equilibrium with the central compartment. The drug is distributed more slowly into a third compartment (compartment 3). The sum of the compartmental volumes is the apparent volume of distribution during steady-state (V_{dSS}) and is proportionally constant, relating the plasma drug concentration at steady-state to the amount of drug in the body [13].

Micro-rate constants, expressed as k_{ij}, define the rate of drug transfer from compartment i to compartment j. Compartment 0 is a compartment outside the model, so k_{10} is the micro-rate constant for those processes acting through biotransformation or elimination that irreversibly remove drug from the central compartment (compartment 1). The intercompartmental micro-rate constants (k_{12}, k_{21}, etc.) describe the exchange of drug between the central and peripheral compartments. Each compartment has at least two micro-rate constants: one for drug entry and one for drug exit. The differential

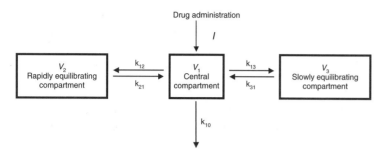

Drug administration

Figure 1.3 The three-compartment pharmacokinetic model.

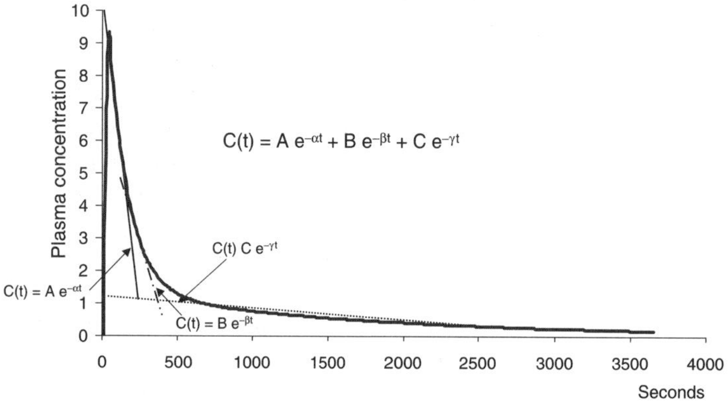

$$C(t) = A\,e^{-\alpha t} + B\,e^{-\beta t} + C\,e^{-\gamma t}$$

$C(t)\,C\,e^{-\gamma t}$

$C(t) = A\,e^{-\alpha t}$

$C(t) = B\,e^{-\beta t}$

Figure 1.4 The triexponential curve representing the time course of a drug plasma concentration after intravenous injection. Each exponential term accounts for a portion of the curve. The individual lines associated with each exponential term are also shown. The triexponential curve represents the algebraic sum of the individual exponential functions. Solid, dashed and dotted lines are used to show how each exponential relates to different portions of the full curve.

equations describing the rate of change for the amount of drugs in compartments 1, 2 and 3, follow directly from the micro-rate constants (note the similarity to the one-compartment model).

For example, for a three-compartment model, the differential equations are:

$$dx_1/dt = I + x_2 k_{21} + x_3 k_{31} - x_1 k_{10} - x_1 k_{12} - x_1 k_{13}$$
$$= I + x_2 k_{21} + x_3 k_{31} - x_1(k_{10} + k_{12} + k_{13}) \qquad (23)$$

$$dx_2/dt = x_1 k_{12} - x_2 k_{21} \qquad (24)$$

$$dx_3/dt = x_1 k_{13} - x_3 k_{31} \qquad (25)$$

where I is the rate of drug input, x is the amount of drug for a specific compartment and k is a micro-rate constant. Each of the above equations can be solved and the complete solution can be found in the literature [14].

How may we explore into how many compartments the pharmacokinetic behaviour of a specific drug fits? This can be done by taking plasma samples at specific time points after a bolus injection and de-

picting the results in a log (plasma concentration) over time graph, as shown in Fig. 1.4.

Three distinct phases can be distinguished. There is a *rapid 'distribution' phase* (solid line) that begins immediately after the bolus injection. This phase is characterized by very rapidly equilibrating tissues. There often is a *slower second distribution phase* (dashed line) that is characterized by a movement of the drug into more slowly equilibrating tissues and a return of the drug from the most rapidly equilibrating tissues (i.e. those that reached equilibrium with the plasma during phase I). The terminal phase (dotted line) is a straight line when plotted on a semi-logarithmic graph. The terminal phase often is called the *elimination phase* because the primary mechanism for decreasing drug concentration during the terminal phase is its elimination from the body [13].

Mathematically, a decreasing curve with a constant slope can be described, as in equation 21. This is for a one-compartmental model. Curves that continuously decrease over time, with a continuously declining slope (Fig. 1.4), can be described by the sum of multiple equations 21, one for each compartment. This is the sum of exponentials describing the decrease of plasma concentration over time:

$$C(t) = A\,e^{-\alpha t} + B\,e^{-\beta t} + C\,e^{-\gamma t} \qquad (26)$$

where t is the time after injection of the bolus, C(t) is the drug concentration after a bolus dose, and A, α, B, β, C and γ are variables of a pharmacokinetic model. A, B, and C are called *coefficients* and express an equivalent of compartmental concentrations. At time 0,

$$C_0 = A + B + C \qquad (27)$$

α, β and γ are called *exponents* (sometimes called *hybrid rate constants*). These exponents express the slope of each exponential decay, as shown in Fig. 1.4.

Equation 26 can be transformed mathematically from the exponential form to the 'compartmental' form (the form using the micro-rate constants). For the three-compartment mammillary model, this interconversion between the exponential form (equation 26) and the micro-rate constant form (equations 23–25) becomes exceedingly complex as more exponents are added. This is because every exponent is a function of every micro-rate constant and vice versa. It is not the purpose of this chapter to explain and solve all the equations. The complete solution of the three-compartment model can be found in the literature [13,14].

Front-end kinetics to optimize compartmental models

In a classical multicompartmental mammalian pharmacokinetic model, intravenously administered drugs are assumed to mix instantaneously in an initial distribution volume (V_c) that includes, at a minimum, the intravascular space. In reality, the volume of distribution of a drug expands with a time course dependent on the physiological environment and chemical characteristics of the drug. As a result, the estimate of V_c will be smaller when earlier blood sampling is applied. Nonetheless, conventional pharmacokinetic models overestimate because they ignore the complexity of intravenous mixing [15].

Recirculatory multicompartmental pharmacokinetic modelling can be applied to describe drug disposition from the moment of rapid intravenous injection. These models retain the relative simplicity of mammalian models, but incorporate descriptions of key physiological processes that have emerged as important determinants of intravenously injected drug disposition. In the fit of the recirculatory model to the data, the concentration at time zero is zero and there is a delay between the time the drug is administered and the time the drug appears at the sampling site. This model fits the early arterial concentrations of samples obtained soon after rapid intravenous input. Pulmonary uptake, injection rate, intravascular mixing and the influence of the cardiac output on this phenomenon are taken into account. First applications of these recirculatory multicompartmental models have recently been published [15,16].

Non-linear compartmental models

When drug behaviour is studied by pharmacokinetic models, it is mostly assumed that distribution and elimination are first-order processes resulting in a linear relationship between concentration at any time and dose. This assumption is only correct if elimination and transport processes never become saturated. When saturation occurs (e.g. saturation of an enzyme system), the rate of drug elimination reaches a maximum and becomes concentration independent [12]. For a single non-linear compartmental model, the elimination rate (ER) can be described as:

$$ER = \frac{V_n C_u(t)}{K_m + C_u(t)} \qquad (28)$$

where $C_u(t)$ is the concentration of the unbound drug at time t and K_m is the Michaelis–Menten constant, which is the concentration at which the rate is half maximum, V_m. When $C_u \ll K_m$, then the process is not saturated and the rate is dependent on the concentration, described as:

$$ER = \frac{V_n}{K_m} \cdot C_u(t) = Cl \cdot C_u(t) \qquad (29)$$

In contrast, when C_u is much greater than K_m, saturation occurs, the elimination rate approaches V_m and is concentration independent (ER = V_m).

Physiological models

The description of physiological drug models depends on the interpretation of drug distribution in terms of anatomical or physiological spaces, which have defined volumes, perfusion characteristics and partition coefficients. Individual compartments may have 'flow-limited' or 'membrane-limited' characteristics (depending on whether blood flow or transmembrane transport is the limiting factor governing drug uptake). This means that the time course of drug or metabolite levels in the various 'physiological' organs or compartments is calculated using blood flow rate through each particular region, diffusion of the drug between blood and tissue, and the relative affinity of drug for blood and the various tissues and organs [17].

These complex physiologically based pharmacokinetic models have been used to describe the disposition of volatile anaesthetics [18]. For intravenously administered agents, however, their application has been sporadic because of the large number of parameters involved in the studies to determine the models. Therefore, their application is justified only when detailed mechanisms of drug metabolism or excretion by liver, kidney, lung or other organs is required or when specific tissue localization should be depicted (e.g. anticancer drugs).

Connecting pharmacokinetics and dynamics

The time course of drug concentration, defined as the pharmacokinetics of the drug, cannot in itself predict the time course or magnitude of drug effect. In clinical practice, a delay is frequently observed between the moment of peak plasma concentration, peak concentration at the effect site and peak drug effect. This delay occurs when the plasma is not the site of drug action, but only a means of transport, and is called counterclockwise or anticlockwise hysteresis. Drugs exert their biological effect at the 'biophase', also called the effect site, which is the immediate area where the drug acts on the body, and includes membranes, receptors and enzymes. The study of the concentration–effect relationship is called pharmacodynamics and is covered elsewhere in this book. Problems resulting from temporal disequilibrium (hysteresis) can be overcome by using

the concept of the effect compartment model [19,20] in which drug response is modelled against drug concentration in a hypothetical effect compartment. The concentration of the drug in this theoretical compartment is directly related to the measured drug effect.

The effect compartment is an additional compartment linked to the central compartment of the mammillary pharmacokinetic model, as shown in Fig. 1.5. The effect compartment receives drug from the central compartment by a first-order process, expressed by a first-order rate constant, k_{e1}. The actual mass of drug reaching the effect compartment is negligible. It is assumed that the effect compartment kinetics do not affect the pharmacokinetic model. Given these assumptions, the effect compartment can be considered a compartmental model with an input defined by a first-order rate constant (k_{e1}) and a first-order rate constant defining the output (k_{e0}). The time to reach a steady-state concentration in this effect compartment is dependent on the elimination from the effect compartment. A clarification of this statement is found in equation 30

$$C_e = C_{SSe} \left(1 - e^{-k_e0t}\right) \tag{30}$$

The term C_e defines the drug concentration in the effect compartment, C_{SSe} refers to the concentration at steady-state or the concentration that will be reached in the effect compartment after equilibration with the concentration in the central compartment of the pharmacokinetic model. The time to reach a steady-state is solely dependent on the k_{e0}. This rate constant can precisely characterize the temporal aspect of equilibration between plasma concentration and drug effect. The rate constant k_{e0} in the pharmacokinetic model, together with a pharmacodynamic model (e.g. the sigmoid E_{max} model) driven by the predicted effect site concentration, allows us to characterize the effect data directly to the plasma concentration using non-linear regression analysis. This step simultaneously yields estimations of the pharmacokinetic and pharmacodynamic variables. The exact equations for the combination of an effect compartment with a three-compartment mammillary model can be found in the literature [19].

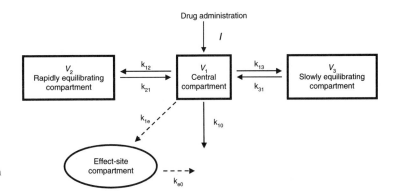

Figure 1.5 The three-compartment pharmacokinetic model enlarged with an effect site compartment.

Population pharmacokinetic analysis

The pharmacokinetic characteristics of a specific drug are usually reported as mean population variables. However, it is crucial to reveal additional information about the magnitude of variability in the population receiving the drug. The analysis of pooled data from many subjects, or summary statistics derived from individual pharmacokinetic studies, are generally considered to be unsatisfactory methods for population analysis. Although this *pooled approach* will describe the observations well most of the time (because the objective function for the regression model is precisely that — to minimize the error between model prediction and the observed value), this pooled approach is 'naïve' and does not take into account specific population variability. Failure to appreciate the magnitude of variability in the pharmacology of a drug can compromise fixed dose clinical trials outcomes by making the drug appear less effective or more toxic [21].

Population pharmacokinetic analysis is crucial during every drug development as it has considerable predictive value. Previously, a *'two-stage' approach* was applied to characterize population variability. In this case, pharmacokinetic data are derived for every individual from the population and then population mean (and standard deviations) are calculated to depict the population and its variability. Although reported frequently in the literature, the major problem of the two-stage approach is that it fails to address the two major sources of population variability: intra- versus interindividual variability [22].

When obtaining multiple blood samples from various patients to calculate the population pharmaco-kinetic model, two problems are faced. First, there is a random intra-individual variability resulting from unavoidable (small) errors in the assay method or individual variability. Secondly, there is an interindividual variability which can be defined as randomized effects (not measurable difference between individuals) or fixed effects (measurable, also defined as covariates). Even after having entered all possible covariates (e.g. age, weight, height, gender, body surface, lean body mass), randomized effects will still exist. To be able to reveal all possible sources and explanations of population variability, sophisticated statistical analysis, called *non-linear mixed effect modelling*, is required. Various commercially available software packages are able to process population data using such modelling [20,23–27].

Pharmacological changes resulting from physiological and pathophysiological alterations

The different pharmacokinetic processes explained above may be altered because of physiological and pathophysiological effects leading to changes in free concentration at the effect site, and eventually to alterations in drug effect. Changes in drug effect may also result from changes in pharmacodynamics such as alterations in intrinsic drug efficacy or end organ sensitivity to the drug. These events make up the pharmacodynamics of a drug. Both pharmacokinetics and pharmacodynamics are susceptible to physiological processes and pathophysiological conditions. The potential impact of age, pregnancy, chronopharmacology, obesity and renal, liver, circulatory and respiratory failure, head injury and cardiopulmonary bypass on the pharmacology of the drug are discussed. The examples used to illustrate this section focus on drugs frequently used during anaesthesia.

Age

With increasing age, multiple physiological and pathophysiological changes occur in the cerebrovascular, cardiovascular, respiratory, renal and hepatic systems, resulting in pharmacological changes such as a reduction in excretion and metabolism, and an increased CNS sensitivity [28]. The changes may result in an increased drug effect, reduced elimination rate and prolonged duration of drug action. The increase in body fat, reduction in muscle mass and decrease in total body water with age may result in an increase of distribution volume for lipophilic drugs, and decrease for hydrophilic drugs.

For most intravenous hypnotic agents, such as midazolam [29] and propofol [30], and for the inhalational anaesthetic agents, the increased sensitivity with age is, at least in part, explained by altered pharmacodynamics. For opioids, the pharmacodynamic involvement is not always clear. The prolonged opioid effect of sufentanil in elderly patients has been attributed to alterations in pharmacodynamics [31], whereas for alfentanil changes in pharmacokinetics have been suggested to account for the lower dose requirement in elderly patients [32]. For neuromuscular agents, the increased effect in the elderly appears to be caused by altered pharmacokinetics resulting in a decreased clearance because of an age-related decrease in renal and hepatic function.

Physiological changes also influence the pharmacokinetics of drugs in children [33]. The neonatal phase is characterized by rapid and dramatic changes of organ function. Changes in body composition and the content of plasma proteins influence volume of distribution, the drug distribution to different compartments and the amount of free drug in plasma. A decrease in extracellular fluid space during the first year of life influences distribution volume of neuromuscular blocking agents which are polar drugs whose distribution is restricted to the extracellular fluid space [34]. Thus, weight-normalized doses of neuromuscular blocking agents yield smaller plasma concentrations in neonates or infants than in children or adults. Pharmacokinetics of propofol in children are characterized by a larger central compartment volume, which is consistent with the higher induction dose requirement reported for children [35]. As a result of the immaturity of the hepatic microsomal systems there is decreased metabolism of agents such as diazepam, midazolam and morphine [33]. In the first year of life, capacity of the enzymatic systems increase, which is accompanied by increased drug clearance. For remifentanil, which is metabolized by tissue and plasma esterases, the opposite is observed, with an increased clearance in young infants compared with older children and young adults [36]. Beyond the neonatal period, the pharmacology of most opioid analgesics are not markedly different from those of adults [37]. Maturational changes may also occur in pharmacodynamics (e.g. increased sensitivity to neuromuscular blocking agents in younger patients) [34].

Pregnancy

Throughout pregnancy there are marked physiological changes that may have a significant influence on the pharmacokinetics of drugs [38]. The increased minute ventilation, decreased functional residual capacity and increased cardiac output may result in increased pulmonary uptake of gases, leading to decreased anaesthetic requirement in pregnancy. However, the rate of induction with inhalational anaesthetic agents is not necessarily faster because this depends on both pulmonary equilibration kinetics and tissue distribution kinetics. Apparent distribution volumes of drugs may increase during pregnancy because of the expansion of fluid volume and the presence of fetal and placental tissues resulting in an increased elimination half-life. However, contrary to what one would expect, these changes in distribution volume are not observed with the polar neuromuscular relaxants, for which distribution volumes are unchanged during pregnancy [39]. The increased cardiac output may accelerate the onset of action of induction agents and neuromuscular blockers. Unbound drug fraction may increase during pregnancy because of reduced albumin concentration and endogenous displacing substances. With regard to metabolism, both inhibition and induction of enzymes have been reported during pregnancy. The increased thiopental clearance during pregnancy has been attributed to hormonal enzyme induction. Hepatic blood flow is thought to be unchanged during pregnancy, although clearance of propofol, which is considered blood flow dependent, has been reported to be increased during pregnancy, and increased extrahepatic clearance can probably account for this observation. Renal plasma flow is increased, resulting in increased renal drug excretion, and the increased clearance of pancuronium during caesarian section has been explained by the increased glomerular filtration rate [39]. Elimination of inhalational anaesthetics is expected to be enhanced by the increased minute ventilation. Apart from pharmacokinetic changes, pharmacodynamics of drugs, although not well investigated in pregnancy, may also be influenced by the physiological processes occurring. For instance, an increased pain threshold during pregnancy, mediated by endorphins, may theoretically influence opioid effects. The prolonged apnoea following large doses of succinylcholine in pregnancy may be explained by decreased plasma pseudocholinesterases [39].

Chronopharmacology

Chronopharmacology is the influence of circadian rhythm on the pharmacology of drugs. Pharmacological parameters are influenced by different physiological functions displaying circadian rhythm [40]. Information regarding circadian rhythms for general anaesthesia remains fragmentary. Barbiturates are more effective in the evening than in the morning, which has been explained by endogenous variation in hepatic drug metabolism and by diurnal changes in GABAergic activity. A temporal pattern in pharmacology has also been observed for midazolam, with a higher clearance after an intravenous dose in the late afternoon than after a morning dose and a circadian fluctuation in the sensitivity of the CNS. No data are currently available regarding circadian changes for propofol or etomidate. Diurnal changes in the efficacy of halothane has been investigated and it was found that its greatest efficacy occurred in the early morning, which may theoretically be explained by circadian rhythmicity in receptor activity

as well as distribution and metabolism. Circadian changes in pancuronium requirements could be explained by time-dependent changes in renal elimination and cholinesterase activity. Diurnal variation in pain perception has been shown to be highly relevant to the daily practice of pain management, leading to variations in the need for analgesics at different times of day.

Obesity

Obesity can significantly alter the tissue distribution and elimination of drugs, and may necessitate modified loading and/or maintenance doses [41]. The altered pathophysiology of the obese body can affect drug distribution because of changes in body composition, regional blood flow and binding to plasma proteins. In obese people, the percentage of fat per kilogram of total body weight is markedly increased, whereas that of lean tissue is reduced. Cardiac performance may be impaired and tissue blood flow per gram of fat can be significantly decreased. There is also uncertainty about the binding of drugs to plasma proteins in obese patients. Increased α_1-acid glycoprotein acid levels may lead to increased protein binding of drugs. The behaviour of molecules with weak or moderate lipophilicity (e.g. vecuronium, rocuronium) is generally rather predictable, as these drugs are distributed mainly in lean tissues, and the dosage of these drugs should be based on the ideal body weight. For highly lipophilic drugs (e.g. remifentanil), there are great discrepancies in distribution in obese individuals, and the size of the distribution volume is not always correlated with the degree of lipophilicity.

Some data suggest that the activities of hepatic cytochrome P450 isoforms are altered in obesity, but no clear overview of drug hepatic metabolism is currently available. Pharmacokinetic studies provide differing data on renal function in obese patients. Clearance and distribution volumes of propofol have been correlated with total body weight in obese patients, so that the values of the elimination half-life in non-obese and obese individuals are similar. This can explain why there are no signs of drug accumulation in obese patients. For sufentanil, clearance and distribution volume corrected per kilogram of total body weight were similar in obese and non-obese patients, whereas for remifentanil these parameters were significantly smaller in obese patients. Accordingly, remifentanil doses for obese patients should be based on ideal body weight.

Liver failure

The liver is the major route for elimination of a wide variety of drugs. Biotransformation, liver blood flow, protein binding and biliary excretion, which can all potentially influence drug pharmacokinetics, depend upon the normal functioning of the liver. Impaired liver function may therefore lead to significant alterations in the pharmacokinetics of many drugs, necessitating dosage adjustment. Most information about the influence of liver insufficiency on the pharmacokinetics of drugs comes from patients with hepatic cirrhosis. However, other disease conditions such as hypothermia, hypotension and sepsis may also be associated with impaired liver function. Studies show that more than 50% of critically ill patients have hepatic dysfunction.

In order to fully understand the impact of liver failure on the pharmacokinetics of a particular drug, the underlying determinants of hepatic drug clearance must be well understood (see above). Measurement of endogenous substances such as bilirubin, bile pigments, albumin and enzymes have been used to assess liver function. However, unlike the assessment of renal function by measuring creatinine clearance, these parameters have not proven to be generally useful. Liver function tests do not generally correlate well with important physiological determinants of drug disposition such as liver blood flow and intrinsic clearance.

The histopathological changes occurring in liver cirrhosis are associated with a reduction in liver blood flow, the presence of portosystemic shunting and a reduction in the number and in the activity of the hepatocytes. The clinical manifestations of cirrhosis such as varices, oedema and ascites may also contribute to alterations in the pharmacokinetic behaviour of many drugs [42]. Impaired albumin production in cirrhotic patients may reduce plasma binding and thus increase the free drug fraction. In addition, drug absorption may be markedly altered in cirrhosis. A decrease in the fraction of the mesenteric blood flow passing through the liver (due to portosystemic shunts) and decreased activity of drug metabolizing enzymes may result in an increased bioavailability of some orally administered drugs, such as midazolam and morphine. Drug distribution of certain drugs in cirrhotic patients may be increased because of reduced plasma protein levels and changes in body composition (ascites, oedema). An increased distribution volume of rocuronium in patients with liver disease results in a longer elimination half-life and a prolonged recovery time [43]. Hepatic clearance of high extraction drugs in cirrhotic patients is expected to be decreased because of impaired hepatic blood flow resulting from extra- and intrahepatic shunts. Morphine clearance was found to be decreased in cirrhosis [44]. However, contrary to what one would expect, there was no reduction in clearance of the high extraction drugs propofol [45,46], fentanyl and sufentanil [47] in cirrhotic patients. Clearance of low extraction drugs may be impaired because of hepatocellular damage, whereas an increase in free drug fraction may facilitate hepatic clearance of these drugs. Oxidative metabolic reactions, catalysed by CYP enzymes, appear to be more affected than glucuronidation in cirrhotic patients; reduced oxidation of alfentanil in patients with cirrhosis resulted in a decreased clearance [48]. Reduced midazolam clearance in cirrhotic patients was also observed [49], which may be explained by a reduced CYP3A4 isoenzyme activity. The pharmacokinetics of remifentanil, which is metabolized by tissue and plasma esterases, appear to be unaffected in liver disease [48]. In liver cirrhosis, extrahepatic metabolism may compensate, at least in part, for the impaired metabolism of the drug by hepatic enzymes. Biliary obstruction in liver cirrhosis may also lead to impaired biliary excretion of drugs and/or their metabolites.

Cardiovascular failure, resulting from, for instance, sepsis, cardiogenic and hypovolaemic shock, may also affect hepatic clearance [50–53]. Inadequate hepatic perfusion during cardiovascular failure is expected to decrease clearance of high extraction drugs, as has been shown for morphine in septic shock patients. Respiratory failure, requiring mechanical ventilation, often develops during cardiovascular failure. The reduction in cardiac output and liver blood flow induced by mechanical ventilation is also expected to decrease clearance of high extraction drugs. The use of vasopressor agents may also alter hepatic blood flow, thereby influencing drug clearance. Hepatocellular enzyme activity is often reduced during cardiovascular failure, leading to decreased clearance of low extraction drugs, and is presumably influenced by factors such as organ perfusion, intracellular oxygen tension and cofactor availability. The CYP enzyme system has been shown to be markedly altered in critical illnesses, and to a greater extent than the phase II enzymes. This may be because the CYP enzyme system is located in the more hypoxic central region of the liver lobule and therefore is more sensitive to hypoxia. Hypoxaemia results in reduced enzyme production in the liver, reduced efficiency of the enzyme present and decreased oxygen available for drug oxidation. Exposure of isolated human hepatocytes to hypoxia for several days resulted in a reduction in the CYP enzymes, with certain CYP families more affected than others. In patients with congestive heart failure, clearance of antipyrine was reduced; this is a low extraction drug independent of hepatic blood flow, often used as a model substrate for microsomal oxidative metabolism [54]. Clearance of midazolam was also found to be decreased in these patients [55]. Hepatic drug metabolism in sepsis may also be reduced by the nitric oxide mediated inhibition of CYP-dependent drug metabolism. *In vitro* experiments using human hepatocytes showed that cytokines may also reduce CYP expression. Temporary failure of midazolam metabolism in patients with sepsis, attributed to changes in hepatic blood flow and/or hepatic enzyme activity, has been reported [56]. Interestingly, serum from septic patients decreased CYP3A4-mediated metabolism of midazolam *in vitro*, which has been attributed to the depressant effects of cytokines.

Renal failure

The kidneys are responsible for the excretion of many drugs, both the parent drug and its metabolites. The urinary excretion of a drug is the net result of filtration, secretion and reabsorption. The causes of renal impairment are numerous and can be divided into prerenal, renal and postrenal causes. Septic shock, for instance, initially results in a prere-

nal type of acute renal failure, which then leads to the full picture of tubular/obstructive acute renal failure. In renal failure, both the parent drug and metabolites may accumulate.

Renal failure may also influence drug distribution [52]. A decrease in albumin concentration, changes in albumin structure, and competition between endogenous substances and drugs at albumin binding sites may increase free drug fraction during renal failure. This may theoretically increase drug effect for intravenously administered high extraction drugs extensively bound to albumin, and drug distribution volume. Both distribution volume and clearance of midazolam were found to be increased in patients with chronic renal failure, which has been attributed to reduced protein binding and a higher free drug fraction [57]. Metabolic acidosis occurring during renal failure may also be expected to affect drug distribution. For drugs that are weak acids, a decrease in pH will result in an increase in the non-ionized fraction, which may theoretically enhance drug distribution, whereas for weak bases the opposite may occur. Fluid retention is also a feature of renal failure, resulting in changes in total body water and the distribution of many drugs.

The kidneys have a modest capacity for autoregulation, and when renal blood flow is moderately reduced (10–20%), the glomerular filtration rate does not fall. Further reductions in blood flow resulting from, for example, cardiovascular failure, may compromise kidney perfusion as part of homeostasis, resulting in decreased glomerular filtration and a reduction in renal drug clearance. Clearance of drugs that are only filtered and not secreted or reabsorbed, is determined by both glomerular filtration rate and the free drug fraction. The pharmacokinetics of morphine and its glucuronide metabolites, morphine-3-glucuronide and morphine-6-glucuronide, have been investigated in intensive care patients with renal failure [58]. The two metabolites are eliminated by renal filtration only, and a linear relationship between renal function and the renal clearances of the two metabolites was found. Renal failure may thus result in higher plasma concentrations of these active metabolites. The latter was confirmed in another study in which the increased susceptibility to morphine in patients with renal failure was explained by the observed accumulation of the active metabolite morphine-6-glucuronide in cerebrospinal fluid. The pharmacokinetics of the synthetic opioids alfentanil, sufentanil and remifentanil have been found to be little changed in patients with renal failure whereas continuous administration of fentanyl, although primarily metabolized in the liver, was found to result in prolonged sedation [59]. Prolonged sedation has also been observed after administration of midazolam in critically ill patients with renal failure, which has been attributed to accumulation of the active conjugate metabolite. No changes in pharmacokinetics of propofol, which is mainly metabolized in the liver, were found in patients with end-stage renal disease [60]. One study even found higher propofol requirements in patients with end-stage renal disease, which has been attributed to the hyperdynamic circulation caused by anaemia in these patients [61]. In patients with chronic renal failure, plasma clearance of vecuronium, which mainly undergoes hepatic elimination [62] resulting in an active metabolite, was found to be decreased. Also for rapacuronium [63], pancuronium and their potent metabolites, decreased clearance was observed in patients with renal failure. However, pharmacokinetics of atracurium were found to be unaffected by renal failure, explained by its spontaneous chemical degradation and ester hydrolysis. However, concern has been expressed about possible accumulation of its principal metabolite laudanosine in patients with renal failure. Renal failure was found to have little impact on the duration of action of rocuronium and cisatracurium [64]. Besides renal filtration, urinary drug secretion may also be part of the renal excretion process for certain drugs. Urinary drug secretion may be influenced by protein binding, depending on the efficiency of the secretion process, and on the contact time at the secretory sites. By analogy with hepatic metabolism, drugs that are almost completely removed from blood within the time they are in contact with the active transport site, secretion is dependent on blood flow but independent of protein binding, and reduced renal blood flow may be expected to slow elimination.

Tubular reabsorption may also occur with certain drugs. During cardiovascular failure, reabsorption may be expected to increase as a consequence of decreased urine flow accompanying a decrease in glomerular filtration rate, but documentation of clinically important decreases in drug excretion as a result of this mechanism is lacking.

Circulatory failure

Circulatory failure caused by, for example, sepsis, cardiac failure or haemorrhage, is a common cause of altered pharmacokinetics [50–53,65,66]. A dramatic illustration of the impact of haemorrhage on the pharmacology of anaesthetics has been provided by Halford [67], who, in 1943, described an increased mortality rate in wounded military personnel during surgery under thiopental anaesthesia at the beginning of the Second World War. Regardless of aetiology, circulatory failure results in a redistribution of cardiac output with blood shunted away from less vital organs such as kidneys, spleen and gut to vital organs such as heart and brain. This may result in a disproportionate fraction of the available cardiac output delivered to the heart and brain. These changes in blood flow during haemodynamic shock may theoretically be expected to influence the pharmacokinetics of a drug by affecting absorption, distribution, metabolism and excretion. The pharmacodynamics may also be altered by changes in, for example, end organ sensitivity.

Circulatory dysfunction results in a decreased perfusion of muscles, skin and splanchnic organs. Absorption of drugs from sites with impaired blood flow is slow, sometimes incomplete, and subject to changes in circulatory status. Thus, the oral, transdermal, subcutaneous and intramuscular routes may not be reliable in critically ill patients, and an intravascular route is preferred. Cardiovascular failure will indeed result in a reduced enteral absorption of drugs not only because of the decreased forward flow (reduced organ perfusion), but also because of the increased back pressure (venous congestion) in the gut circulation. Gut hypoperfusion and poor absorption of drugs may theoretically also be worsened by mucosal oedema caused by hypoproteinaemia. Moreover, gastrointestinal failure is often present in the critically ill patient because of gut hypomotility (e.g. after surgery) caused by the constellation of organ failure associated with sepsis or as a result of the administration of opioids for analgesia.

The rate and extent of distribution of a drug is determined by cardiac output, regional blood flow, the drug permeability of the tissue membranes and the relative distribution of the drug between tissue and blood. The latter is dependent on the binding of the drug in blood and tissues, the tissue mass, the lipid solubility of the drug and, for ionizable drugs, the pKa and the pH of the environment. All these determinants of distribution may change during circulatory failure, thereby altering the drug distribution volume.

Cardiovascular failure with a reduction of cardiac output may result in decreased drug distribution resulting in the homeostatic redistribution of blood flow away from less vital organs with preservation of blood flow to heart and brain. This phenomenon may be important for rapidly intravenously administered drugs with a high degree of lipid solubility, such as anaesthetics, and may result in an increased risk of CNS effects. Benowitz *et al.* [68] illustrated this principle by using a computer simulation of lidocaine kinetics for a 70-kg person in normal and hypovolaemic conditions following simulated removal of 30% of the blood volume. Following lidocaine administration, the amount of drug in the blood pool is higher during haemorrhage because the blood volume is smaller and because perfusion of other tissues is decreased. As a result of the higher blood concentrations and the autoregulation of brain blood flow, lidocaine content in the brain is much higher in early phases, explaining why CNS toxicity may result when standard lidocaine doses are administered to patients with circulatory failure. The slower and decreased distribution of lidocaine to the muscles during haemorrhage results from the homoeostatic vasoconstriction in this organ.

Systemic inflammatory response syndrome has a widespread effect on the endothelium leading to increased capillary permeability which may result in accumulation of fluids in the interstitial space. This so-called 'third spacing' phenomenon may affect the distribution of drugs, particularly those with a small distribution volume. Endothelial barrier disruption may also lead to leakage of proteins away from the blood pool thereby influencing drug distribution. Sepsis may also be expected to influence other tissue membranes, and meningeal inflammation, for instance, has been shown to increase the permeability of the blood–brain barrier. This is important for hydrophilic drugs, whereas penetration of more lipophilic compounds was found to be less dependent on the function of the blood–brain barrier.

Changes in the plasma protein binding of drugs during circulatory failure may be caused by changes in the concentration of the plasma proteins to which they are bound, by competition of endogenous substances for binding sites or by changes in the binding characteristics. Critical illness can cause increased concentrations of acute phase reactant proteins like α_1-acid glycoprotein which is a major binding protein for basic drugs such as alfentanil. Increases in the concentration of α_1-acid glycoprotein will decrease the unbound fraction of drugs that bind to this protein in the plasma, and result in a decreased distribution volume. In contrast, reduction in the level of serum albumin during critical illness because of reduced dietary protein intake, increased capillary permeability, haemodilution, renal loss and/or reduced hepatic synthesis may increase the free drug fraction of drugs that bind to albumin resulting in an increased distribution volume. For midazolam, which is extensively bound to albumin, a negative correlation was found between its distribution volume and the plasma albumin concentration in intensive care patients [69].

Fluid retention, as part of the homeostasis in response to a failing heart and as a result of fluids administered during resuscitation, may increase the volume of distribution. Alterations in distribution volume may also be expected from changes in tissue volume. Changes in general lean body mass and total body fat are likely to be of importance for the drug distribution volume. For instance, total body fat will decrease during sepsis because of stimulation of lipolysis and reduction of lipogenesis.

Reduced organ perfusion causes anaerobic metabolism and metabolic acidosis which may alter the distribution of ionizable drugs. The latter may also result from pH changes resulting from respiratory and kidney failure. No data are available on the influence of changes in pH on drug distribution during circulatory failure. For drugs that are weak acids, a decrease in pH will result in an increase in the non-ionized fraction, which may theoretically enhance drug distribution, whereas for weak bases the opposite may occur.

Respiratory failure

Respiratory disorders induce several pathophysiological changes involving gas exchange and acid–base balance, regional haemodynamics, and alterations of the alveolar-capillary membrane which may affect absorption, distribution and elimination of drugs [70]. Changes in blood pH are expected to alter plasma protein binding and volume of distribution. Decreased cardiac output and hepatic blood flow in patients resulting from right ventricular failure or mechanical ventilation are expected to cause an increase in the plasma concentration of drugs with a high hepatic extraction ratio (see above). The same mechanisms may be responsible for a decreased renal elimination of drugs during respiratory failure. Acute and chronic lung disease can result in hypoxia, which may have significant effects on the enzymes responsible, leading to decreased biotransformation of drugs with a low extraction ratio [51]. However, clinical data on the effects of lung disease on the clearance of drugs are lacking.

Head injury

Patients with head injury may develop profound metabolic changes resulting in a hypermetabolic, hypercatabolic and hyperdynamic state. These changes may be expected to alter pharmacokinetics. Hepatic oxidative and conjugative metabolism have indeed been shown to be significantly increased over time in patients after acute head injury [71], resulting in increased metabolism of, for instance, pentobarbital, thiopental and lorazepam [72]. Hypoalbuminaemia and a rise in α_1-acid glycoprotein accompanying the acute phase response in patients with head injury are expected to alter both drug distribution and metabolism.

Cardiopulmonary bypass

Cardiopulmonary bypass is accompanied by profound changes that may alter the pharmacokinetics of drugs [73,74]. For many drugs, such as mida-

zolam, propofol, etomidate, pancuronium, fentanyl, alfentanil and sufentanil, an abrupt decrease in serum concentration has been observed upon initiation of bypass which is explained by haemodilution and an increase in distribution resulting from decreased protein binding. For opiates, adsorption to the bypass apparatus was shown to be important. The gradual increase in serum concentrations seen during cardiopulmonary bypass after the initial fall as has been observed for midazolam, etomidate and sufentanil is usually explained by redistribution of the drug from tissues to the serum and/or a decrease in its elimination. The latter can be caused by impairment of renal or hepatic clearance resulting from lowered perfusion and hypothermia. The same phenomena are thought to explain why in the post-bypass period a concentration increase occurs, or at least a slower decrease than expected; this has been observed for drugs such as midazolam, etomidate and fentanyl.

Acknowledgements

The authors thank Professors Eric Mortier, Walter Buylaert and Frans Belpaire for their help during the realization of this chapter.

References

1 Peck TE, Hill SA, Williams M. Drug passage across the cell membrane. In: Peck TE, Hill SA, Williams M, eds. *Pharmacology for Anaesthesia and Intensive Care*, 2nd edn. London: Greenwich Medical Media, 2003: 3–10.

2 Karp G. The structure and function of the plasma membrane. In: Karp G, ed. *Cell and Molecular Biology: Concepts and Experiments*, 3rd edn. New York: John Wiley and Sons, 2002: 122–82.

3 McGeown JG. Cardiovascular physiology. In: McGeown JG, ed. *Physiology: A Clinical Core Text of Human Physiology with Self-assessment*, 2nd edn. Edinburgh: Churchill Livingstone, 2002: 49–82.

4 Hudson RJ. Basic principles of clinical pharmacology. In: Barash PG, Cullen BF, Stoelting RK, eds. *Clinical Anesthesia*, 3rd edn. Philadelphia: Lippincott-Raven, 1997: 221–42.

5 Welling PG. Parenteral routes of drug administration. In: Welling PG, ed. *Pharmacokinetics: Processes, Mathematics and Applications*. Washington: American Chemical Society, 1997: 19–42.

6 Rang HP, Dale MM, Ritter JM. Absorption and distribution of drugs. In: Rang HP, Dale MM, Ritter JM, eds. *Pharmacology*, 5th edn. Edinburgh: Churchill Livingstone, 2003: 91–105.

7 Evers AS. Inhalational anesthetics. In: Evers AS, Maze M, eds. *Anesthetic Pharmacology, Physiologic Principles and Clinical Practice*. Pennsylvania: Churchill Livingstone, 2004: 369–93.

8 Calvey TN, Williams NE. Drug absorption, distribution and elimination. In: Calvey TN, Williams NE, eds. *Pharmacology for Anaesthetists*, 4th edn. Oxford: Blackwell Science, 2001: 1–21.

9 Hull CJ. General principles of pharmacokinetics. In: Prys-Roberts C, Hug Jr CC, eds. *Pharmacokinetics of Anaesthesia*. Oxford: Blackwell Scientific Publications, 1984: 1–24.

10 Stanski DR, Watkins WD. Pharmacokinetic principles. In: Stanski DR, Watkins WD, eds. *Pharmacology*, 5th edn. New York: Grune and Stratton, 1982: 1–46.

11 Wilkinson GR, Shand DG. Commentary: a physiological approach to hepatic drug clearance. *Clin Pharmacol Ther* 1975; **18**: 377–90.

12 Schnider TW, Minto CF. Pharmacokinetic and pharmacodynamic principles of drug action. In: Evers AS, Maze M, eds. *Anesthetic Pharmacology: Physiologic Principles and Clinical Practice*. Edinburgh: Churchill Livingstone, 2003.

13 Shafer SL. Principles of pharmacokinetics and pharmacodynamics. In: Longnecker DE, Tinker JH, Morgan GE, eds. *Principles and Practice of Anesthesiology*, 2nd edn. New York: Mosby-Year Book, 1998: 1159–210.

14 Hull CJ. Compartmental models. *Anaesthetic Pharmacology Review* 1994; **2**: 188–203.

15 Avram MJ, Krejcie TC. Using front-end kinetics to optimize target-controlled drug infusions. *Anesthesiol* 2003; **99**: 1078–86.

16 Upton RN. The two-compartment recirculatory pharmacokinetic model: an introduction to recirculatory pharmacokinetic concepts. *Br J Anaesth* 2004; **92**: 475–84.

17 Welling PG. Physiological pharmacokinetic models. In: Welling PG, ed. *Pharmacokinetics: Processes, Mathematics and Applications*. Washington: American Chemical Society, 1997: 297–310.

18 Eger E. A mathematical model of uptake and distribution. In: Papper EM, Kitz RJ, eds. *Uptake and Distribution of Anesthetic Agents*. New York: McGraw-Hill, 1963.

19 Holford NH, Sheiner LB. Pharmacokinetic and pharmacodynamic modeling *in vivo*. *CRC Crit Rev Bioeng* 1981; **5**: 273–322.

20 Sheiner LB, Stanski DR, Vozeh S, Miller RD, Ham J. Simultaneous modeling of pharmacokinetics and pharmacodynamics: application to d-tubocurarine. *Clin Pharmacol Ther* 1979; **25**: 358–71.

21 Levy G. Predicting effective drug concentrations for individual patients: determinants of pharmacodynamic variability. *Clin Pharmacokinet* 1998; **34**: 323–33.

22 Kataria BK, Ved SA, Nicodemus HF, *et al.* The pharmacokinetics of propofol in children using three different data analysis approaches. *Anesthesiol* 1994; **80**: 104–22

23 Beal SL, Sheiner LB. Estimating population kinetics. *Crit Rev Biomed Eng* 1982; **8**: 195–222.

24 Sheiner LB, Beal SL. Evaluation of methods for estimating population pharmacokinetics parameters. I. Michaelis–Menten model: routine clinical pharmacokinetic data. *J Pharmacokinet Biopharm* 1980; **8**: 553–71.

25 Sheiner LB, Beal SL. Bayesian individualization of pharmacokinetics: simple implementation and comparison with non-Bayesian methods. *J Pharm Sci* 1982; **71**: 1344–8.

26 Sheiner LB. The population approach to pharmacokinetic data analysis: rationale and standard data analysis methods. *Drug Metab Rev* 1984; **15**: 153–71.

27 Smith MK. Software for non-linear mixed effects modelling: a review of several packages. *Pharm Stat* 2003; **2**: 69–75.

28 Dodds C. Anaesthetic drugs in the elderly. *Pharmacol Ther* 1995; **66**: 369–86.

29 Kanto J, Aaltonen L, Himberg JJ, Hovi-Viander M. Midazolam as an intravenous induction agent in the elderly: a clinical and pharmacokinetic study. *Anesth Analg* 1986; **65**: 15–20.

30 Schnider TW, Minto CF, Shafer SL, *et al.* The influence of age on propofol pharmacodynamics. *Anesthesiol* 1999; **90**: 1502–16.

31 Matteo RS, Schwartz AE, Ornstein E, Young WL, Chang WJ. Pharmacokinetics of sufentanil in the elderly surgical patient. *Can J Anaesth* 1990; **37**: 852–6.

32 Lemmens HJ, Bovill JG, Hennis PJ, Burm AG. Age has no effect on the pharmacodynamics of alfentanil. *Anesth Analg* 1988; **67**: 956–60.

33 Roper A, Lauven PM. Pharmacokinetics in newborns and infants. *Anaesthesiol Intensivmed Notfallmed Schmerzther* 1999; **34**: 616–25.

34 Fisher DM. Neuromuscular blocking agents in paediatric anaesthesia. *Br J Anaesth* 1999; **83**: 58–64.

35 Saint-Maurice C, Cockshott ID, Douglas EJ, Richard MO, Harmey JL. Pharmacokinetics of propofol in young children after a single dose. *Br J Anaesth* 1989; **63**: 667–70.

36 Ross AK, Davis PJ, Dear Gd GL, *et al.* Pharmacokinetics of remifentanil in anesthetized pediatric patients undergoing elective surgery or diagnostic procedures. *Anesth Analg* 2001; **93**: 1393–401.

37 Olkkola KT, Hamunen K, Maunuksela EL. Clinical pharmacokinetics and pharmacodynamics of opioid analgesics in infants and children. *Clin Pharmacokinet* 1995; **28**: 385–404.

38 Gin T. Pharmacokinetic optimisation of general anaesthesia in pregnancy. *Clin Pharmacokinet* 1993; **25**: 59–70.

39 Guay J, Grenier Y, Varin F. Clinical pharmacokinetics of neuromuscular relaxants in pregnancy. *Clin Pharmacokinet* 1998; **34**: 483.

40 Chassard D, Bruguerolle B. Chronobiology and anesthesia. *Anesthesiology* 2004; **100**: 413–27.

41 Cheymol G. Effects of obesity on pharmacokinetics: implications for drug therapy. *Clin Pharmacokinet* 2000; **39**: 215–31.

42 Verbeeck RK, Horsmans Y. Effect of hepatic insufficiency on pharmacokinetics and drug dosing. *Pharm World Sci* 1998; **20**: 183–92.

43 Magorian T, Wood P, Caldwell J, *et al.* The pharmacokinetics and neuromuscular effects of rocuronium bromide in patients with liver disease. *Anesth Analg* 1995; **80**: 754–9.

44 Hasselstrom J, Eriksson S, Persson A, *et al.* The metabolism and bioavailability of morphine in patients with severe liver cirrhosis. *Br J Clin Pharmacol* 1990; **29**: 289–97.

45 Servin F, Cockshott ID, Farinotti R, *et al.* Pharmacokinetics of propofol infusions in patients with cirrhosis. *Br J Anaesth* 1990; **65**: 177–83.

46 Servin F, Desmonts JM, Haberer JP, *et al.* Pharmacokinetics and protein binding of propofol in patients with cirrhosis. *Anesthesiol* 1988; **69**: 887–91.

47 Hohne C, Donaubauer B, Kaisers U. Opioids during anesthesia in liver and renal failure. *Anaesthesist* 2004; **53**: 291–303.

48 Tegeder I, Lotsch J, Geisslinger G. Pharmacokinetics of opioids in liver disease. *Clin Pharmacokinet* 1999; **37**: 17–40.

49 Pentikainen PJ, Valisalmi L, Himberg JJ, Crevoisier C. Pharmacokinetics of midazolam following intravenous and oral administration in patients with chronic liver disease and in healthy subjects. *J Clin Pharmacol* 1989; **29**: 272–7.

50 Bodenham A, Shelly MP, Park GR. The altered pharmacokinetics and pharmacodynamics of drugs commonly used in critically ill patients. *Clin Pharmacokinet* 1988; **14**: 347–73.

51 Park GR. Pharmacokinetics and pharmacodynamics in the critically ill patient. *Xenobiotica* 1993; **23**: 1195–230.

52 Power BM, Forbes AM, van Heerden PV, Ilett KF. Pharmacokinetics of drugs used in critically ill adults. *Clin Pharmacokinet* 1998; **34**: 25–56.

53 De Paepe P, Belpaire FM, Buylaert WA. Pharmacokinetic and pharmacodynamic considerations when treating patients with sepsis and septic shock. *Clin Pharmacokinet* 2002; **41**: 1135–51.

54 Prescott LF, Adjepon-Yamoah KK, Talbot RG. Impaired lignocaine metabolism in patients with myocardial infarction and cardiac failure. *Br Med J* 1976; **1**: 939–41.

55 Patel IH, Soni PP, Fukuda EK, *et al.* The pharmacokinetics of midazolam in patients with congestive heart failure. *Br J Clin Pharmacol* 1990; **29**: 565–9.

56 Shelly MP, Mendel L, Park GR. Failure of critically ill patients to metabolise midazolam. *Anaesthesia* 1987; **42**: 619–26.

57 Vinik HR, Reves JG, Greenblatt DJ, Abernethy DR, Smith LR. The pharmacokinetics of midazolam in chronic renal failure patients. *Anesthesiol* 1983; **59**: 390–4.

58 Milne RW, Nation RL, Somogyi AA, Bochner F, Griggs WM. The influence of renal function on the renal clearance of morphine and its glucuronide metabolites in intensive-care patients. *Br J Clin Pharmacol* 1992; **34**: 53–9.

59 Davies G, Kingswood C, Street M. Pharmacokinetics of opioids in renal dysfunction. *Clin Pharmacokinet* 1996; **31**: 410–22.

60 Ickx B, Cockshott ID, Barvais L, *et al.* Propofol infusion for induction and maintenance of anaesthesia in patients with end-stage renal disease. *Br J Anaesth* 1998; **81**: 854–60.

61 Goyal P, Puri GD, Pandey CK, Srivastva S. Evaluation of induction doses of propofol: comparison between end-stage renal disease and normal renal function patients. *Anaesth Intensive Care* 2002; **30**: 584–7.

62 Lynam DP, Cronnelly R, Castagnoli KP, *et al.* The pharmacodynamics and pharmacokinetics of vecuronium in patients anesthetized with isoflurane with normal renal function or with renal failure. *Anesthesiol* 1988; **69**: 227–31.

63 Szenohradszky J, Caldwell JE, Wright PM, *et al.* Influence of renal failure on the pharmacokinetics and neuromuscular effects of a single dose of rapacuronium bromide. *Anesthesiol* 1999; **90**: 24–35.

64 Agoston S, Vandenbrom RH, Wierda JM. Clinical pharmacokinetics of neuromuscular blocking drugs. *Clin Pharmacokinet* 1992; **22**: 94–115.

65 Pentel P, Benowitz N. Pharmacokinetic and pharmacodynamic considerations in drug therapy of cardiac emergencies. *Clin Pharmacokinet* 1984; **9**: 273–308.

66 Jellett LB, Heazlewood VJ. Pharmacokinetics in acute illness. *Med J Aust* 1990; **153**: 534–41.

67 Halford FJ. A critique of intravenous anesthesia in war surgery. *Anesthesiol* 1943; **4**: 67–9.

68 Benowitz N, Forsyth RP, Melmon KL, Rowland M. Lidocaine disposition kinetics in monkey and man. II. Effects of hemorrhage and sympathomimetic drug administration. *Clin Pharmacol Ther* 1974; **16**: 99–109.

69 Vree TB, Shimoda M, Driessen JJ, *et al*. Decreased plasma albumin concentration results in increased volume of distribution and decreased elimination of midazolam in intensive care patients. *Clin Pharmacol Ther* 1989; **46**: 537–44.

70 Taburet AM, Tollier C, Richard C. The effect of respiratory disorders on clinical pharmacokinetic variables. *Clin Pharmacokinet* 1990; **19**: 462–90.

71 Boucher BA, Kuhl DA, Fabian TC, Robertson JT. Effect of neurotrauma on hepatic drug clearance. *Clin Pharmacol Ther* 1991; **50**: 487–97.

72 Boucher BA, Hanes SD. Pharmacokinetic alterations after severe head injury: clinical relevance. *Clin Pharmacokinet* 1998; **35**: 209–21.

73 Buylaert WA, Herregods LL, Mortier EP, Bogaert MG. Cardiopulmonary bypass and the pharmacokinetics of drugs: an update. *Clin Pharmacokinet* 1989; **17**: 10–26.

74 Hiraoka H, Yamamoto K, Okano N, *et al*. Changes in drug plasma concentrations of an extensively bound and highly extracted drug, propofol, in response to altered plasma binding. *Clin Pharmacol Ther* 2004; **75**: 324–30.

CHAPTER 2
Pharmacodynamics

Susan Hill

Introduction

Pharmacodynamics describes the way in which a drug effects change in the body. There is a number of ways in which this can happen: as a result of physico-chemical interaction, such as the acid-neutralizing effect of sodium citrate or as a result of enzyme inhibition, such as the anti-inflammatory effects of aspirin on cyclo-oxygenase enzymes. However, many drugs interact specifically with endogenous receptors, macromolecules that act as signal transducers between drug binding and response. The term 'receptive substance' was first used by Langley at the end of the 19th century. Many drugs of importance to the anaesthetist interact with receptors; for example propofol and isoflurane act at central $GABA_A$ receptors and neuromuscular blocking agents prevent the action of acetylcholine (ACh) at the nicotinic cholinergic receptors at the motor endplate. With modern technological advances both in X-ray crystallography and gene sequencing, we now know the three-dimensional structure and amino acid sequences of many receptors. Some are multisubunit transmembrane proteins that are associated with very rapid response signalling due to ion channel opening, as are the nicotinic ACh and $GABA_A$ receptors. There is also a very large number of heptahelical transmembrane receptors that require coupling with secondary proteins, G-proteins, before signal transduction can be effected: opioid drugs such as morphine act through such G-protein-coupled receptors (GPCRs). Still other transmembrane proteins have integral enzyme activity associated with their cytosolic face that is activated by extracellular ligand binding; for example, the tyrosine kinase activity associated with the receptor for insulin. Although we

understand the three-dimensional structure of many such receptors, we must also be able to describe the dynamics of drug–receptor interaction.

As we will see later, there may be very different effects observed for transient compared with chronic exposure of a receptor to a given drug concentration. This chapter first briefly describes the nature of the chemical interactions between drug and receptor, then discusses the classic model for drug–receptor interaction and concludes with more recent developments in drug–receptor models that take into account such phenomena as constitutive activity, inverse agonism and agonist signal trafficking.

Nature of the interaction between drug and receptor

Any pharmacodynamic model must be based on permitted chemical interaction(s) between the drug and its receptor. Most drug–receptor interactions are reversible, which implies that the chemical forces responsible for this association must also be reversible. A typical receptor may be thought of as one or more large proteins each folded into a characteristic three-dimensional conformation; the shape adopted and the interaction between subunits will be determined by thermodynamic principles. Successful binding of a drug molecule implies a change in energy state with a new conformation that has a different thermodynamic equilibrium.

In chemical terms, there are several possible types of bonds that can exist within and between molecules. Biological systems are based on carbon compounds, and receptors and enzymes are organic molecules whose atoms are held together by strong covalent bonds that require a large energy input in order to break them. Covalent bonds are rarely involved in drug–receptor interaction although enzymes provide the catalytic energy to overcome energy barriers to break and remake such bonds. Drugs acting as enzyme inhibitors may form a transient intermediate product involving covalent links between enzyme and substrate such as carbamylation of acetylcholinesterase by neostigmine. Ionic bonds are responsible for the electrostatic interaction between atoms that carry opposite charge. Certain amino acids such as histidine and serine have additional carboxylic acid or amine groups that become ionized at pH 7.4 and if present at the receptor site will be available for ionic bond formation. An example is the binding of edrophonium, which carries a permanent charge, to the anionic site of acetylcholinesterase.

A less strong electrostatic interaction known as hydrogen bonding commonly occurs between organic molecules. Hydrogen bonds arise when a hydrogen bond donor and a hydrogen bond acceptor are found in such close proximity that they can form a bridge. A hydrogen bond acceptor is a group possessing a lone pair of electrons such as an amine and a hydrogen bond donor is an electronegative atom that has a hydrogen atom attached to it, such as a hydroxyl group. Each hydrogen bond is much weaker than an ionic bond but often several exist in close proximity so producing an additive effect. With specific arrays of amino acids, specialized three-dimensional structures can be stabilized by hydrogen bonds; in G-protein-coupled receptors the three-dimensional conformation of the seven transmembrane domains is stabilized by hydrogen bonds in the form of α-helices long enough to span the membrane.

The weakest form of association between organic molecules is the van der Waals bond, which is only effective over a very short distance. Random fluctuations in the electron clouds around non-polar groups, particularly neutral hydrocarbon regions, result in areas with a transient excess or deficit of electrons. As a result, weak electrostatic attraction is possible between an area with a transient electron deficit and a similar region on a ligand that has a transient excess of electrons. This type of interaction explains why alkyl groups and aromatic rings are common components of drug molecules. Alkyl groups may be able to fit into hydrophobic pockets and aromatic rings into hydrophobic slots through van der Waals bonds. Many neurotransmitters have such a structure; norepinephrine, the natural ligand for adrenoceptors, has an aromatic ring and an ethylamine side chain. Dipole–dipole interactions exist if there is a tendency for the electron cloud of a molecule to be asymmetrical along its axis, where one end of the molecule becomes relatively negative compared with the other. Molecules with dipole moments will therefore line-up in parallel.

The association of the drug with its receptor involves several of these bonds. The initial interaction is often electrostatic, which brings the drug close to the receptor site. Dipole–dipole interactions may influence the orientation with which the drug closely approaches the binding site. The initial interaction is then strengthened by the formation of hydrogen and van der Waals bonds; the greater the area of contact between drug and active site the greater the density of these weaker, stabilizing bonds. The drug will not be held so tightly that dissociation is prevented, but will be held long enough to distort the three-dimensional arrangement of the peptide sequences in close proximity to the binding site. Such small changes are then sufficient to allow a conformational change that triggers the chain of events leading to the response. The new conformation will be in thermodynamic equilibrium, depending on the continued presence of the drug. The closer the correlation between the three-dimensional conformation of the receptor site and the ligand, the closer the drug can approach the active site. This is the lock-and-key concept often discussed with reference to substrate suitability for enzymes. Because stereoisomers differ in their three-dimensional configuration, often just one isomer will activate the receptor.

Occupancy theory: the law of mass action

Early studies on whole tissue preparations identified a saturable relationship between drug concentration and response, which resembled the hyperbolic Michaelis–Menten kinetics for enzyme activity. Later studies showed that drug binding was both specific and non-specific. Once non-specific low-affinity high-capacity binding is subtracted from overall binding a characteristic hyperbolic curve is revealed, which reflects specific high-affinity low-capacity binding. The similarity of binding and response curves for agonist drugs supported early theories of drug receptor interaction based on the law of mass action, as for enzyme kinetics.

$$D + R \leftrightarrow DR \rightarrow\rightarrow\rightarrow\rightarrow Response$$

One of the first models of drug–receptor interaction was Clark's occupancy theory [1], which assumed that physiological response (E) was linearly related to fractional receptor occupancy (f) with a maximum response when all receptors were occupied. In this model, receptors are analogous to switches that can be turned on and off and it is assumed there is a fixed total number of receptors:

$$f = [D]/(K_D + [D])$$

A plot of fractional response, f, against concentration of agonist drug, [D], is hyperbolic, as required.

When f = ½, the drug concentration is equal to the equilibrium dissociation constant (i.e. $[D] = K_{D)}$. For agonist drugs this concentration is also known as the effective dose producing 50% response ($ED_{50)}$; it is a measure of the potency of the drug and allows us to compare drugs acting on the same receptor system. The semi-logarithmic plot of log (dose) against response, which is sigmoid with an almost linear central region, allows for better comparison of ED_{50} for different agonists in a given system (Fig. 2.1b). The assumption of a linear relationship between receptor occupancy and response predicts a linear relationship between 1/E and 1/[D], which can be demonstrated in a Lineweaver–Burk plot (Fig. 2.1c).

If more than one drug molecule binds to a receptor:

$$nD + R \leftrightarrow D_nR \rightarrow\rightarrow\rightarrow\rightarrow Response$$

then for the resulting linear relationship:

$$\log(f/(1 - f)) = n \log [D] + \log K_D$$

a plot of log (f/(1 – f)) against log [D], a Hill plot (Fig. 2.1d), will give a straight line with gradient n. If n is non-integer, then cooperative binding is present where the binding of the second and subsequent molecule to the receptor is easier than for the first, as

first described for the binding of oxygen to haemoglobin.

Developments of the classic occupancy model

Although some early experimental evidence supported the assumptions made in Clark's model, anomalies arose. Not all agonists elicited the same maximum physiological responses; the switch was not simply 'on' or 'off', but could be partly on. Those drugs that failed to elicit the maximum response associated with full agonist activity were known as partial agonists. In the 1950s, modifications to Clark's model made independently by Ariëns [1] and Stephenson [2] introduced an empirical constant of proportionality between response and fractional occupancy. Ariëns regarded 'intrinsic activity' as a property of the agonist, whereas Stephenson described 'efficacy' as a property of the tissue. Partial agonists were proposed to have an efficacy above 0 but less than 1. Furchgott [3] realized that both agonist- and tissue-dependent factors can influence response, accounting both for partial agonism and 'spare receptors' — the observation that an agonist can exhibit maximal effect with submaximal occupancy. All these models retained the assumption of a linear relationship between receptor occupancy and response, with affinity and efficacy being independent properties.

Antagonists

So far, we have discussed agonists, drugs that produce a positive tissue response. Drugs that can inhibit the response to agonists are known as antagonists or inhibitors; they have affinity but exert no response themselves so in classic terms their efficacy is 0. Antagonists can be either reversible or irreversible, depending on whether the inhibitor is temporarily or permanently bound to the receptor. Some inhibitory drugs bind irreversibly to the receptor; an example in clinical practice is the use of phenoxybenzamine in the treatment of thyrotoxicosis.

Reversible antagonists

Classically, there are two types of reversible antagonists: competitive and non-competitive.

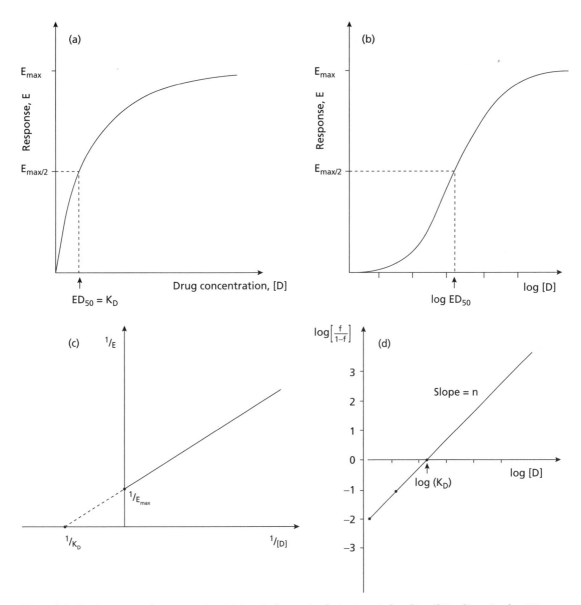

Figure 2.1 Classic receptor theory: agonists. (a) A typical hyperbolic dose–response curve. (b) A semi-logarithmic transformation gives a log(dose)–response curve, which is sigmoid. The drug concentration at which 50% of the maximum response is obtained is the ED_{50}. (c) Lineweaver–Burk plot: a double reciprocal plot that is linear if there is a linear relationship between receptor occupancy and response. (d) The Hill plot, see Appendix for derivation. A plot of $\log(f/(1-f))$ against $\log[D]$, where f is fractional response, gives a straight line. The slope of the line will be more than 1 if positive cooperativity is present (i.e. if two or more drug molecules bind then the binding of the second occurs more readily than the first). The intercept on the x-axis gives $\log(K_D)$. For further information on classic theories see Bowman and Rand [30].

Competitive antagonists bind to the same site on the receptor as the agonist; non-competitive antagonists bind at a separate site. In the presence of a fixed dose of a competitive inhibitor the log(dose)–response curve is shifted to the right in a parallel fashion, without altering the maximum response (Fig. 2.2a). An example in anaesthetic practice is the competitive non-depolarizing blockade produced by vecuronium at the nicotinic acetylcholine receptor at the neuromuscular junction. The apparent K_D of the agonist is therefore increased in the presence of a competitive antagonist: its apparent affinity has been reduced. The extent of that reduction in affinity is determined by the dose of inhibitor and its dissociation constant for the receptor (K_I), which can be found from the Schild equation (Fig. 2.2d; see Appendix for derivation):

$$\log(\text{dose ratio} - 1) = \log[I] - \log(K_I)$$

Partial agonists and inhibition

In the presence of full agonists, partial agonists can apparently act as competitive inhibitors. With a fixed submaximal dose of a partial agonist at low dose of full agonist we see just the effects of the partial agonist. On increasing the dose of the full agonist an additive effect is seen, but at higher doses of full agonist we encounter competition and the partial agonist acts like a competitive antagonist (Fig. 2.2d). It is also possible to elicit a series of log(dose)–response curves for a partial agonist in the presence of different fixed doses of full agonist (Fig. 2.2e). In this case, with a high initial concentration of full agonist, the response falls as the concentration of partial agonist is increased, until the competitive effect of the partial agonist overwhelms that of the full agonist and the observed response is equal to that for the partial agonist alone.

Non-competitive inhibitors

A reversible non-competitive antagonist interferes with the series of events responsible for the response to an agonist at a site distant from the agonist binding site but does not affect the affinity of the receptor for the drug, so K_D is unaffected. However, its presence reduces the maximum possible effect so reducing the efficacy of the drug (Fig. 2.2b). This has the effect of

reducing the slope rather than the position of the log(dose)–response curve. An example of non-competitive inhibition is the action of ketamine at the N-methyl-D-aspartate (NMDA) receptor, where the agonist is glutamate. In more recent classifications of ligand activity, non-competitive antagonism has been included with negative allosteric mechanisms [4].

An operational model

A major development in receptor theory was made by Black and Leff [5], who challenged the classic assumption of a linear relationship between occupancy and response. They argued that a hyperbolic relationship between concentration of occupied receptors and response would also fit the observed relationship between drug concentration and response. Their model gives the relationship:

$$E/E_{max} = [D]\,\tau/\{[D](\tau+1) + K_D\}$$

This describes a hyperbolic response curve with $ED_{50} = K_D/(1+\tau)$, which distinguishes the model from one where a linear relationship between occupancy and response occurs. The ratio $K_E/[R_T]$ is the transducer ratio, τ, where K_E is the equilibrium dissociation constant of the stimulus–response event and $[R_T]$ the total receptor concentration. The transducer ratio reflects the efficiency of coupling between stimulus and response, a measure of efficacy, whereas K_D reflects the strength of binding of drug to receptor. In highly coupled tissues τ will be small, because a small number of occupied receptors will produce a large response. The magnitude of τ determines both potency and maximal response observed for a given tissue. For two agonists with different efficacies, the ratio of their efficacies will translate from one tissue to another although the absolute values of their efficacies are tissue-dependent (Fig. 2.3).

The operational model has been widely accepted as the model of choice for functional receptor pharmacology, because it separates binding from effect therefore accounting for both agonist and antagonist actions without recourse to the empirical constant, ε, used in earlier models. Receptor theory now refers to 'ligands' binding to receptors, with action determined by τ and K_D, which allows for inhibitors that

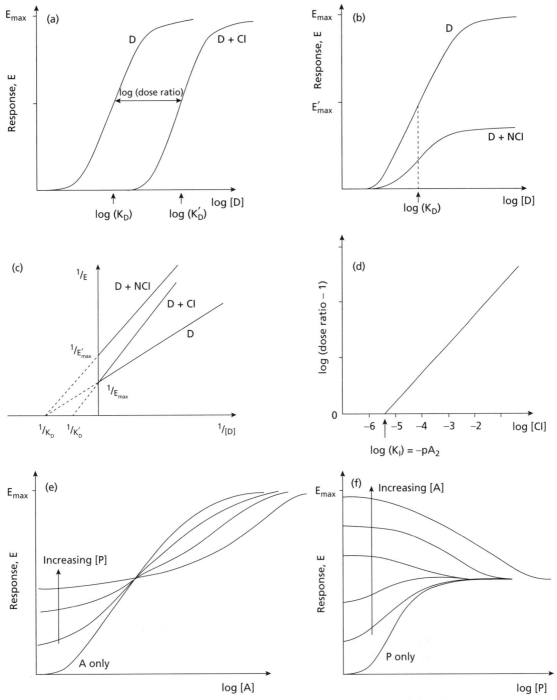

Figure 2.2 Classic receptor theory: antagonists. Typical log(dose)–response curve for a competitive antagonist, CI, E_{max} is unaffected, but there is an increase in the apparent dissociation constant; K_D increases to K_D'. (b) Typical log(dose)–response curve for a non-competitive antagonist, NCI, here K_D is unaffected, but E_{max} is reduced. (c) Theoretical Lineweaver–Burk plots for competitive and non-competitive antagonists. (d) A Schild plot for obtaining K_I, the equilibrium dissociation constant for a competitive inhibitor; derivation of the Schild equation

log(dose ratio – 1) = log [I]—log (K_I) is given in the Appendix. When the dose ratio is 2, the intercept on the x-axis is log K_I, sometimes referred to as $-pA_2$. (e) The inhibitory actions of a partial agonist; log(dose)–response curves for full agonist, A, in the presence of different fixed concentrations of partial agonist (P). (f) Log(dose)–response curves for partial agonist (P) in the presence of different fixed concentrations of full agonist (A). For further information on classic theories see Bowman and Rand [30].

(a)

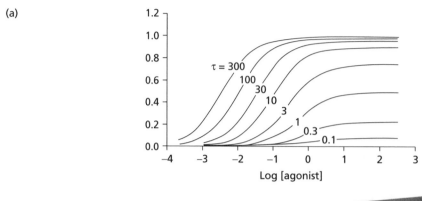

(b)

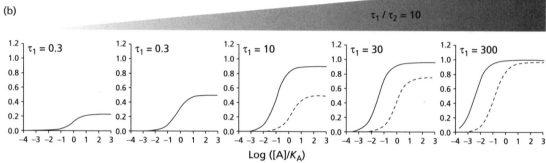

Figure 2.3 The operational model. This shows log(dose)–response curves as predicted for different tissues with different efficacies (τ). (a) In this model, τ determines both maximum response and potency, each curve represents a different value for τ. The model also predicts that relative activity is preserved from tissue to tissue. (b) The relative efficacies of the two tissues is constant $(\tau_1)/(\tau_2) = 10$, but the value of the most efficacious, τ_1, is increased on going from left to right, which represents increased efficiency of tissue-receptor coupling. (Modified from Kenakin [20] with permission.)

alter both affinity and efficacy of an agonist–receptor interaction. Such agents are known as allosteric modulators and may increase (positive allosteric modulators) or decrease the response (negative allosteric modulators) to agonist.

Receptor conformations and pharmacodynamic models

Black and Leff's model separates drug binding from signal transduction. The discovery of GPCRs and G-proteins allowed further investigation of the operational model because there was a clear distinction between binding of ligand to receptor and the necessary interaction with a separate entity, the G-protein, before a response cascade could be triggered. Developments in molecular techniques have al-

lowed study of genetically modified receptors, *in vitro* manipulation of the subunit composition of G-proteins and effects of varying GPCR–G-protein stoichiometry.

Conformational theories of G-protein-coupled receptor action

Before the discovery of G-proteins, excess guanine nucleotides were known to reduce agonist binding to many receptors. Initially it was proposed that two separate binding sites on a single receptor protein were responsible for these observations, but De Lean *et al.* [6] described the ternary complex model, which predicted the existence of G-proteins as entities separate from the receptor–ligand complex (Fig. 2.4a). The model proposed that two conformations of the receptor exist: a high affinity and low affinity form. Association of agonist (A) with receptor (R) forms a binary complex, AR, which increases the rate of association with a third element, now known to be a G-protein, and stabilizes this complex in the high affinity form. The high affinity ternary complex, ARG, then triggers the response cascade. The presence of guanine nucleotides stabilizes the precoupled receptor–G-protein complex, RG, with low affinity for agonist. In this model the proportion of receptors in the high affinity form correlates with the intrinsic activity of the agonist for the receptor as was initially demonstrated for the β_2-adrenergic system [7] but also confirmed in other systems such as D_2-dopaminergic receptors [8].

In 1982, Braestrup *et al.* [9] published evidence of convulsant activity by a ligand binding to the benzodi-

azepine receptor on the $GABA_A$ ionophore complex. The ligand β-carboline-3-carboxylate (β-CCE) acted as an inverse or negative agonist, producing an effect opposite to that of an agonist. In classic terms, a negative agonist has an efficacy between -1 and 0. It was proposed that the negative agonist 'locked' the receptor into a conformation that reduced the ability of GABA to open the channel described by a two-state model [9,10]. The first description of inverse agonism in a G-protein-coupled system was for the δ opioid receptor. Costa and Herz [11] reported a small but consistent response in the absence of ligand binding and provided evidence that this background activity could itself be inhibited. The ternary complex model could not explain this constitutive activity in the absence of ligand binding, which led Samama *et al.* [12] to propose the extended ternary model (Fig. 2.4b)

Figure 2.4 Two-state models. These models are dependent upon the native receptor existing in two distinct conformations. (a) *Ternary complex model.* K_A is the equilibrium affinity constant of ligand for R, α is the differential affinity of ligand for the RG complex, K_G is the equilibrium affinity constant of R for G-protein. (b) *Extended ternary complex model.* This includes an additional activated unbound receptor state, R_a different from the inactive state, R_i. L is the allosteric constant $[R_a]/[R_i]$, K_A now refers to the equilibrium affinity constant of A for R_i and K_G is the equilibrium affinity constant of R_a for G-protein. β is differential affinity of ligand for the activated receptor and α is the differential affinity of AR_a for G-protein. (c) *Cubic ternary complex model.* This model introduces the possibility of G-protein interaction with the inactive receptor. K_A, K_G and L are defined as for the extended ternary complex, α, β, γ and δ are constants that modify the affinity constants as shown.

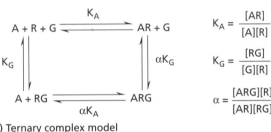

(a) Ternary complex model

(b) Extended ternary complex model

(c) Cubic ternary complex model

that includes an allosteric transformation between inactive (R_i) and active (R_a) receptor forms. In this model agonists have a higher affinity for the active over the inactive receptor, but in addition an inverse agonist has a higher affinity for the inactive receptor, R_i, so can sequester the receptor in a form less responsive to an agonist. An inverse agonist will increase the proportion of receptors in the inactive state so reducing any constitutive activity associated with the active binary complex, R_aG. Neutral antagonists will not favour either form of receptor, binding equally to both. Thus, an antagonist should inhibit the activity of both agonists and inverse agonists equally, which has been shown to be the case both in G-protein-coupled systems and ionophore complexes.

Experimental evidence now suggests that at least 85% of those antagonists that were thought to be neutral antagonists can act as inverse agonists in certain recombinant systems [13]. Not all native GPCRs display constitutive activity and in the absence of such activity inverse agonists will behave exactly like neutral antagonists. There is some debate over the importance of constitutive activity *in vivo* and the therapeutic importance of inverse agonism. The delayed onset of antipsychotic drugs has been attributed to their inverse agonist activity at D_2-dopamine receptors [14]. It has been suggested that up-regulation is associated with inverse agonism, which could arise as a result of reduced internalization and recycling of receptors (normally associated with agonist activity; see below). After long-term use of inverse agonists, true agonists would then exert a greater effect corresponding to an increase in receptor numbers and hence tolerance. This may account for tolerance seen with chronic use of the histamine H_2-antagonists cimetidine and ranitidine [15]. Neutral antagonists are not expected to alter receptor recycling as they have equal affinity for both active and inactive form of the receptor.

More recent studies have provided evidence that not only can the G-protein associate with active receptor, but also with the inactive form, although this in itself will not produce a response. The cubic extended ternary model [16] incorporates this possibility; it is thermodynamically more complete but more complex than the extended ternary model (Fig. 2.4c). Experimentally, it can be difficult to distinguish between these two models, although certain inverse agonists have been shown to sequester the CB_1 cannabinoid receptor as a non-signalling ternary complex [17], suggesting the model may be valid for some receptor systems.

The extended ternary model shows that producing a physiological effect is potentially complex and dependent upon several factors. Effect site concentration of ligand will influence the concentration of occupied receptors and the type of ligand determines the observed response. Any ligand for which $\beta > 1$ will be an agonist; one with $\beta < 1$ may act as an inverse agonist and one where $\alpha = \beta = 1$ will be a pure antagonist. Tissues that have receptors or G-proteins with different subunit composition may display different orders of potency for a series of ligands. In the presence of constitutive activity, it is theoretically possible for a ligand to be an agonist in one system but an inverse agonist in another. This is referred to as protean agonism and was first demonstrated experimentally in the β_2-adrenoceptor system [18]. Such activity has been demonstrated *in vitro* with recombinant systems, but its therapeutic relevance *in vivo* is yet to be established.

Probability models

The models described above are often referred to as 'two-state models' because they assume two distinct receptor conformations: active and inactive. In reality they describe an infinite number of receptor–ligand conformations because the thermodynamic equilibrium conformation in the presence of one ligand will be different from that with another [19,20], although both may elicit a maximum physiological response.

It is clear that although the extended ternary model is useful when describing the potency and efficacy of a physiological response, there are other responses associated with drug–receptor interaction, which have been described as ligand-specific receptor responses. The efficacy of these secondary responses does not necessarily correspond with the efficacy of the primary physiological response and cannot be accounted for by the two-state linkage models described above [21]. Study of the interaction of ligand-coupled GPCRs with multiple G-proteins and the regulation of these interactions has shown a number of secondary cellular responses triggered by agonists. Many of these secondary responses affect physiological response and are often referred to as agonist signal trafficking. The extent to which these secondary responses occur may depend on the duration of the agonist signal and so are determined by the pharmacokinetics of drug administration and effect site concentration. The observed effect in the presence of chronic exposure to an agonist may not be the same as in acute exposure; chronic exposure may be associated with the development of tolerance. These time-dependent phenomena cannot be explained by simple two-state models.

There are several possible mechanisms involved in signal modification: desensitization; up- and down-regulation of receptor numbers; internalization; phosphorylation, interaction with receptor activity-modifying proteins [22] and dimerization or oligomerization [20,21].

Desensitization describes a reduction in receptor response to excess administration of ligand. The rate at which desensitization develops differs among receptor systems; it occurs rapidly in opioid GPCR systems. There are several mechanisms whereby desensitization may occur; receptor numbers may be reduced by internalization or signal-coupling may become less efficient. This is either associated with a reduction in receptor numbers (down-regulation) or by a reduction in signal transduction such as that associated with receptor phosphorylation. One mechanism for internalization is covalent association with ubiquitin, a 76 amino acid polypeptide, which 'tags' a protein for removal from its membrane site by endocytosis for lysosomal degradation [23]. It has been shown that the β_2-adrenoceptor is polyubiquitinated in response to agonist stimulation [24]. Up-regulation is also seen in many neurotransmitter systems when the concentration of natural ligand is chronically reduced; it is an adaptive mechanism aimed at restoring the normal level of neuronal traffic. An example is seen in motor nerve damage, where the neural supply to a muscle group is reduced resulting in an increase in the number of nicotinic cholinergic receptors on the postsynaptic muscle membrane,

both at the neuromuscular junction and extrajunctionally. Interestingly, these receptors are of the fetal type, where the ε subunit seen in adults is replaced by the fetal γ subunit. Fetal receptors have a longer channel-opening time than the adult type, which explains the hyperkalaemia observed after suxamethonium use in patients with denervation injuries [25]. Although desensitization and internalization are usually associated with agonist activation of receptors, these two effects can sometimes be separated, particularly with chronic exposure, such as in the μ-opioid system. Methadone produces much greater desensitization than morphine [26] and morphine fails to trigger rapid receptor internalization compared with etorphine [27]. Such agonist-dependent differences in signal trafficking could be exploited therapeutically.

The operational model does not explain the observation that efficacy of primary physiological response and efficacy of secondary response can differ. This has been referred to as a difference in quality of agonist action or 'ligand-specific agonism'. Kenakin [20] suggests these differences may be explained by considering a probabilistic model of protein conformations, with several possible ensembles each associated with a given response [28,29]. The probability distribution of the conformations permitted change upon interaction with ligand. Each agonist will induce a slightly different distribution of microconformations, all of which permit signal transduction, but the exact probability distribution in response to each agonist is different; some will overlap with conformations that induce internalization or dimerization for example, whereas others will not (Fig. 2.5).

Other transmembrane signalling systems

Thus far we have concentrated on membrane-bound GPCRs as a means of signal transduction. There are several other mechanisms through which agonist-induced responses may be triggered such as ionophore complexes and integral transmembrane protein–enzyme systems. In terms of pharmacodynamic models, those that have been developed for GPCRs can also be adapted to these other systems.

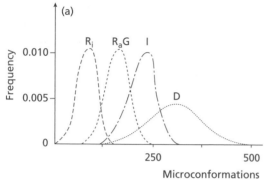

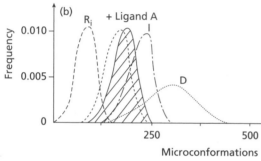

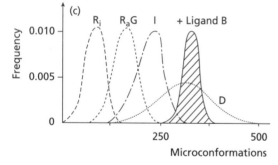

Figure 2.5 Probability model for ligand-specific agonism. Probability distributions of microconformations associated with primary (R_aG) and secondary responses in a hypothetical receptor system forming ligand ensembles. R_i is the distribution of conformations associated with inactive receptor, I is the distribution of conformations associated with internalization of receptors and D is the distribution of conformations associated with dimerization of the receptor. Each ligand-bound receptor can assume a different distribution of conformations. (a) Hypothetical distributions of microconformations producing primary and secondary responses. (b) Ligand A will signal and trigger internalization. (c) Ligand B will not signal but causes dimerization. (Modified from Kenakin [18] with permission.)

Conclusions

In this chapter, receptor theory has been introduced as the underlying mechanism for drug-induced physiological responses. The crucial link between pharmacokinetics and pharmacodynamics is the effect site concentration, which determines the extent of this response. Classic occupation theory failed to account adequately for efficacy and operational theory has become the accepted two-state model for describing the primary response to agonist binding. Further work involving GPCRs, allowing separation of ligand binding and signal coupling, has led to the extended ternary complex model for GPCR activation. This model explains partial, inverse and protean agonists by the inclusion of both allosteric (receptor-dependent) and coupling (tissue-dependent) factors with the possibility of constitutive as well as ligand-induced activation. A probabilistic approach to the distribution of microconformations of receptor proteins has been proposed to account for ligand-dependent differences in the triggering of secondary, regulatory, responses to drug binding such as desensitization, receptor internalization and phosphorylation. The newly discovered complexity of receptor formation, activation and regulation should provide new avenues for target-specific drug development.

References

1 Ariëns EJ. Affinity and intrinsic activity. *Arch Int Pharmacodyn Ther* 1954; **99**: 32–49.

2 Stephenson RP. A modification of receptor theory. *Br J Pharmacol* 1956; **11**: 379–93.

3 Furchgott RF. The use of β-haloalkylamines in the differentiation of receptors and in the determination of dissociation constants of receptor-agonist complexes. *Adv Drug Res* 1966; **3**: 21–55.

4 Onaran HO, Costa T. Agonist efficacy and allosteric models of receptor action. *Ann N Y Acad Sci* 1997; **812**: 98–115.

5 Black JW, Leff P. Operational models of pharmacological agonists. *Proc R Soc Lond B Biol Sci* 1983; **220**: 141–62.

6 De Lean A, Stadel JM, Lefkowitz RJ. A ternary complex model explains the agonist-specific binding properties of the adenylate cyclase-coupled β-adrenergic receptor. *J Biol Chem* 1980; **255**: 7108–17.

7 Chidiac P, Nouet S, Bouvier M. Agonist-induced modulation of inverse agonist efficacy at the β_2-adrenergic receptor. *Mol Pharmacol* 1996; **50**: 662–9.

8 Wreggett KA, De Lean A. The ternary complex model: its properties and application to ligand interactions with the D_2-dopamine receptor of the anterior pituitary gland. *Mol Pharmacol* 1984; **26**: 214–27.

9 Braestrup C, Schmiechen R, Neef G, Nielsen M, Petersen EN. Interaction of convulsive ligands with benzodiazepine receptors. *Science* 1982; **216**: 1241–3.

10 Ehlert FJ, Roeske WR, Gee KW, Yamamura HI. An allosteric model for benzodiazepine receptor function. *Biochem Pharmacol* 1983; **32**: 2375–83.

11 Costa T, Herz A. Antagonists with negative intrinsic activity at δ-opioid receptors coupled to GTP-binding proteins. *Proc Natl Acad Sci USA* 1989; **86**: 7321–5.

12 Samama P, Cotecchia S, Costa T, Lefkowitz RJ. A mutation-induced activated state of the β_2-adrenergic receptor: extending the ternary complex model. *J Biol Chem* 1993; **268**: 4625–36.

13 Kenakin TP. Inverse, protean, and ligand-selective agonism: matters of receptor conformation. *FASEB J* 2001; **15**: 598–611.

14 Hall DA, Strange PG. Evidence that antipsychotic drugs are inverse agonists at D_2-dopamine receptors. *Br J Pharmacol* 1997; **121**: 731–6.

15 Nwalko CU, Smith JTL, Sawyer AM, Pounder RE. Rebound intragastric hyperacidity after abrupt withdrawal of histamine H_2-receptor blockade. *Gut* 1991; **32**: 1455–60.

16 Weiss JM, Morgan PH, Lutz MW, Kenakin TP. The cubic ternary complex receptor-occupancy model. I. Model description. *J Theoret Biol* 1996; **178**: 151–67.

17 Bouaboula M, Perrachon S, Milligan L, *et al.* A selective inverse agonist for central cannabinoid receptor inhibits mitogen-activated protein kinase activation stimulated by insulin or insulin-like growth factor. *J Biol Chem* 1997; **272**: 22330–9.

18 Kenakin TP. Drug efficacy at G-protein coupled receptors. *Ann Rev Pharmacol Toxicol* 2002; **42**: 349–79.

19 Kenakin TP, Onaran O. The ligand paradox between affinity and efficacy: can you be there and make a difference? *Trends Pharmacol Sci* 2002; **23**: 275–80.

20 Kenakin T. Principles: receptor theory in pharmacology. *Trends Pharmacol Sci* 2004; **25**: 186–92.

21 Yu Y, Zhang L, Yin X, *et al.* μ Opioid receptor phosphorylation, desensitization and ligand efficacy. *J Biol Chem* 1997; **272**: 28869–74.

22 Wojcikiewicz RJH. Regulated ubiquitination of proteins in GPCR-initiated signaling pathways. *Trends Pharmacol Sci* 2004; **25**: 35–41.

23 Shenoy SK, McDonald PH, Kohout TA, Lefkowitz TA. Regulation of receptor fate by ubiquitination of activated β_2-adrenergic receptor and β-arrestin. *Science* 2001; **294**: 1307–13.

24 Morfis M, Christopoulos A, Sexton P. RAMPs: 5 years on, where to now? *Trends Pharmacol Sci* 2003; **24**: 596–601.

25 Scheutze S. Embryonic and adult acetylcholine receptors: molecular basis of developmental changes in ion channel properties. *Trends Neurosci* 1986; **9**: 386–8.

26 Strange PG. Mechanisms of inverse agonism at G-protein-coupled receptors. *Trends Pharmacol Sci* 2002; **23**: 89–95.

27 Keith DE, Murray SR, Zaki PA, *et al.* Morphine activates opioid receptors without causing their rapid internalization. *J Biol Chem* 1996; **271**: 19021–4.

28 Hilsier VJ. Modeling the native state ensemble. In: Murphy K, ed. *Protein Structure, Stability and Folding: Methods in Molecular Biology.* Totowa, NJ: Humana Press, 2001: 93–115.

29 Kenakin TP. Pharmacological proteus? *Trends Pharmacol Sci* 1995; **16**: 256–8.

30 Bowman WC, Rand MJ. Principles of drug action. In: *Textbook of Pharmacology,* 2nd edn. Oxford: Blackwell Scientific Publications, 1980: 39.1–39.69.

Appendix

The following sections give more detailed derivations of some of the classic receptor models; for further information see Bowman and Rand [30]. The derivation of the mathematical expressions of the two-state models is not expanded here, although the definitions given in Fig. 2.4 are readily derived. For a more detailed review see Kenakin [20].

Simple mass action

For a drug [D] interacting with a receptor [R] according to the law of mass action, the equation relating the rates of the forward and reverse reactions at equilibrium is given by:

$$[D] \cdot [R] \cdot k_f = [DR] \cdot k_b \tag{1}$$

An expression for [DR] in terms of the equilibrium dissociation constant from (1) gives:

$$[DR] = [D][R]/K_D \tag{2}$$

We do not know [R], but we know the number of receptors is finite. If R_T is the total number of receptors and we assume that maximum response occurs when all receptors are occupied, $[R] = [R_T] - [DR]$. Substituting this into the equation above gives:

$$[DR] = [D] \cdot ([R_T] - [DR])/K_D \qquad (3)$$

Rearrangement gives:

$$[DR]/[R_T] = [D]/(K_D + [D]) \qquad (4)$$

Fractional response, f, is the ratio of occupied receptors to the total number of receptors (1) so from (4):

$$f = [D]/(K_D + [D])$$

The Hill plot

The mass action equation for n drug molecules per single receptor:

$$nD + R \leftrightarrow D_nR \rightarrow \rightarrow \rightarrow Response$$

This will give a different expression for K_D:

$$K_D = [D]^n[R]/[D_nR]$$

So we now can find expressions for the fraction of occupied (f) and unoccupied (1 − f) receptors:

$$f = [D]^n/([D]^n + K_D)$$

$$1 - f = 1 - [D]^n/([D]^n + K_D) = K_D/([D]^n + K_D)$$

If we take the ratio of occupied to unoccupied receptors we end up with a simple expression:

$$f/(1 - f) = [D]^n/K_D$$

If we take logarithms of both sides, we have the equation of a straight line:

$$\log(f/(1 - f)) = n \log[D] + \log K_D$$

A plot of log $(f/(1 - f))$ against log $[D]$ will give a straight line with gradient n. When n is non-integer, cooperativity of binding should be suspected.

The Schild equation for finding K_I for competitive antagonists

Let $[D1]$ be agonist drug concentration before adding antagonist and $[D2]$ after the addition of a competitive antagonist; $[D1]$ and $[D2]$ exert the same response. Let $[I]$ be the concentration of antagonist added to the system. Before adding inhibitor:

$$D + R \leftrightarrow DR \rightarrow \rightarrow \rightarrow Response$$

and it was shown in the text that fractional occupancy is given by:

$$f = [D_1]/([D_1] + K_D) = 1/(1 + K_D/[D_1]) \qquad (1)$$

After addition of competitive inhibitor:

$$D + R + I \leftrightarrow DR + DI \rightarrow \rightarrow \rightarrow Response$$

we now have two equilibrium reactions:

$$D + R \leftrightarrow DR \qquad (2)$$

$$I + R \leftrightarrow IR \qquad (3)$$

Thus:

$$K_D = [D_2][R]/[DR] \quad \text{and so} \quad [R] = K_D[DR]/[D_2] \qquad (4)$$

but if K_I is the dissociation constant for the inhibitor at concentration $[I]$:

$$K_I = [I][R]/[IR] \quad \text{and so} \quad [R] = K_I[IR]/[I] \qquad (5)$$

The fractional occupancy in each case is $[DR]/[R_T]$, because they produce the same response. Now:

$$[R_T] = [R] + [DR] + [IR] \qquad (6)$$

from (4) and (5):

$$K_D[DR]/[D_2] = K_I[IR]/[I]$$

so we can write $[IR]$ as:

$$[IR] = [I] K_D[DR]/[D_2] K_I \qquad (7)$$

Substituting for $[R]$ from (4) and $[IR]$ from (7), we can now write fractional response after adding inhibitor as:

$$[DR]/[R_T] = [DR]/(K_D[DR]/[D_2] + [DR] + [I]K_D[DR]/[D_2] K_I)$$

After rearrangement this gives:

$$[DR]/[R_T] = 1/(1 + (K_D/D_2)\{1 + ([I]/K_I)\})$$

because this is the same response seen without inhibitor present, from (1):

$$1/(1 + K_D/[D_1]) = 1/(1 + (K_D/[D_2])\cdot(1 + ([I]/K_I)))$$

Thus:

$$K_D/[D_1] = (K_D/[D_2])\cdot(1 + ([I]/K_I))$$

so we now have:

$$[D_2]/[D_1] = 1 + ([I]/K_I) \qquad (8)$$

Therefore the dose ratio, $[D_2]/[D_1]$, is related in a simple way to the concentration of inhibitor present and the dissociation constant for the inhibitor.

If we rearrange and take logarithms:

$$\log(\text{dose ratio} - 1) = \log[I] - \log(K_I)$$

the Schild plot log (dose ratio − 1) against log [I] which is linear and K_I can be found. When the dose ratio is 2, the intercept on the *x*-axis is log (K_I), which is sometimes known as $-pA_2$ (i.e. the negative logarithm of the dose of inhibitor that requires the agonist concentration to be doubled in order to overcome the inhibition and return to the original response).

Mathematical representation of the extended ternary model

By extension of the mass action equations to the increased number of receptor species present, it can be shown that in the presence of agonist, the response produced is given by:

$$E = \{L[G]/K_G(1 + \beta\alpha\,[A]/K_A)\}/\{[A]/K_A(1 + \beta L\,(1 + \alpha\,[G]/K_G)) + 1 + L\,(1 + [G]/K_G)\}$$

This model is shown in Fig. 2.4b. Note the use of K_A rather than K_D to emphasize the importance of association with rather than dissociation from the receptor; K_G is the equilibrium association constant for inactive receptor (R_i) with G-protein. The constants L, α and β are as defined in Fig. 2.4b. In the absence of agonist, A = 0, but if constitutive activity is present there will still be a response given by:

$$E_0 = (L\,[G]/K_G)/\{1 + L\,(1 + [G]/K_G)\}$$

The maximum response occurs when [A] is effectively infinite. The response is then:

$$E_{max} = (\alpha\beta L\,[G]/K_G)/\{1 + \beta L(1 + \alpha\,[G]/K_G\}$$

Thus, the ratio of response in the presence and absence of agonist is given by E_0/E_{max}:

$$E_0/E_{max} = ((L\,[G]/K_G)/\{1 + L\,(1 + [G]/K_G)\})/((\alpha\beta L\,[G]/K_G)/\{1 + \beta L\,(1 + \alpha\,[G]/K_G\})$$

This simplifies to:

$$= \{\alpha\beta\,(1 + L\,(1 + [G]/K_G)\}/\{1 + \beta L\,(1 + \alpha\,[G]/K_G)\}$$

In some systems *in vivo* this is zero, because constitutive activity is not observed.

CHAPTER 3
Pharmacogenomics

Amr Mahdy

Introduction

There is a great heterogeneity in the way individuals respond to medication, in terms of both toxicity and therapeutic effects. This difference in response has almost always been attributed to a variety of non-genetic factors such as age, sex and race, the pathogenesis and severity of the disease being treated, drug interactions, hepatic and renal function, nutritional status and the presence of concomitant illness. Despite the importance of these factors, it is now recognized that inherited differences in metabolism and disposition of drugs, and genetic polymorphisms in the targets of drug therapy, can have an even greater influence on the efficacy and toxicity of medications. Such genetic determinants of drug disposition and effects remain stable for a person's lifetime and can have marked effects, independent of the non-genetic factors.

In 510 BC, Pythagoras noted that ingestion of fava beans resulted in a potentially fatal reaction in some individuals [1]. Two and half millennia later, during the Second World War, it was noted that some black soldiers who were given primaquine as prophylaxis against malaria developed haemolytic anaemia. Subsequently, it was recognized that interindividual differences in the activity of the enzyme glucose-6-phosphate dehydrogenase were responsible for the reactions noted by Pythagoras as well as those noted with primaquine [2].

In the 1950s, clinical evidence of inherited differences in drug effects continued to emerge. Prolonged muscle relaxation after suxamethonium was explained by an inherited deficiency of a plasma cholinesterase [3]; similarly, peripheral neuropathy of isoniazid was explained by inherited differences in the acetylation of this medication [4].

In 1959, Vogel was the first to use the term 'pharmacogenetics' [5]. Subsequently, Kalow [6] covered the whole field for the first time in 1962 in his book *Pharmacogenetics — Heredity and the Response to Drugs*.

In the late 1980s, the occurrence of diplopia and blurred vision after administration of the anti-arrhythmic/oxytocic drug, sparteine, and severe orthostatic hypotension after treatment with the antihypertensive agent, debrisoquine, led to the discovery of a genetic polymorphism that affects the drug-metabolizing enzyme cytochrome P450 2D6 (CYP2D6) [7]. This was a major breakthrough towards understanding the molecular genetic basis for inherited differences in drug disposition and metabolism.

Pharmacogenetics and pharmacogenomics

Pharmacogenetics has been defined as the study of variability in drug response resulting from heredity. More recently, the term 'pharmacogenomics' has been introduced. The latter is a broader based term that encompasses all genes in the genome that may determine drug response [8]. However, at present, there is no consensus in the literature and the two terms are often used interchangeably.

In 2002, the Committee for Proprietary Medicinal Products (CPMP) of the European agency for the Evaluation of Medicinal Products (EMEA) introduced a 'position paper on terminology in pharmacogenetics'. The committee defined pharmacogenetics as 'the study of individual variations in DNA sequence related to drug response', whereas pharmacogenomics was defined as 'the study of the variability of the expression of individual genes relevant to disease susceptibility as well as drug response at cellular, tissue, individual or population level' [9].

Basic genetics

Much of what makes us unique individuals is that the DNA sequence in each of us is different from that of other people. Data from the Human Genome Project (HGP) indicate that on average any two people have 99.9% identical DNA sequences. Yet that 0.1% difference is spread over 3.2 billion bases of DNA and thus amounts to a significant number of distinct genetic traits that uniquely distinguish the genome of every person. In fact, the HGP now estimates that there are just 32 000 functional genes in the human genome. For each of these genes, there exist many different variant forms in the human population, and each person has a unique combination of these forms [10].

The simplest definition of a gene is a string of nucleotides that ultimately determines the structure of a protein, and in molecular terms it is the entire nucleic acid sequence that is necessary for the synthesis of a functional polypeptide. With the exception of genes occurring on the X or Y chromosomes (sex-linked genes), every individual carries two copies of each gene. Copies of a specific gene present within a population may not have identical nucleotide sequences and hence is said to exhibit genetic polymorphism [11].

The word polymorphism comes from the Greek *poly*, meaning several, and *morphe*, meaning form. Thus, a polymorphism is something that can take one of several forms [12]. In genes in which polymorphisms have been detected, alternative forms of the gene are called alleles. When the alleles at a particular gene locus are identical on both chromosomes, a homozygous state exists, whereas heterozygous refers to the situation in which different alleles are present at the same gene locus. The term genotype refers to the genetic constitution of an individual, whereas the observable characteristics or physical manifestations constitute the phenotype, which is the net consequence of genetic and environmental effects [13].

To end confusion between genotypic and phenotypic definitions of polymorphism and to clarify the relationship between genetic concepts and the clinical relevance of a given phenotype, Meyer [14] proposed that pharmacogenetic polymorphism be defined as a monogenic trait caused by the presence in the same population of more than one allele at the same locus and more than one phenotype regarding drug interaction with the organism with the frequency of the least common allele being greater than 1%.

Genetic polymorphism, although taking many forms, arises mainly from two types of genetic mutation events, the simplest of which results from a single base mutation that substitutes one nucleotide for another. This mutation event accounts for the most common form of variation and is known as single nucleotide polymorphisms (SNP; pronounced 'snip'). The other type of mutation results from the insertion or deletion of a section of DNA. At the simplest level this can result in the insertion or deletion of one or more nucleotides, so-called insertion/deletion polymorphisms. The most common insertion/deletion events occur in repetitive sequence elements, where repeated nucleotide patterns, so-called 'variable number tandem repeats' (VNTRs), expand or contract as a result of insertion or deletion events. The rarest insertion/deletion events involve deletions or duplications of regions ranging from a few kilobases to several megabases [15].

SNPs have received more attention than other sequence variants because they are probably responsible for most phenotypic differences and are particularly suitable for pharmacogenetic studies, being more frequent, dense and stable and more amenable to high-throughput genotyping strategies. SNPs are common, occurring in the human genome at a frequency of 10% or higher. They may be located in coding regions (cSNPs), non-coding regions (perigenic SNPs), introns (intronic SNPs) or between genes (intergenic SNPs). A SNP in a coding region that changes the amino acid sequence is called a non-synonymous SNP, whereas a SNP that does not change an amino acid sequence is called a synonymous SNP. The estimated number of cSNPs in the human genome that result in alterations in amino acid sequence is around 50 000–100 000. However, the relative importance of SNPs in altering regulatory regions (e.g. promoter elements, splice sites) is difficult to predict and should not be underestimated [16].

The main bulk of SNP data generated over the past few years can primarily be traced to two major overlapping sources: the SNP Consortium [17] and members of the Human Genome Sequencing Consortium, particularly the Sanger Institute and Washington University. The predominance of SNP data from these sources has facilitated the development of a central SNP database — dbSNP at the NCBI [18,19].

However, it should be noted that the association of a SNP with an altered therapeutic response might have no functional explanation but instead might be caused by a type 1 error (i.e. an association is accepted as real when it is actually false). In the setting of multiple testing, with many loci in a candidate gene or a few loci in many genes, erroneous associations are likely to be made because of statistical artefacts. By correcting for multiple comparisons and using relatively conservative thresholds of significance, type 1 error can be avoided. Moreover, a SNP can be associated with a particular phenotype in the absence of an obvious functional effect because of linkage disequilibrium (i.e. two or more alleles at different loci occur together more often than expected by chance because of their close proximity in the genome and infrequent recombination). The non-functional SNP is associated with altered drug response because it is in linkage disequilibrium with a functional SNP that is the true pharmacogenetic locus [20].

These issues are complicated further by the inheritance of families of SNPs together in a given narrow chromosomal region; the group of linked SNPs is known as a SNP haplotype. A pharmacogenetic phenotype can require the interaction of two or more SNPs within a gene or among several genes. Experience with the SNP haplotypes suggests that they are more useful than single SNPs for predicting drug response; however, large study populations are necessary to identify all the common haplotypes and to achieve adequate statistical power [16].

Another common cause of an erroneous association is the use of poorly chosen populations. There might be an ethnic or racial imbalance between drug responders and non-responders such that a SNP that is more frequent in one group reflects ethnic or racial differences and not the genetic basis of the altered drug response. Such confounding factors can be avoided by choosing cases and controls carefully; however, stratification is not always obvious, especially in ethnically and racially diverse populations [16].

Not all pharmacogenetic polymorphisms of drug disposition and action are clinically relevant. However, the likelihood of a clinically significant event is enhanced if the drug is used widely in clinical practice; if the drug displays a narrow therapeutic range; if the defective metabolic pathway is quantitatively significant in determining the overall fate of the compound in the body; and if therapeutic alternatives are limited or absent [13].

Most of the current understanding of pharmacogenetic polymorphisms involves enzymes responsible for drug biotransformation. However, genetic polymorphisms have also been reported in transporter proteins and drug targets and receptors.

Genetic polymorphism influencing drug disposition and action

Polymorphisms in drug metabolizing enzymes

There are over 30 families of drug metabolizing enzymes in humans, and essentially all have genetic variants, many of which cause functional changes in the proteins encoded, and thereby change the metabolism of drugs [21]. Phenotypically, individuals are classified as being extensive, rapid, or ultra-rapid metabolizers at one end, and slow or poor metabolizers at the other end of a spectrum that may also include an intermediate metabolizer group. Patients who express dysfunctional or inactive enzymes are considered poor metabolizers (PM). Pro-drugs, which require biotransformation to an active metabolite, are often not effective in these patients. Drug toxicity may also be observed in this group of patients as a result of impaired drug clearance. Intermediate metabolizers are patients who express decreased enzyme activity and have diminished drug metabolism. Extensive metabolizers (EM) are patients who express enzymes that have normal (extensive) activity, in whom the anticipated medication response would be seen with standard doses of drugs. Ultra-rapid metabolizers are patients who have higher quantities of expressed enzymes because of gene duplication. Normal doses of drugs in this group of patients may result in reduced or no efficacy of some drugs, or toxicity with pro-drugs [22].

Thiopurine methyltransferase (TPMT) polymorphism

Although thiopurine *S*-methyltransferase (TPMT) substrates, such as azathioprine and mercaptopurine, are not commonly used in anaesthesia and intensive care, TPMT is the best example to date of the potential value of pharmacogenetics applied to clinical medicine. Thiopurines are commonly used for a diverse range of medical indications, including leukaemia, rheumatic diseases, inflammatory bowel disease and organ transplantation. The principal cytotoxic mechanism of these agents is mediated via the incorporation of thioguanine nucleotides into DNA. Thus, thiopurines are inactive pro-drugs that require metabolism to thioguanines to exert cytotoxicity [23].

Thiopurines are principally metabolized via oxidation by xanthine oxidase or via methylation by TPMT. However, in haematopoietic tissues, xanthine oxidase is negligible, leaving TPMT as the only inactivation pathway. Approximately 89% of the white and black populations have high TPMT activity, 11% have intermediate activity and 0.3% are completely devoid of TPMT activity [13].

Interest in TPMT pharmacogenetics has been fuelled by the finding that the TPMT genotype identifies patients who are at risk of toxicity from mercaptopurine or azathioprine. A total of nine TPMT alleles have been characterized to date, three of which (TPMT*2, TPMT*3A, TPMT*3C) account for approximately 95% of intermediate or low enzyme activity cases. All three alleles are associated with lower enzyme activity, because of increased rates of proteolysis of the mutant enzyme. Patients with a homozygous mutant or compound heterozygous genotype are TPMT deficient and hence at a very high risk of developing severe haematopoietic toxicity if treated with conventional doses of thiopurines. Moreover, patients who are heterozygous at the TPMT gene locus are at intermediate risk of dose-limiting toxicity [23].

The molecular bases of TMPT genetic polymorphism is not yet clear. However, recently, a polymorphic locus consisting of 3–9 repeats of a specific nucleotide sequence in tandem (VNTR) has been identified in the promoter region of the TPMT gene. This polymorphism seems to modulate TPMT activity to a modest degree *in vitro* and *in vivo* [24].

TPMT genotyping is now available as a molecular diagnostic test from reference laboratories, representing the first certified pharmacogenetic test for individualizing drug treatment based on an individual patient's genotype. The test has been well documented in the effective clinical management of patients with acute lymphoblastic leukaemia; reducing the dose of 6-mercaptopurine by 10–15-fold compared with conventional doses makes the drug as tolerable and effective in TPMT-deficient patients as it is in patients with normal enzyme activity [25].

N-acetyltransferase-2 polymorphism

The arylamine *N*-acetyltransferases (NATs) are found in nearly all species from bacteria to humans. They catalyse the acetyl-transfer from acetyl-coenzyme A to an aromatic amine (e.g. heterocyclic amine or hydrazine compound). In humans, acetylation is a major route of biotransformation for many arylamine and hydrazine drugs, as well as for a number of known carcinogens present in the diet, cigarette smoke and the environment. Two NAT isoenzymes have been identified in humans, NAT1 and NAT2, which are the products of two distinct genes, designated *NAT1* and *NAT2*, respectively. Sequencing of *NAT1* and *NAT2* revealed a number of allelic variants that affect activity of both genes *in vivo*, providing a genetic understanding for the long-known functional polymorphism in NAT2 activity and, more recently, in NAT1 activity [26].

In 1991, the human *NAT2* locus was established as the site of the classic acetylation polymorphism. Since then, the study of *NAT2* allelic variation has been an area of intense investigation. To date, more than 25 different *NAT2* alleles have been detected in human populations, each of which is the result of between one and four nucleotide substitutions located in the protein-encoding region of the gene, with several studies showing clear correlations between

NAT2 genotype and acetylator phenotype: individuals homozygous for a loss of function *NAT2* allele display a slow acetylator phenotype; individuals heterozygous for a loss of function allele are intermediate acetylators; and individuals homozygous for the wild-type allele are rapid acetylators [27]. The frequency of the slow acetylator phenotype varies considerably among ethnic groups, ranging from 40% to 70% in Caucasian and African populations, and 10–30% in Asian populations.

The association between acetylator status and the risk of various diseases has been extensively reported and reviewed in detail. Altered risk with either the slow or rapid phenotype has been observed for bladder, colon and breast cancer, systemic lupus erythematosus, diabetes, Gilbert's disease, Parkinson's disease and Alzheimer's disease. These associations imply a role for environmental factors that are metabolized by the *NATs*, in particular *NAT2*, in each disorder. However, identifying those factors has remained elusive [28].

In addition to its association with disease status, the acetylator status contributes to the polymorphic metabolism of several drugs including isoniazid, hydralazine, procainamide, endralazine, nitrazepam, dapsone, and a number of sulphonamides. Fortunately enough, the incidence of failed or less effective clinical response as a consequence of acetylation polyphorphism is uncommon. This is because most drugs that are metabolized by the NATs have a wide therapeutic window or because acetylation is a minor metabolic pathway. An exception is hydralazine. Early studies showed that the antihypertensive activity of hydralazine was less in rapid acetylators and that a 40% higher dose was necessary for a similar therapeutic effect compared with slow acetylators. This difference appeared to be because of a change in the bioavailability of the drug, which decreased from 33% in slow acetylators to less than 10% in rapid acetylators. A more common consequence of the polymorphic acetylation of therapeutic agents is an increase in the frequency and severity of side-effects associated with the acetylator state. Slow acetylators are at a greater risk of sulphonamide-induced toxicity, hydralazine and procainamide-induced lupus, isoniazid-induced renal toxicity and dapsone-induced neurotoxicity [29].

Polymorphisms in cytochrome P450

The cytochrome P450 system is a group of enzymes that are responsible for metabolizing up to 40–50% of all medications into more hydrophilic substances. CYP is the standard abbreviation for mammalian cytochrome P450 isoenzymes. Families of these isoenzymes share greater than 40% protein sequence homology with each other and are designated by the first number following CYP (e.g. CYP2). Subfamilies share greater than 55% homology with each other and are differentiated by the letter following the family designation (e.g. CYP2D). Single members of subfamilies represent a particular gene and are designated by the number following the subfamily description (e.g. CYP2D6) [30]. The main cytochromes relevant to drug metabolism are CYP3A4, CYP2D6, CYP2C9, CYP2C19, CYP1A2, CYP2E1 and CYP2B6, which metabolize 34%, 19%, 16%, 8%, 8%, 4% and 3% of current therapeutics, respectively [31].

Alleles that cause defective, qualitatively altered, diminished or enhanced rates of drug metabolism have been identified for many of the P450 enzymes and the underlying molecular mechanisms elucidated. Descriptions of the alleles, as well as the nomenclature and relevant references are continuously updated at the web page (http://www.imm.ki.se/ CYPalleles/). To be assigned as a unique P450 allele, newly identified alleles must contain nucleotide changes that have been shown to have significant effects on enzyme activity or result in at least one amino acid change. Individual alleles are designated by the gene name followed by an asterisk and an Arabic number (e.g. CYP2D6*2). The normal version of each gene, designated wild-type, is always given the number 1, thus CYP2D6*1 is the wild-type CYP2D6 allele while CYP2D6*4 is the third identified variant. Alleles that display only minor differences thought to be of no functional significance are given the same numerical designate but differentiated by letter (e.g. CYP2D6*3A and CYP2D6*3B).

The clinical relevance of genetic variability in cytochrome P450 genes is dependent upon many factors including the alleles present, clinical state of the patient, therapeutic index of the administered drug, smoking status and concomitantly administered drugs. Given that many drugs are metabolized by multiple P450s, the percentage of total drug metabolized by a genetically variant P450 is also a major consideration [31].

Variability in cytochrome P450 genes may be assessed at the level of phenotype (by investigating enzyme activity) or genotype (by determining which alleles are present). Phenotypic assessment generally involves the collection of urine after the administration of an appropriate substrate and determination of a relevant metabolic ratio. Poor metabolizers would typically have a much lower ratio of metabolite to drug in urine. This method provides an indication of enzyme activity but does not identify if variability is a result of genetic or other causes. Within a population, the appearance of a clear bimodal or trimodal distribution of the metabolite ratio (reflecting enzyme activity) is strongly suggestive of the presence of genetic polymorphism. Genotyping provides direct information on which cytochrome P450 alleles are present but accurate interpretation requires an understanding of the relationship between any given genotype and the resultant phenotype.

In the following paragraphs a brief discussion of common polymorphisms in CYP3A4, CYP2D6, CYP2C9, CYP2C19 and CYP1A2 is given, together with any relevant clinical applications.

Debrisoquine hydroxylase (CYP2D6) polymorphism is probably the most well-characterized genetic polymorphism in cytochrome P450 enzymes. It is, in fact, the first human polymorphic drug-metabolizing enzyme to be cloned and characterized at the molecular level [7]. It was initially discovered when a principal investigator developed marked hypotension during participation in a pharmacokinetic study of debrisoquine, an antihypertensive [32]. Family studies subsequently showed that he had an inherited deficiency of debrisoquine hydroxylase, an enzyme deficiency that was discovered independently with sparteine [33].

The CYP2D6 gene locus is highly polymorphic, with more than 80 allelic variants having been described to date (http://www.imm.ki.se/CYPalleles/cyp2d6.htm). Allelic variants are a consequence of point mutations, single base pair deletions or additions, gene rearrangements, or deletion of the entire gene. A genetic lack of CYP2D6 'PM phenotype' is now known to occur in approximately 5–10% of white people and 1–2% of the Asian population, and can result in either exaggerated drug effects when CYP2D6 is the major inactivation pathway, or diminished effects when CYP2D6 is required for activation of a pro-drug [34]. Another CYP2D6 phenotype is known as ultra-rapid metabolizer and is caused by the occurrence of duplicated, multiduplicated or amplified CYP2D6 genes. At present, alleles with two, three, four, five and 13 gene copies in tandem have been reported and the number of individuals carrying multiple CYP2D6 gene copies is highest in Ethiopia and Saudi Arabia, where up to one-third of the population displays this genotype [35].

CYP2D6 is responsible for the metabolism of a wide range of therapeutic agents including anti-arrhythmics, β-blockers, antidepressants, antipsychotics and morphine derivatives. It is therefore not surprising that genetic variations affecting this enzyme would account for some clinically important interindividual variability in drug response.

Codeine is an alkaloid obtained from opium or prepared from morphine by methylation. It is a pro-drug that requires demethylation to morphine before it can exert any analgesic effects, a reaction that is catalysed by CYP2D6. In patients who are CYP2D6 poor metabolizers, lack of CYP2D6 enzymatic activity leads to inefficient analgesia and increased side-effects from the parent drug. On the other hand, high doses of codeine can generate extensive formation of morphine and trigger adverse effects in CYP2D6 ultra-rapid metabolizers [12].

Tramadol is another pro-drug that depends on CYP2D6 for producing an active metabolite. It is a synthetic opioid with a proven analgesic efficacy in postoperative pain management. Tramadol is formulated as a racemic mixture that produces analgesia by synergistic action of its two enantiomers and their metabolites. CYP2D6 metabolizes tramadol to 11-desmethylated compounds, of which *O*-desmethyl-tramadol predominates and possesses analgesic properties. (+) *O*-desmethyl-tramadol has been demonstrated to have an affinity to μ-opioid receptors that is approximately 200 times greater than that of the parent compound. Thus, it is largely responsible for opioid receptor mediated analgesia, whereas (+)- and (−)-tramadol inhibits reuptake of the neurotransmitters serotonin and noradrenaline providing a second analgesic mechanism. Experimental pain studies on volunteers showed reduced analgesic efficacy of tramadol in CYP2D6 poor metabolizers. Moreover, in patients receiving tramadol patient-controlled analgesia, poor metabolizers display a lower response rate compared with extensive metabolizers. It is therefore clear that CYP2D6 pharmacogenetics may explain some of the varying response to this medication in the postoperative period [36].

Tricyclic antidepressants (TCAs) are still one of the major classes of antidepressants prescribed today. TCAs are metabolized to pharmacologically active amines by the cytochrome P450 system. Subsequent hydroxylation of these amines by CYP2D6 produces pharmacologically inactive metabolites. Consequently, TCA users who are CYP2D6 poor metabolizers may experience cardiotoxicity and increased adverse effects, such as tachycardia, dry mouth, constipation and fatigue, as a result of drug concentrations above the therapeutic range. Alternatively, TCAs may be ineffective or subtherapeutic in patients who are CYP2D6 ultra-rapid metabolizers [12,37,38]. The effect of CYP2D6 polymorphism on antidepressant therapy is best exemplified by nortriptyline. In most patients, a daily dose of 75–150 mg is usually optimum. In poor 2D6 metabolizers, however, the effective tolerable dose can be as low as 10–20 mg. On the other hand, ultra-rapid metabolizers may require a dose in excess of 500 mg to achieve therapeutic effect. It should be noted, however, that many antidepressants that undergo biotransformation by 2D6 produce pharmacologically active metabolites, and this tends to complicate the interpretation of toxicity–efficacy relationships [38].

Propafenone is an antiarrhythmic that is metabolized extensively by CYP2D6. Patients who are poor metabolizers are more likely to have visual blurring, dizziness and paraesthesias in association with higher concentrations of propafenone in the blood than are those who are extensive metabolizers (67% versus 14%). Moreover, these patients have a higher incidence of nausea, vomiting and arrhythmias because of slower drug metabolism [39].

The CYP3A subfamily of cytochrome P450 consists of four members (CYP3A4, -3A5, -3A7 and -3A43) and is quantitatively the most important group of CYPs in terms of hepatic drug biotransformation. CYP3A enzymes catalyse the oxidation of many different therapeutic entities, several of which are of potential importance in anaesthesia and intensive care. CYP3A4 is the major isoform expressed in adult liver and also is expressed abundantly in intestine, where it contributes significantly to the first-pass metabolism of substrates such as midazolam [13].

About three-quarters of the white population and half of the black population have a genetic inability to express functional CYP3A5 [40]. However, the lack of functional CYP3A5 may not be readily evident, because many medications metabolized by CYP3A5 are also metabolized by the universally expressed CYP3A4. For medications that are equally metabolized by both enzymes, the net rate of metabolism is the sum of that due to CYP3A4 and that due to CYP3A5. The existence of this dual pathway partially obscures the clinical effects of genetic polymorphism of CYP3A5 but contributes to the large range of total CYP3A activity in humans [41]. The CYP3A pathway of drug elimination is further confounded by the presence of single-nucleotide polymorphisms in the CYP3A4 gene that alter the activity of this enzyme for some substrates but not for others [42, 43].

Recently, the genetic basis for polymorphic CYP3A5 expression was discovered; a SNP in intron 3 creates an abnormal splice site causing >130 nucleotides of intronic sequence to be inserted into the mRNA. This additional mRNA sequence introduces an early stop codon that encodes a truncated nonfunctional CYP3A5 protein [23].

Although it is now possible to determine which patients express both functional enzymes (i.e. CYP3A4 and CYP3A5), the clinical importance of these variants for the many drugs metabolized by CYP3A remains unclear [41].

Cytochrome P450 2C9 (CYP2C9) is responsible for the metabolism of several drugs with narrow therapeutic indices, such as phenytoin, warfarin and tolbutamide. Independent single-nucleotide polymorphisms result in two defective allelic variants of CYP2C9 (CYP2C9*2 and -*3 alleles). The resultant

CYP2C9*2 and -*3 enzymes are associated with approximately 5.5- and 27.0-fold decreased intrinsic clearance relative to the wild-type (CYP2C9*1) enzyme, giving rise to a poor metabolizer phenotype. Clinical and experimental data indicate that the consequences of the CYP2C9*3 allele are likely to be more dramatic than those associated with CYP2C9*2. Approximately 0.2–1% of white people and 2–3% of Asians are homozygous for the -*3 alleles (CYP2C9*3/*3) and hence at risk for severe toxicity if exposed to normal doses of substrates with narrow therapeutic indices [13].

Glipizide is a CYP2C9 substrate used for the treatment of non-insulin dependent diabetes mellitus. Patients who are homozygous for the CYP2C9*3 alleles are hence at an increased risk of drug-induced life-threatening hypoglycaemia even after normal doses of glipizide. Such a reaction has been reported in the literature [43].

Biotransformation of phenytoin to (S)-5-(4-hydroxyphenyl)-5-phenylhydantoin by CYP2C9 and subsequent conjugation with glucuronic acid represents the principal metabolic pathway by which the drug is eliminated from the body. Therefore, patients expressing dysfunctional CYP2C9 enzyme are likely to experience toxicity at 'standard' therapeutic doses and will require lower doses to maintain therapeutic concentrations [43].

Associations between the CYP2C9 genotype and sensitivity to warfarin have been reported, particularly among patients with the CYP2C9 poor metabolizer phenotype who are at increased risk of haemorrhage following administration of 'standard' doses of the drug [44]. The clearance of S-warfarin among subjects homozygous for the CYP2C9*3 allele has been shown to be reduced by 90% compared with subjects homozygous for the wild-type allele. It has also been shown that patients prescribed low-dose (<2 mg/day) warfarin were six times more likely to possess a variant allele, coding for reduced CYP2C9 activity, which decreased warfarin metabolism. Additionally, the CYP2C9 genotype has been associated with the risk of over anticoagulation and bleeding events [44,45].

Cytochrome P450 2C19 (CYP2C19) deficiency is present in 3–5% of the white population and in approximately 20% of the Asian population. A poor-metabolizer phenotype is conferred by inheritance of two recessive loss-of-function alleles. At least five defective alleles have been identified to date. The two most common variant alleles, CYP2C19*2 and -*3, result from single base substitutions that introduce premature stop codons and, consequently, truncated polypeptide chains that possess no functional activity [13].

Omeprazole is a well-known CYP2C19 substrate and hence poor metabolizers have a better response to omeprazole when used for the eradication of *Helicobacter pylori* than do extensive metabolizers. In one study, CYP2C19 poor metabolizers had 100% eradication rates of *H. pylori* after 1 week of treatment with omeprazole and amoxicillin, compared with an eradication rate of 41% in intermediate metabolizers. The improved efficacy was most likely a result of higher omeprazole concentrations because of reduced drug metabolism [46]. However, this advantage is not without some drawbacks. Long-term high serum omeprazole concentrations in CYP2C19 poor metabolizers may cause cobalamin deficiency and result in haematological and neuropsychiatric abnormalities. This deficiency most probably results from the lack of protein-bound dietary cobalamin resulting from omeprazole-induced hypochlorhydria or achlorhydria. Additionally, high omeprazole concentrations increase the activity of CYP1A2. Substrates of CYP1A2, such as theophylline and amitriptyline, when taken concomitantly, may need to be given in larger doses to provide continued therapeutic benefit during omeprazole treatment in patients with poor metabolism [22].

Diazepam is another CYP2C19 substrate. However, it is also metabolized by CYP2D6. The differences in diazepam pharmacokinetic parameters are notable between CYP2C19 extensive metabolizers and poor metabolizers, but minimal between CYP2D6 extensive metabolizers and poor metabolizers. CYP2C19 poor metabolizers displayed an elimination half-life twice that of extensive metabolizers, which could lead to prolonged sedation [47].

Cytochrome P1A2 (CYP1A2) is involved in the metabolism of many drugs including theophylline, caffeine and tacrine. Significant interindividual variability in human CYP1A2 enzyme levels and/or activity has been observed in several human populations. In a study using caffeine as a model, CYP1A2 substrate, a trimodal distribution of enzyme activity consistent with high, low and intermediate metabolizer phenotypes was observed [48]. However, a more recent study provided no indication of polymorphic enzyme activity [49]. Smoking and dietary factors (e.g. consumption of charcoal-broiled beef and cruciferous vegetables) have been shown to increase CYP1A2 activity; such modulatory extrinsic factors confound analysis and may account for the discrepancy between different studies [50]. Regardless of this, CYP1A2 expression shows considerable variability in humans as much as 100-fold for some activities, and some of this variability may be attributed to a recently described polymorphism in the regulatory region of the CYP1A2 gene, affecting inducibility in response to smoking and possibly other inducers [51].

Polymorphisms in drug transport proteins

Most drugs or drug metabolites enter the cells by passive diffusion. However, some drugs are actively transported by transporter proteins, of which membrane transporters may play a key part. The adenosine triphosphate (ATP) binding cassette (ABC) family of membrane transporters comprise an extensively studied group of transporters influencing drug disposition. P-glycoprotein (PGP), a member of the ABC family, is involved in the energy dependent efflux of substrates, including bilirubin, several anticancer drugs, cardiac glycosides, immunosuppressive agents and glucocorticoids (Table 3.1) [52].

Table 3.1 Substrates of P-glycoprotein relevant to anaesthesia.

Drug type	Example(s)
Antibiotics	Cefotetan, cefazolin
Analgesics	Morphine
Antiarrhythmics	Amiodarone, quinidine
Antiemetics	Ondansetron
Calcium blockers	Diltiazem, verapamil
Cardiac stimulants	Digoxin, nicardipine

PGP expression differs markedly among individuals, the molecular basis of which has not been fully elucidated. Recently, a synonymous SNP was reported to be associated with a loss of function PGP allele; patients homozygous for the loss function allele had more than twofold lower duodenal PGP expression compared with those homozygous for the wild-type allele [53]. Clinical pharmacokinetic studies of digoxin, a PGP substrate, demonstrated significantly higher bioavailability in patients with the latter group of patients.

Polymorphisms of drug receptors and targets

The majority of drug receptors and targets are proteins. Proteins are gene products and, as such, their quality and quantity are subject to genetic regulation and hence genetic variation. Polymorphisms in the genes encoding enzymes or receptors (drug targets) relevant to drug treatment of different diseases cause widespread variation in sensitivity to many drugs. The reaction to drugs includes lack of effect, reduced effect, normal effect, increased effect or adverse effect.

Malignant hyperthermia is one such example of a very dramatic interaction between a drug and a mutated receptor. Exposing an individual with a certain mutation in the skeletal muscle ryanodine receptor gene (RYR1 gene) to a triggering agent (e.g. halothane, suxamethonium) may lead to a life-threatening condition where a pathophysiological cascade sets in as a result of uncontrolled release of calcium from sarcoplasmic reticulum in skeletal muscle cells. Today more than 20 mutations in the RYR1 gene on chromosome 19 are known to cause susceptibility to malignant hyperthermia (MHS phenotype). In addition, several other gene loci on chromosomes 17, 7, 5, 3 and 1 are positional candidate genes [12].

Genetic polymorphism of the μ-opioid receptor is another example of a receptor polymorphism that may prove to be of relevance to clinical anaesthesia. Recently published data indicate that there are differences between individuals in levels of μ-opioid receptor gene expression, responses to painful stimuli and responses to opioid drugs, probably because of a genetic polymorphism in the transcription-regulating region of this gene. A SNP in the human μ-opioid receptor gene at position 118 (A118G transition) results in a receptor variant that binds β-endorphin approximately three times more tightly than the most common allelic forms of the receptor. This makes β-endorphin nearly three times more potent than in persons without the mutation [54,55].

Genetic polymorphism of the $β_2$-adrenoceptor (B2AR) exemplifies another well-characterized and clinically relevant polymorphism in a drug receptor. The $β_2$-adrenoceptor is a G-protein-coupled receptor that interacts with various medications and endogenous catecholamines. These receptors are widely expressed in humans and play an important part in regulating cardiac, vascular, pulmonary and metabolic functions. Studies of such physiological functions of the human $β_2$-adrenoceptor have revealed substantial interpatient differences in receptor function and responsiveness to stimulation [56]. Insights into the molecular basis for inherited differences in the $β_2$-adrenoceptor have been illuminated by the discovery of several SNPs in the B2AR gene, and their association with altered expression, down-regulation or coupling of the receptor [57]. A SNP resulting in an arginine to glycine amino acid change at codon 16 is relatively common and being extensively investigated for its clinical importance.

In a study of $β_2$-agonist-mediated vasodilatation and desensitization, subjects who were homozygous for Arg16 (arginine at codon 16) had nearly complete desensitization after continuous infusion of isoproterenol, with venodilatation decreasing from 44% at baseline to 8% at 90 minutes. Homozygous Gly16 (glycine at codon 16) patients had no significant change in venodilatation [56].

These results were consistent with the reported effects of B2AR genotype on bronchodilator response to acute or chronic $β_2$-agonist therapy. The forced expiratory volume in 1 second (FEV_1) response to a single dose of oral albuterol was more than sixfold higher in patients homozygous for Arg16 compared with patients homozygous for Gly16, even though similar plasma drug concentrations were achieved [58]. Interestingly, the influence of this genotype was different in patients on long-term $β_2$-agonist therapy. It was noted that Arg16 homozygous patients on regularly scheduled $β_2$-agonist therapy display a gradual decline in morning peak expiratory flow over time, while no change in this parameter was observed in Gly16 homozygous patients. Moreover, it was also noted that morning peak expiratory flow deteriorates substantially after cessation of treatment in Arg16 homozygous patients, an effect not seen in Gly16 homozygotes [59]. These data suggest that Arg16 homozygous patients may be at risk for deleterious or non-beneficial effects of regularly scheduled inhaled β-agonist therapy and may be candidates for alternative treatment or dosing schedules and/or earlier initiation of anti-inflammatory drugs. It is also possible that tachyphylaxis can be prevented in this group of patients by using $β_2$-agonists on an as-needed schedule instead of on a regular-use schedule [16].

Angiotensin converting enzyme (ACE) and its sensitivity to ACE inhibitors is yet another clinical example of the impact of genetic polymorphisms in drug targets. It has been recently suggested that ACE inhibitors might be less effective in black than white populations, with a significant reduction of risk of hospitalization and mortality from heart failure when ACE inhibitors were used in the latter group [60]. Although the exact explanation for this variation in response to ACE inhibitors is unclear, it is well known that variability in ACE activity is in large part determined by the genetic profile of the patient and has been ascribed to a common bi-allelic polymorphism in intron 16 of the ACE gene. The two alleles differ in the presence (insertion, I allele) or absence (deletion, D allele) of a 287-base section of DNA. The D allele is generally associated with either higher ACE activity or angiotensin II levels in normal subjects, people with hypertension or chronic heart failure. This insertion/deletion polymorphism results in three genotypes: DD, ID and II, which affect serum and tissue ACE activity. However, there is a controversy in the literature with respect to the association of this polymorphism with response to ACE inhibitor therapy [21].

Polymorphisms in genes encoding proteins that are neither direct targets of medications nor involved in their disposition have been shown to alter the response to treatment in certain situations. For example, inherited differences in coagulation factors can predispose women taking oral contraceptives to deep-vein or cerebral-vein thrombosis [61], whereas genetic polymorphism in the apolipoprotein E gene appears to have a role in predicting responses to therapy for Alzheimer's disease and to lipid-lowering drugs including HMG-CoA reductase inhibitors (statins) [62].

Genetic variation in cellular ion transporters can also have an indirect role in predisposing patients to the toxic effects of drugs. For example, patients with variant alleles for potassium transporters may have substantial morbidity or mortality in response to a given medication. A mutation in the HERG gene (human ether-a-go-go-related gene) has been associated with drug-induced long QT syndrome and *torsade de pointes* after quinidine and cisapride. Another mutation in KCNE2 (the gene for an integral membrane subunit that assembles with HERG to form I_{Kr} potassium channels) was identified in a patient who had cardiac arrhythmia after receiving clarithromycin [63]. Moreover, KCNE2 variants have been associated with the development of a very long QT interval after therapy with co-trimoxazole. KCNE2 variants occur in about 1.6% of the population and their effect on drug actions can cause death; they are therefore excellent candidates for pharmacogenetic strategies to prevent serious drug-induced toxic effects [64].

Pharmacogenomics and personalized medicine

The past 50 years has seen major improvements in the length and quality of life. However, the efficiency of drug treatment is far from being satisfactory. The response rates in the treatment of diseases such as Alzheimer's disease, cardiac dysrhythmias, depression, incontinence, osteoporosis, schizophrenia and rheumatoid arthritis are still in the range of 30–60%, and optimal therapy is relatively elusive for current major killers such as coronary artery disease, cerebral vascular events and many cancers [65,66]. Moreover, adverse drug reactions are becoming more of a problem than previously thought. A recent meta-analysis revealed that serious adverse drug reactions occur in 6.7% of all hospitalized patients and that 0.32% of all hospitalized patients develop fatal adverse reactions, causing more than 100 000 deaths annually in the USA [67]. In the UK, such reactions

cause up to 7% of all hospital admissions [68] and in Sweden 13% of all admissions to internal medicine clinics are caused by drug reactions [69]. There is also clear evidence of significant heterogeneity in the efficacy and toxicity of most therapeutic agents, when viewed across the population.

In view of this relatively low efficacy and serious consequences of adverse drug reactions, and reaction of the observed heterogeneity in drug response, the scope of personalized medicine is becoming a reality and notions like 'one drug fits all' or 'one dose fits all' can no longer hold true. Moreover, in the last few years we have seen the completion of the HGP, the maturation of the SNP database, the introduction of DNA array technology and high-throughput screening systems, and the advancement in bioinformatics. It is anticipated that, in the near future, these advances will be utilized in the field of personalized medicine.

It is clear that the information we have today is substantial and allows provision of data that could facilitate an individualized therapy both with respect to the choice and dosage of drug therapy. However, pharmacogenetics still has a way to go; knowledge about genetic variation at the level of drug metabolism is extensive, whereas the knowledge about interindividual differences in the function of drug transporters and drug targets is scarce. In addition, some of the results in this field are incomplete, conflicting and sometimes difficult to interpret.

Knowledge about the genetic structure of a targeted population will, in the future, lead to the use of variants of each drug specially tailored to subgroups of populations, making it necessary to genetically test patients in order to match genotype to the most suitable therapy. It is probable that pharmaceutical companies in the future will demand a pretreatment genetic test of the patient in order to choose the right drug variant for this particular person.

Gene expression arrays and pharmacogenomics

While DNA is the basic genetic material that carries information from one generation to the next, its effects on the characteristics of the cell requires first copying into RNA (transcription) and then the transformation of mRNA into a polypeptide by ribosomes.

In other words, transcription and translation are the processes through which genes express their content of genetic information (become functional).

The first methods that were developed for the study of gene expression allowed investigators to study the expression of a specific RNA or a specific protein. Gradually, methods became available that also made it possible to compare increasingly complex mixtures of gene products. The most dramatic change has been the introduction of arrays for the simultaneous assessment of multiple genes. The improvement in robotics and fluid physics is such that up to 64 000 gene clones can be evaluated on a single 1 × 1 cm slide. The gene expression arrays have enabled a degree of genomic analysis not previously feasible. It is estimated that the quantity of data available from a single array would have taken a researcher over 20 years to complete by northern blot analysis [21].

In addition to microarray technology, strategies such as fluorescence energy transfer detection, fluorescence polarization, kinetic polymerase chain reaction (PCR), mass spectrometry, oligonucleotide ligation/flow cytometry, high performance liquid chromatography (HPLC) fragment analysis and mini-sequencing have all been used to increase the throughput of genotype information from genomic DNA. In addition, computational biology, or bioinformatics, has been instrumental in the development of pharmacogenomics. The gene expression arrays and high-throughput genotyping techniques generate a large amount of data in a single experiment, much more than can be evaluated using commonly available spreadsheets. Therefore, software has been developed that not only captures the experimental data, but includes comparison of results with existing genome databases. This provides the investigator with a powerful and comprehensive output on which rapid interpretation and implementation of data can be made [21].

In pharmacogenomics, DNA microarray technology can be used as a diagnostic tool to identify an individual's genotype prior to drug selection and dosage, to monitor changes in gene expression in response to drug treatment and can prove invaluable in new drug discovery in the near future.

The AmpliChip™ (Roche Molecular Diagnostics, Almeda, CA, USA) is an example of widescale application of diagnostic microarray technology in pharmacogenomics. The chip can identify naturally occurring genetic variations in CYP2D6 and CYP2C19. Common variations in these genes have a crucial role in determining how an individual can process or metabolize many commonly prescribed drugs. With such technology, drug metabolism genotyping in the future could be used to assist in therapeutic decision making with the goal of prescribing drugs that are optimally effective and safe for the individual [70].

Gene expression arrays can also be applied to define the mechanism of action of new compounds or to screen for direct influence of an agent on a specific pathway. By using this technology, a profile of genes altered after drug exposure can be generated and may thereby yield a greater understanding of mechanisms of action. Gene expression arrays can also be used during screening of candidate compounds. By constructing arrays for genes involved in a pathway of interest, *in vitro* and or *in vivo* gene dynamics can be used as a functional map for drug activity.

The most attractive application of microarrays is in the study of differential gene expression in disease. Diversion from normal physiology is frequently accompanied by changes in gene expression patterns. The up- or down-regulation of gene activity can either be the cause of the pathophysiology or the result of the disease. Targeting disease-causing gene products is desirable to achieve disease modification, whereas interfering with genes that are expressed as a consequence of disease may be exploited to alleviate symptoms. The opportunity to compare the expression of thousands of genes between 'disease' and 'normal' tissues and cells will allow the identification of multiple potential targets. Such examples of monitoring differential gene expression by microarrays are beginning to appear in the literature.

It is clear therefore that with the aid of microarray technology and bioinformatics, pharmacogenomics will have a lot to offer in the near future; optimizing the efficiency and reducing the adverse reactions of current therapeutics, helping with understanding the mechanisms of action of new agents and offering a smart solution for efforts to discover new therapeutic targets for disease.

Gene therapy

Until the latter part of the last century, the possibility of actually changing faulty genetic blueprints was beyond the imagination of the realistic medical scientist. In 1972, Friedmann and Roblin [71] argued that defective genes could be replaced by those with the correct sequence. Since then a great deal of effort has been expended to bring such a therapeutic manipulation to clinical practice, so far with limited success. Genetic therapy may be divided into two main strategies: germ line cell-targeted genetic therapy and somatic cell genetic therapy. Germ line cell-targeted genetic therapy refers to genetic engineering of germ line cells or fertilized ova. Disease genes may be replaced with 'normal' genes, making the genetically engineered organism and its potential offspring free of the particular disease. Somatic cell gene therapy refers to introduction of nucleic acids (gene/s) to an organism's somatic cells in order to obtain a therapeutic effect. These added nucleic acids will then be taken up by the cells and be expressed to proteins by the cells' gene expressing systems. Nucleic acids may be presented to the cells as naked DNA or in virus or plasmid vectors. This type of genetic modification is not heritable, and will most often have a transient effect. However, new technology may lead to systems making it possible to switch expression of genes delivered on or off [12].

Ethical considerations

Clearly, pharmacogenetics/pharmacogenomics has the potential to improve both the safety and efficacy of current and future therapeutic agents. However, this is bound to raise important ethical, legal, social and regulatory issues.

Arguments have been advanced that genotype determinations for pharmacogenetic characterization, in contrast to 'genetic' testing for primary disease risk assessment, are less likely to raise potentially sensitive issues with regard to patient confidentiality, the misuse of genotyping data and the possibility of stigmatization. However, two lines of reasoning may actually indicate an increased potential for ethical issues with respect to pharmacogenetic data. First, the very nature of pharmacogenetic data calls for a rather more liberal position regarding use if this information is to serve its intended purpose. Thus, the prescription for a drug that is limited to a group of patients with a particular genotype will inevitably disclose the receiving patient's genotype to any one of a large number of individuals involved in the patient's care. Secondly, for any given disease risk, patients less likely to respond to treatment would be seen as a more unfavourable insurance risk, particularly if non-responder status is associated with chronic and/or costly illness rather than with early mortality. The pharmacogenetic profile may thus, under certain circumstances, even become a more important (financial) risk-assessment parameter than primary disease susceptibility, and should therefore be treated with similar weight as other genetic and environmental risk factors [72].

Conclusions

The application of pharmacogenomics principles in drug development will raise several other issues, as drug companies might direct treatment at individuals or specific ethnic groups who have higher response rates with the result that some groups in the society are being disadvantaged. This raises ethical issues because it would potentially exacerbate inequalities. In addition, we should question whether incentives should be offered to encourage pharmaceutical companies to develop medicines to only a small number of patients.

It should be noted, however, that the great potential gains from pharmacogenomics, in terms of both patient wellbeing and cost of health care, heavily outweigh any risks. There is therefore an urgent need for the establishment of a dialogue among relevant parties within society to develop and endorse a set of criteria to ensure that inappropriate exploitation does not preclude the vast public good that will emerge from the field of pharmacogenomics.

References

1 Nebert DW. Pharmacogenetics and pharmacogenomics: why is this relevant to the clinical geneticist? *Clin Genet* 1999; **56**: 247–58.

2 Carsen PE, Flanagan CL, Iokes CE. Enzymatic deficiency in primaquine-sensitive erythrocytes. *Science* 1956; **124**: 484–5.

3 Kalow W, Staron N. On distribution and inheritance of atypical forms of human serum cholinesterase, as indicated by dibucaine numbers. *Can J Med Sci* 1957; **35**: 1305–20.

4 Evans DA, Manley KA, McKusick KV. Genetic control of isoniazid metabolism in man. *Br Med J* 1960; **5197**: 485–91.

5 Vogel F. Moderne Probleme der Humangenetik. *Ergeb Inn Med Kinderheilkd* 1959; **12**: 65–126.

6 Kalow W. *Pharmacogenetics: Heredity and the Response to Drugs*. London: W.B. Saunders, 1962.

7 Gonzalez FJ, Skoda RC, Kimura S, *et al.* Characterization of the common genetic defect in humans deficient in debrisoquine metabolism. *Nature* 1988; **331**: 442–6.

8 Pirmohamed M. Pharmacogenetics and pharmacogenomics. *Br J Clin Pharmacol* 2001; **52**: 345–7.

9 Anonymous. Position paper on terminology in pharmacogenetics: The European Agency for the Evaluation of Medicinal Product, 2002.

10 Brown SM. Human genetic variation. In: Brown SM, ed. *Essentials of Medical Genomics*. New Jersey: John Wiley & Sons, 2003: 99–118.

11 Sweeney BP. Watson and Crick 50 years on: from double helix to pharmacogenomics. *Anaesthesia* 2004; **59**: 150–65.

12 Fagerlund TH, Braaten O. No pain relief from codeine . . . ? An introduction to pharmacogenomics. *Acta Anaesthesiol Scand* 2001; **45**: 140–9.

13 Leeder JS. Pharmacogenetics and pharmacogenomics. *Pediatr Clin North Am* 2001; **48**: 765–81.

14 Meyer UA. Genotype or phenotype: the definition of a pharmacogenetic polymorphism. *Pharmacogenetics* 1991; **1**: 66–7.

15 Barnes MR. Human genetic variation: databases and concepts. In: Barnes MR, Gray IC, eds. *Bioinformatics for Geneticists*. West Sussex: John Wiley & Sons, 2003: 40–70.

16 Hjoberg J, Drazen JM, Palmer LJ, Weiss ST, Silverman ES. The pharmacogenetics of asthma and allergic disease. *Immunol Allergy Clin North Am* 2002; **22**: 223–33.

17 Altshuler D, Pollara VJ, Cowles CR, *et al.* An SNP map of the human genome generated by reduced representation shotgun sequencing. *Nature* 2000; **407**: 513–6.

18 Sherry ST, Ward MH, Kholdov M, *et al.* dbSNP: the NCBI database of genetic variation. *Nucleic Acids Res* 2002; **29**: 308–11.

19 Vieux E, Marth G, Kwok P. SNP discovery and PCR-based assay design: from in silico data to the laboratory experiment. In: Barnes MR, Gray IC, eds. *Bioinformatics for Geneticists*. West Sussex: John Wiley & Sons, 2003: 203–15.

20 Silverman EK, Palmer LJ. Case–control association studies for the genetics of complex respiratory diseases. *Am J Respir Cell Mol Biol* 2000; **22**: 645–8.

21 Evans WE, Relling MV. Pharmacogenomics: translating functional genomics into rational therapeutics. *Science* 1999; **286**: 487–91.

22 Rogers JF, Nafziger AN, Bertino JS Jr. Pharmacogenetics affects dosing, efficacy, and toxicity of cytochrome P450-metabolized drugs. *Am J Med* 2002; **113**: 746–50.

23 Evans WE. Pharmacogenomics: marshalling the human genome to individualise drug therapy. *Gut* 2003; **52**(Suppl 2): 10–8.

24 Yan L, Zhang S, Eiff B. Thiopurine methyltransferase polymorphic tandem repeat: genotype–phenotype correlation analysis. *Clin Pharmacol Ther* 2000; **68**: 210–9.

25 Relling MV, Hancock ML, Rivera GK. Mercaptopurine therapy intolerance and heterozygosity at the thiopurine *S*-methyltransferase gene locus. *J Natl Cancer Inst* 1999; **23**: 1983–5.

26 Butcher NJ, Boukouvala S, Sim E, Minchin RF. Pharmacogenetics of the arylamine *N*-acetyltransferases. *Pharmacogenomics J* 2002; **2**: 30–42.

27 Cascorbi I, Drakoulis N, Brockmoller J, *et al.* Arylamine *N*-acetyltransferase (NAT2) mutations and their allelic linkage in unrelated Caucasian individuals: correlation with phenotypic activity. *Am J Hum Genet* 1995; **57**: 581–92.

28 Meyer UA, Zanger UM. Molecular mechanisms of genetic polymorphisms of drug metabolism. *Annu Rev Pharmacol Toxicol* 1997; **37**: 269–96.

29 Spielberg SP. *N*-acetyltransferases: pharmacogenetics and clinical consequences of polymorphic drug metabolism. *J Pharmacokinet Biopharm* 1996; **24**: 509–19.

30 Nelson DR, Koymans L, Kamataki T. P450 superfamily-update on new sequences, gene mapping, accession numbers and nomenclature. *Pharmacogenetics* 1996; **6**: 1–42.

31 Rendic S, Di Carlo FJ. Human cytochrome P450 enzymes: a status report summarizing their reactions, substrates, inducers, and inhibitors. *Drug Metab Rev* 1997; **29**: 413–580.

32 Mahgoub A, Idle JR, Dring LG. Polymorphic hydroxylation of Debrisoquine in man. *Lancet* 1977; **ii**: 584–6.

33 Eichelbaum M, Bertilsson L, Sawe J, Zekorn C. Polymorphic oxidation of sparteine and debrisoquine: related pharmacogenetic entities. *Clin Pharmacol Ther* 1982; **31**: 184–6.

34 Dahl ML, Iselius L, Alm C, *et al*. Polymorphic 2-hydroxylation of desipramine: a population and family study. *Eur J Clin Pharmacol* 1993; **44**: 445–50.

35 Johansson I, Lundqvist E, Bertilsson L, *et al*. Inherited amplification of an active gene in the cytochrome P450 CYP2D locus as a cause of ultrarapid metabolism of debrisoquine. *Proc Natl Acad Sci USA* 1993; **90**: 11825–9.

36 Stamer UM, Lehnen K, Hothker F, *et al*. Impact of CYP2D6 on postoperative tramadol analgesia. *Pain* 2003; **105**: 231–8.

37 Rusnak JM, Kisabeth RM, Herbert DP, McNeil DM. Pharmacogenomics: a clinician's primer on emerging technologies for improved patient care. *Mayo Clin Proc* 2001; **76**: 299–309.

38 Ingelman-Sundberg M, Oscarson M, McLellan RA. Polymorphic human cytochrome P450 enzymes: an opportunity for individualized drug treatment. *Trends Pharmacol Sci* 1999; **20**: 342–9.

39 Chow MS, White CM, Lau CP. Evaluation of CYP2D6 oxidation of dextromethorphan and propafenone in a Chinese population with atrial fibrillation. *J Clin Pharmacol* 2001; **41**: 92–6.

40 Kuehl P, Zhang J, Lin Y. Sequence diversity in CYP3A promoters and characterization of the genetic basis for polymorphic CYP3A5 expression. *Nat Genet* 2001; **27**: 383–91.

41 Evans WE, McLeod HL. Pharmacogenomics: drug disposition, drug targets, and side effects. *N Engl J Med* 2003; **348**: 538–49.

42 Sata F, Sapone A, Elizondo G. CYP3A4 allelic variants with amino acid substitutions in exons 7 and 12: evidence for an allelic variant with altered catalytic activity. *Clin Pharmacol Ther* 2000; **67**: 48–56.

43 Kidd RS, Straughn AB, Meyer MC. Pharmacokinetics of chlorpheniramine, phenytoin, glipizide and nifedipine in an individual homozygous for the CYP2C9*3 allele. *Pharmacogenetics* 1999; **9**: 71–80.

44 Aithal GP, Day CP, Kesteven PJ, Daly AK. Association of polymorphisms in the cytochrome P450 CYP2C9 with warfarin dose requirement and risk of bleeding complications. *Lancet* 1999; **353**: 717–9.

45 Higashi MK, Veenstra DL, Kondo LM. Association between CYP2C9 genetic variants and anticoagulation-related outcomes during warfarin therapy. *JAMA* 2002; **287**: 1690–8.

46 Tanigawara Y, Aoyama N, Kita T. CYP2C19 genotype-related efficacy of omeprazole for the treatment of infection caused by *Helicobacter pylori*. *Clin Pharmacol Ther* 1999; **66**: 528–34.

47 Bertilsson L, Henthorn TK, Sanz E. Importance of genetic factors in the regulation of diazepam metabolism relationship to *S*-mephenytoin, but not debrisoquin, hydroxylation phenotype. *Clin Pharmacol Ther* 1989; **45**: 348–55.

48 Tang BK, Zhou Y, Kalow W. Caffeine as a probe for CYP1A2 activity: potential influence of renal factors on urinary phenotypic trait measurements. *Pharmacogenetics* 1994; **4**: 117–24.

49 Welfare MR, Aitkin M, Bassendine MF, Daly AK. Detailed modelling of caffeine metabolism and examination of the CYP1A2 gene: lack of a polymorphism in CYP1A2 in Caucasians. *Pharmacogenetics* 1999; **9**: 367–75.

50 Eaton DL, Gallagher EP, Bammler TK. Role of cytochrome P4501A2 in chemical carcinogenesis: Implications for human variability in expression and enzyme activity. *Pharmacogenetics* 1995; **5**: 259–74.

51 Nakajima M, Yokoi T, Mizutani M. Genetic polymorphism in the 5-flanking region of human CYP1A2 gene: effect on the CYP1A2 inducibility in humans. *J Biochem (Tokyo)* 1999; **125**: 803–8.

52 Brinkmann U, Roots I, Eichelbaum M. Pharmacogenetics of the human drug-transporter gene MDR1: impact of polymorphisms on pharmacotherapy. *Drug Discov Today* 2001; **6**: 835–9.

53 Sakaeda T, Nakamura T, Horinouchi M. MDR1 genotype-related pharmacokinetics of digoxin after single oral administration in healthy Japanese subjects. *Pharm Res* 2001; **18**: 1400–4.

54 Uhl GR, Soar I, Wang Z. The mu opiate receptor as a candidate gene for pain: polymorphisms, variations in expression, nociception, and opiate responses. *Proc Natl Acad Sci USA* 1999; **96**: 7752–5.

55 Bond C, LaForge KS, Tian M. Single-nucleotide polymorphism in the human mu opioid receptor gene alters beta-endorphin binding and activity: possible implications for opiate addiction. *Proc Natl Acad Sci USA* 1998; **95**: 9608–13.

56 Dishy V, Sofowora GG, Xie HG. The effect of common polymorphisms of the beta2-adrenergic receptor on agonist-mediated vascular desensitization. *N Engl J Med* 2001; **14**: 1030–5.

57 Liggett SB. Beta(2)-adrenergic receptor pharmacogenetics. *Am J Respir Crit Care Med* 2000; **161**: S197–201.

58 Lima JJ, Thomason DB, Mohamed MH. Impact of genetic polymorphisms of the beta2-adrenergic receptor on albuterol bronchodilator pharmacodynamics. *Clin Pharmacol Ther* 1999; **5**: 519–25.

59 Israel E, Drazen JM, Liggett SB. Effect of polymorphism of the beta(2)-adrenergic receptor on response to regular use of albuterol in asthma. *Int Arch Allergy Immunol* 2001; **124**: 183–6.

60 Baliga RR, Narula J. Pharmacogenomics of congestive heart failure. *Med Clin North Am* 2003; **87**: 569–78.

61 Martinelli I, Battaglioli T, Mannucci PM. Pharmacogenetic aspects of the use of oral contraceptives and the risk of thrombosis. *Pharmacogenetics* 2003; **13**: 589–94.

62 Siest G, Bertrand P, Herbeth B, *et al*. Apolipoprotein E polymorphisms and concentration in chronic diseases and drug responses. *Clin Chem Lab Med* 2000; **38**: 841–52.

63 Abbott GW, Sesti F, Splawski I, *et al*. MiRP1 forms IKr potassium channels with HERG and is associated with cardiac arrhythmia. *Cell* 1999; **97**: 175–87.

64 Sesti F, Abbott GW, Wei J, *et al*. A common polymorphism associated with antibiotic-induced cardiac arrhythmia. *Proc Natl Acad Sci USA* 2000; **97**: 10613–8.

65 Ingelman-Sundberg M. Pharmacogenetics: an opportunity for a safer and more efficient pharmacotherapy. *J Intern Med* 2001; **250**: 186–200.

66 McLeod HL, Evans WE. Pharmacogenomics: unlocking the human genome for better drug therapy. *Annu Rev Pharmacol Toxicol* 2001; **41**: 101–21.

67 Lazarou J, Pomeranz BH, Corey PN. Incidence of adverse drug reactions in hospitalized patients: a meta-analysis of prospective studies. *JAMA* 1998; **279**: 1200–5.

68 Green CF, Mottram DR, Rowe PH, Pirmohamed M. Adverse drug reactions as a cause of admission to an acute medical assessment unit: a pilot study. *J Clin Pharm Ther* 2000; **25**: 355–61.

69 Adverse drug reactions as a cause for admission to a clinic of internal medicine. Joint 3rd Congress of the European Association for Clinical Pharmacology and Therapeutics/4th Jerusalem Conference on Pharmaceutical Sciences and Clinical Pharmacology, Jerusalem, 1999.

70 Microarray ('DNA' CHIP) and Roche AmpliChip™ CYP450 backgrounder: Roche Diagnostics, 2004.

71 Friedmann T, Roblin R. Gene therapy for human genetic disease? *Science* 1972; **175**: 949–55.

72 Lindpaintner K. Pharmacogenetics and the future of medical practice. *Br J Clin Pharmacol* 2002; **54**: 221–30.

CHAPTER 4

Receptors and second messenger systems

Thomas Engelhardt

Receptors

Receptors in biochemical terms are proteins on the cell membrane or within the cytoplasm that bind specific factors (ligands) and initiate a cellular response to the ligand. They can therefore be divided into transmembrane and intracellular receptors. The transmembrane receptors are relevant to anaesthesia.

Transmembrane receptors

Transmembrane receptors are integral membrane proteins that bind to a signalling molecule on one side of the membrane and initiate a response on the other side. They are often composed of two or more subunits and classified based on their known or hypothesized membrane topology. In its simplest structure, a polypeptide chain crosses the lipid bilayer only once, but more commonly it crosses it as many as seven times. Principally, transmembrane receptors may be divided according to its function (metabotropic or ionotropic) or its structure (domains), as shown in Fig. 4.1.

Ionotropic receptors

Ionotropic receptors are a subclass of transmembrane receptors and their activity is regulated by either the membrane potential (voltage-gated) or ligands (ligand-gated). Voltage-gated ion channels are usually closed at the resting membrane potential of the cell. A change in the membrane potential causes conformational changes resulting in the opening of the pore followed by a transitional change to an inactivated state. The channel may not be able

to conduct ions in this state until a recovery period has taken place. Voltage-gated ion channels such as sodium, potassium or calcium channels are mainly involved in fast synaptic transmission but are unlikely to be involved in modulating the effects of general anaesthesia.

Ligand-gated ion channels have been identified as primary targets for anaesthetic agents. They contain an intrinsic ion channel and an extracellular binding site(s) for the ligand(s). Ligand binding causes a conformational change with an increase in the opening probability of the ion pore. The ion channel may be closed when the ligand is attached. All ligand-gated ion channels are characterized by a pentameric arrangement of subunits and can be subdivided into excitatory and inhibitory ligand-gated channels (Fig. 4.2).

GABA$_A$ and GABA$_C$

GABA (γ-aminobutyric acid) is the major inhibitory neurotransmitter and GABA receptors are classified into GABA$_A$, GABA$_B$ and GABA$_C$ receptors. GABA$_A$ are hetero-oligomeric chloride channels generally leading to hyperpolarization of the cell membrane and thus inhibition. They are composed of five subunits arranged around the ion channel with a diameter of approximately 8 nm. The subunits are selected from four principal families α, β, γ and δ although others have been identified. Each of the subunit isoforms is encoded by a single gene with additional heterogeneity produced through alternative splicing. The most common mammalian central nervous system (CNS) GABA$_A$ receptor appears to comprise two α_1, two β_2 and a single γ_2 subunit. Each GABA$_A$ receptor isoform appears to display characteristic

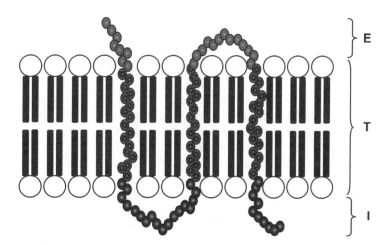

Figure 4.1 Simplified illustration of receptor structure with (E) extracellular, (T) transmembrane and (I) intracellular domain.

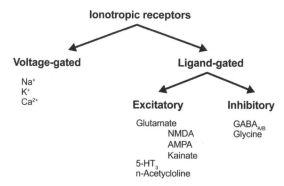

Figure 4.2 Ligand-gated ion channels are characterized by a pentameric arrangement of subunits and can be subdivided into excitatory and inhibitory ligand-gated channels. AMPA, α-amino-3-hydroxy-5-methylisoxazole-4-propionic acid; GABA, γ-amino-butyric-acid; 5-HT, 5-hydroxytryptamine; NMDA, N-methyl-D-aspartate.

distribution in the brain suggesting specific physiological functions.

GABA$_C$ receptors appear to represent a relatively simple form of ligand-gated chloride channel made up of ρ (rho) subunits. GABA$_C$ receptors are insensitive to bicuculline and baclofen and are mostly prominent at the retina and are not modulated by barbiturates or benzodiazepines.

Glutamate receptors

The ion channel family of glutamate receptors are divided based on their pharmacology and protein structure into three major subtypes: N-methyl-D-aspartate (NMDA), α-amino-3-hydroxy-5-methyl-isoxazole-4-propionic acid (AMPA) and kainate. The glutamate receptors mediate fast excitatory neurotransmission in mammals and are principally calcium ion channels although they also conduct sodium and potassium ions.

NMDA receptors

The NMDA subtype is a hetero-oligomer consisting of an NR1 subunit combined with one or more NR2 (A–D) subunits. Two ligand recognition sites must be occupied for channel opening — one for glutamate and one for glycine. The channel is permeable to calcium and blocked by magnesium ions. The neuronal form of nitric oxide synthase (nNOS or type I NOS) is coupled to the NMDA receptor. This close coupling allows tight regulation of calcium influx and regulation of type I NOS activity (see also second messenger systems).

The hippocampus is particularly rich in NMDA synapses and appears to have a central role in learning and memory. Plasticity within the hippocampus is mediated in part through changes in synaptic strength and revealed by long-term potentiation (LTP) and long-term depression (LTD). NMDA receptors are crucial for inducing these plastic changes, and blocking these receptors reduces plasticity and impairs learning. Intravenous and volatile anaesthetic agents appear to impair LTP and enhance LTD development.

AMPA receptors

The AMPA subtype is a hetero-oligomer formed from combinations of GluR1–4 subunits. AMPA receptors appear to regulate calcium influx under resting conditions although a functional cross-talk between the NMDA and AMPA receptors types is likely. NMDA receptors are crucial in mediating synaptic plasticity by LTP and are thought to be involved in memory and learning. However, silent synapses, in which LTP rapidly switches on AMPA receptor function at NMDA-receptor-only synapses, provides a postsynaptic mechanism, whereby NMDA receptor activation results in the rapid recruitment of AMPA receptors as well as a covalent modification of synaptic AMPA receptors.

Kainate receptors

The kainate receptor subtype consists of hetero-oligomers comprising the GluR5–7 and KA1 and KA2 subunits. The role of kainate receptors is less clear but there is evidence for a presynaptic location in the hippocampus. Antagonists of kainate, NMDA and AMPA receptors are thought to be of therapeutic benefit in stroke, head injuries, epilepsy and pain.

Nicotinergic acetylcholine receptors

The neurotransmitter acetylcholine exerts its postsynaptic effects on muscarinergic and nicotinergic receptors. Neuronal nicotinic acetylcholine receptors (nAChR) are ubiquitously distributed in various regions of the brain. They are principally a family of ligand-operated cation channels (calcium, sodium and potassium) and are thought to modulate the activity of various transmitter systems through a cascade of multisynaptic events. The pentameric channels are formed from α ($\alpha1$–$\alpha10$), β ($\beta1$–$\beta4$), γ, δ and ϵ subunits with each subunit having four transmembrane spanning domains (M1–M4) and M2 lining the channel pore. The acetylcholine binding site is located on an α subunit; thus, homomers have five putative binding sites while heteromers typically have two binding sites. In addition to the acetylcholine binding site, nAChR have associated modulatory sites for neurosteroids and acetylcholine esterase inhibitors. The predominant neuronal nAChR (also neuronal nicotinic receptors) are composed of the subunits $\alpha4\beta2$ and $\alpha7$ with the latter forming a pentameric homomer. The nAChR may be involved in Parkinson's and Alzheimer's disease and the pathophysiology of schizophrenia.

Glycine receptor

Glycine is a major inhibitory neurotransmitter in the CNS, with glycinergic synapses abundant in the spinal cord and brainstem. The postsynaptic glycine receptor is a hetero-oligomeric ligand-gated chloride channel and consists of three α and two β subunits. Four α subunit genes ($\alpha1$–$\alpha4$) are expressed and co-expression of the β subunits is essential for targeting the receptor to the synapse. Strychnine is a major glycine receptor antagonist, whereas β-alanine and β-aminobutyric acid and taurine are full or partial agonists.

Metabotropic receptors

Metabotropic receptors are a subclass of transmembrane receptors commonly thought of as a group of seven membrane-spanning domains organized much like a basket. Their signal is amplified through G-proteins, which are linked to the receptor, and the signalling unit is referred to as G-protein-linked receptors (GPLR). They constitute the largest family of cell-surface receptors.

G-protein cycle

G-proteins are a family of 'molecular switches' that transduce a signal to an amplifying enzyme whose activity produces a second messenger resulting in the activation or inhibition of an enzyme or ion channel. Figure 4.3 illustrates the G-protein cycle.

G-proteins comprise three subunits: α, β and γ. Agonists bind to specific receptors, which activate G-proteins through the release of guanosine 5' diphosphate (GDP) bound to the α subunit. Guanosine triphosphate (GTP) binding, which leads to dissociation of the heterotrimer into its component subunits, follows release of GDP. The GTP-ase activity of the α subunit determines the lifetime of this dissociated, now active G-protein. Hydrolysis of GTP back to GDP leads to reassociation of the heterotrimer. Both the α and $\beta\gamma$ subunits can transduce signals and regulate a range of second messengers. G-proteins can be divided into four classes according to the four types of α subunits: α_s, α_i, α_q and $\alpha_{12/13}$

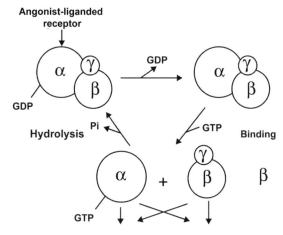

Figure 4.3 Heterotrimeric G-protein cycle. The figure illustrates the activation and deactivation of G-proteins. GDP, guanosine 5′ diphosphate; GTP, guanosine triphosphate.

and their main functions are summarized in Table 4.1.

Principally, $G\alpha_s$ stimulates adenylate cyclase activity and regulates calcium channels; $G\alpha_i$ inhibits adenylate cyclase, activates cyclic GMP-specific phosphodiesterase (PDE) in the retina and regulates K^+/calcium channels. The $G\alpha_q$ family contains G-proteins insensitive to cholera and pertussis toxin and activates phospholipase β (PLC-β) with a preference for the PLC-β_2 family. The function of $G\alpha_{12/13}$ is probably to regulate Cl^- ion channels but remains uncertain. The βγ subunits were long regarded as inactive but have now been shown to interact with other G-protein subunits, adenylyl cyclase, PLC-β and calmodulin.

Individual receptors can activate more than one G-protein and variation in different stages of G-protein activation and deactivation can affect the regulation of intracellular signalling. The GTP hydrolysis and binding properties vary for individual $G\alpha$ subunits, and accessory and regulatory protein also affect these processes. General G-protein function can be studied in *in vivo* and *in vitro* experiments,

Table 4.1 Classification and effects of Gα subunits.

Class	Members	Toxin	Distribution	Main functions
$G\alpha_s$	$G\alpha_s$	Cholera	Wide	Adenylyl cyclase stimulation
	$G\alpha_{olf}$	Cholera	Brain/olfactory	Adenylyl cyclase stimulation
$G\alpha_i$	$G\alpha_{i-1}$	Pertussis	Wide	Adenylyl cyclase inhibition
	$G\alpha_{i-2}$	Pertussis	Wide	Adenylyl cyclase inhibition
	$G\alpha_{i-3}$	Pertussis	Wide	Adenylyl cyclase inhibition
	$G\alpha_{oA,B}$	Pertussis	Brain	Potassium channel regulation
	$G\alpha_{t1, t2}$	Pertussis	Retina	Cyclic GMP specific PDE activation
	$G\alpha_z$			Not known
$G\alpha_q$	$G\alpha_q$		Wide	PLC-β regulation
	$G\alpha_{11}$		Wide	PLC-β regulation
	$G\alpha_{14,15,16}$			PLC-β regulation
$G\alpha_{12/13}$	$G\alpha_{12}$		Wide	? Chloride channels regulation
	$G\alpha_{13}$		Wide	

GMP, guanosine monophosphate; PDE, phosphodiesterase; PLC, phospholipase C.

utilizing the sensitivity to cholera and pertussis toxin for $G\alpha_s$ and $G\alpha_i$ classes, respectively. The effects of the $G\alpha_q$ classes are more difficult to study and generally use inhibitors of their effectors.

α_2-Adrenoceptors

α_2-Adrenoceptors are members of the G-protein-coupled family of membrane receptors and mediate the actions of the endogenous catecholamines epinephrine and norepinephrine. They are widely distributed and are located at pre- or postsynaptic and non-synaptic (platelets) sites. Activation of the pre-synaptic receptors results in sympatholytic action, whereas postsynaptic activation in the brainstem leads to an inhibition of sympathetic outflow. Three α_2-adrenoceptor proteins have been cloned and are designated α_{2a}, α_{2b} and α_{2c}, with α_{2a} being responsible for most of the α_2-adrenoceptor mediated actions. The α_2-receptor agonists exert their effects via coupled $G\alpha_i$ proteins by inhibiting adenylyl cyclase and modifying K^+/calcium channel activity. Selective α_2-adrenoceptor agonists are used for the treatment of hypertension, sedation and analgesia although no *in vitro* selective agonists for α_2-adrenoceptor subtypes exist.

Muscarinic acetylcholine receptors

The neurotransmitter acetylcholine exerts its post-synaptic effects on muscarinergic and nicotinergic receptors. Muscarinergic receptors are metabotropic receptors and currently five receptor subtypes have been cloned (m1–m5). 'Odd' numbered subtypes (m1, m3, m5) signal through increases in calcium mediated by $G\alpha_q$ and $G\alpha_o$ facilitated PLC-β activation. Activation of the m1 and m3 receptors often mediate 'slow' neuronal excitability involving inhibition of calcium-regulated potassium channels leading to inhibition after hyperpolarization. Cortical and hippocampal muscarinic receptors may be important in cognition. The 'even' numbered subtypes (m2 and m4) signal through $G\alpha_i$, resulting in a decrease in adenylyl cyclase activity. The m2 muscarinic receptors activate cardiac potassium channels leading to hyperpolarization and reduced heart rate. Besides their coupling to second messenger systems, muscarinic receptors may also couple with serine/threonine protein kinases from which modulation of gene expression results.

Metabotropic glutamate receptors

Metabotropic glutamate receptors are widely distributed throughout the CNS. They contain eight receptors which have been classified into three groups according to their amino acid homology, linkage to signalling pathways and pharmacology. The receptors contained in group 1 (m1 and m5) may play an important part in regulating calcium release from internal stores via $G\alpha_q$ G-proteins. The receptors from the other two groups modulate adenylyl cyclase via $G\alpha_i$ G-proteins. Quisqualate is the most potent agonist for group 1 receptors. Group 1 receptors may augment neurodegeneration, whereas group 2 and 3 receptor agonists may be neuroprotective.

$GABA_B$ receptors

The $GABA_B$ are hetero-oligomeric receptors composed of three receptor proteins ($GABA_BR1_{a/b}$ and $GABA_BR2$). Synaptic activation produces a slow inhibitory postsynaptic potential (IPSP) in contrast to fast IPSP produced by $GABA_A$. $GABA_B$ are metabotropic receptors and activate PLC-β, calcium and potassium channels. Baclofen is a selective agonist and used as an antispastic and analgesic agent. $GABA_B$ antagonist (phaclofen) may suppress absence epilepsy and improve cognitive function.

Serotonin receptors

Serotonin (5-hydroxytryptamine; 5-HT) is a major neurotransmitter in the CNS and synthesized from l-tryptophan in enterochromaffin cells as well as in serotonergic neurones. Thirteen human subtypes are subdivided into seven different classes (5-HT$_1$–5-HT$_7$) with further subdivisions. The 5-HT$_1$ receptors transduce their effects via $G\alpha_i$-mediated adenylyl cyclase modulation. The 5-HT$_{1A}$ receptors are involved in depression and anxiety and selective serotonin reuptake inhibitors (SSRIs) are widely used, whereas the 5-HT$_{1B/D}$ receptors have emerged as targets for migraine treatment (sumatriptan). The 5-HT$_2$ receptors signal via $G\alpha_q$, leading to an increase in PLC-β activity. Several receptor subtypes may present future targets for treatment of schizophrenia and obesity.

The 5-HT$_3$ subclass does not contain metabotropic receptors but ligand-gated cation channels and include commonly used anti-emetics such as ondansetron and granisetron.

Intracellular receptors

In contrast to transmembrane receptors, intracellular receptors are located within the cytoplasm or nucleus of the target cell. Lipid-soluble ligands such as steroid hormones cross the cell membrane by simple diffusion, whereas thyroid hormones enter the cell by facilitated diffusion. Steroid and thyroid hormone receptors are transcription factors; the mechanism of action is to modulate gene expression in target cells. Intracellular receptors are composed of a single polypeptide chain with at least three distinct domains.

The amino-terminus is involved in the interaction with other transcription factors and is highly variable between receptors. The DNA-binding domain and the ligand-binding domain are responsible for binding to a specific DNA sequence and hormone binding, respectively. Other receptor regions variably expressed are the nuclear localization sequence, which targets the protein to the nucleus, and a dimerization domain. Drugs that act on intracellular receptors are slow acting and their effects may persist after their elimination. Intravenous and volatile anaesthetic agents are therefore unlikely to signal via intracellular receptors.

Second and third messenger systems

Second messengers are low weight diffusible molecules that relay signals within a cell. They are synthesized or released as a result of an external signal received by a transmembrane receptor and serve to greatly amplify signal strength, with the strength of the signal being proportional to the concentration of the second messenger. Their half-life is very short and subcellular localizing and their water solubility enables the cell to limit duration and spread of the signal activity. There are three major classes of second messengers relevant to anaesthesia: cyclic nucleotides, lipids and calcium.

Cyclic nucleotides

Water-soluble molecules such as the cyclic nucleotides cyclic adenosine monophosphate (AMP) and cyclic guanosine monophosphate (GMP) are usually located within the cytosol. They are formed from adenosine triphosphate (ATP) and GTP, respectively,

through the action of the enzymes adenylyl and guanylyl cyclase and rapidly inactivated by PDEs.

Cyclic AMP is the major and best characterized second messenger and is involved in regulating neuronal, cardiovascular, metabolic and other functions. Principally, cyclic AMP is synthesized from ATP by adenylyl cyclases (ACs) following binding of hormones such as epinephrine, glucagons and luteinizing hormone to their respecive GPLR. The adenylyl cyclases are activated by $G\alpha_s$ and inhibited by $G\alpha_i$.

$$\text{ATP/GTP} \xrightarrow{\text{AC/GC}} \text{cyclic AMP/GMP} \xrightarrow{\text{PDE}} \text{5'AMP/GMP}$$

Adenylyl cyclases integrate the activity of a variety of signalling pathways and are susceptible to many modes of regulation. Currently, there are nine membrane-bound and one soluble AC known. The ACs are differentiated by their response to calcium, the $G_{\beta\gamma}$ subunits and $G\alpha_i$. Most tissues express more than one AC but all calcium/calmodulin stimulated species are restricted to neuronal and secretory tissues; AC5 is concentrated in striate and cardiac tissue.

Adenylyl cyclases possess five major domains: an N-terminus, two transmembrane clusters and a duplicated catalytic domain. The latter is further subdivided into a highly conserved C1a and C2a, which dimerize to form the catalytic site, and the less conserved C1b and C2b domains. An intracellular compartmentalization by co-localization of ACs with capacitative calcium entry channels in caveolae and organization in microdomains, allows a regulation of cyclic AMP production within the cell.

Cyclic GMP has long been recognized as a second messenger but its importance in signal transduction was not recognized for more than 20 years in the absence of a recognized 'first messenger'. Also, its relatively low intracellular concentrations when compared with cyclic AMP have made the investigations of its biological role more technically challenging. Cyclic GMP is formed from GTP through the action of the enzyme ghanylate cylcase (GC), which exists in either soluble or particulate forms, with the soluble form being located within the cytosol and the particulate form within the cell membrane. In general, particulate GCs are activated through natriuretic peptide receptors or intestinal peptide-binding receptors, binding at their extracellular domain and resulting in production of cyclic GMP.

Soluble GC is the most abundant form in the CNS. It exists as a heterodimer consisting of α and β subunits and is activated by interaction of nitric oxide, resulting in up to 400-fold activation. Carbon monoxide can also activate soluble GC, resulting in a four- to sixfold increase in activation. Clinically used activators of soluble GC are described as nitric oxide donors and include glycerol trinitrate, nitroprusside or *S*-nitrosothiols. Methylene blue has been described as an inhibitor of soluble GC but has also been shown to inhibit nitric oxide synthase directly.

Cyclic AMP mediates a variety of short- and long-term responses with its main effects in activating protein kinase A (PKA) and regulating gene transcription. The release of cyclic GMP has effects at three levels: by affecting cyclic GMP kinases (PKG), cyclic GMP regulated ion channels and PDE activity.

The duration of cyclic nucleotide signalling is not only dependent on the rate of cyclic nucleotide formation, but also on its rate of breakdown. The cyclic nucleotides cyclic AMP and cyclic GMP are hydrolysed by PDE of which there are currently 11 isoforms described. PDEs possess a central catalytic domain with both the N- and C-terminus having regulatory properties. The N-terminus is thought to be involved in allosteric regulation and membrane targeting, whereas the C-terminus may be involved in dimerization and targeted for PDE-specific kinases. The human PDE isoform distribution and selective inhibitors are summarized in Table 4.2. Apart from the selective PDE inhibitors listed in Table 4.2, there are several well-known non-isoform specific inhibitors such as caffeine, theophylline and pentoxifylline. Most PDEs utilize both cyclic nucleotides (PDE 1, 2, 3, 10 and 11), whereas PDE 5, 6 and 9 are specific for cyclic GMP. PDE 5 is cyclic GMP specific and is a well-established and important regulator of cyclic GMP function. The activity of the PDE enzymes is regulated by cyclic AMP and cyclic GMP and is subject to feedback activation and inhibition of PDE.

Lipid signalling

Phospholipases are enzymes that catalyse cleavage of acyl- or phosphoacyl groups from glycerophospholipids. They are implicated in the rearrangement of phospholipids and in the release of arachidonic acid in the eicosanoid metabolism (phospholipase A2). Other phospholipases such as PLC-β isoforms function as effector enzymes for $G\alpha_q$ proteins and βγ-subunits typically released from $G\alpha_i$. This leads to an increase in its catalytic activity and amplification of the initial receptor stimulus. PLC-β isozymes hydrolyse phosphatidylinositol 4,5-bisphosphate, generating two intracellular products: inositol 1,4,5-trisphosphate (IP$_3$), a universal calcium-mobilizing second messenger, and diacylglycerol (DAG), an activator of PKC PLC-β isoenzymes, are strongly associated with membranes via scaffolding proteins and plasma membrane lipids forming microdomains similar to ACs.

IP$_3$ is a small water-soluble molecule that diffuses through the cytosol and binds to receptors on the endoplasmic and sarcoplasmic reticulum, resulting in the release of calcium into the cytosol. DAG stimulates membrane-bound protein PKC by greatly increasing the affinity for calcium and phosphatidyl serine. A conformational change pulls a pseudosubstrate sequence from the catalytic core facilitating binding and phosphorylation of target proteins.

Calcium

Calcium ions are critical and probably the most widely used intracellular messengers. Calcium ions are involved in signal transduction, metabolic regulation, exocytosis, muscle contraction, apoptosis and immune regulation. Intracellular calcium concentrations are tightly controlled, with resting cytoplasmic concentrations of 10–100 nmol in non-excitable cells compared with extracellular calcium concentrations of 2 mmol. In stimulated cells, intracellular calcium concentrations can rise to 1–2 µmol. There are two main calcium depots: the extracellular fluid and the endoplasmic reticulum. Calcium is released into the cytoplasm from the extracellular fluid by voltage-gated calcium channels in response to plasma membrane depolarization and ligand-gated calcium channels. Calcium ions are also released from the endoplasmic reticulum via IP$_3$-gated channels and ryanodine receptors. Ryanodine receptors are found in most cells but are concentrated in striate muscle and show sequence homology with IP$_3$-gated channels. Caffeine is a very effective activator of the ryanodine receptor, whereas heparin is used as an inhibitor. Calcium ions are returned by energy

Table 4.2 Human phosphodiesterase (PDE) characteristics, tissue distribution and selective inhibitors.

Family	Characteristics	Primary tissue distribution	Selective inhibitors
PDE 1	Calcium/calmodulin-stimulated	Heart, brain, lung, smooth muscle	Vinpocetine
PDE 2	Cyclic GMP-stimulated	Adrenal gland, heart, lung	EHNA
PDE 3	Cyclic GMP-inhibited, cyclic AMP-selective	Heart, lung, liver, platelets	Milrinone
PDE 4	Cyclic AMP-specific, cGMP-insensitive	Sertoli cells, kidney, brain	Rolipram
PDE 5	Cyclic GMP-specific	Lung, brain, smooth muscle	Sildenafil
PDE 6	Cyclic GMP-specific	Photoreceptors	Zaprinast
PDE 7	Cyclic AMP-specific	Skeletal muscle, heart, brain	None
PDE 8	Cyclic AMP-selective, IBMX insensitive	Testes, eye, liver, heart	None
PDE 9	Cyclic GMP-specific, IBMX insensitive	Kidney, liver, lung, brain	None
PDE 10	Cyclic GMP-sensitive, cAMP-selective	Testes, brain	None
PDE 11	Cyclic GMP-sensitive, dual specificity	Skeletal muscle, prostate	None

AMP, adenosine monophosphate; EHNA, erythro-9- (2-hydroxy-3-nonyl) adenine hydrochloride; GMP, guanosine monophosphate; IBMX, 3-isobutyl-L-methylxanthine .

dependent active transport systems such as calcium-ATPase and sodium–calcium exchangers to the extracellular fluid and endoplasmic reticulum (Fig. 4.4).

'Third' messenger systems

Third messengers are dependent on second messenger systems and represent events down the signalling cascades. These systems now possess substantial receptor reserve and complicated feedback mechanisms and are integrated with numerous intracellular pathways. Most second messenger systems, however, activate protein kinases as their primary target and are considered here. Protein kinases catalyse phosphoryl transfers from ATP to serine, tyrosine, threonine and histidine residues of regulatory proteins. They are allosterically controlled and depend on the concentrations of intracellular messengers. The protein kinases are named based on their primary activators such as PKC for calcium dependent, PKA for cyclic AMP dependence and PKG for cyclic GMP activation.

Protein kinase C are a family of membrane-bound kinases that phosphorylate specific serine and threonine residues in target proteins including ligand- and voltage-gated ion channels and metabotropic receptors. Known target proteins include calmodulin, β-adrenergic receptors, glucose transporter, HMG-CoA reductase and cytochrome P450. PKC can be classified based on their sensitivity to calcium and DAG and phorbol ester. Many PKC isoforms have their own distinct tissue distribution, implying unique regulatory roles for each class. They are laterally organized within the plasma membrane and bound to proteins known as receptors for activated C kinases (RACKs) which are also capable of

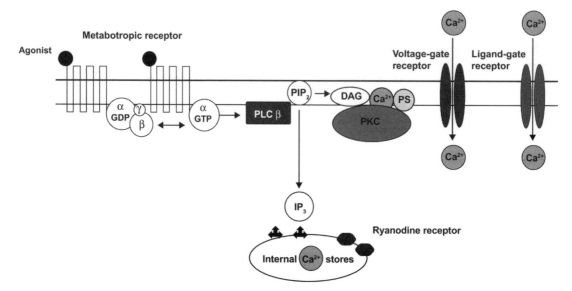

Figure 4.4 Calcium regulation. DAG, diacylglycerol; GDP, guanosine 5′ diphosphate; GTP, guanosine triphosphate; IP_3, inositol 1,4,5-trisphosphate; PKC, protein kinase C; PLC-β, phospholipase C-β; PS, phosphatidylserine.

binding components of other signalling pathways and could serve therefore as sites of signal integration.

Cyclic AMP exerts almost all of its actions through the activation of a single enzyme, PKA. Cyclic AMP-dependent protein kinase is one of the simplest members of the protein kinase family and its kinetic properties as well as crystal structure have been well characterized. The catalytic subunit is regulated by four different regulatory subunits that target PKA to scaffolding proteins (A kinase anchoring proteins; AKAP) to achieve close proximity to specific substrates within the cell. The catalytic subunit has a small amino terminal domain for ATP binding and a larger carboxyl terminal domain as a docking site for the protein substrate. The regulatory subunit inhibits the catalytic subunit activity and serves as primary receptor for cyclic AMP.

There are two major types of cyclic GMP dependent protein kinases: a soluble cyclic GMP kinase, defined as type 1 (PKG1) which exists as a dimer, and secondly a particulate membrane-bound monomeric form termed type 2 (PKG2). Cyclic GMP kinases are serine/threonine protein kinases and are most abundant in smooth muscle, platelets and cerebellum. Recently, immunocytochemistry studies demonstrated that cerebral PKG1 is almost restricted to Purkinje cells but may exert its main role at the neuromuscular endplate. PKG2 is a ubiquitous brain protein kinase and responsible for most cyclic GMP-mediated protein phosphorylation.

PKG has been implicated in a number of biologically important processes ranging from regulation of intracellular calcium to gene regulation and cell proliferation. Its primary function, however, appears to be the control of intracellular calcium concentration within a narrow range through non-specific voltage-gated and metabotropic calcium channels. This effect is mediated through calcium-activated potassium channels, which increase the opening probability leading to an inward potassium flux in exchange for calcium. Cyclic GMP may exert a degree of feedback inhibition of its formation through the action of PKG on these channels, leading to a decrease in calcium influx and reduced nitric oxide release. There is also some evidence that 5′ GMP, a metabolite of cyclic GMP, rather than PKG, is the activating compound for the potassium–calcium exchanger. PKG has also been reported to phosphorylate AMPA receptors in cerebellar slices, although the expected feedback inhibition of AMPA may be primarily caused by cyclic GMP rather than PKG. In addition to these channel modulations, cyclic GMP and PKG may also reduce intracellular calcium through sodium–calcium exchange, calcium ATPase and G-protein modulation. However, it is unlikely that a single mechanism is responsible for the effects of cyclic GMP on calcium homoeostasis.

Receptors and messenger systems relevant to anaesthesia

The first general anaesthetic was administered more than 150 years ago but a generally accepted hypothesis for the mechanisms involved in general anaesthesia remains elusive. There are several theories for the mechanisms of anaesthesia, ranging from the Meyer–Overton theory suggesting the importance of a lipid-like phase, to more recent theories of proteins as anaesthetic targets. Clinical concentrations of anaesthetic agents can enhance the effects of inhibitory, or block the actions of excitatory, ligand- and voltage-gated ion channels. Given the diverse molecular structure of anaesthetic agents, ranging from noble gases such as xenon to the more complex structure of amino steroids, it appears unlikely that all anaesthetic agents act on one target only. More likely, they act on a number of targets and complex systems. In tracing a cascade of events towards the response elements, the further one gets away from agonist binding, the more likely it gets that intracellular systems integrate and provide feedback mechanisms, making firm conclusions about cause and effect difficult. This is particularly true for interpretation of *in vitro* and *in vivo* investigations and should be borne in mind in the following discussion of the effects of anaesthetic agents.

Ionotropic receptors
Inhibitory ligand-gated ion channels

Volatile and intravenous anaesthetic agents enhance the currents through $GABA_A$ and glycine chloride channels, resulting in a reduction in the excitability of neurones and anaesthetic depressant actions. *In vitro* studies suggest that volatile and intravenous anaesthetic agents directly activate $GABA_A$ receptors or potentiate GABA actions by increasing the opening probability of $GABA_A$ receptors. *In vivo* studies using a point mutation of the β_3 subunit of the $GABA_A$ receptor suggest a critical role of the $GABA_A$ receptor in mediating the effects of propofol and etomidate for immobility and to a lesser extent for hypnosis. However, this is not necessarily proven for inhalational anaesthetic agents.

Glycine is a major inhibitory neurotransmitter in the spinal cord. The glycine receptor antagonist increases the minimum alveolar concentration (MAC) of volatile anaesthetic agents in *in vivo* studies and anaesthetic agents prolong the glycinergic duration of miniature postsynaptic currents *in vitro*. With the spinal cord being the prime candidate for mediating the immobility actions of volatile anaesthetic agents, glycinergic receptors are likely to be involved in mediating the effects of anaesthetic agents.

Excitatory ligand-gated ion channels

Several volatile anaesthetics can block NMDA receptors at clinically relevant concentrations and NMDA receptor blockade dose dependently decreases MAC in *in vivo* studies. However, ketamine, nitrous oxide and xenon have greater *in vitro* effects than potent volatile anaesthetics on NMDA receptors. These results suggest that NMDA receptors may have a significant role in mediating the effect of anaesthetic agents. Although AMPA and kainate receptor antagonists reduce MAC and anaesthetic agents inhibit AMPA and kainate-mediated excitatory postsynaptic currents, genetically modified mice absent in AMPA receptors have normal MAC values. In addition, kainate receptors require anaesthetic concentrations in excess of clinically relevant, suggesting that both kainate and AMPA receptor systems might not be relevant during anaesthesia.

Small concentrations of volatile anaesthetic agents and ketamine inhibit nicotinergic transmission in *in vitro* studies but neither agonists nor antagonists of nicotinic receptors in *in vivo* studies decrease MAC for volatile anaesthetics. Non-immobilizers (i.e. volatile agents predicted to have anaesthetic activity but do not cause or add to anaesthetic effects) inhibit nicotinergic receptors *in vitro*, suggesting that nicotinergic transmission is not involved in modulating the effects of anaesthesia.

The 5-HT$_3$ receptor ligand-gated cation channel possesses a considerable sequence homology to other ionotropic channels such as GABA$_A$, glycine and nicotinergic channels and displays an increase in pro-excitatory effects in response to anaesthetic agents. In addition, the absence of *in vivo* effects in response to antagonism suggests that 5-HT$_3$ receptors do not have a role in anaesthesia.

Metabotropic receptors

The α_2-receptor agonists clonidine and dexmedetomidine decrease anaesthetic requirements via inhibition of the locus coeruleus with the resulting disinhibition of the ventrolateral pre-optic nucleus (GABAergic) and inhibition of tuberomammillary nucleus. This suggests a convergence on endogenous sleep-promoting pathways. Recent *in vivo* studies using genetically modified mice indicate that possibly α_{2A}-receptors are responsible for hypnotic effects and α_{2B}-receptor for analgesic properties (? nitrous oxide) of α_2-receptor agonists.

Volatile anaesthetic agents inhibit muscarinergic signalling through activation of PKC *in vitro*. However, *in vivo* studies with muscarinergic antagonists alone or in combination with nicotinic blocking drugs do not change MAC, suggesting that cholinergic inhibition is not a primary target for anaesthetic agents.

Second and 'third' messenger systems

The glutamate–nitric oxide cyclic GMP pathway has been identified as a potential major target for general anaesthetic agents, because acute inhibition of this pathway using non-isoform specific nitric oxide synthase inhibitors reduces the anaesthetic requirements in most animal studies by either reducing the minimum anaesthetic concentration for volatile anaesthetic agents or increasing sleep times for intravenous anaesthetic agents. However, chronic administration of NOS inhibitors and the genetic absence of the neuronal NOS isoform (type I NOS or nNOS) do not reduce the anaesthetic requirements in *in vivo* experiments, suggesting alternative or compensatory mechanisms. Glutamate stimulates NMDA receptors, resulting in an influx of calcium and subsequent stimulation of type I NOS coupled to the NMDA receptor via PSD95. Cerebral cyclic GMP concentrations change during anaesthesia in ani-

mals and similar changes have been observed in human plasma. Cyclic GMP may therefore represent a potential biochemical marker for anaesthesia. Very little is known about the effects of anaesthesia on the hydrolysis of cyclic nucleotides.

Early *in vivo* experiments suggested an important role for protein kinases in anaesthesia, because non-specific inhibitors cause behavioural changes similar to anaesthesia. *In vitro* experiments implicate PKC in the actions of anaesthetic agents, suggesting that an activation of PKC results in receptor and channel phosphorylation and dampening of the agonist response. It is unclear, however, if anaesthetics change the cellular levels of activators such as DAG or calcium or even simply change the phosphorylation sites of their targets.

G-proteins themselves may be primary targets for anaesthetic agents because the receptor–G-protein coupling is sufficiently sensitive to a wide range of anaesthetics. For example, an *in vitro* study investigating the effects of volatile anaesthetic agents on purified Gα subunits demonstrated an inhibition in GTP binding in Gα_{i-1-3} subunits and minimally in Gα_s subunits for all volatile anaesthetic agents, whereas Gα_o subunits were completely insensitive to volatile anaesthetic agents. GTP hydrolysis was also unaffected by volatile anaesthetic agents. More work is needed to provide definitive answers on the role of G-proteins during anaesthesia.

Further reading

Alderton WK, Cooper CE, Knowles RG. Nitric oxide synthase: structure, function and inhibition. *Biochem J* 2001; **357**: 593–615.

Cooper DMF. Regulation and organisation of adenylyl cyclases and cAMP. *Biochem J* 2003; **375**: 517–29.

Jurd R, Arras M, Lambert S, *et al.* General anesthetic actions *in vivo* strongly attenuated by a point mutation in the GABA(A) receptor beta3 subunit. *FASEB J* 2003; **17**: 250–2.

Rebecchi MJ, Pentyala SN. Anaesthetic actions on other targets: protein kinase C and guanine nucleotide-binding proteins. *Br J Anaesth* 2002; **89**: 62–78.

Sonner JM, Antognini JF, Dutton RC, *et al.* Inhaled anesthetics and immobility: mechanisms, mysteries, and minimum alveolar anesthetic concentration. *Anesth Analg* 2003; **97**: 718–40.

CHAPTER 5

Anaphylaxis

Michael Rose and Malcolm Fisher

Introduction

An anaphylactic reaction describes an immunological response generated by the body towards a molecule recognized as being hostile, and involves type I hypersensitivity mediated by immunoglobulin E (IgE) or immunoglobulin G (IgG) antibodies (Fig. 5.1). The term anaphylaxis has also been widely used to describe a set of clinical signs and symptoms that resemble type I hypersensitivity, regardless of the mechanism.

Anaphylactoid reactions are those reactions that clinically resemble antibody-mediated, immunologically driven anaphylaxis, but which are caused by other mechanisms, such as the direct effect of drugs on vessels, drug interactions or drug-mediated direct release of mediators such as histamine (Fig. 5.2). The lack of an immunological cause for an event may be confused with an inability to detect an immunological cause because of technical reasons. An anaphylactic reaction may then be labelled an anaphylactoid reaction, resulting in a drug being administered to a sensitive patient because a direct lack of causation was not determined. For this reason, the term *anaphylactoid* should be reserved for those cases in which no chance of an immunological mechanism exists, *clinical anaphylaxis* to the clinical syndrome, and *anaphylaxis* to those situations in which true type I hypersensitivity is suspected or has been demonstrated. Until causation of an event is established it is best to assume that an immune mechanism is present, and subsequent exposure to possible precipitating agents avoided.

Incidence of anaphylaxis in anaesthesia

The incidence of anaphylaxis under anaesthesia var-ies between series and countries. In all series, true anaphylaxis during anaesthesia is rare. It would require approximately 30 million patients to be studied to establish a true incidence within 5% confidence limits [1] which is, of course, impractical. However, estimates of incidence have been made, and the Boston Collaborative Drug Surveillance Study [2] estimated the incidence of in-hospital reactions as 3 in 10 000 patients. The incidence of anaphylaxis during anaesthesia in Australia is thought to be 1 in 10 000–20 000 [1] and in France as 1 in 13 000 cases, or 6500 cases where a neuromuscular blocker was used [3]. Anaphylaxis to neuromuscular blocking drugs (NMBDs) is more common in females, with approximately 55–73% of reactions in women reported in several international studies [4–7].

Aetiology, pathogenesis and clinical features of anaphylaxis

Anaphylaxis is an example of type I hypersensitivity according to the classic description by Coombes and Gell [8]. The major immunoglobulin involved in anaphylaxis is IgE. Sensitization occurs following exposure to an allergenic substance either alone or after combination with another protein or hapten. The result is the production of IgE against this allergen, some of which binds to the surface of mast cells and basophils. At a later time when the patient is again exposed to the allergen, an antigen–antibody reaction occurs on the surface of the cell during which two molecules of IgE are cross-linked. The result is degranulation of mast cells and basophils and release of histamine and other inflammatory mediators such as platelet activating factor (PAF), proteases and proteoglycans [9]. An inflammatory cascade is generated, resulting in the release of

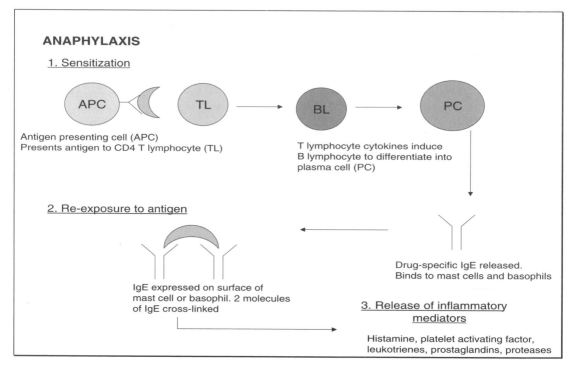

Figure 5.1 Mechanism of anaphylactic reactions.

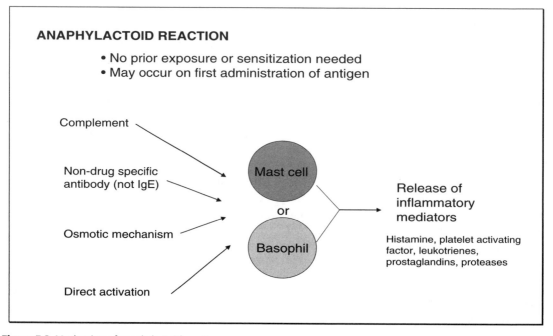

Figure 5.2 Mechanism of anaphylactoid reactions.

leukotrienes (LTC4, LTE4 and LTD4) and prostaglandins (PGD2).

Histamine, PGD2 and LTC4 are mediators involved in vascular permeability and have been implicated in the vascular phenomena associated with anaphylaxis. While histamine is involved in many of the early symptoms and signs of the reaction, it is rapidly cleared from the plasma [10]. The overall result of the sudden release of inflammatory mediators is vasodilatation, smooth muscle contraction, glandular secretion and increased capillary permeability, both locally and systemically.

Histamine may also be released directly from mast cells by some drugs and this may result in clinical symptoms and signs. These are related to dose of drug and rate of infusion. There is some evidence that histamine release varies in different groups of mast cells. While the relevance of these laboratory studies to the intact patient is controversial, they provide an attractive explanation for some of the clinical effects of drugs that stimulate histamine release. The site of histamine release may be important in the clinical effects produced. Drugs such as morphine stimulate release of histamine from skin alone [11] and have little propensity for systemic symptoms such as asthma, whereas drugs such as atracurium and propofol, which produce histamine release from lung mast cells, may be more likely to induce bronchospasm [12]. For the most part, direct stimulation of histamine release produces transient symptoms, although severe reactions may occur in some patients, especially with vancomycin and Haemaccel® (Syner-Med).

True anaphylactoid reactions are triggered by mechanisms other than by direct histamine release. These include activation of the complement system (e.g. some intravenous drugs, X-ray contrast media), non-IgE antibody already present in the patient's plasma or osmotic mechanisms (e.g. dextrose, mannitol).

Clinical manifestations of anaphylaxis

The syndrome of clinical anaphylaxis (either truly anaphylactic or anaphylactoid) usually (in 95% of cases) begins within 5 min of administration of the allergen if it has been administered intravenously. The onset of anaphylaxis may be slower and progression less rapid if the trigger is not parenteral (e.g. food or latex). Reactions vary in severity from mild to fatal (mortality 4% and a further 2% sustaining brain damage in a large series) [1].

Clinical features involve multiple organ systems and are variable. The incidences of clinical features of anaphylaxis to drugs given intravenously in the perioperative period are presented in Table 5.1. It can be seen that the most common manifestations are cardiovascular manifestations (hypotension, including collapse), cutaneous manifestations (rash, erythema, urticaria), respiratory compromise (bronchospasm) and angioedema. Cardiovascular collapse is the most common manifestation to present alone and is most likely to be the most severe feature. A recent survey in France [3] graded the severity of anaphylactic reactions, ranging from I to IV. Grade I was defined as presence of cutaneous signs; grade II as presence of measurable but not life-threatening symptoms including cutaneous effects, arterial hypotension (defined as more than 30% decrease in arterial blood pressure associated with unexplained tachycardia); grade III as presence of a life-threatening reaction

Table 5.1 Clinical features of anaphylaxis in 774 patients.

	Number	Sole feature	Worst feature
Cardiovascular collapse	662	81	607
Bronchospasm	283	35	133
Transient	113		
Asthmatics	100		
Cutaneous			
Rash	116		
Erythema	328		
Urticaria	62		
More than 1	40		
Angioedema	179	10	29
Generalized oedema	45		
Pulmonary oedema	19	1	3
Gastrointestinal	40		

such as cardiovascular collapse, tachycardia or bradycardia, arrhythmias or severe bronchospasm; and grade IV was defined as circulatory insufficiency and cardiac and/or respiratory arrest. Of the 477 cases examined in this case review, the most common severity was grade III (62.6%) followed by grade II (22.9%), grade I (10.1%) and finally grade IV (4.4% of cases).

The diagnosis of anaphylaxis is usually made at a time when the reaction is well advanced. This is demonstrated by the timing of the first clinical feature noted in a series of 750 patients (Table 5.2). Since 1990, when the use of pulse oximetry was widespread, the most common presenting feature has been desaturation or loss of pulse oximetry waveform, or transient difficulty in lung inflation. It is worth noting that asthmatics experiencing anaphylaxis virtually always have bronchospasm. When bronchospasm is severe it is extremely difficult to treat. Pulmonary oedema is rarely associated with anaphylaxis and the mechanism involved is a noncardiogenic oedema, associated with low venous pressures and a large volume deficit. However, reactions to protamine, blood products and venoms may produce severe pulmonary vasoconstriction and right ventricular failure [13–15].

Differential diagnosis of anaphylaxis

The diagnosis of anaphylaxis may be obvious in the setting of cardiovascular collapse, urticaria and bronchospasm following the administration of an intravenous medication, particularly if the patient is known to be sensitive. The cardinal symptoms and signs that anaphylaxis may be severe include rapidity of onset, dyspnoea, stridor, facial swelling and hypotension.

The diagnosis may not be so apparent if the reaction is low grade or if concomitant events cause confusion over the genesis of signs (such as hypotension and tachycardia as a result of excessive blood loss during surgery). During general anaesthesia, early symptoms of anaphylaxis such as tongue swelling, itch, breathing difficulty and wheeze will obviously not be reported. Signs such as rash or urticaria may not be noted until drapes are removed, leading to delay in diagnosis or possibly even failure of a diagnosis of clinical anaphylaxis being considered.

The unusual reactions involving only one organ system, such as bronchospasm, also may lead to an anaphylactic cause being overlooked and a delay in treatment, especially in patients known to suffer from asthma. Other causes of hypotension and bronchospasm during anaesthesia are more common than allergic reactions. Cardiovascular collapse may result from inherent cardiac causes such as cardiac failure and acute myocardial infarction, and pulmonary embolism of blood clot or other matter. Distinction of these from a diagnosis of anaphylaxis may be difficult, but is aided by the presence of low venous pressure, vasodilatation and the presence of supraventricular tachycardia as the predominant rhythm in established anaphylaxis [16]. Vasovagal reactions may also simulate anaphylaxis in the awake patient and are often misdiagnosed as allergic, particularly with local anaesthesic blocks for surgery. Signs that aid the diagnosis are initial bradycardia and sweating, hyperventilation and initial bradycar-

Table 5.2 First clinical feature noted during anaphylactic reactions in 750 patients.

Symptom	Number
Subjective	17
Cough	46
No pulse	197
No bleeding	2
Swelling	13
Difficult to inflate	177
ECG abnormality	14
Rash	37
Flush	124
Urticaria	15
Other	21
Desaturation	87
Total records	589

dia and hypotension followed by the return of normal pulse rate and blood pressure without the need for treatment.

Factors altering risk of anaphylaxis

Females are more likely to experience anaphylaxis than males. This preponderance persists even after the increased rate of anaesthesia in women is taken into account [17]. In a comprehensive review of risk factors, Fisher and Doig [18] found few valid risk factors. Those that did appear to be significant included previous anaphylaxis or an unexplained adverse event during anaesthesia. In addition, patients with spina bifida or allergy to some fruits were at increased risk of latex allergy and those with IgA deficiency were at risk from blood products and their derivatives (including some colloid solutions). However, it is important to remember that in spite of an increased incidence of a history of allergy, atopy and asthma in patients who have anaphylaxis during anaesthesia, the overwhelming majority of patients with such a history have uneventful anaesthesia and that such a history does not constitute a valid predictor of risk [19].

Factors affecting severity of anaphylaxis

Health

Anaphylaxis is a condition generally seen in fit patients. It is less commonly seen in critically ill patients on the intensive care unit. It is thought that the response to stress (release of both steroid hormones and adrenaline) acts to 'pre-treat' such patients, antagonizing the release and effects of the mediators of anaphylaxis.

Asthma

Patients who suffer from asthma are more likely to develop severe bronchospasm, which is difficult to treat [20]. In addition, patients with asthma have a reduced catecholamine response [21].

β-Adrenergic blockade

Patients treated with β-adrenergic antagonists may experience more severe anaphylaxis, with features of severe hypotension, bronchospasm and paradoxical bradycardia [22]. Such patients are more likely to be refractory to treatment, and massive doses of adrenaline (epinephrine) may be needed. Consideration should also be given to the use of drugs with prominent α-adrenergic agonist properties such as metaraminol or noradrenaline (norepinephrine). Glucagon may also have a role.

Epidural blockade

The sympathectomy induced by epidural blockade may exacerbate cardiovascular collapse during anaphylaxis and may necessitate higher doses of adrenaline and greater volumes of fluid resuscitation. The risk of death from anaphylaxis to dextrans is increased in patients with epidural blockade [23].

Anaphylaxis under anaesthesia — most common triggers

In contrast to anaphylaxis in the community, which tends to be triggered by foodstuffs (especially nuts), *Hymenoptera* (e.g. bees, wasps) plants and drugs, the most common anaesthetic triggers for anaphylaxis occurring during anaesthesia are intravenous drugs. Of these, neuromuscular blocking drugs are the most common cause in most countries with available data. In Sweden, however, reactions to latex and chlorhexidine are more common than reactions to NMBDs. Reactions to NMBDs are rarely described in the USA and rarely seen in South Africa. Antibiotics, colloids and protamine are the next most common triggers. Recently, there have been increasing reports of intraoperative anaphylaxis to chlorhexidine [24, 25], patent blue dye and aprotinin. Latex is also becoming a relatively frequent cause of adverse reaction under anaesthetic. In some patients, sensitization to more than one agent administered is found during subsequent testing. Volatile agents are not known to cause anaphylactic reactions.

Neuromuscular blocking drugs

Anaphylaxis resulting from NMBDs is brought about

by IgE antibodies binding to the NMBD-substituted paired tertiary or quaternary ammonium ions, which are inherent to the structure of the NMBD molecule. The NMBD most likely to cause anaphylaxis is suxamethonium, possibly because its structure is flexible, making cross-linking of two IgE molecules relatively easy [26,27]. Cross-sensitivity between NMBD is approximately 60% [28] but is not entirely predictable on the basis of relationships of structure and class between drugs, with the exception of cisatracurium and atracurium which are antigenically isomers [29]. Cross-sensitivity to NMBDs can be identified by skin testing or radioimmunoassay. Historically, the most common pairs of drugs to cross-react are suxamethonium and gallamine, alcuronium and D-tubocurarine and pancuronium and vecuronium [1]. Data on cross-sensitivity is dependent on whether it is detected by skin testing or radioimmunoassay.

A particularly unusual feature of anaphylaxis to NMBDs is that sensitization via previous exposure to these agents does not appear to be evident in many cases. The reason for this is unclear, but may relate to the fact that many other compounds found in foodstuffs and other pharmaceutical preparations (e.g. morphine, neostigmine) contain tertiary or quaternary ammonium ions that could potentially sensitize patients to subsequent NMBD exposure.

Antibiotics

Allergy to antibiotics is a growing problem in an era when routine use of such drugs during anaesthesia is common. A history of antibiotic allergy should always be clarified carefully prior to anaesthesia in order either to avoid administration of drugs likely to be antigenic in a patient, or not to avoid the most appropriate antibiotic when symptoms of so-called allergy are simply minor gastrointestinal upset.

Penicillin allergy is perhaps the most common quoted allergy reported by patients and often the history of the inciting event is poorly remembered. The only way to clarify the patient's status in questionable cases (after exclusion of clear positives and negatives from history) is to perform skin prick and intradermal testing. It is important to note that the predictive value of a negative skin test to penicillin is 97% (approximately 3% of those with a negative

test will develop a limited skin rash with penicillin administration) [30]. When allergy to penicillin is established, or insufficient time exists for clarification, other antibiotics must be chosen for antibacterial therapy. Traditionally, cross-reactivity between penicillins and cephalosporins was thought to occur in approximately 10% of cases on the basis of the shared antigenicity of the β-lactam ring common to both groups of antibiotics. Debate continues as to whether there is true cross-reactivity between the groups, as reactions to early generation cephalosporins in penicillin-allergic patients have since been attributed to traces of penicillin present, or to rashes of non-immunological cause. Post-marketing studies of second and third generation cephalosporins have demonstrated no increase in allergic reactions in patients with histories of penicillin allergy [31].

Opioids

Adverse reactions to opioids (including morphine, pethidine, fentanyl and congeners or codeine) are commonly described by patients, but are usually adverse effects such as nausea and vomiting, hallucinations or dysphoria, drowsiness or apnoea. Anaphylaxis to this group of drugs is possible but is rare [32]. Non-immunological histamine release in response to morphine and pethidine is more commonly encountered.

Latex

Adverse reactions to latex (a natural rubber compound produced from the sap of the *Hevea brasiliensis* tree) can occur, in decreasing order of severity and increasing order of frequency, as type I mediated hypersensitivity reaction (anaphylaxis), a type IV mediated hypersensitivity reaction, delayed-onset hypersensitivity, allergic contact dermatitis and, most commonly, irritant contact dermatitis.

High-risk groups for latex reactions include those frequently exposed to latex antigens such as healthcare workers and spina bifida patients (many of whom have undergone frequent urinary catheterization) as well as atopic individuals and those sensitive to certain fruits that may share a 30-kd epitope with latex (avocados, pears, bananas, kiwifruit, strawberries, guavas, peaches and citrus fruits). Type

I hypersensitivity to latex has become a very important cause of anaphylaxis during anaesthesia. Universal precautions became widespread in the 1980s, and the resulting demand for rubber gloves saw production of rubber rapidly increase, with a subsequent decrease in purity of the product (more antigenic latex proteins). Latex sensitivity has since become a major cause of anaphylaxis under anaesthesia, second only to NMBDs in the survey conducted by Laxenaire et al. [33] in France between 1994 and 1996 (16.6% of cases). Since then, increased awareness of latex allergy combined with alternatives to latex products (e.g. neoprene, vinyl, silicone) has seen reports of the incidence of latex sensitivity decline, and a follow-up survey revealed a fall to 12.1% of cases in 1997–98 [34].

Type IV hypersensitivity to latex results from T-cell mediated sensitization to additives in the latex product. This reaction begins 2–3 days after exposure and may cause erythema, with scales and vesicles [34]. Irritant contact dermatitis is a non-immunological reaction that may occur on first or subsequent exposure to latex products, and is caused by chemical irritation of the gloves and their high pH. It results in hands feeling itchy or sore and looking red and usually resolves with discontinuation of exposure and treatment with moisturizers [34].

Local anaesthetics

Genuine allergic reactions to local anaesthetic agents are extremely rare, despite reports of such allergy. The most common causes for adverse reactions after local anaesthesia administration are vasovagal reactions, palpitations secondary to adrenaline administered as a local anaesthetic additive, toxicity from overdosage of local anaesthesia used for regional blocks or facial swelling caused by trauma from dental injections. Cases in which true anaphylaxis is suspected can be confirmed by skin testing or excluded by progressive challenge. Some cross-reactivity between amide local anaesthetics and, less commonly, between amide and ester local anaesthetics has been described [35].

Induction agents

The incidence of reactions to this induction of agents is low. Propofol was originally formulated in a vehicle containing Cremophor® EL but was reformulated as a lipid emulsion following reports of severe allergic reactions. The current preparation is an uncommon cause of anaphylaxis and contains soybean oil, glycerol and egg lecithin. Concerns about reactions to the egg lecithin component of the preparation in patients known to be allergic to egg have led to the recommendation from manufacturers of propofol that patients known to have allergy to egg should not receive this drug. While this would seem sensible, there has been no evidence to date to corroborate or refute these concerns. Anaphylaxis to the thiobarbiturate thiopental has also been described, but is uncommon. Interestingly, although IgE reactions to thiobarbiturate are documented, no incidences of such a reaction have been attributed to its close relative methohexital, an oxybarbiturate.

Colloids

Clinical anaphylaxis to all groups of colloids is possible, including gelatins (such as Haemaccel® and Gelofusine®), albumin, dextrans and starches. Of these, dextrans are the only group to which antibodies have been demonstrated and anaphylaxis has been proven. Reactions to these fluids accounted for 2.9% of intraoperative anaphylaxis in a French survey [33]. Gelatins and dextrans seem to be more likely to produce reactions than albumin or hetastarch [36].

Testing of patients following reactions to gelatins may demonstrate elevated mast cell tryptases and positive skin tests, but antigelatin antibodies are yet to be demonstrated in these patients. Gelatins are also potent direct histamine releasers and may produce adverse effects purely from the direct effects of histamine. As a result of anaphylactic events to the Dextran 40 or 70 preparations, Promit® (Dextran 1) has been developed as a monovalent hapten to be administered within 15 min of the larger molecule. This decreases the likelihood of anaphylaxis, but may generate anaphylaxis itself. As such, patients known to be sensitive to dextrans should not be given colloids altogether.

Methylmethacrylate

No allergic mechanism has been demonstrated for

reported episodes of hypotension and systemic reactions observed after the use of bone cement intraoperatively.

Treatment of anaphylaxis during anaesthesia

As the clinical manifestations of anaphylaxis are extremely varied, from single organ signs (e.g. bronchospasm) to cardiorespiratory arrest, treatment in each individual case should be tailored accordingly. There are no randomized controlled trials of treatment approaches in anaphylaxis, so the following is derived more from accepted practice and consensus than evidence.

In broad terms, management should include:

1 Removal or discontinuation of likely causative agents

2 Calling for help

3 Resuscitation following standard guidelines (airway, breathing, circulation, etc.) and in particular the use of adrenaline and intravenous fluid

4 Prevention of further inflammatory mediator release

5 Provision of an adequate environment for post-event monitoring and care (intensive care unit)

6 Investigation of the event to confirm a diagnosis of anaphylaxis and identify a likely inciting cause.

Non-specific measures

High concentration (100%) oxygen should be administered immediately. The airway should be secured with an endotracheal tube if the patient is unconscious, to enable ventilation in the event of severe bronchospasm and also to ensure a patent airway in the case of ensuing airway oedema. Determination of adequacy of cardiac output will dictate commencement of external cardiac compressions if necessary. Large-bore intravenous access should be secured as a priority to enable the administration of fluid and pharmacological agents. Full monitoring should be established, with an emphasis on electrocardiography as this increases the safety of administration of adrenaline. A venous tourniquet above a suspected site of injection of antigen may decrease its absorption. Documentation of the reaction including symptoms and signs, drugs and treatment given along with accurate timing of these will become ex-

tremely important in follow-up of the incident at a later date.

Specific therapy
Adrenaline

The primary pharmacological antagonist of anaphylactic mediator release and end-organ effects are sympathomimetics. The most likely of these to produce a response is adrenaline, which also has the advantage of being useful in the treatment of various clinical manifestations of anaphylaxis: hypotension, bronchospasm and angioedema [16,37,38].

Adrenaline should be administered intramuscularly if the reaction is not immediately life threatening or if no intravenous access or cardiovascular monitoring are available. The initial dose should be 0.3–0.5 mg in an adult, which may be repeated after 5–10 min if there is no clinical improvement. The intramuscular dose for children is 0.01 mg/kg.

Intramuscular injection of adrenaline into the thigh (vastus lateralis) in adults has been shown to produce higher plasma concentrations of adrenaline than either subcutaneous or intramuscular adrenaline injections into the deltoid muscle, neither of which elevated the plasma adrenaline levels higher than endogenous levels associated with the injection of saline [39]. The lateral thigh is thus the preferred site for the intramuscular injection of adrenaline in anaphylaxis. Subcutaneous injection may result in erratic and delayed absorption of adrenaline in shocked patients [38] and is no longer recommended.

As the intravenous administration of adrenaline is potentially hazardous, this route is appropriate only when intravenous access has been established, cardiovascular monitoring is present (electrocardiography, blood pressure monitoring — preferably invasive) and when the anaphylaxis is severe, the patient poorly perfused and the situation is life threatening. Severe hypertension may occur, resulting in cerebrovascular haemorrhage, arrhythmias or coronary ischaemia, especially with large doses of adrenaline given quickly, poor blood pressure surveillance or when given to patients without compromised blood pressure. Although adverse effects have been noted after the administration of intravenous adrenaline, these are often after excessive doses were administered and/or in patients suffering mild reactions that were unlikely to represent true anaphylaxis [38]. The value of adrenaline given intravenously in true severe anaphylaxis should be emphasized.

The dose of adrenaline to be given intravenously is 1–5 ml of a 1:10 000 solution (0.1–0.5 mg) over 5 min. It is important that concentrated adrenaline (1:1000) should never be given intravenously in anaphylaxis other than in cardiac arrest. Continuous infusion of adrenaline intravenously may become necessary (1–4 µg/min).

α-Adrenergic agonists and other agents to treat hypotension

It is worth noting that β-adrenoceptor blocked patients and those with epidurals *in situ* may be relatively resistant to the effects of adrenaline and may require massive doses. In these situations and in other cases of severe anaphylaxis, where hypotension is refractory to adrenaline therapy, agents with prominent α-adrenergic activity such as metaraminol and noradrenaline should be tried. Dopamine administered intravenously at a rate of 2–20 µg/min (400 mg in 500 ml 5% dextrose) may also be tried for refractory hypotension [22]. Similarly, glucagon has been used successfully for the treatment of refractory hypotension, especially in patients on β-blocker therapy [22,40]. Glucagon may be administered as a 1–5 mg (20–30 µg/kg in children, maximum 1 mg) dose over 5 min followed by an infusion of 5–15 µg/min [22]. Recently, vasopressin has been recommended in refractory anaphylaxis [41].

Fluid therapy

A large volume deficit will often accompany a severe anaphylactic reaction, characterized by cardiovascular collapse or pulmonary oedema. This is best counteracted by rapid infusion of an initial bolus of 1–2 L intravenous fluid initially (20 mL/kg initially in children) before reassessment. Adults may require 2–5 L. While there are neither outcome studies nor randomized controlled trials showing superiority of colloid over crystalloid, what limited evidence there is favours the use of colloid.

Inhaled and intravenous bronchodilators

Salbutamol, a β₂-agonist, may be useful in cases where bronchospasm is prominent and has proven resistant to adrenaline. Salbutamol may be given to awake subjects by nebulizer (2.5–5 mg), but in intubated patients salbutamol may be given as 100 µg doses via aerosol into the breathing circuit by a connector into the endotracheal tube. Administration should be timed with inspiration, and titrated to effect.

In the event of failure of response to β₂-agonists, aminophylline may be tried via infusion. A dose of 6 mg/kg lean bodyweight should be administered to adults over 20–30 min to achieve a target serum concentration of 10 µg/mL.

Steroids

Intravenous corticosteroids are not helpful acutely in anaphylaxis but may be useful for cases that are prolonged or in relapse, especially in asthmatics and those already on steroids. Hydrocortisone 5 mg/kg, which can be repeated every 6 hours, is appropriate.

Antihistamines

Although not drugs of first choice and no proof of efficacy of these drugs in the treatment of human anaphylaxis exists, there are anecdotal reports of improvement in refractory cases after administration of antihistamines. H₁ and/or H₂ receptor antagonists may be tried, such as 25 mg diphenhydramine by slow intravenous infusion, 300 mg cimetidine i.v. or i.m., or 50 mg ranitidine [22]. H₃ receptor antagonists have been shown to improve cardiac function in a model of canine anaphylaxis [42].

Investigation of suspected anaphylactic episodes

Once a suspected anaphylactic episode has occurred, investigation and follow-up are mandatory.

Immediate investigation
Mast cell tryptase

Tryptase is a protease found in mast cell granules. Release of this substance in large quantities into the serum follows degranulation as a result of an anaphylactic or anaphylactoid reaction. Levels peak at 1 hour after the reaction [43] and stay elevated for up to 5 hours, which allows for the immediate treatment of the reaction to occur before investigation takes place [44]. All patients with raised mast cell tryptase levels should be assumed to have had an anaphylactic or anaphylactoid reaction and referral for further follow-up and testing to identify the causing agent is mandatory. Further, an elevated mast cell tryptase result indicates that follow-up skin testing is likely to be successful. A negative mast cell tryptase result means that follow-up skin testing is unlikely to reveal sensitivity to agents administered and that another cause for the observed reaction is likely [44].

The mast cell tryptase assay itself is quite a robust one, requiring no special collection techniques. Specimens should be separated and the serum transported frozen. Postmortem collection of samples for assay is also possible [45]. Samples should be collected in 5–10 mL volume tubes immediately following resuscitation of the patient, then 1 hour after the reaction began: this is the most valuable specimen. A further specimen obtained 6–24 hours after the reaction began may also be helpful. Each tube should clearly identify the patient and the time of sample collection. Serum obtained from samples should be stored at 4°C if the sample can be analysed within 48 hours, or –20°C if analysis is to occur at a later time.

Other immediate tests

Measurement of histamine levels, serum complement levels, drug-specific IgE levels and urinary methylhistamine levels have been used to assess the likelihood of anaphylactic or anaphylactoid reactions. These tests are not routinely performed in most centres, are less reliable and more difficult to interpret than the mast cell tryptase assay and are not recommended for routine use.

Follow-up testing

It is the responsibility of the primary responsible anaesthetist present at the time of the initial reaction to ensure that appropriate follow-up and testing of the patient occurs. The patient should be referred to a specialist allergist, accompanied by results of mast cell tryptase assays, photocopies of anaesthetic charts from the incident and a letter describing observations of the event, including signs of anaphylaxis noted and their temporal relationship to drugs administered.

History

The history is of vital importance in the establishment of a diagnosis of allergy to a specific agent. Information should be sought as to previous exposure to all drugs possibly implicated in the current reaction, history of exposure to latex, history of previous anaesthetics, both eventful and otherwise (along with procurement of copies of the anaesthetic records associated with these), as well as past medical history with specific questioning about asthma, atopy and a current list of medications taken.

Skin testing

Skin testing should be performed 4–6 weeks after a reaction has occurred. Two types of skin tests are used: skin prick tests (where the drug is introduced into the dermis by pricking the patient's skin through a drop of undiluted drug) and intradermal testing (where the drug is diluted and injected into the dermis). Both these types of skin test look for IgE antibodies to drugs being tested and comparative studies show little difference between the two, with skin prick testing tending to produce false negatives and intradermal testing tending to produce false positives [45]. The tests will agree on the identity of the drug likely to have caused the reaction in approximately 90% of cases [45,46]. The risk of precipitating anaphylaxis is higher with intradermal testing; accordingly, skin prick testing is usually used first line. Intradermal testing requires the use of appropriate published dilutions of drugs in order to avoid false negatives and false positives.

Testing in both types of skin tests involves the use of negative (saline) and positive controls (morphine, codeine or histamine) and will include all agents used in the anaesthetic (except volatile anaesthetics) including agents for skin preparation and latex. These tests are of little use in identifying reactions to blood products, colloid solutions and contrast media [47].

There has been recent controversy over skin testing, with studies suggesting that the usual concentrations employed may be too concentrated and produce false positives, may overdiagnose reactions to NMBDs, and produce skin lesions that are not wheal and flare reactions [48–51]. The studies produce conflicting results and have all been performed in non-reacting patients. While skin testing has limited value in mechanisms other than IgE-mediated anaphylaxis and possibly idiosyncratic exaggerated direct histamine release, large studies have demonstrated diagnostic efficacy, correlation with mast cell tryptase and radioimmunoassay, and the safety of subsequent anaesthesia based on skin tests. False positive tests are less relevant to the safety of subsequent anaesthesia than false negative tests.

Radioimmunoassay testing

Radioimmunoassay tests are capable of identifying drug-specific IgE antibodies *in vitro*. For detection to be possible, tests must have been developed for the specific antigen responsible for the reaction. Testing is available for propofol, thiopental, NMBDs, latex, penicillin and morphine. Commercial testing kits for suxamethonium and penicillin antibodies are also available.

Radioimmunoassay testing will identify the drug responsible for a reaction with approximately the same frequency as skin testing so long as a radioimmunoassay test is available for that drug. When both skin testing and radioimmunoassay testing are combined, the likelihood of detecting the drug responsible is greater than with either test alone. As with skin testing, radioimmunoassay testing produces both false negatives and false positives [26,27].

Other tests

Leucocyte and basophil histamine release tests have been used and give similar results to radioimmunoassay. Unfortunately, few laboratories have the expertise to perform such tests at the present time. In practice, combinations of skin testing and radioimmunoassay testing are used in specialized allergy testing centres. When results of these tests differ, it is prudent to advise the patient against receiving any of the drugs to which they tested positive.

Given the limitations in accuracy of currently available tests there is no evidence to suggest routine screening of patients before anaesthesia [18].

Preventing subsequent anaphylaxis

Avoidance of allergen administration

Those people who have experienced anaphylaxis should take all possible precautions to avoid further exposure to antigens that may result in a subsequent reaction:

1 *Medic alert bracelet* — stating the nature of reaction, for example, and the names of identified triggers. This enables such information to be transferred to health professionals even if the patient is unable to do so (e.g. dementia, trauma) and may aid in diagnosis and establishment of treatment if the patient is found unconscious.

2 *Letter* — offering greater detail about the nature of the reaction and implicated drugs, including results of testing carried out and recommendations from the allergists about drugs to be avoided. This allows the anaesthetist to evaluate the evidence of allergy more critically than relying on patient information or medic alert bracelet alone. Subsequent uneventful anaesthesia and drugs given can be noted on attached documents at later times.

3 *Other forms of anaesthesia* — local or regional anaesthesia may be used when testing fails to identify a cause for an anaphylactic reaction under general anaesthesia. Anaesthetists should remain cognizant that major regional anaesthesia such as epidural blockade may predispose the patient to a severe reaction poorly responsive to therapy if anaphylaxis occurs to the agents used on this subsequent occasion (such as antibiotics or local anaesthetics).

4 *Avoidance of cross-reactive agents* — drugs antigenically related to the demonstrated cause of a previous reaction should be avoided.

Avoidance of agents that may predispose to a severe reaction

This may include avoidance of some medications such as β-adrenergic antagonists (may exaggerate cardiovascular collapse and hinder treatment), angiotensin converting enzyme (ACE) inhibitors (may antagonize compensatory responses to hypotension), monoamine oxidase (MAO) inhibitors and tricyclic antidepressants (may increase the danger of administration of adrenaline by retarding its degradation).

Desensitization

Desensitization may be necessary when no satisfactory alternative to a known antigen exists and may be needed at a future time (e.g. penicillins), or where exposure to the antigen at a future time is likely despite precautions (e.g. latex, insect stings). Reactions must be IgE mediated (i.e. anaphylactic) for desensitization to be effective. Successful blocking has been shown with a monovalent quaternary ammonium salt (tiemonium) in one case [52]. Theoretically, morphine may block reactions to NMBDs because of its strong affinity for the NMBD antibody [53].

References

1 Fisher M, Baldo BA. Anaphylaxis during anaesthesia: current aspects of diagnosis and prevention. *Eur J Anaesth* 1994; **11**: 263–84.

2 Boston Collaborative Drug Surveillance Survey. Drug-induced anaphylaxis. *JAMA* 1973; **224**: 613–5.

3 Laxenaire MC, Mertes PM, Groupe d'Etudes des Reactions Anaphylactoides Peranesthesiques. Anaphylaxis during anaesthesia: results of a two-year survey in France. *Br J Anaesth* 2001; **87**: 549–58.

4 Laxenaire MC, Moneret-Vautrin DA, Vervloet D. The French experience of anaphylactoid reactions. *Int Anesthesiol Clin* 1985; **23**: 145–60.

5 Galletly DC, Treuren BC. Anaphylactoid reactions during anaesthesia: seven years' experience of intradermal testing. *Anaesthesia* 1985; **40**: 329–33.

6 Fisher MM, Baldo BA. The incidence and clinical features of anaphylactic reactions during anesthesia in Australia. *Ann Fr Anesth Reanim* 1993; **12**: 97–104.

7 Rose M, Fisher M. Rocuronium: high risk for anaphylaxis? *Br J Anaesth* 2001; **86**: 678–82.

8 Coombs RRA, Gell PGA. Classification of allergic reactions responsible for clinical hypersensitivity and disease. In: Gell PGA, Coombs RRA, Lachman PJ, eds. *Clinical Aspects of Immunology*. Oxford: Blackwell, 1975: 761–81.

9 Bach MK. Mediators of anaphylaxis and inflammation. *Annu Rev Microbiol* 1982; **36**: 371–413.

10 Lorenz W. Histamine release in man. 1975 [classical article]. *Agents Actions* 1994; **43**: 117–31.

11 Tharp MD, Kagey-Sobotka A, Fox CC, *et al.* Functional heterogeneity of human mast cells from different anatomic sites: *in vitro* responses to morphine sulfate. *J Allergy Clin Immunol* 1987; **79**: 646–53.

12 Stellato C, de Paulis A, Cirillo R, *et al.* Heterogeneity of human mast cells and basophils in response to muscle relaxants. *Anesthesiol* 1991; **74**: 1078–86.

13 Lakin J, Blocker T, Strong D, Yocum L. Anaphylaxis to protamine sulphate mediated by a complement de-pendent IgG antibody. *J Allergy Clin Immunol* 1978; **61**: 102–6.

14 Raper RF, Fisher MM. Profound reversible myocardial depression after anaphylaxis. *Lancet* 1988; **ii**: 386–7.

15 Horrow JC. Protamine: a review of its toxicity. *Anesth Analg* 1985; **64**: 348–61.

16 Fisher MM. Clinical observations on the pathophysiology and treatment of anaphylactic cardiovascular collapse. *Anaesth Intensive Care* 1986; **14**: 17–21.

17 Clergue F, Auroy Y, Pequignot F, *et al.* French survey of anesthesia in 1996. *Anesthesiol* 1999; **91**: 1509–20.

18 Fisher MM, Doig GS. Prevention of anaphylactic reactions to anaesthetic drugs. *Drug Saf* 2004; **27**: 393–410.

19 Fisher MM, Outhred A, Bowey CJ. Can clinical anaphylaxis to anaesthetic drugs be predicted from allergic history? *Br J Anaesth* 1987; **59**: 690–2.

20 Fisher MM, More DG. The epidemiology and clinical features of anaphylactic reactions in anaesthesia. *Anaesth Intensive Care* 1981; **9**: 226–34.

21 Ind PW, Causon RC, Brown MJ, Barnes PJ. Circulating catecholamines in acute asthma. *Br Med J* 1985; **290**: 267–9.

22 Kemp SF, Lockey RF. Anaphylaxis: a review of causes and mechanisms. *J Allergy Clin Immunol* 2002; **110**: 341–8.

23 Ljungstrom KG, Renck H, Strandberg K, *et al.* Adverse reactions to dextran in Sweden 1970–1979. *Acta Chir Scand* 1983; **149**: 253–62.

24 Garvey LH, Roed-Petersen J, Husum B. Anaphylactic reactions in anaesthetised patients: four cases of chlorhexidine allergy. *Acta Anaesthesiol Scand* 2001; **45**: 1290–4.

25 Garvey LH, Roed-Petersen J, Menne T, Husum B. Danish Anaesthesia Allergy Centre: preliminary results. *Acta Anaesthesiol Scand* 2001; **45**: 1204–9.

26 Baldo BA, Harle DG, Fisher MM. *In vitro* diagnosis and studies on the mechanism(s) of anaphylactoid reactions to muscle relaxant drugs. *Ann Fr Anesth Reanim* 1985; **4**: 139–45.

27 Baldo BA, Fisher MM. Anaphylaxis to muscle relaxant drugs: cross-reactivity and molecular basis of binding of IgE antibodies detected by radioimmunoassay. *Mol Immunol* 1983; **20**: 1393–400.

28 Fisher MM, Munro I. Life-threatening anaphylactoid reactions to muscle relaxants. *Anesth Analg* 1983; **62**: 559–64.

29 Fisher MM. Cisatracurium and atracurium as antigens. *Anaesth Intensive Care* 1999; **27**: 369–70.

30 Hepner DL, Castells MC. Anaphylaxis during the perioperative period. *Anesth Analg* 2003; **97**: 1381–95.

31 Anne S, Reisman RE. Risk of administering cephalosporin antibiotics to patients with histories of penicillin allergy. *Ann Allergy Asthma Immunol* 1995; **74**: 167–70.

32 Fisher MM, Harle DG, Baldo BA. Anaphylactoid reactions to narcotic analgesics. *Clin Rev Allergy* 1991; **9**: 309–18.

33 Laxenaire MC, Mertes PM, Groupe d'Etudes des Reactions Anaphylactoides Peranesthesiques. Anaphylaxis during anaesthesia: results of a two-year survey in France. *Br J Anaesth* 2001; **87**: 549–58.

34 Hepner DL, Castells MC. Latex allergy: an update. *Anesth Analg* 2003; **96**: 1219–29.

35 Fisher MM, Bowey CJ. Alleged allergy to local anaesthetics. *Anaesth Intensive Care* 1997; **25**: 611–4.

36 Ring J, Messmer K. Incidence and severity of anaphylactoid reactions to colloid volume substitutes. *Lancet* 1977; **1**: 466–9.

37 Soreide E, Buxrud T, Harboe S. Severe anaphylactic reactions outside hospital: etiology, symptoms and treatment. *Acta Anaesthesiol Scand* 1988; **32**: 339–42.

38 Pumphrey RS. Lessons for management of anaphylaxis from a study of fatal reactions. *Clin Exp Allergy* 2000; **30**: 1144–50.

39 Simons FE, Gu X, Simons KJ. Epinephrine absorption in adults: intramuscular versus subcutaneous injection. *J Allergy Clin Immunol* 2001; **108**: 871–3.

40 Zaloga GP, DeLacey W, Holmboe E, Chernow B. Glucagon reversal of hypotension in a case of anaphylactoid shock. *Ann Intern Med* 1986; **105**: 65–6.

41 Kill C, Wranze E, Wulf H. Successful treatment of severe anaphylactic shock with vasopressin: two case reports. *Int Arch Allergy Immunol* 2004; **134**: 260–1.

42 Schwartz JC, Morisset S, Rouleau A, *et al.* Therapeutic implications of constitutive activity of receptors: the example of the histamine H_3 receptor. *J Neural Transm Suppl* 2003; **20**: 1–16.

43 Payne V, Kam PC. Mast cell tryptase: a review of its physiology and clinical significance. *Anaesthesia* 2004; **59**: 695–703.

44 Fisher MM, Baldo BA. Mast cell tryptase in anaesthetic anaphylactoid reactions. *Br J Anaesth* 1998; **80**: 26–9.

45 Fisher MM, Baldo BA. The diagnosis of fatal anaphylactic reactions during anaesthesia: employment of immunoassays for mast cell tryptase and drug-reactive IgE antibodies. *Anaesth Intensive Care* 1993; **21**: 353–7.

46 Fisher MM, Bowey CJ. Intradermal compared with prick testing in the diagnosis of anaesthetic allergy. *Br J Anaesth* 1997; **79**: 59–63.

47 Leynadier F, Sansarricq M, Didier JM, Dry J. Prick tests in the diagnosis of anaphylaxis to general anaesthetics. *Br J Anaesth* 1987; **59**: 683–9.

48 Fisher MM. Intradermal testing in the diagnosis of acute anaphylaxis during anaesthesia: results of five years experience. *Anaesth Intensive Care* 1979; **7**: 58–61.

49 Berg CM, Heier T, Wilhelmsen V, Florvaag E. Rocuronium and cisatracurium-positive skin tests in non-allergic volunteers: determination of drug concentration thresholds using a dilution titration technique. *Acta Anaesthesiol Scand* 2003; **47**: 576–82.

50 Levy JH. Anaphylactic reactions to neuromuscular blocking drugs: are we making the correct diagnosis? *Anesth Analg* 2004; **98**: 881–2.

51 Dhonneur G, Combes X, Chassard D, Merle JC. Skin sensitivity to rocuronium and vecuronium: a randomized controlled prick-testing study in healthy volunteers. *Anesth Analg* 2000; **98**: 986–9.

52 Thomas H, Eledjam JJ, Macheboeuf M, *et al.* Rapid preoperative immunotherapy in a patient allergic to muscle relaxants. *Eur J Anaesth* 1988; **5**: 385–9.

53 Fisher MM, Baldo BA. Immunoassays in the diagnosis of anaphylaxis to neuromuscular blocking drugs: the value of morphine for the detection of IgE antibodies in allergic subjects. *Anaesth Intensive Care* 2000; **28**: 167–70.

CHAPTER 6
Reflections on chirality

Daniel Burke

Introduction

Many compounds in the natural world exhibit chirality and their isomers can have quite different biological activity. For example, (*S*)-limonene smells of lemons while the mirror image compound (*R*)-limonene smells of oranges. A basic understanding of chiral chemistry is necessary to explain why one or more stereoisomers of a drug, identical in many respects, can produce different therapeutic effects. This chapter aims to provide an overview of stereochemical nomenclature, a historically confusing topic, together with some new theories on chiral recognition processes, plus an illustration of how single isomer drugs are produced in the pharmaceutical industry today. For more detailed information on isomer-specific differences between anaesthetic agents, references are provided.

Chirality is a fundamental characteristic of nature and is seen throughout the living world. Most proteins, for example, are formed of L-amino acids while carbohydrates are composed of natural sugars, all D-isomers. Biological receptor systems comprise a complex structural organization of helices and sheets and display 'handedness'. There is thus a resultant profound effect on drug-receptor interactions at the molecular level.

The subject has a long and fascinating history. In the latter half of the 17th century the phenomenon of light polarization had been observed, Biot noting that a plate of quartz cut perpendicular to its axis rotated plane-polarized light. However, the realization that chirality was present in the organic world was made by Pasteur. Following on earlier work by de la Provostaye, he undertook crystallographic studies on tartaric acid and its salts and demonstrated the presence of hemihedral facets. In some instances these were orientated to the left, in others to the right. By handpicking the crystals he divided them into two groups and found that the solutions rotated light in equal yet opposite directions. Pasteur recognized that the cause of this phenomenon lay in the molecular structure, and by extending these ideas evolved the theory of the asymmetric carbon atom.

Why is chirality relevant to anaesthesia? Advances in chiral technology are allowing the commercial synthesis of single isomer compounds hitherto of academic interest only. By understanding the role of these stereoisomers in biological systems, the next logical step is the application of this knowledge to human physiology and pharmacology.

Terminology

Two non-identical molecules with the same molecular formula are called isomers. If these isomers have different atomic connectivity then they are called constitutional isomers. Constitutional isomers are easily separated as they have different physical and chemical properties. For example, both isoflurane and enflurane have the same molecular formula ($C_3H_2ClF_5O$) but differ in their boiling points, partition coefficients, etc. Constitutional isomers may have similar pharmacological effects or these may differ.

A stereoisomer has the same molecular formula *and* atomic connectivity. Stereoisomers have identical physicochemical properties and are consequently difficult to separate. They also exhibit optical activity.

A stereoisomer can either be superimposed on its mirror image or not. If not, this results in two or more mirror images which are called enantiomers (Fig. 6.1). In contrast, if the mirror images of a stere-

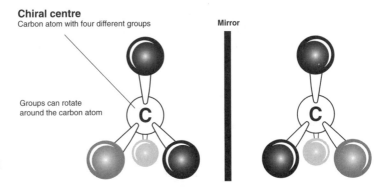

Chiral centre
Carbon atom with four different groups

Mirror

Groups can rotate
around the carbon atom

Figure 6.1 General depiction of a chiral molecule.

oisomer can be superimposed then the molecules are termed diastereoisomers. For example, in a molecule with two chiral centres, the L,L- and D,D- forms are enantiomers while the L,D- and D,L- forms are diastereoisomers. Diastereoisomerism may be due to either the presence of more than one chiral centre or to geometric isomerism.

The term chiral derives from the Greek *chiros*, meaning 'handed' and was introduced into the English language towards the end of the 19th century by Lord Kelvin. An object is described as being 'chiral' if its image in a plane cannot be superimposed on the original. This can arise in a number of ways and examples of chirality are found commonly both in nature (e.g. the helical direction of mollusc shells) and in manufactured objects (e.g. propellers, screws). Of more relevance to anaesthetic practice is the fact that approximately 60% of the drugs in daily use are chiral. They are administered either as a mixture of two or more stereoisomers (e.g. bupivacaine) or as a single isomer (e.g. ropivacaine). In addition, many of the naturally occurring drugs used in anaesthesia are chiral (e.g. morphine, adrenaline (epinephrine)) as their formation by natural enzymes and proteins is stereoselective.

Chiral molecules exhibit optical activity. This phenomenon is seen with some crystalline substances (e.g. quartz) and also by some liquids (most noticeably sugar solutions) and vapours. For solutions, the rotation of light (natural rotation) is proportional to the concentration and path length.

A chiral molecule in its most familiar form can be represented by a central carbon or sulphur atom attached to four different groups, thus producing a tetrahedron. This concept was first proposed by Van't Hoff in 1874 and enables the existence of two non-superimposable mirror images or enantiomers (Greek *enantios*, meaning 'opposite', *meros* meaning 'form') that share identical physicochemical properties (e.g. identical melting points, boiling points, density) but differ in their rotation of plane-polarized light. Only the *direction* of optical rotation differs; the magnitude of rotation is identical. Importantly, they can also differ in their pharmacological profile, owing to highly stereospecific interactions at the receptor interface.

A mixture of two enantiomers is called a racemate, as popularized by Beilstein. Racemates have different physical properties from those of their pure enantiomers. A racemate is designated by the prefix (±), rac- or by the symbols RS or SR and has no optical activity.

The body responsible for standardization of stereochemical nomenclature is the International Union of Pure and Applied Chemistry (IUPAC) [1]. Widespread adoption of terms suggested by this organization has helped clarify what has historically been a confusing subject.

Relative descriptors

The most common way to refer to the chirality of a molecule is still based on the effect it has on the rotation of optical light, with the descriptors (+) and (−) applied when the rotation is clockwise and anticlockwise respectively. This is synonymous with the terms *dextrorotatory* and *levorotatory*.

To measure optical activity plane-polarized light is used. This is light whose vibrations take place in only one plane. Nicol prisms have been used to produce plane-polarized light, containing crystals of Iceland spar (calcium carbonate) cut and cemented together in a specific manner. This technique has been largely replaced by the use of thermoplastic Polaroid sheets, which contain an optically active compound that acts as a filter for visible light, giving either plane-polarized or circularly polarized light on transmission (Fig. 6.2).

To measure optical rotation, an optically inactive sample (e.g. air) is placed in a light beam. Light polarized by the first polarizer passes through the sample and the analyser is turned to establish a dark field (the second polarizer has its axis of polarity perpendicular to the first and no light passes). This defines the zero of optical rotation. The measuring sample is then placed in the light beam and the number of degrees that the analyser has to be turned in order to re-establish the dark field is the optical rotation of the sample. Optical rotation is a quantitative measure of activity and the observed rotation is proportional to the concentration, c (g/mL) of the optically active compound plus length, l (dm) of sample container, i.e. $\alpha = [\alpha]\,cl$, where $[\alpha]$ is the constant of proportionality. The specific rotation is the observed rotation at a concentration of 1 g/mL and a path length of 1 dm and is used as a standard measure of optical activity. It is conventionally reported with a subscript indicating the wavelength of light used (see below) and a superscript indicating temperature.

Optical rotation, although an unambiguous physical property, varies with measurement conditions and these are therefore standardized. The degree of rotation is measured using yellow light from the sodium arc (the sodium D line with wavelength 589.3 nm at 254 nm). The actual property measured is an electronic transition between the orbitals in the molecule under study. The complete spectrum, the circular dichroism (CD) spectrum, differs from the ultraviolet spectrum in being both positive and negative. Rotation is determined by both electronic and magnetic moments. Achiral molecules, having no magnetic moment, do not rotate plane-polarized light. At very low rotation strengths, errors can occur because of the presence of contaminants. The type of solvent used and pH changes can also produce dramatic changes in the CD spectrum.

Absolute descriptors

The D, L system is an older system still used in amino acid and carbohydrate chemistry. With this exception, the R, S system (Sequence Rule Notation) has gained virtually universal acceptance. This notation, proposed by Cahn et al. [2], is based on attaching an order of priority to substituent ligands attached to the central chiral atom. In this model, the ligands around the chiral centre are 'sized' according to their atomic number, placing the smallest to the back and looking at the remainder in terms of relative size (Fig. 6.3). Consider a molecule Cabcd, where a, b, c,

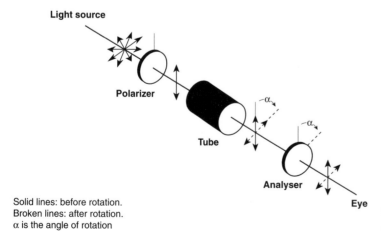

Solid lines: before rotation.
Broken lines: after rotation.
α is the angle of rotation

Figure 6.2 Measurement of optical activity using a polarimeter.

d are groups placed around a central atom C. If the sequence of the ligands in terms of size (largest to smallest) produces a clockwise progression then the arrangement is termed 'R' from the Latin *rectus*, meaning 'right'. Conversely, an anticlockwise order is termed 'S' from the Latin *sinister*, meaning 'left'. Any chiral molecule can be designated in this way. In a situation when two or more ligands are of equal size, the next atom along a chain is examined.

Thus, a full description of a chiral compound may be given by an expression combining terms for the absolute descriptor, the relative descriptor and the chemical or generic name, e.g. S (−) bupivacaine, S (+) ketoprofen. (Note that there is no simple relationship between the sign of optical rotation and the absolute configuration.)

The theory of chiral recognition

Intermolecular reaction occurs at a particular site on the cellular surface, the bioreceptor. The discriminatory nature of this interaction is pivotal to the subsequent biological response. How does this discrimination arise?

Molecular interaction

Various analogies have been proposed to describe stereospecific interactions at the bioreceptor. Fischer suggested a 'lock and key' mechanism to describe enzyme specificity and the 'close relationship in configuration obtained between the enzyme and the substance which it attacks'. In 1929, Macht (commenting on the synergistic effects of the diastereoisomers of adrenaline) was the first to use the 'glove' analogy, whereby two hands or feet may be identical in shape and symmetry, yet neither hand nor foot of the one side would fit into the glove or shoe belonging to the other. Easson and Stedman (1933) [3] and Ogston (1948) [4] proposed new models, subsequently called 'three-point attachment' models, a phrase coined by Dalgleish. A chiral molecule is conceptualized as being tetrahedral, with a central point C and four groups in space (abcd) surrounding this point. When such a molecule interacts with a receptor it does so with its complementary pairing sites ABC on the surface of the receptor (Fig. 6.4).

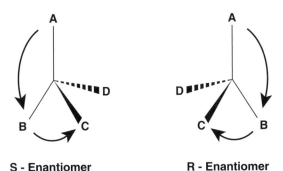

S - Enantiomer   **R - Enantiomer**

Figure 6.3 Sequence rule notation (see text for details).

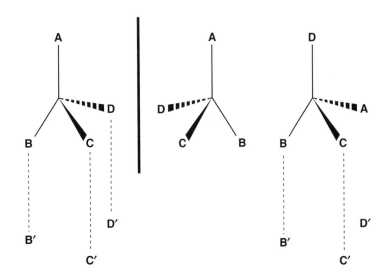

Figure 6.4 The Easson–Stedman model (see text for details).

Note that some assumptions are made in this model. First, it is assumed that these sites are topographically lying in a plane and that the drug approaches from one direction only. It is also assumed that maximal interaction results when like areas bind like (i.e. Aa, Bb and Cc). The more each of the interactions tend to the maximum possible, the greater the complementarity of drug and receptor and the greater the affinity of the relationship. These interactive bonds need not solely be the result of attractive forces (e.g. covalent linkages, ionic bonding, hydrogen binding); Wilcox noted the possibility of repulsive interactions in the early 1950s.

The constraints in the above model implies that it only holds true if it assumed that the ligand can approach a flat protein surface from the top. If the binding sites on the protein molecule are in a cleft or on protruding residues, the three-point model will not be sufficient to allow discrimination. It is therefore suggested that a fourth point, whether a binding site or location, is essential to distinguish between enantiomers in an actual protein structure. Topiol and Sabio, using distance matrix analysis, first made this suggestion in 1989 and showed that in the general case, and in the absence of constraints on imposing a specific orientation on the approaching molecule, a minimum of four locations (i.e. eight chiral centres) were required for discrimination. Mesecar and Koshland [5] elaborately described a new four-location model of protein stereospecificity in 2000, using the enzyme isocitrate dehydrogenase (IDH) to gain insight into ligand binding restraints and specificity (Fig. 6.5).

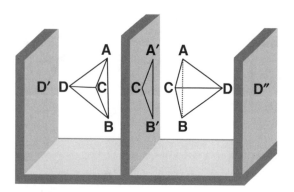

Figure 6.5 The four-location model (see text for details).

The crystalline structure of this enzyme was examined using electron density mapping in the presence or absence of Mg^{2+}. When metal-free crystals of IDH are presented with rac-IDH, only the L-isomer binds to the active site. In contrast, in the presence of Mg^{2+}, only the D-isomer is seen at this site. A fourth group, the hydroxyl of the C2 atom, varies its association dependent upon conditions and stabilizes the interaction between the enzyme and the D-isomer more powerfully than the L-isomer. The conclusion is that a minimum of four designated locations are needed in order to explain a protein's ability to discriminate between enantiomers. The four locations can be four attachment sites or three attachment sites and a direction, but a minimum of four designated locations are needed.

Chirality and pharmacokinetics

Given the fact that enantiomers differ in their pharmacological effects, it is to be expected that differences are also possible in pharmacokinetic parameters. For passive processes, such as transport across cell membranes, differences between enantiomers are likely to be negligible owing to their identical physical characteristics (e.g. lipophilicity). However, when active processes are involved (e.g. enzymatic conversion, protein binding) stereo-selective differences become apparent and affect intercompartmental rate constants. The different effect of the bupivacaine isomers on vascular tone is well known and this influences the rate of systemic absorption. Additionally, the plasma levels of the bupivacaine isomers differ. Following intravenous administration of the racemate the concentration of S (−) and R (+) bupivacaine can be measured using high performance liquid chromatography. Burm *et al.* found that, in general, *total* plasma concentrations of S (−) bupivacaine were higher than those of R (+) bupivacaine while unbound concentrations of S (−) bupivacaine were lower [6]. In the unbound state the volume of distribution did not differ, suggesting that the systemic disposition of the isomers is determined by their degree of protein binding. The absorption of drugs onto plasma proteins is essentially the same as interaction with receptor systems and can be expected to be stereoselective.

The importance of determining the specific pharmacokinetic profile of each isomer is therefore emphasized by drug regulatory authorities such as the US Food and Drug Administration (FDA) who state that techniques to quantify individual isomers in samples should be developed at an early stage in drug development. Some examples of techniques used to achieve this include chiral high performance liquid chromatography (HPLC), chiral gas chromatography, nuclear magnetic resonance, optical rotatory dispersion and X-ray crystallography.

In essence, each isomer is regarded as a distinct entity in its own right. *In vivo* sampling will detect any potential for interconversion of the isomers following administration as a racemate. For example, the R (−) enantiomers of some of the 2-arylpropionic acid non-steroidal anti-inflammatory drugs undergo metabolic chiral inversion to their opposite isomer (antipode). The process is drug and species dependent and usually unidirectional. When rac-ibuprofen is administered to humans, the enantiomeric ratio excreted is 70% S (+) and 30% R (−). Facts such as these are important to know, because toxicological side-effects may lie in only one isomer or an isomer-specific metabolite. Granulocytopenia is related to the D-isomer of levodopa; while for prilocaine, the two isomers are roughly equipotent as local anaesthetics but the (−) R isomer undergoes metabolism to *o*-toluidine and other aminophenols, which can cause methaemoglobinaemia. Similarly, after administration of rac-methadone to humans, the recovery of the (+) S enantiomer is greater than after administration of only the (+) S form, suggesting that the (−) R enantiomer produces an inhibitory effect on the metabolism of the (+) S enantiomer.

The enantiomer of most importance for a desired pharmacological effect is called the eutomer while the other is called the distomer. For any particular racemate and any specific pharmacological action the ratio of the activity between the two is called the eudismic ratio. This ratio is large if the eutomer is highly potent, a phenomenon known as Pfeiffer's rule.

The eudismic proportion is the concentration ratio [eut]/[dist] in, for example, the plasma. Following initial administration of the drug as a racemate (1 : 1

ratio by definition) the proportions change as a result of stereoselective metabolism until a steady state is reached. This can only be detected by chiral assays and may differ in different body compartments. If non-chiral assays are used then only the sum of the isomers is quantified and this has no direct relationship with the pharmacological effect seen. Chiral assays have allowed the influence of disease states, genetic polymorphism, age- and gender-related differences in pharmacokinetics to become apparent.

In addition to the above considerations, use of single isomer drugs allows dose reduction, results in less intersubject variability and a clearer dose–response relationship. The distomer is viewed as an unwanted component. While there are still instances where synthetic manufacture of a racemate is still justified, production of a drug in which only 50% of the excipients produce the desired pharmacological effect is uneconomical.

Single isomer drug development

Of the synthetic drugs in existence, more than 50% have at least one stereogenic centre. However, only approximately 11% of these are marketed as a single enantiomer. In contrast, of those drugs on the market derived from natural sources (e.g. morphine, adrenaline, hyoscine), almost all are chiral and, with only eight exceptions, they are marketed as a single enantiomer. Given the differences in pharmacological properties between enantiomers the desirability of asymmetric synthesis is self-evident, but historically the technology for their separation either did not exist or was prohibitively expensive. Industrial companies are obviously concerned about inefficiency and costs involved in any chemical processes whereby production of a racemate yields lower than 50% of the desired end product.

Chiral switching [7], whereby an existing racemate (e.g. rac-bupivacaine) is split into its component isomers, which are then viewed as distinct entities, can only introduce a limited number of 'new' compounds into the market place. However, this can be an attractive option for drug companies, as drug regulatory submission data on the original racemate can be used and bolstered by 'bridging studies'. However, there is limited potential in the market place for the degree of therapeutic benefit obtained to justify the degree of investment in many cases.

The real benefit of chiral technology lies in its application into the research of novel chemical entities. Regarding enantiomers as chemically distinct entities at an early stage in the research and development process is a valuable aid towards our understanding of drug mechanisms. An illustration of the interplay between drug design (based on an increased understanding of biological receptor systems) and chiral technology is illustrated in Fig. 6.6.

Finding new methods of asymmetric synthesis has in the past 20 or 30 years become a key activity for organic chemists, with research efforts focused on generating a range of 'chiral technologies' that aim to exert ultimate control over a chemical reaction by diverting its enantioselectivity.

For example, in a catalytic asymmetric reaction, a chiral catalyst is used to produce large quantities of an optically active compound from a precursor that may be chiral or achiral. A small amount of material can ultimately generate a large amount of product. Such reactions are thus highly productive and economical, and, when applicable, they make the waste resulting from racemate resolution (i.e. 'isomeric ballast') obsolete.

The fact that the pharmaceutical industry is now increasingly moving toward the development of single isomer drugs, either *de novo* compounds or those

derived from a racemate parent compound (a 'chiral switch'), has been influenced by several factors. These have occurred independently and in parallel with a quest in the industry as a whole to develop more potent, selective and specific drugs.

The drug regulatory authorities have realized the importance of the different pharmacological and toxicological profile of enantiomers. The FDA policy statement for the development of stereoisomeric drugs in 1992 made it more difficult to obtain approval for racemates. It emphasized that approval could not be granted for a drug containing more than one isomer, unless the pharmacokinetic and pharmacodynamic properties of each could be both described *and* justified. In addition, the FDA offers a shortened approval process for the single isomer version of approved drugs, with the promise of patent protection.

While it is unlikely that many racemates will be approved in future as a result of this, there are still indications where their production is justified, including the following:

1 The enantiomers are configurationally unstable *in vitro* or undergo racemization *in vivo*
2 The enantiomers have similar pharmacokinetic, pharmacodynamic and toxicological properties
3 It is not technically feasible to separate the enantiomers in sufficient quantity and/or quality.

Situations also exist where an enantiomeric ratio other than one may be justified if the ratio is expected to improve the therapeutic profile, as there

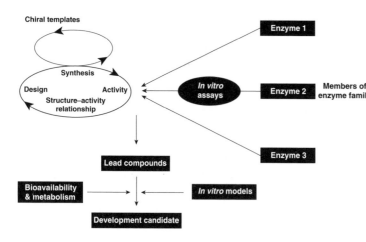

Figure 6.6 An illustration of the interplay between drug design (based on an increased understanding of biological receptor systems) and Chiral technology.

is no reason necessarily to expect the optimum eudismic ratio to be 1 : 1.

The second reason why there has been an explosion in the release of single isomer drugs is a result of the improvement in the methods allowing their manufacture. These are discussed below.

Chiral drug manufacture

Isomer separation

This falls into three main categories.

Separation by chromatography (e.g. simulated moving bed, SMB)

Chromatography is the only method applicable to all stages of the pharmaceutical development chain, from discovery to full-scale process. The first application of a countercurrent chromatographic process, of which SMB is an example, was based on Broughton's patent from 1961 and was widely adopted in the petrochemical industry. Since the 1990s, the problems of scaling down the multi-ton systems used in this industry have been overcome, enabling laboratory-scale systems to be developed for application to medicinal chemistry.

The basic concept of SMB technology is the continuous countercurrent movement of stationary and mobile phases in which the movement of a stationary phase is simulated. The small particles in this component are packed into single columns and connected to form a circle. Four external valves allow for the addition and subtraction of feed and effluent. The mobile phase is pumped through the circle and when it passes the stationary phase, a slight separation occurs with the less absorbable compound running in front and the more absorbable staying behind. When steady state is reached, the system can be continually operated. An example of a pharmaceutical compound separated by SMB chromatography is tramadol.

Crystallization

Two methods predominate. First, where the racemic product or a simple chiral salt of the product (e.g. hydrochloride) will under specific conditions crystallize to give only one isomer. This methodology has been used in the resolution of α-methyl-L-dopa,

methadone, asparagine and glutamic acid and these compounds are known as conglomerates; however, relatively few compounds (approximately 7%) exhibit this behaviour.

The second crystallization method is to form a diastereomeric salt (i.e. the racemate is mixed with a chirally pure compound). Again, under the correct conditions, only one diastereomer will crystallize out. This technique relies upon the ability of the two components to form a salt; however, a covalent bond could also be formed with a chiral auxillary. This last example is not widely used in the manufacture of chiral drugs.

Enzymic resolution (biotransformation)

Enzyme-mediated reactions are appealing to the developmental chemist as they produce a diverse range of transformations and avoid extreme reaction conditions with their concomitant inflated manufacturing costs and potential hazards. Enzymes have been used not only in the resolution of racemates, but also to allow the introduction of new stereogenic centres. Their use for the preparation of chiral pharmaceuticals has increased relatively recently as the methodologies employed have been adapted to commercial production. Enzyme resolution allows the separation of a racemic drug or drug derivative (e.g. an ester) into its two enantiomers because the enzyme only reacts with one isomer. Two general approaches are used.

The first technique involves incorporating in the synthetic design of the desired compound an enzyme resolution stage as a means of separating and recovering the isomer. Alternatively, the diversity of biotransformations that enzymes can produce is considered and synthesis is designed around that transformation, which results in the desired chiral centre(s).

As the use of enzyme transformations in the pharmaceutical process expands, these two approaches may ultimately converge in creation of the desired product. Enzymatic resolution has been used in preparation of benzodiazepines (e.g. S-14 lotrafiban, SmithKline Beecham), antibacterial drugs (e.g. levofoxacin) and anti-inflammatory drugs (e.g. the S isomers of 2-aryl propionic acids, S naproxen, S suprofen).

Asymmetric synthesis

Asymmetric synthesis refers to the process of taking an achiral drug (i.e. containing no chiral centre) and synthetically converting it by one of a number of routes to one isomer of a compound with a chiral centre. These methods include asymmetric hydrogenation (asymmetric catalysis), asymmetric dihydroxylation, hydroxamination, etc. Computational tool kits for molecular design, visualization and analysis (e.g. SYBYL, created by Astra-Zeneca) can assist the process.

Chiral pools

The term 'chiral pool' refers to the many naturally available chiral molecules that exist in high enantiomeric purity and frequently at low cost. The most versatile chiral starting materials in order of their industrial production per annum are: carbohydrates, α-amino acids, terpenes, hydroxy acids and alkaloids. Other inexpensive chiral natural products are ascorbic acid, dextrose, ephedrine, limonene, quinidine and quinine. Naturally occurring amino acids are readily available from bulk fermentation processes and these constitute the most important class within the chiral pool, with amounts ranging between 10 and 10^5 tons per year. These compounds can be incorporated into the molecule to provide the desired chiral centre (e.g. synthetic peptides) or to induce the desired chiral centre during synthesis (chiral induction or diastereoselective synthesis). The latter term involves the formation of a new chiral centre into a single enantiomer where only one new isomer is formed. Chiral starting materials such as amino acids can be converted into antibacterials, cytotoxic agents and protease inhibitors (e.g. ritonavir) by using this technology.

A practical example

The manufacture of ropivacaine [8] provides an example of single isomer drug synthesis, the technique being based on a resolution method published 30 years ago by Tullar in which it was found that (±)-2′,6′-pipecoloxylide could be resolved by using (−)-dibenzoyl-L-tartaric acid (a natural isomer), thereby making virtually any member of the series of N-substituted enantiomeric derivatives available via a subsequent alkylation step. Ropivacaine HCL.H_2O can be synthesized in three steps:

1 *Resolution.* This is achieved using fractional crystallization. Optical purity and enantiomeric yield are dependent on both the crystallization time and water content in the solvent.

2 *Alkylation.* N-alkylation of the resolved pipecoloxylidide base is then performed and the HCl salt precipitated from the organic phase by adding hydrochloric acid.

3 *Final optical purification.* A final recrystallization of the crude hydrochloride from acetone/water (10 : 1) gives ropivacaine HCL.H_2O. Using this process generates an overall yield of 50% and an optical purity of >99.5%.

Conclusions

The natural world contains an abundance of enantiopure organic molecules owing to the stereospecificity inherent in its enzyme systems. The molecular chemists are catching up.

The pharmaceutical industry has undergone a strategic shift and embraced the wide spectrum of asymmetric synthetic methods now available. The use of these processes in development syntheses and large-scale manufacturing has provided new challenges in drug discovery, motivated by a desire to improve industrial efficacy and decrease the time from new drug concept to marketplace. The economic impact of industrial production of chiral drugs is now huge, with more than 50% of the 500 top selling drugs being single enantiomers.

The advantages of producing single isomer drugs to target specific receptors offers the potential to gain a better understanding of physiological processes, while at the same time potentially minimizing unwanted drug side-effects. The ability to provide chiral templates and attack the key targets of selectivity and specificity will potentially accrue great benefits, while research into new chemical entities that can interact specifically with enzyme families may potentially lead to new therapies for complex disease processes.

References

1 IUPAC Commission on nomenclature of organic chemistry. *Rules for the Nomenclature of Organic Chemistry*, Section E; *Stereochemistry*, Pergamon Press, Oxford, 1974.

2 Cahn RS, Ingold SC, Prelog V. Specification of molecular chirality. *Agnew Chem Internat Ed Eng* 1966; **5**: 385–415.

3 Easson LH, Stedman E. Studies on the relationship between chemical constitution and physiological action. *Biochem J* 1933; **27**: 1257–66.

4 Ogston AG. *Nature* 163, 963 (1948) 8.

5 Mesecar AD, Koshland DE. Sites of binding and orientation in a four-location model for protein stereospecificity. *Life* 2000; **49**: 457–66.

6 Burm AG, Van der Meer AD, Van Kleef JW *et al*. Pharmacokinetics of the enantiomers of bupivacaine following intravenous administation of the racemate. *Br J Clin Pharmacol* 1994; **38**: 125–129.

7 Tucker GT. Chiral switches. *Lancet* 2000; **355**: 1085–7.

8 Federsel H-J, Jaksch P, Sandberg R. An efficient synthesis of a new chiral 2′,6′-pipecoloxylidide local anaesthetic agent. *Acta Chem Scand* 1987; **41**(Series B): 757–61.

Further reading

Bentley R. From optical activity in quartz to chiral drugs: molecular handedness in biology and medicine. *Perspect Biol Med* 1995; **38**: 188–227.

Burke D, Henderson DJ. Chirality: a blueprint for the future. *Br J Anaesth* 2002; **88**: 563–76.

Calvey TN. Isomerism and anaesthetic drugs. *Acta Anaesthesiol Scand* 1995; **39**: 83–90.

Hutt AJ, Tan SC. Drug chirality and its clinical significance. *Drugs* 1996; **52**(Suppl. 5): 1–12.

CHAPTER 7
Ion channels

George Lees, Leanne Coyne and Karen M. Maddison

Introduction

Over 100 years ago, Meyer [1] and Overton [2] proposed a model for anaesthetic action derived from the lipid solubility–potency relationship of diverse anaesthetic drugs. It was believed that anaesthetics produced their effects by increasing the fluidity of lipid membranes [3]. More recent work has produced strong evidence to show that anaesthetics produce their effects by binding to proteinaceous molecular targets within the neuronal membranes, rather than disrupting the lipid bilayer itself [4]. This chapter presents the relatively recent evidence for the existence of chiral (stereoselective) receptor sites on fast ligand-gated ion channels (LGIC), which may constitute the molecular sensors for anaesthetic action. We also profile the ion channel superfamilies that exhibit sensitivity at or around clinical concentrations to both anaesthetics and drugs commonly used in the perioperative arena.

Mode of action of general anaesthetics

Although inhalational and induction anaesthetics have been in use for over 100 years, their mechanism of action remains unclear. The high concentrations of these lipid-soluble drugs needed to exert their effects suggested they were non-selective membrane disruptors for a number of years. Even today, this dogma has been at the core of most teaching on the subject and is still rehashed in many textbooks of pharmacology. This has been forcefully challenged in recent years based on some key observations and huge technological developments in molecular neuropharmacology (most notably, gene cloning, transgenic animals and cellular electrophysiology).

Increasing or decreasing body temperature by a degree or two has no anaesthetic effect but does exert tangible effects on bilayer fluidity and/or volume [5,6]. However, cooling to less than 24°C is often used to induce and maintain a state of anaesthesia but concurrently stops the heart so relies on extracorporeal perfusion. The effects of barbiturates, which modulate neuronal function in the low micromolar range, have long been known to be stereoselective (i.e. the isomers probably bind differentially to chiral sites on proteins); but even here, many pharmacologists taught that in this concentration range the effects of such drugs could not be receptor-active).

The seminal work of Franks' group in a variety of preparations demonstrated that isomers of isoflurane are similarly differentially active at LGIC *in vitro* [4]. In general, several groups had highlighted that LGIC were responsive to anaesthetic drugs at concentrations required to produce general anaesthesia [7]. Most researchers in this field now suggest that the preferential targets are LGIC [4,8,9]. Certainly anaesthetics do disrupt LGIC function in the clinical concentration range but they can hardly be described as 'high affinity' effectors. LGIC modulation by inhalational agents is exerted at concentrations in the 0.2–0.4 mm range which equates to "MAC (minimum alveolar concentration) equivalent" concentrations in patient cerebrospinal fluid. Receptors bearing an integral ion channel are composed of several aggregated 'subunits', with five subunits surrounding the membrane spanning channel lumen. Because each functional channel is made up of a heteromeric assembly of distinct subunits there are potentially thousands of possible isomeric assemblies of LGIC. The 'cloners' and electrophysiologists have now discerned that when the channel subunits are differentially expressed in an invariant lipid membrane, there are major changes in their pharmacology. With the advent of molecular medicine, drug designers are keen to profile the changes in the expression of disease-associated changes in the expression of specific channel isoforms.

The anaesthetist also exploits fast ion channel modulators in the form of suxamethonium and curareform muscle relaxants (see review by Prior [10]) but we focus on centrally acting drugs in this overview. The role of voltage-gated channels as targets for anticonvulsant and analgesic drugs has been highlighted recently [11].

Fine structure and physiology of ligand-gated ion channels

Ligand-gated ion channels are the favoured target for anaesthetic action, particularly the cys-loop family (see: http//www.pasteur.fr/recherche/banques/LGIC/LGIC.html) and are vital in cellular communication. The fact that they open in response to chemical stimuli confers upon them the versatility of either exciting or inhibiting the postsynaptic cells. When a neurone is activated, a chemical neurotransmitter is released from the presynaptic cell into the synapse. The neurotransmitter then binds to postsynaptically located LGIC, causing them to open, allowing the influx of ions. In the anionic LGIC (activated by GABA or glycine), influx of negatively charged Cl^- ions causes hyperpolarization of the postsynaptic cell. Cationic LGIC (activated by acetylcholine or L-glutamate) allow the influx of positively charged ions, resulting in cellular depolarization. Because of their bifunctional signalling capacity, LGIC are crucial regulators of excitability in neuronal networks and are exploited as drug targets in the treatment of anxiety, sleep disturbance, epilepsy and spasticity.

There are several families of LGIC, which can be categorized according to their structure and pharmacology. Our focus here is on the cys-loop (or nicotinic acetylcholine receptor [nAChR]) superfamily.

Nicotinic acetylcholine or 'cys-loop' receptor superfamily

There are both cationic and anionic members of the nAChR superfamily. The cation selective channels (excitatory) are nAChR and 5-hydroxytryptamine $(5-HT)_3$ receptors. The anion selective channels (inhibitory) are γ-aminobutyric acid $(GABA)_A$ receptors and glycine receptors. All members of this family are structural homologues. They are all believed to have a pentameric structure, made up from five separate subunits (Fig. 7.1). Each subunit contains four hydrophobic transmembrane regions (M1–M4), a long N-terminal and a large intracellular loop between M3 and M4. The second of these transmembrane domains, M2, is thought to line the pore of the ion channel. This region is important in ion selectivity, because of the charged amino acids. Rings of amino acids at the inner and outer end of the M2 domain contain amino acids that carry the opposite charge to the permeant ion (i.e. a cation channel will contain an M2 selective filter with a ring of negative charge), which will attract the positive cations. A cysteine–cysteine bond in the N-terminal (i.e. a cysteine loop) gives rise to the superfamily name.

The greatest insight into LGIC structure comes from the seminal work of Brisson and Unwin [12] and is based on electron microscopic analysis of nicotinic receptor dimers, which are highly enriched in fish electric organs. The high resolution of this technique (currently circa 0.6 nm) confirms that the five subunits surround a centrally located channel pore. This pore is lined with hydrophilic hydroxylated amino acids on one face of a kinked amphiphilic helix. At the apex of this kinked rod there is an amino acid residue (leucine) that is conserved throughout all LGIC [13] and which may be important in channel gating. When the channel is activated, a conformational change results in the subunits 'twisting' to open the pore (Fig. 7.1) allowing a rapid signal to be transmitted across the cell membrane. Further work on Torpedo electroplax [14] suggests that the intracellular end of the nicotinic acetylcholine channel pore contains narrow 'tunnels' which filter ions through the receptor. It has been postulated that counter-ionic charged amino acids here might explain the virtually undetectable single channel currents through $5-HT_3$ receptor isoforms [15,16]. The binding pocket for acetylcholine (ACh) is thought to be inside the channel vestibule rather than on the outside, with ACh entering the vestibule before it can reach its binding site. When the channel is closed,

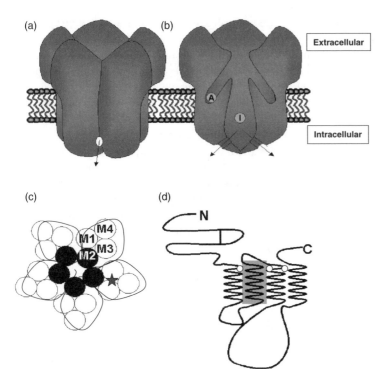

Figure 7.1 Nicotinic acetylcholine receptor superfamily structure. (a) 65-kD subunits assemble to produce a pentameric structure within the cell membrane. Note that the extracellular segments constitute the bulk of the quaternary structure, which has been confirmed by electron microscopy. (b) Cross-section indicating agonist binding site (A), and pores that ions pass through (I). (c,d) Each subunit has four transmembrane regions (M1–M4) of which M2 lines the pore. Each subunit bears a large amino terminal and a short carboxyl terminal, which are both extracellular.

the pore is blocked close to the centre of the membrane by branches from the chain of amino acids which make up the subunits [14].

Nicotinic acetylcholine receptors

Nicotinic acetylcholine receptors (nAChRs) are the most studied of all LGIC. They are mainly located on the postsynaptic membranes of muscle cells at the neuromuscular junction, but different subtypes of this receptor (mainly $\alpha_4\beta_2$) are also centrally located [13]. Although there are many subtypes of the nAChR, agonists (e.g. nicotine, lobeline and decamethonium) show little selectivity, whereas antagonists can be extremely specific. For example, α-bungarotoxin specifically targets ACh receptors located at the neuromuscular junction and central α_7 receptors [17]. Other antagonists are specific for central nicotinic receptors, such as mecamylamine. Volatile anaesthetics may also produce a weak blocking effect on various subtypes of the nAChR [18] but they synergize with relaxant drugs in the operating theatre. nAChRs in the brain differ from those on muscle membranes in that they are more diverse in

terms of subunit combination. Some of these may have a role in generating a state of consciousness. For example, nicotinic receptor titres are abnormal in Loewi body dementia; patients drift in and out of consciousness [19]. Central nicotinic receptors may be involved in the therapeutic actions and in the production of several of the side-effects of anaesthetics such as amnesia and delirium [18]. Mutations in the α_4 subunit result in autosomal dominant nocturnal frontal lobe epilepsy, which again results in transient alterations in consciousness [20]. A mutation in the β_2 subunit also causes hyperactivity disorders [20]. Centrally located nAChRs isoforms are certainly modulated by anaesthetics at clinically relevant concentrations. The $\alpha_4\beta_2$ isoform is the most widely distributed in the brain and is highly sensitive to inhalational anaesthetics and propofol [21], such that sensitivity is about 35 times greater than at receptors at the neuromuscular junction. Others report that volatile anaesthetics and ketamine both inhibit central nAChRs at clinically relevant doses, but higher concentrations of barbiturates are required to produce the same effect [18]. Moreover, there are also suggestions that nACh receptors are involved in nociception, another vital component of general anaesthesia. This evidence is derived from knockout mice, lacking genes for α_3, α_4, α_7, α_9, β_2 and β_4 subunits [20].

5-HT$_3$ receptors

The 5-HT$_3$ receptor is the only member of the serotonergic receptor family that is ionotrophic. This receptor contains an integral fast ion channel and all other 5-HT receptor families exert their effects by indirect coupling to G-proteins. These receptors are excitatory (they are selectively permeant to cations). The 5-HT$_3$ receptor has a limited distribution in the central nervous system (CNS) but is expressed in the gastrointestinal tract and in brainstem vomiting centres and almost certainly has a role in anaesthetic-induced nausea [22]. Compared with other cys-loop family members, the single channel behaviour of these pores has been very difficult to interpret. Elegant studies by Lambert's group on recombinant/chimaeric receptors suggests that key residues on the inner aspects of the pore-forming domains regulate channel conductance in certain receptor isoforms [15]. Several reports suggest that these excitatory receptors are blocked by anaesthetics, as one would probably expect, based on the homology to nicotinic receptors. Volatile anaesthetics enhance 5-HT$_3$ mediated currents [22], whereas barbiturates inhibit currents in 5-HT$_{3A}$ receptors in HEK 293 cells [23].

Glycine receptors

Glycine receptors are ligand-gated anion channels with an inhibitory role at fast synapses. Predominantly found in the brainstem and spinal cord [24], they are also distributed throughout the brain [25]. Glycine receptors are activated by glycine itself and the structural congener taurine. They have distinct pharmacology to GABA$_A$ receptors, but with a similar subunit structure, but both inhibitory transmitters are used at the same synaptic sites, notably in the spinal cord [26]. Like GABA$_A$ receptors, they can be modulated by a range of depressant drugs, such as volatile anaesthetics and barbiturates. Glycine receptors are blocked by strychnine [27]. The glycine receptor also shows sensitivity to ethanol [28], although until recently there has been limited

research. Glycine increases ethanol-induced loss of the righting reflex, whereas the glycine receptor antagonist strychnine has the opposite effect. The M2 region of the α_1 subunit may have an important role in glycine sensitivity to ethanol and enflurane. Mutation of the amino acid at position 267 caused receptors to become insensitive to modulation by ethanol and enflurane.

GABA$_A$ receptors

The final member of the cys-loop family is the anionic GABA$_A$ receptor. Many hypnotic agents, such as barbiturates and benzodiazepines, are potentiators of the GABA$_A$ receptor [29–33]. GABA$_A$ receptors appear to be pentameric, and hence are broadly consistent with the nicotinic template we have already described [32]. GABA is thought to bind to the N-terminal region [33]. Thus far, eight classes of subunit, based on sequence homology, have been discovered, with most classes containing further subtly different variants (α_{1-6}, β_{1-3}, γ_{1-3}, δ, ε, ρ_{1-2}, π and θ). Random pentameric assembly from such a large list of subunits means that theoretically, hundreds of thousands of GABA$_A$ isoforms may be expressed in the CNS. However, the list of functionally expressed receptors is likely to be a lot shorter than this. First, the ρ subunit forms receptors only with other ρ subunits, although they may be made from a combination of ρ_1 and ρ_2. Also, other than the ρ subunit, the other subunits cannot form functional receptors unless there is an α and a β subunit present. The γ subunit can be replaced by π, ε and δ, and the θ subunit requires $\alpha\beta$ and γ to be present to form a functional receptor [34]. There are likely to be no more than 20 naturally occurring combinations in the CNS according to recent evidence based on ribonucleic acid (RNA) expression or immunoprobing [35].

Expression of different subtypes of receptor in different parts of the brain gives rise to the possibility that different physiological or pathological roles are regulated by different receptor types. It also allows the pharmaceutical industry to target specific subunits of the GABA receptor, which can now be screened for sensitivity to a bewildering number of combinatorial chemical ligands using high throughput assays, to treat a variety of neurological conditions including anxiety, insomnia, epilepsy and neuropathic pain. For example, specifically targeting the α_1 subunit would result in sedation, or α_2 would result in anxiolytic effects [36,37]. The most commonly expressed subtype is thought to consist of 2α, 2β and 1γ subunits [38]. $\alpha_1\beta_2\gamma_2$ make up approximately 40% of all GABA$_A$ receptors, $\alpha_3\beta\gamma_2$ make up approximately 20%; $\alpha_2\beta\gamma_2$ make up approximately 20%; $\alpha_2\beta\gamma_1$ contribute to around 10% and other combinations make up the remaining 10% [33]. Although certain isoforms are specifically located in certain brain regions (e.g. α_6 is found exclusively in the cerebellum), $\alpha_1\beta_2\gamma_2$ is distributed throughout the CNS.

Pharmacology of GABA$_A$

Both the α and β subunits are involved in GABA binding and activation of the ion channel [33]. When GABA binds to its receptor, this causes a conformational change that results in a localized rotation of the M2 α-helix, causing the receptor to open [39].

Benzodiazepines

Benzodiazepines are a group of hypnotic/anticonvulsant/anxiolytic drugs introduced to clinical practice in 1960 [40]. These, in the form of midazolam and related compounds, are now widely used as anaesthetic synergists and premedication agents. They produce their physiological effects via the GABA$_A$ receptor by an allosteric action on the receptor protein [41]. By binding to a site independent of the GABA binding site, this gives some diversity in the actions produced by benzodiazepines. Benzodiazepines can be agonists (i.e. potentiate GABA currents), antagonists (i.e. have no effect on GABA currents) or inverse agonists (i.e. inhibit GABA currents) [42]. When benzodiazepine agonists bind to the benzodiazepine site, they increase the affinity of GABA for its receptor, ultimately resulting in a sedative effect. The most likely mechanism for this is via changing the structure of the ion channel slightly, therefore making it easier for GABA to bind (Fig. 7.2) [41]. Antagonists of the benzodiazepine site bind to the receptor and have no effect on the GABA current, but do prevent agonists of that site from binding.

The selective antagonist flumazenil is extremely useful in the poisons clinic, although benzodiazepines are relatively safe drugs in acute overdose. In healthy individuals who have not ingested exogenous benzodiazepines, flumazenil does not produce an overt pharmacological response on arousal and is not anxiogenic, suggesting that there is no endogenous ligand for the benzodiazepine site [43]. However, others have demonstrated cognitive changes in human volunteers and hence contest this conclusion [44,45].

Different combinations of subunits of the GABA$_A$ receptor show varying sensitivities to benzodiazepines. A histidine residue in the N-terminal of α subunits is important for diazepam sensitivity, such

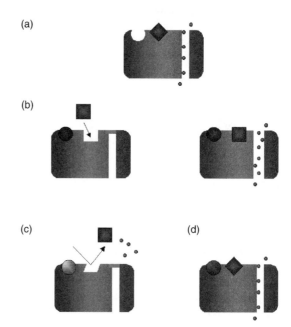

Figure 7.2 (a) In the absence of a benzodiazepine, GABA binds to the receptor, allowing Cl$^-$ influx. (b) When a benzodiazepine binds to a receptor, it causes a conformational change, allowing GABA to bind to the receptor more readily, thus allowing GABA to activate more current through the ion channel. (c) Inverse agonists, such as the β-carbolines, bind to the benzodiazepine site and cause a conformational change that reduces the chance of GABA binding to the receptor. (d) Neutral antagonists of the benzodiazepine site prevent benzodiazepines from binding, but have no effect on the affinity of GABA for the receptor or the ionic current.

that if this residue is converted to arginine, it renders the receptor insensitive [46]. α_4 and α_6 subunits, which are insensitive to diazepam in wild-type receptors, become sensitive if the amino acid at position 99 in α_4 or 100 in α_6 is mutated to arginine. Receptors containing α_1 subunits show high sensitivity to diazepam, flumazenil, zolpidem and DMCM (methyl 6,7,-dimethoxy-4-ethyl-β-carboline-3-carboxylate which is a very potent convulsant with high affinity for specific benzodiazepine binding sites), whereas α_2, α_3 and α_5 containing receptors show reduced sensitivity to flumazenil, but are highly sensitive to diazepam, zolpidem and DMCM. However, α_4 and α_6 containing receptors are insensitive to diazepam, zolpidem and DMCM but are sensitive to flumazenil [45]. In the absence of the γ subunit (i.e. in αβ only combinations), benzodiazepines have no effect [42,47], suggesting that benzodiazepines bind at the α–γ interface [48]. Replacement of the γ subunit with ε, δ and π also renders receptors insensitive to benzodiazepines, suggesting that the γ subunit is crucial for benzodiazepine binding [34]. The π subunit can coassemble with the α, β and γ subunits, but these receptors are also insensitive to modulation by benzodiazepines [34]. However, incorporation of the θ subunit, to produce an αβγθ combination does show sensitivity to benzodiazepines [34].

Barbiturates

Barbiturates are a group of drugs whose clinical effects range from sedation to anaesthesia. Their clinical usefulness has diminished as a result of their side-effects, such as physical dependence and tolerance [49], but thiopental is still widely used as an induction agent by anaesthetists. Unlike benzodiazepines, barbiturates produce profound respiratory depression and in overdose have been frequently used to commit suicide, usually in combination with alcohol. Although barbiturates are hypnotic, they do not produce physiological sleep and cycles of rapid eye movement (REM) and slow wave sleep (SWS) are abnormal, leading to sleep that is not restful [50]. Like benzodiazepines, they are well known to modulate $GABA_A$ receptors, but they also have a blocking effect on voltage-gated sodium channels [51]. The $GABA_A$ receptor is again the primary site of action for the barbiturates [16]. Barbiturates have three differ-

ent effects at the $GABA_A$ receptors: (i) a positive modulatory effect at low concentrations (approximately 1–300 μmol); (ii) a direct activation of GABA receptors at mid-high concentrations (approximately 60 μmol–3 mmol); and (iii) a blocking effect at high concentrations [16,52]. These effects are produced by barbiturates binding at distinct sites on the $GABA_A$ receptor [30]. The site of direct activation by barbiturates is unlikely to be at the same site as the GABA binding site, because threonine and tyrosine residues in the β subunit are crucial for channel activation by GABA, but not by barbiturates [48].

Like other drugs that interact with the $GABA_A$ receptor, the subunit composition determines the effects of barbiturates. Homomeric ρ_1 receptors are insensitive to barbiturates [53], but a mutation of a single amino acid residue in the M2 region leads to the sensitivity of ρ_1 to pentobarbital [54]. Different isoforms of the α subunit show different sensitivities to barbiturates. α_6 is three times more sensitive to direct activation by barbiturates than the other α subunits [16]. The β subunit is important in the effects of barbiturates on the $GABA_A$ receptor and replacing an alanine residue with a proline residue in the M1 region of the β_1 subunit decreases barbiturate sensitivity [48]. A glycine residue in the M1 region of the β and α subunits is vital for enhancement by pentobarbital [48], while a mutation in the M2 region of the β_3 subunit eliminates sensitivity to pentobarbital. Although there is not much variation between different β subunits in their sensitivity to barbiturates, β_3 is usually the most sensitive [16].

Anticonvulsants

Anticonvulsants that exert their effect via the $GABA_A$ receptor block paroxysmal depolarizing shifts *in vitro* and ictal seizures *in vivo*. Several different anticonvulsants exert their effects in different ways. Some anticonvulsant drugs such as tiagabine and vigabatrin work by increasing the levels of GABA in the brain. Others, like diazepam, produce their effects by binding directly to the $GABA_A$ receptor [31]. The anticonvulsant loreclezole exerts its effects on the $GABA_A$ receptor by binding to the β subunit, and does not need the α or γ subunit to be present. However, its effects are absolutely dependent on which β subunit is expressed: only $GABA_A$ receptors containing the $\beta_{2/3}$ subunits are sensitive to loreclezole [31]. Further mutations in the M2 and M3 domains reveal that a single amino acid in M2 (serine residue in β_1 and asparagine in β_2) is crucial in determining β_1 insensitivity and β_2 sensitivity to etomidate and loreclezole [55,56]. In addition, β_2 knockout mice show markedly reduced sensitivity to etomidate [37].

Neurosteroids

Neurosteroids are endogenous steroids found in the CNS and are vital to the normal functioning of the human brain. For example, decreased levels of allopregnenolone are found in depressed patients [57] and changes in steroid titres are likely to underpin the associated anxiogenic, psychological and mood swings seen in premenstrual syndrome. The steroidal anaesthetic alphaxalone was the first shown to act upon the $GABA_A$ receptor and since then several neurosteroids have been found to mimic this effect [58]. Steroids have a number of behavioural effects, such as anxiolytic, hypnotic, anaesthetic and anticonvulsant, all of which are hallmarks of drugs that modulate the $GABA_A$ receptor [58]. Neurosteroids can inhibit (excitatory/convulsive effects) or enhance (inhibitory/sedative effects) the $GABA_A$ Cl^- currents. For example, 3α-OH-DHP (3α-hydroxy-5α-pregnan-ol-20-one) potentiates GABA activity, whereas pregnenolone sulphate depresses the receptors [59].

Like anaesthetic agents, neurosteroids bind to multiple recognition sites on the $GABA_A$ receptor. Most neurosteroids will only modulate GABA receptors composed of a combination of α_1, $\beta_{1/2}$, and γ_2. Although the presence of the γ subunit is not necessary for neurosteroid modulation, replacing the γ_2 subunit for a γ_1 subunit significantly reduces sensitivity [31,60]. As well as having a positive modulatory effect on exogenous GABA responses, steroids also increase the duration of spontaneous inhibitory postsynaptic currents (sIPSC), although there is no change in the amplitude [58]. This is an effect analogous to barbiturate actions on $GABA_A$ receptors and, like benzodiazepines, neurosteroids also increase the frequency of channel openings [58]. Neurosteroids can directly activate the $GABA_A$ receptor. Although this may associate neurosteroids with barbiturates, they are known to bind to distinct sites on the $GABA_A$ receptor [61].

The state of phosphorylation of the $GABA_A$ receptor is an important contributing factor to neurosteroid action [62]. The effect of neurosteroids on the duration of the IPSC can be abolished by blockade of G-protein coupled receptors and protein kinase C (PKC) [62]. However, activation of G-proteins and PKC in the absence of a neurosteroid fails to mimic the neurosteroid effects. This suggests that the neurosteroid binds to the $GABA_A$ receptor, not to PKC or the G-protein directly [62].

Neurosteroids do not specifically target $GABA_A$ receptors; depending on the subunit combination, neurosteroids can either enhance or inhibit N-methyl-D-asparate (NMDA) receptors [57]. Some neurosteroids such as hydrocortisone enhance glycine-mediated currents, although none of the neurosteroids modulates both GABA and glycine receptors [58]. Furthermore, voltage-gated Ca^{2+} channels are inhibited by nanomolar concentrations of 5α-pregnan-3α,11β,21-triol-20-one [58].

Non-steroidal anti-inflammatory drugs

Non-steroidal anti-inflammatory drugs (NSAIDs) include aspirin, ibuprofen and mefenamic acid (MFA). MFA has been found to have a subunit-dependent effect on the $GABA_A$ receptor [63] and currents produced by $GABA_A$ receptors ($\alpha_1\beta_2\gamma_2$) were positively modulated by this drug. Replacement of β_2 with β_1 rendered receptors insensitive to modulation by MFA [63] and, furthermore, in the presence of a γ_{2L} subunit (rather than γ_{2S}), MFA is inhibitory at β_1-containing receptors [64]. These observations may contribute to the analgesic profiles of such drugs, but also represent an exciting new target for anxiolytic, hypnotic and anticonvulsant drug discovery [35].

Phosphorylation

$GABA_A$ receptor function can be modulated by the phosphorylation secondary to kinase or phosphatase action. There are numerous sites susceptible to phosphorylation by PKA and PKC (Fig. 7.3). These sites are located between M3 and M4 of α, β, γ, ϵ, π and ρ subunits [65]. PKA injection decreases the frequency of channel opening in neurones and reduces re-

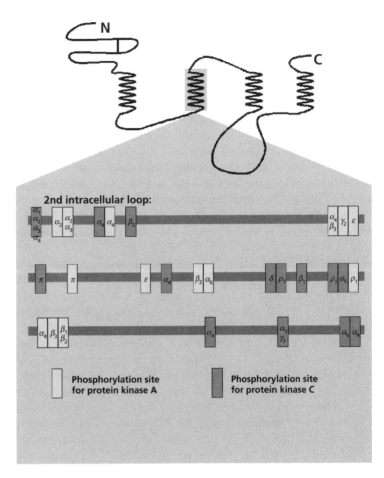

Figure 7.3 Predicted sites for phosphorylation of GABA receptor subunits by protein kinase A (PKA) and protein kinase C (PKC).

sponses to GABA in oocytes and these effects are also shown by PKC [32]. It has been suggested that a site on the γ_{2L} subunit is essential for GABA sensitivity of ethanol [66], although other papers report that phosphorylation of γ_{2L} is not important for ethanol sensitivity [67].

There are many types of protein kinases, including PKA and PKC, each of which has several isoforms. There are at least eleven known classes of PKC, α, β_I, β_{II}, γ, δ, ϵ, ζ, η, θ, μ and λ [68] and these subtypes can be further divided into three groups. Conventional PKC (cPKC) isoforms (α, β_I, β_{II} and γ) require activation by diacylglycerol (DAG) and Ca^{2+}. These isoforms are expressed throughout the brain and are associated with phospholipase C activation [68]. Novel PKC (nPKC) isoforms (δ, ϵ, η, θ and μ) are similar to cPKC isoforms in their structure, but they can

be activated independently of Ca^{2+}; however, they require activation by DAG. Atypical PKC (aPKC) isoforms (ζ and λ) differ from cPKC and nPKC isoforms in structure and require neither Ca^{2+} nor DAG for activation [68]. PKC is subject to autophosphorylation, when Ca^{2+} levels are increased for a length of time [68].

There is another subtype of PKC which is insensitive to autophosphorylation, called protein kinase M (PKM). PKC activation results in inhibition of GABA$_A$ receptors expressed in *Xenopus laevis* oocytes [69], but this has not been replicated in neurones, with some laboratories reporting that activation of PKC causes potentiation of GABA receptor currents [70,71]. Different *in vitro* expression systems are probably the cause of these contradictory results. Alternatively, it is possible that the different cell or species types express different isoforms of PKC, resulting in the different effect of PKC in different expression systems.

Data from experiments in *Xenopus* oocytes have shown that PKC activated inhibition of ρ_1 receptors is caused by internalization of the receptor, rather than phosphorylation of individual residues [72]. There is evidence to suggest that certain drugs can modulate PKC and a recent article has shown that the volatile anaesthetic halothane increases the translocation of PKC to the cell surface [73]. Neurosteroid modulation of the GABA$_A$ receptor appears to be dependent upon the phosphorylation state [62]. Other anaesthetics and alcohol have also been shown to inhibit PKC. Modulation of the GABA receptor by phosphorylation allows a diverse range of changes to GABA receptor function. PKA is activated by cyclic adenosine monophosphate (cAMP) and high levels of PKA are found in the hypothalamus [70]. Activation of PKA causes an increase in GABA release [74]. Other work has shown that the PKA activator, forskolin, can increase the amplitude of sIPSC as well as miniature inhibitory postsynaptic current (mIPSC) frequency [70]. The role of PKC and PKA in the sensitivity of GABA$_A$ receptors to a variety of drugs remains unclear but may represent novel drug targets.

General anaesthetics and GABA$_A$ receptors

The discovery that the ρ subunit was absolutely insensitive to inhalational anaesthetics was a pivotal finding. Lengths of protein from a sensitive subunit were spliced at the appropriate segment into copy DNA (cDNA) for the ρ homologue to produce chimeras. This showed that segments that span the membrane were crucial. This seminal work has shown that the M2 domain on both α and β subunits are vital for the binding of certain anaesthetics and alcohol [75]. For example, isoflurane sensitivity can be eliminated by mutating certain residues on the α_2 and/or β_1 subunits [76]. In addition, a mutation in the β_1 subunit abolished the ability of propofol to potentiate the GABA receptor,

although direct activation at high doses was still possible [76].

Further elegant work focusing on mutations in the M2 and M3 domains revealed that a single amino acid in M2, which is serine in β_1 and asparagine in β_1, confers insensitivity to etomidate and loreclezole in the β_1 subunit compared with the sensitive β_2 subunit [55,56]. Mutation of Gly219 in the M1 region of the β_2 subunit almost eliminates sensitivity to intravenous anaesthetics including pentobarbital, propofol, etomidate and alphaxalone [77]. As well as the type of amino acid present at these key sites, the size of the anaesthetic molecule also determines the sensitivity of various mutations [63]. This suggests that there is a 'pocket' where anaesthetics bind, and slight variations in the amino acids creating this pocket could lead to differential anaesthetic sensitivity. Further evidence to support the binding pocket theory was produced by Belelli *et al.* [54] in 1999. They showed that mutation of a single amino acid in the ρ subunit produced sensitivity to pentobarbital in a previously insensitive subunit [54]. Clearly, different types of anaesthetics bind to different parts of the GABA$_A$ receptor, although it is unknown which of these sites is important physiologically for the binding of endogenous substances.

Although the GABA$_A$ receptor is the consensus molecular target for anaesthetic effects based on the recent literature, the fact remains that such drugs exhibit relatively low affinity for a variety of neuronal targets, which probably accounts for their diverse pharmacological and cardiovascular safety profiles and also making it unlikely that a single receptor underpins their diverse pharmacological profiles. The importance of GABA$_A$ receptor isomerism is now being examined in whole animals using recombinant techniques and transgenic laboratory strains or gene knockouts. Because of the importance of inhibitory GABAergic transmission, GABA$_A$ knockouts can be lethal [37]. However, deletion of subunits believed to be important in anaesthesia is feasible. GABA sensitivity to some anaesthetics is absolutely dependent on certain subunits. By eliminating these subunits, these animals could, if modulation of GABA$_A$ is the key step for anaesthesia, be insensitive to these anaesthetics. Until recently, the only major subunit to be deleted was γ_2, which proved to be lethal. However, more recently, α_1 and β_2 knockout mice were produced [37]; α_1 null mice showed an 80% reduction in the loss of the righting reflex in response to zolpidem and β_2-knockouts showed a 50% reduction in response to etomidate. In addition, knock-in mice, with the mutation β2N265S, had reduced sensitivity to etomidate with improved motor coordination and reduced postanaesthetic sedation [78]. Drugs that do not modulate β_2-containing receptors offer the possibility of anaesthesia with improved recovery, which would be particularly beneficial for short-stay patients. In addition to its importance in postanaesthetic recovery, Cirone *et al.* [78] have also shown that the β_2 subunit is important in hypothermia during anaesthesia. The β2N265S knock-in mice described above had a smaller hypothermic response to etomidate than wild-type mice and also returned a normal body temperature more rapidly [78]. Other workers have focused on β_3 subunit knockouts and have shown a marked shift in sensitivity to anaesthetics. The length of time of the loss of the righting reflex induced by etomidate and midazolam was reduced in these mice, but not that induced by halothane, pentobarbital, ethanol and enflurane. However, the immobilizing action, as tested in a tail clamping assay, of halothane and enflurane were decreased. Thus, the β_3 subunit may be involved in the anaesthetic effects of these agents [79]. Interestingly, β_3-containing GABA receptors may have an important role in REM sleep, which is considerably reduced during anaesthesia [80].

Conclusions

Ligand-gated ion channels have a major signalling role in the CNS and are important molecular targets for anaesthetics; particularly the $GABA_A$ receptor. Anaesthetics were discovered by serendipity rather than an enlightened and rational research programme based on activity at ion channel targets. Many anaesthetists would argue, with justification, that their mode of action is irrelevant and that a single molecular target may never be able to explain their efficacy and diverse *in vivo* pharmacological profiles. However, it is now widely acknowledged that fast ligand-gated channels represent one of the

better model targets to explain anaesthetic action. The data reviewed here have radically transformed our perceptions of how anaesthetic drugs may exert their effects at the cellular level, and there is growing evidence for the role of $GABA_A$ isoforms in transducing the effects of anaesthetics in the living brain. However, it is doubtful whether this will, even in the mid-term future, be able to impact on rational design of novel and safer anaesthetic agents.

References

1 Meyer H. *Harvey Lectures.* 1905; **1**: 11–7.

2 Overton E. *Studien uber die Narkose, Zugleich ein Beitrag zur Allgemeinen Pharmakologie.* Jena, Germany: Gustav Fischer, 1901.

3 Miller KW. The nature of the site of general anaesthesia. *Int Rev Neurobiol* 1985; **27**: 1–61.

4 Franks NP, Lieb WR. Molecular and cellular mechanisms of anaesthesia. *Nature* 1994; **367**: 607–13.

5 Antognini JF. Hypothermia eliminates isoflurane requirements at 20 degrees C. *Anesthesiology* 1993; **78**: 1152–6.

6 Wollenek G, Honarwar N, Golej J, Marx M. Cold water submersion and cardiac arrest in treatment of severe hypothermia with cardiopulmonary bypass. *Resuscitation* 2002; **52**: 255–63.

7 Hall AC, Lieb WR, Franks NP. Stereoselective and non-stereoselective actions of isoflurane on the $GABA_A$ receptor. *Br J Pharmacol* 1994; **112**: 906–10.

8 Mihic SJ, Ye Q, Finn SE, *et al.* Molecular mechanisms of inhalation anesthetic action: regulation of the human glycine receptor is independent of the cytoplasmic loop. *Anesthesiol* 1996; **85**: A675.

9 Pistis M, Belelli D, Peters JA, Lambert JJ. The interaction of general anaesthetics with recombinant GABA(A) and glycine receptors expressed in *Xenopus laevis* oocytes. *Br J Pharmacol* 1997; **122**: 1707–19.

10 Prior C. Muscle relaxants: past, present and future. *Curr Anaesth Crit Care* 2003; **14**: 38–46.

11 Errington AC, Stohr T, Lees G. Voltage gated ion channels: targets for anticonvulsant drugs. *Curr Top Med Chem* 2005; **5**: 15–30.

12 Brisson A, Unwin PNT. Tubular crystals of acetylcholine receptor. *J Cell Biol* 1984; **99**: 1202–11.

13 Itier V, Bertrand D. Neuronal nicotinic receptors: from protein structure to function. *FEBS Lett* 2001; **504**: 118–25.

14 Miyazawa A, Fujiyoshi Y, Stowell M, Unwin N. Nicotinic acetylcholine receptor at 4.6 angstrom resolution:

transverse tunnels in the channel wall. *J Mol Biol* 1999; **288**: 765–86.

15 Peters JA, Kelley SP, Dunlop JI, *et al.* The 5-hydroxy-tryptamine type 3 (5-HT3) receptor reveals a novel determinant of single-channel conductance. *Mol Struct Ligand-gated Ion Channel Function* 2004; **32**: 547–52.

16 Thompson SA, Whiting PJ, Wafford K. Barbiturate interactions at the human GABA$_A$ receptor: dependence on receptor subunit combination. *Br J Pharmacol* 1996; **117**: 521–7.

17 Albuquerque EX, Pereira EFR, Braga MFM, Alkondon M. Contribution of nicotinic receptors to the function of synapses in the central nervous system: the action of choline as a selective agonist of α_7 receptors. *J Physiol (Paris)* 1998; **92**: 309–16.

18 Tassonyi E, Charpantier E, Muller D, Dumont L, Bertrand D. The role of nicotinic actylcholine receptors in the mechanisms of anaesthesia. *Brain Res Bull* 2002; **57**: 133–50.

19 Teaktong T, Graham A, Court J, *et al.* Alzheimer's disease is associated with a selective increase in α7 nicotinic acetylcholine receptor immunoreactivity in astrocytes. *Glia* 2003; **41**: 207–11.

20 Changeux J, Edelstein SJ. Allosteric mechanisms in normal and pathological nicotinic acetylcholine receptors. *Curr Opinion Neurobiol* 2001; **11**: 377.

21 Violet JM, Downie DL, Nakisa RC, Lieb WR, Franks NP. Differential sensitivities of mammalian neuronal and muscle nicotinic acetylcholine receptors to general anesthetics. *Anesthesiol* 1997; **86**: 866–74.

22 Machu TK, Harris RA. Alcohols and anaesthetics enhance the function of 5-hydroxytryptamine 3 receptors expressed in *Xenopus laevis* oocytes. *J Pharmacol Exp Ther* 1994; **271**: 898–905.

23 Barren M, Meder W, Dorner Z *et al.* Recombinant human 5HT3A receptors in outside out patches of HEK 293 cells: basic properties and barbiturate effect. *Naunyn Schmiedebergs Arch Pharmacol* 2000; **362**: 255–65.

24 Betz H. Glycine receptors: heterogeneous and widespread in the mammalian brain. *Trends Neurosci* 1991; **14**: 458–61.

25 Betz H, Kuhse J, Schmieden V, *et al.* Structure and functions of inhibitory and excitatory glycine receptors. *Annals N Y Acad Sci* 1999; **868**: 667–76.

26 Jonas P, Bischofberger J, Sandkühler J. Corelease of two fast neurotransmitters at a central synapse. *Science* 1998; **281**: 419–24.

27 Rang HP, Dale MM, Ritter JM. *Pharmacology*, 3rd edn. Edinburgh: Churchill Livingstone, 1995.

28 Kalluri HSG, Ticku MK. Role of the GABA$_A$ receptors in the ethanol-mediated inhibition of extracellular signal-regulated kinase. *Eur J Pharmacol* 2002; **451**: 51–4.

29 Mihic SJ. Acute effects of ethanol on GABA$_A$ and glycine receptor function. *Neurochem Int* 1999; **35**: 115–23.

30 Robertson B. Actions of anaesthetics and avermectin on GABA$_A$ chloride channels in mammalian dorsal root ganglion neurones. *Br J Pharmacol* 1989; **98**: 167–76.

31 Mehta AK, Ticku MK. An update on GABA$_A$ receptors. *Brain Res Rev* 1999; **29**: 196–217.

32 Nayeem N, Green TP, Martin IL, Barnard EA. Quaternary structure of the native GABA$_A$ receptor determined by electron microscopic image. *J Neurochem* 1994; **62**: 815–8.

33 Mohler H, Fritschy JM, Luscher B, *et al.* The GABA$_A$ receptors: from subunits to diverse functions. *Ion Channels* 1996; **4**: 89–113.

34 Costa E, Auta J, Grayson DR, *et al.* GABA$_A$ receptors and benzodiazepines: a role for dendritic resident subunit mRNAs. *Neuropharmacol* 2002; **43**: 925–37.

35 McKernan RM, Whiting PJ. Which GABA$_A$ receptor subtypes really occur in the brain? *Trends Neurosci* 1996; **19**: 139–43.

36 Johnstone TBC, Hogenkamp DJ, Coyne L, *et al.* Modifying quinolone antibiotics yield new anxiolytics. *Nat Med* 2004; **10**: 31–2.

37 Blednov YAS, Alva JH, Wallace D, *et al.* Deletion of the α1 or β2 subunit of GABA$_A$ receptors reduces actions of alcohol and other drugs. *J Pharmacol Exp Ther* 2003; **304**: 30–6.

38 Farrar SJ, Whiting PJ, Bonnert TP, McKernan RM. Stoichiometry of a ligand-gated ion channel determined by fluorescence energy transfer. *J Biol Chem* 1999; **274**: 10100–4.

39 Smith GB, Olsen RW. Functional domains of GABA(A) receptors. *Trends Pharmacol Sci* 1995; **16**: 162–8.

40 Doble A, Martin IL. Multiple benzodiazepine receptors: no reason for anxiety. *Trends Pharmacol Sci* 1992; **13**: 76–81.

41 Tecott LH. Designer genes and anti-anxiety drugs. *Nat Neurosci* 2000; **3**: 529–30.

42 Lüddens H, Korpi ER. GABA(A) receptors: pharmacology, behavioral roles, and motor disorders. *Neuroscientist* 1996; **2**: 15–23.

43 Mathieu-Nolf M, Babe MA, Coquelle-Couplet V, *et al.* Flumazenil use in an emergency department: a survey. *J Toxicol Clin Toxicol* 2001; **39**: 15–20.

44 Neave N, Reid C, Scholey AB, *et al.* Dose-dependent effects of flumazenil on cognition, mood, and cardio-

respiratory physiology in healthy volunteers. *Br Dent J* 2000; **189**: 668–74.

45 Smith TAD. Type A γ-aminobutyric acid (GABA$_A$) receptor subunits and benzodiazepine binding: significance to clinical syndromes and their treatment. *Br J Biomed Sci* 2001; **58**: 111–21.

46 Benson JA, Low K, Keist R, Mohler HRU. Pharmacology of recombinant γ-aminobutyric acid$_A$ receptors render diazepam-insensitive by point mutated α-subunits. *FEBS Lett* 1998; **431**: 400–4.

47 Malherbe P, Draguhn A, Multhaup G, Beyreuther K, Möhler HRU. GABA$_A$ receptors expressed from rat brain α and β subunit cDNAs display potentiation by benzodiazepine receptor ligands. *Mol Brain Res* 1990; **8**: 199–208.

48 Greenfield LJ, Zaman SH, Sutherland ML, *et al*. Mutation of the GABA$_A$ receptor M1 transmembrane proline increases GABA affinity and reduces barbiturate enhancement. *Neuropharmacol* 2002; **42**: 502–21.

49 Weitzel KW, Wickman JM, Augustin SG, Strom JG. Zaleplon: a pyrazolopyramidine sedative-hypnotic agent for the treatment of insomnia. *Clin Ther* 2000; **22**: 1254–67.

50 Lancel M. Role of GABA(A) receptors in the regulation of sleep: initial sleep responses to peripherally administered modulators and agonists. *Sleep* 1999; **22**: 33–42.

51 Rehberg B, Xiao YH, Duch DS. Central nervous system sodium channels are significantly suppressed at clinical concentrations of volatile anesthetics. *Anesthesiology* 1996; **84**: 1223–33.

52 Michaelis EK. Molecular biology of glutamate receptors in the central nervous system and their role in excitotoxicity, oxidative stress and ageing. *Prog Neurobiol* 1998; **54**: 369–415.

53 Korpi ER, Gründer G, Lüddens H. Drug interactions at GABA$_A$ receptors. *Prog Neurobiol* 2002; **67**: 113–59.

54 Belelli D, Pau D, Cabras G, Peters JA, Lambert JJ. A single amino acid confers barbiturate sensitivity upon the GABA rho 1 receptor. *Br J Pharmacol* 1999; **127**: 601–4.

55 Belelli D, Lambert JJ, Peters JA, Wafford K, Whiting PJ. The interaction of the general anaesthetic etomidate with the γ-aminobutyric acid type A receptor is influenced by a single amino acid. *Proc Natl Acad Sci U S A* 1997; **94**: 11031–6.

56 McGurk KA, Pistis M, Belelli D, Hope AG, Lambert JJ. The effect of a transmembrane amino acid on etomidate sensitivity of an invertebrate GABA receptor. *Br J Pharmacol* 1998; **124**: 13–20.

57 Puia G, Belelli D. Neurosteroids on our minds. *Trends Pharmacol Sci* 2001; **22**: 266–7.

58 Lambert JJ, Belelli D, Hill-Venning C, Peters JA. Neurosteroids and GABA$_A$ receptor function. *Trends Pharmacol Sci* 1995; **16**: 295–303.

59 Zaman SH, Shingai R, Harvey RJ, Darlison MG, Barnard EA. Effects of subunit types of the recombinant GABA$_A$ receptor on the response to a neurosteroid. *Eur J Pharmacol* 1992; **225**: 321–30.

60 Belelli D, Casula A, Ling A, Lambert JJ. The influence of subunit composition on the interaction of neurosteroids with GABA$_A$ receptors. *Neuropharmacol* 2002; **43**: 651–61.

61 Peters JA, Lambert JJ. Anaesthetics in a bind? *Trends Pharmacol Sci* 1997; **18**: 454–5.

62 Fancsik A, Linn DM, Tasker JG. Neurosteroid modulation of GABA IPSCs is phosphorylation dependent. *Neuroscience* 2000; **20**: 3067–75.

63 Halliwell RF, Thomas P, Patten D, *et al*. Subunit-selective modulation of GABA(A) receptors by the nonsteroidal anti-inflammatory agent, mefenamic acid. *Eur J Neurosci* 1999; **11**: 2897–905.

64 Coyne L, Lees G, Nicholson RA, Zheng J, Neufield KD. The sleep hormone oleamide modulates inhibitory ionotropic receptors in mammalian CNS *in vitro*. *Br J Pharmacol* 2002; **135**: 1977–87.

65 Brandon NJ, Delmas P, Hill J, Smart TG, Moss SJ. Constitutive tyrosine phosphorylation of the GABA$_A$ receptor γ$_2$ subunit in rat brain. *Neuropharmacol* 2001; **41**: 745–52.

66 Wafford KA, Whiting PJ. Ethanol potentiation of GABA$_A$ receptors requires phosphorylation of the alternatively spliced variant of the γ$_2$ subunit. *FEBS Lett* 1992; **313**: 113–7.

67 Zhai J, Stewart RR, Friedberg MW, Li C. Phosphorylation of the GABA$_A$ receptor γ$_{2L}$ subunit in rat sensory neurones may not be necessary for ethanol sensitivity. *Brain Res* 1998; **805**: 116–22.

68 Hemmings Jr HC. General anaesthetic effects on protein kinase C. *Toxicol Lett* 1998; **101**: 89–95.

69 Leidenheimer NJ, McQuilkin SJ, Hahner LD, Whiting PJ, Harris RA. Activation of protein kinase C selectively inhibits the γ-aminobutyric acid$_A$ receptor: role of desensitization. *Mol Pharmacol* 1992; **41**: 1116–23.

70 Capogna M, Gähwiler BH, Thompson SM. Presynaptic enhancement of inhibitory synaptic transmission by protein kinases A and C in the rat hippocampus *in vitro*. *J Neurosci* 1995; **15**: 1249–60.

71 Xu TL, Pang ZP, Li JS, Akaike N. 5-HT potentiation of the GABA(A) response in the rat sacral dorsal commissural neurones. *Br J Pharmacol* 1998; **124**: 779–87.

72 Filippova N, Sedelnikova A, Zong Y, Fortinberry H, Weiss DS. Regulation of recombinant γ-aminobutyric acid $(GABA)_A$ and $(GABA)_C$ receptors by protein kinase C. *Am Soc Pharmacol Exp Ther* 2000; **57**: 847–56.

73 Gomez RS, Barbosa J, Guatimosim C, *et al.* Translocation of protein kinase C by halothane in cholinergic cells. *Brain Res Bull* 2002; **58**: 55–9.

74 Sciancalepore M, Cherubini E. Protein kinase A dependent increase in frequency of miniature GABAergic currents in rat CA3 hippocampal neurones. *Neurosci Lett* 1995; **187**: 91–4.

75 Mihic SJ, Ye Q, Wick MJ, *et al.* Sites of alcohol and volatile anaesthetic action on GABA and glycine receptors. *Nature* 1997; **389**: 385–8.

76 Krasowski MD, Koltchine VV, Rick CE, *et al.* Propofol and other intravenous anesthetics have sites of action on the gamma-aminobutyric acid type a receptor distinct from that for isoflurane. *Mol Pharmacol* 1998; **53**: 530–8.

77 Chang CS, Olcese R, Olsen RW. A single M1 residue in the β2 subunit alters channel gating of $GABA_A$ receptor in anesthetic modulation and direct activation. *J Biol Chem* 2003; **278**: 42821–8.

78 Cirone J, Rosahl TW, Reynolds DS, *et al.* Gamma-aminobutyric acid type A receptor beta 2 subunit mediates the hypothermic effect of etomidate in mice. *Anesthesiol* 2004; **100**: 1438–45.

79 Qunilan JJ, Homanics GE, Firestone LL. Anesthesia sensitivity in mice that lack the beta3 subunit of the gamma-aminobutyric acid type A receptor. *Anesthesiol* 1998; **88**: 775–80.

80 Wisor JP, DeLorey TM, Homanics GE, Edgar DM. Sleep states and sleep electroencephalographic spectral power in mice lacking the β3 subunit of the GABA receptor. *Brain Res* 2002; **955**: 221–8.

CHAPTER 8

Immunosuppression

Roxanna Bloomfield and David Noble

Introduction

Multicellular organisms require mechanisms to distinguish between self and non-self so that invading microbial and parasitic pathogens or rogue cells, such as tumour cells or virally infected cells, are eliminated. This task is performed by the immune system, which comprises a complex network of humoral and cellular factors that are orchestrated to defend the organism against such invaders. These defences are also intimately linked with other systems or pathways such as inflammation and coagulation (see Chapter 11). However, the integrity and vigour of these immune mechanisms can be affected by disease or as a consequence of therapeutic interventions. Management of autoimmune diseases, immune hypersensitivity, bone marrow and solid organ transplantation have also resulted in a variety of strategies to suppress or modulate immune processes for the benefit of individual patients. Drugs developed to facilitate organ transplantation have also been utilized in other disease processes such as prevention of stent-associated stenosis [1].

An overview of the immune system

A brief overview of the immune system allows insights into causes and targets of immunosuppression [2–4]. The immune system organizes responses against invaders by way of humoral factors and cellular responses. Although immune responses can be compartmentalized into innate and adaptive systems, they are overlapping and interdependent.

Physical barriers

Prior to engagement with immune defences, external pathogens must breach hostile barriers such as integument and mucosal surfaces to gain access to the host. However, this is frequently the case in patients encountered in the operating theatre and in intensive care units (ICUs) with the use of peripheral and central vascular devices, intracranial monitoring or drainage systems, artificial airways, urinary catheters and surgical wounds. These factors in concert with reduced conscious level, impaired swallowing reflexes, reduced ciliary clearance and alterations to epithelial cell secretions that can also occur in these patients, contribute to impairment of this first line of defence.

Innate immunity

On first encounter with a pathogen, the adaptive or specific immune response requires proliferation and clonal expansion of cell lines, a process that may take days to complete. Effectors of the innate system, which include antimicrobial peptides, phagocytes and the alternative pathway of complement, can be activated immediately. Thus, innate immunity allows containment of the new invader before the complementary adaptive immune system becomes fully functional [3–4]. This in part is achieved by germ-line encoded receptors that recognize highly conserved moieties found in large groupings of microorganisms. The latter are called pathogen-associated molecular patterns. Examples include lipopolysaccharide, peptidoglycan, lipoteichoic acid, mannans, bacterial DNA, double-stranded RNA and glucans. The receptors that recognize them are called pattern-recognition receptors. The mannose receptor of macrophages is one example. Resulting activation of signal-transduction pathways leads to expression of a variety of immune response genes as well as inflammatory cytokines. Cytokines can up-regulate innate immune responses.

For example, interleukin-12 (IL-12) up-regulates natural killer (NK) cells to more active lymphokine activated killer (LAK) cells. γ-Interferon (IFN-γ) increases resistance to viral replication as well as enhancing several aspects of cellular immunity. Molecules synthesized by the liver as part of the acute phase response, such as mannan-binding lectin, which similarly are activated by pathogen-associated molecular patterns, initiate the complement cascade which can lead to microbial cell lysis or increase the ability of neutrophils and macrophages to phagocytose and kill the complement-coated invaders. Toll receptor molecules found in *Drosophila* flies have become a focus of interest as similar receptors are also found in mammals and have been named Toll-like receptors (TLRs). Studies in mice suggest that TLR4, through the nuclear factor κB (NK-κB) pathway, may be involved in innate responses to lipopolysaccharide. Mice deficient in this TLR gene are profoundly susceptible to Gram-negative bacterial infections. The significance of human TLR polymorphisms in disease currently is an active area of research [3–5].

The innate immune system not only provides an immediate response to non-self pathogens, but is also vital for appropriate T-cell activation. T cells require multiple signals to initiate a full response. This may be viewed as a safety mechanism to prevent activation and inappropriate responses to the host itself. Thus, in normal circumstances, full expression of the adaptive immune response is modulated by dendritic and other antigen presenting cells of the innate immune system through antigen presentation by major histocompatibility complex (MHC) peptide antigen complexes, other co-stimulatory surface molecules and by cytokines such as IL-1, IL-6 and IL-12. Mutations of mannose receptors and mannose-binding lectin have been associated with increased susceptibility to infections. Mutations that leave the innate system constitutively active may predispose to autoimmune, hypersensitivity and inflammatory diseases [3].

Specific or adaptive immunity

Various subpopulations of lymphocytes are the principal players in adaptive immunity. These bone marrow derived cells differentiate into B and T cells, the former lineage being primarily responsible for antibody production and antigen presentation and the latter for cellular immune responses.

In contrast to the innate immune response, somatic hypermutation allows the host to generate a vast repertoire of complementary antigen receptors. However, the stimulated cell clone has to proliferate and differentiate to be fully effective. This process may take days on first presentation of a foreign antigen. Fundamental to generation of the adaptive immune response is clonal selection and deletion. This ensures that foreign antigens induce expansion and improved affinity while self antigens result in non-response through anergy or apoptosis.

B cells differentiating through B1, B2, mature B cells to plasma cells produce immunoglobulins of various classes. Mature plasma cells survive from a few days to weeks. On second exposure to antigen, memory B and T cells ensure a better secondary immune response in terms of greater rapidity and affinity. Most, but not all, foreign antigens will only stimulate a B-cell response with the aid of T helper cells. The interaction of these two types of cell through MHC class II molecules, other co-stimulatory surface molecules and cytokine such as IL-2, IL-4 and IL-5 result in somatic hypermutation with production of higher affinity antibodies, immunoglobulin class switching from IgM to other classes of antibody, and the generation of memory B cells. Immunoglobulins may neutralize toxins, kill pathogens indirectly through complement activation and by priming a number of different effector cells such as macrophages, neutrophils, NK cells and cytotoxic lymphocytes by bound antibody via Fc receptors. This is termed antibody dependent cellular cytotoxicity.

T cells mature from stems cells from bone marrow but develop within the thymus. Like B cells but through different mechanisms, they too undergo positive and negative selection to ensure that cells recognizing foreign antigens develop and proliferate but those recognizing self antigens do not. Developing T cells initially express the cell surface molecules CD4 and CD8. However, eventually they express only one or other of these molecules. CD4 positive cells usually act as helper T cells in cellular and humoral immune responses while CD8 positive T cells are usually cytotoxic. Mature T cells migrate out of the thymus and recirculate between secondary lymphoid tissue such as lymph nodes and the blood stream. Within lymph nodes they interact with antigen presenting cells such as activated dendritic cells which present antigenic peptides on the MHC class II molecule to the T-cell receptor. T-cell receptor activation is insufficient in the absence of other co-stimulatory signals. These are provided by other cell surface molecules or cytokines and in their absence T-cell activation and proliferation will not occur. Activated dendritic cells express large amounts of these co-stimulatory molecules and are potent activators of T cells. If T cells do not encounter specific antigen then the lymphocytes return to the circulation and continue trafficking between lymphoid tissue and the circulation. Lymphocytes spend approximately 30 min in the blood during each cycle around the body. They enter lymph nodes via specialized venules which express specific adhesion molecules. T helper cells are subdivided into T helper 1 (Th1) and T helper 2 (Th2) cells. In this paradigm, Th1 cells promote cellular responses to antigens in part through release of a combination of cytokines that include IL-2, IL-12, IFN-γ and tumour necrosis factor β (TNF-β), whereas Th2 cells promote humoral responses in part through release of cytokines that include IL-4, Il-5, IL-6 and IL-13 [6]. In different animal models of disease different types of helper response can have a survival advantage.

Cytotoxic (CD8) T cells recognize virally infected cells through recognition of viral peptides on MHC class I molecules. Cell death is achieved by injection of granzymes through the infected cell membrane which activates caspases to induce cell death [7]. In this brief overview of the immune system, the complexity and integrated nature of this system suggests there may be many ways of disrupting this system, either inadvertently or targeted for therapeutic gain (Fig. 8.1). However, there is also great redundancy which may defeat some approaches to successful immune modulation.

Incidental or inadvertent immunosuppression

Incidental or inadvertent immunosuppression is documented in a variety of settings. However, the significance of these investigations to clinical outcome is not always apparent.

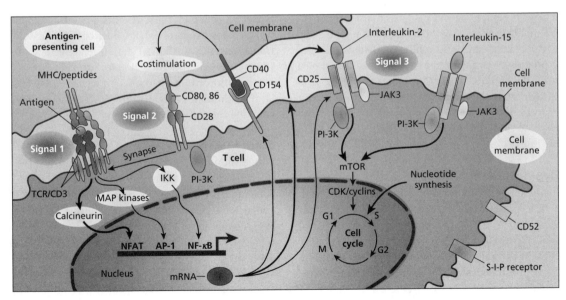

Figure 8.1 The three different signals required for full T-cell activation. From Halloran [62].

Ageing

Ageing is associated with a reduction in immune responses in many but not all elderly individuals. Ageing is associated with decreased delayed hypersensitivity, reduced IL-2 production, decreased lymphocyte response to mitogens and antigens, low rate of seroconversion and decreased antibody titre after vaccination [8].

Genetics

In addition to primary immunodeficiencies, which are well described in standard textbooks [7], investigation of genetic polymorphisms is an active research field. For example, overexpression of TNF-α may predispose to poor outcome for some diseases [9]. Deficiencies in some components of the innate system may predispose to infection [5,10].

Hypothermia

Mild hypothermia can occur during anaesthesia [11], is not uncommon in critically ill patients on admission to hospital and is now increasingly being used as a therapeutic tool [12,13]. Hypothermia can be expected to reduce the effectiveness of many aspects of host defences as the rate of enzymatic reactions and also cellular metabolism are reduced. Hypothermia inhibits release of pro-inflammatory cytokines and suppresses chemotactic migration of leucocytes and phagocytosis [13]. It also impairs T-cell-mediated antibody production and non-specific bacterial killing by neutrophils. This bacterial killing is progressively impaired as temperature is reduced from 41 to 26°C [11]. Clinical studies have also shown increased incidence of infections. This may be as a result of the effects of hypothermia on tissue hypoxia, immune function or its effect on wound healing [11,13].

Hyperglycaemia

It is increasingly appreciated that hyperglycaemia in a variety of clinical situations is associated with adverse outcome [14]. One large randomized clinical trial of patients admitted to ICUs has shown clear benefits of stringent glucose control [15]. It has also been postulated that the adverse outcomes associated with early studies of parenteral nutrition could in part be explained by poor glycaemic control in stressed patients receiving large glucose loads. Complement-mediated mechanisms such as opsonization and impairment of chemotaxis and phagocytosis in acute hyperglycaemia has been reported. The formation of reactive oxygen species as a marker of neutrophil function is also depressed [14]. Some of the adverse effects described may result from the effects of acute hyperglycaemia on the innate immune system [14].

Hypoxaemia

Hypoxaemia is prevalent in critically ill patients both outside and inside the ICU environment and may reduce resistance to infection. Not only does animal model data support this concept, at least one large human outcome study of wound infections also describes benefit of supplemental oxygen to aid adequate oxygen tension in the wound [16–19]. Both innate and adaptive immunity may be affected. Bactericidal activity of neutrophils is mediated by oxidative killing, which is dependent on production of superoxide radicals from molecular oxygen. Oxidative killing by these cells depends on the partial pressure of oxygen in the range 0 to more than 300 mmHg [19]. Hypoxia also affects superoxide production and release of mediators from macrophages [20]. IL-2 production by T lymphocytes appears to be reduced by severe hypoxia [17]). Hypoxaemia can be a mechanism by which loss of gastrointestinal mucosal integrity leads to loss of barrier defence with bacterial translocation into the circulation leading to sepsis [21], although the clinical relevance of bacterial translocation in humans has been questioned. Hypoxia also stimulates production of pro-inflammatory cytokines from intestinal epithelial cells lines [22].

Transfusion

Transfusion of allogeneic blood is immunosuppressive. Depression of NK function for up to 30 days has been observed in patients receiving whole blood [23] and defects in cell-mediated immunity have also been documented [24,25]. These immunosuppressive effects have in the past been exploited to increase survival of renal transplants [23,26]. Transfusion has also been associated with increased rates of infection and a debatable decreased survival after surgery for some types of cancer. Although the effects of blood transfusion on tumour recurrence have not been convincingly demonstrated in clinical practice, animal models clearly demonstrate adverse effects of transfusion of unmodified allogeneic blood [26].

Interpretation of outcomes is complicated by various pretreatments the donor blood receives prior to transfusion [27,28]. The immunosuppressive effects of blood are attenuated by prestorage leucodepletion. Recent data support the former association and the effects of benefits of leucodepletion in reducing infection risks compared with buffy-coat-poor blood [28]. Another randomized trial of leucodepleted blood has demonstrated a reduction in the length of hospital stay and the incidence of multiorgan failure, although infection rates were not reduced when compared with non-filtered blood [29]. Importantly, the seminal Canadian trial of transfusion in critically ill patients did not use leucodepleted blood [30] which is now universally employed in the UK and some other European countries [27]. This may limit the applicability of the results of the study.

Trauma and surgery injury

Numerous studies document that incidental trauma, surgical trauma and burn injury cause immunosuppression. In general, the extent and duration of immunosuppression is proportional to the severity of the traumatic insult. Defects in innate immunity, cell-mediated immunity and humoral immunity have been identified [31–33]. Cell-mediated immune mechanisms appear to be consistently impaired after injury with a variety of demonstrable mechanisms or defects. These include changes in suppressor to helper T-cell ratios and a milieu that favours expression of Th2 cells over Th1 cells with depression of cell-mediated immunity. Antigen presentation to T cells by monocytes may be impaired and reduced stimulation of cell-mediated immunity secondary to altered cytokine responses and prostaglandin E_2 production, together with impaired intracellular signal transduction, may all have a role. Depression of cell-mediated immunity has been shown to be strongly associated with adverse outcomes in surgical patients and ICU and trauma patients are recognized as a particularly high-risk group [34]. Some promise in reducing injury-associated immunosuppression has been seen with the use of

immune modulators such as non-steroidal analgesics [35], granulocyte colony-stimulating factor [31] and dehydroepiandrosterone [36]. Although manipulation of immune defences is an appealing and potentially promising approach, such strategies are experimental at present [37].

Drug effects

Many drugs have a spectrum of action beyond their primary indication. For example, erythromycin, a macrolide antibiotic, is a motilin antagonist. This secondary pharmacological property is now used therapeutically in surgical and intensive care practice to improve gastrointestinal motility. This drug also has effects on the innate immune system though modulation of neutrophil function [38]. Other antibiotics also have immune modulating effects, which appear to have net immunosuppressive effects and others net immunostimulatory effects [39]. Histamine-2 receptor antagonists have immunostimulatory effects that have been exploited therapeutically [40]. In contrast, proton pump inhibitors may exert suppressive effects [41]. Both types of acid suppressant are associated with an increased risk of community-acquired pneumonia but the effects of proton pump inhibitors appear greater, particularly at high dosage [42]. The preferred drug class may not just depend on primary pharmacology but the secondary immune effects may affect choice of drug for stress ulcer prophylaxis in intensive care [41].

Adrenergic agonists such as dobutamine not only have haemodynamic and thermogenic effects, but also have anti-inflammatory and immune effects which are in part a consequence of its action on inhibiting the activation of NF-κB [43]. Paradoxically, adrenergic agents may activate NK cells [44]. Dopamine has many potentially important effects beyond its haemodynamic role [45]. Although in most instances proof is lacking, secondary pharmacological and immunological effects of drugs can be important determinants of clinical outcome in some circumstances.

Nutrition

Severe nutritional deficits have effects on the immune system [46]. Marasmus (protein calorie deficiency) and kwashiorkor (protein deficiency) are both associated with immunodeficiency, most notably cell-mediated immunity. Micronutrient deficiencies of trace elements and vitamins are also associated with impaired host defences. These findings may also be of relevance to poorly nourished, catabolic, critically ill patients in the ICU setting.

Psychological stress

Psychological stress can depress some aspects of immune function through a variety of mechanisms, such as a shift in balance of Th1 to Th2 responses, as well as depression of NK cells and mucosal immunity [47–49]. This can result in increased susceptibility to infections [49].

Anaesthesia, sedation and analgesia

The effects of anaesthesia, sedatives and analgesics have been extensively studied by a variety of techniques over many years [50–56]. In general, many anaesthetic and sedative drugs cause depression of immune responses to some degree. These changes include depression of chemotaxis, phagocytosis and respiratory burst of leucocytes, depression of mitogen-induced proliferation of T cells, and depression of cytokine production by immune cells (reviewed in Galley *et al.* [56]). Opioids depress NK cell function, particularly in high dosage. These immune effects are generally short lived after discontinuation of the sedative or analgesic agent and, given the more prolonged immunodepression of surgical trauma, are considered by many to be of limited clinical significance [56].

However, some animal models suggest that even short-lived anaesthetic-induced immunosuppression may have deleterious consequences. Halothane and isoflurane increased the number of pulmonary metastases of melanoma tumour in a murine model [57]. In a recently published rat tumour model, NK cell activity was decreased by ketamine, thiopental and halothane, but not by propofol [58]. This reduced NK cell activity was associated with increased pulmonary metastases, reinforcing the possibility that perioperative immune effects of anaesthetic agents may indeed be relevant. Indeed, a package of measures to reduce perioperative immunosuppression in cancer patients has been suggested [59].

Anaesthetic agents, other sedatives and opioid analgesics are used extensively in ICUs, often for prolonged periods of time. It remains a plausible, but unproven, concern that depression of immune competence may predispose to nosocomial infection and mortality. There are similar concerns for immunosuppression in critically ill cancer patients. Claude Bernard stated in 1875, 'An anaesthetic is not just a special poison of the nervous system, it anaesthetizes all cells, benumbing all the tissues and temporarily stopping their irritability' [60]. This early observation could still be pertinent over a century later.

Intentional immunosuppression

Many immunosuppressive drugs have been identified and developed in recent years to supplement a few older drugs that still remain in use. The main indications for these drugs are to enable organ or tissue transplantation and suppression of autoimmune processes [61–64]. These agents include corticosteroids, radiation therapy, antiproliferative or cytotoxic drugs, other 'small molecule drugs' such as ciclosporin, a calcineurin inhibitor (sirolimus), a mammalian target of rapamycin inhibitor (mTOR), or protein drugs such as immune cell depleting antibodies, non-depleting antibodies and fusion proteins. Individual drug choice and therapeutic combinations are extensive, with more drugs under development targeting different components of the immune response. The interest in drug combinations results from the desire to obtain immunosuppression while avoiding drug-induced adverse effects from potentially highly toxic drugs.

Glucocorticoids

Corticosteroids are used for a variety of immunopathological and inflammatory conditions. Their pleiotrophic effects are mediated genomically and, at high doses, non-genomically [64–66]. These drugs are used so extensively in clinical medicine that detailed understanding of their mechanisms of action, pharmacokinetics and pharmacodynamics is warranted [64,65]. The most commonly used corticosteroids are hydrocortisone, prednisolone, methylprednisolone and dexamethasone (Table 8.1).

Table 8.1 Basic properties of commonly used systemic corticosteroids.

Corticosteroid	GC potency	MC potency	Duration of action	Comments
Hydrocortisone	1.0	1.0	Short	Unwanted MC effects at high dosages
Prednisolone	4	0.8	Medium	Most commonly used oral systemic corticosteroid
Methylprednisolone	5	0.5	Medium	Better lung penetration compared with prednisolone
Dexamethasone	25	0	Long	Negligible MC effects; good CNS penetration

CNS, central nervous system; GC, glucocorticoid; MC, mineralocorticoid.

Relative potencies depends on the biomarker used; for example, although tables of relative potency in standard textbooks list prednisolone and methylprednisolone with similar potencies, their mean concentrations producing half-maximum effect (EC_{50}) for T helper cell suppression are approximately 10-fold different. However, the broad potencies of corticosteroids are subdivided into glucocorticoid effects which are responsible for immune, anti-inflammatory and metabolic effects, and mineralocorticoid activity which promotes sodium retention and potassium excretion.

Two enzymes are important in the metabolism of corticosteroids. 11β hydroxysteroid dehydrogenase type 1 (11β-HSD1) is widely distributed in glucocorticoid target tissues and liver. It is a reductase that converts inactive cortisone to cortisol which binds to the intracellular glucocorticoid (GR) or mineralocorticoid (MR) receptors. However, mineralocorticoid target cells possess 11β hydroxysteroid dehydrogenase type 2 (11β-HSD2) which oxidizes cortisol to inactive cortisone, thus preventing the mineralcorticoid from occupation by cortisol. Activity of 11B-HSD2 varies with the type of glucocorticoid and this partially explains the different mineralocorticoid activity of glucocorticoids. Unwanted mineralocorticoid effects, such as hypernatraemia, fluid retention and hypokalaemia, occur when capacity of 11B-HSD2 is exceeded. These are common problems in critically ill patients.

Corticosteroids are highly lipophilic pro-drugs, usually solubilized as esters of phosphate or succinate. The drugs are converted into their active forms over a period of 5–30 min. Renal excretion of unchanged drug only accounts for 1–20% of elimination. Oxidation or reduction followed by glucuronidation or sulphation is the major means of elimination.

Hydrocortisone (cortisol) and prednisolone bind to transcortin which has high affinity but low capacity for these molecules, as well as albumin which has low affinity but high capacity. As it is the free drug that determines biological effect, this results in non-linear pharmacokinetics and dynamics when higher dosages of these drugs are used. Transcortin is saturated by hydrocortisone or prednisolone at concentrations of approximately 400 µg/L. These concentrations are reached after administration of doses of hydrocortisone or prednisolone of greater than 20 mg. The normal endogenous production of cortisol is approximately 10 mg/day with a maximum adrenal stress response of approximately 200–400 mg/day.

In contrast, methylprednisolone and dexamethasone bind only to albumin, not transcortin, and their kinetic and dynamics behave in a linear fashion. Low plasma albumin concentrations have been associated with adverse effects during prednisolone therapy and makes interpretation of adrenal gland responsiveness in patients with low albumin levels difficult, unless free concentrations of cortisol are measured [67].

Pharmacokinetic interactions with other drugs can reduce or increase drug concentrations and interactions with other drug enzyme inducers has been associated with decreased graft survival. Inhibitors of cytochrome P450 (CYP) 3A4 decrease the clearance of methylprednisolone and dexamethasone.

Dexamethasone is itself an inducer of CYP3A4 and can increase its own clearance at high doses. Other immunosuppressants also have potentially clinically important interactions [64,68].

Glucocorticoids exert their actions through a variety of genomic and non-genomic effects. Genomic effects mediated through the monomeric or dimeric glucocorticoid receptor (GR) results in trans-activation, trans-repression, post-transcriptional, translational and post-translational effects. Genomic effects require hours or days for the end effect and it is estimated that 100–1000 genes may be up-regulated or down-regulated (Table 8.2). Important effects are mediated through activation of the glucocorticoid response elements as well as through repression of the transcription factors activator protein-1 (AP-1) and NF-κB [65,66]. Non-genomic effects, which can manifest more quickly and which occur at high corticosteroid doses, may occur through GR or non-GR mechanisms. They include phospholipase A_2 inhibition through effects on annexin-1 (lipocortin-1), apoptosis and non-specific membrane effects.

The immune system effects of corticosteroids include modulation of antigen processing and presentation, activation of macrophages and dendritic cells, effects on antigen recognition and activation of T cells, interference with T helper cell responses, inhibition of the production of pro-inflammatory cytokines such as IL-1, IL-2, IL-6, IL-12, IFN-γ and TNF-α from various cells, down-regulation of adhesion molecules and chemokine receptors, inhibition of rejection effector mechanisms, inhibition of cell migration and increased apoptosis.

With these vast array of effects, glucocorticoids would be a powerful method of ensuring adequate suppression of the immune and closely linked systems to deal with autoimmune diseases and transplantation of allografts. However, at the high dosages needed, patients would suffer considerable and unacceptable adverse effects. These include massive weight gain, fat redistribution, glucose intolerance, diabetes mellitus, hypertension, dyslipidaemias, suppression of the hypothalamic-pituitary-adrenal axis, growth retardation in children, infection, reactivation of latent infection, osteoporosis, avascular bone necrosis, skin thinning, gastrointestinal ulcers, cataract, glaucoma, myopathy and psychosis.

Regimens vary with condition but have been classified in terms of daily prednisolone dosage as low (≤7.5 mg), medium (>7.5 but ≤30 mg), high (>30 but ≤100 mg), very high (>100 mg) and pulse therapy (≥250 mg for 1 to a few days). Low, medium and high regimens are associated with <50%, 50–100% and 100% GR saturation.

At modest doses twice a day, dosing is likely to produce desired immunosuppression at lower total dosage as recovery of some effects and even rebound recovery effects occur at less frequent dosing. This has been demonstrated for T helper cell suppression

Table 8.2 Effects of glucocorticoids on gene transcription.

Increased transcription
Annesin-1 (lipocortin-1, phospholipase A_2 inhibitor)
β2-adrenergic receptor
Secretory leucocyte inhibitory protein
Clara cell protein (CC10, phospholipase A_2 inhibitor)
IL-1 receptor antagonist
IL-1R2 (decoy receptor)
IκBα (inhibitor of NF-κB)
IL-10 (indirectly)

Decreased transcription
Cytokines
IL-1–IL-6, IL-9, IL-11, IL-12, IL-13, IL-18, TNF-α, GM-CSF, SCF

Chemokines
IL-8, RANTES, MIP-1α, MCP-1, MCP-3, MCP-4, eotaxin

Adhesion molecules
ICAM-1, VCAM-1, e-selectin

Inflammatory enzymes
Inducible nitric oxide synthetase
Inducible cyclo-oxygenase
Cytoplasmic phospholipase A_2

Inflammatory receptors
Tachykinin NK-1 receptors, NK-2 receptors
Bradykinin B2 receptors

Peptides
Endothelin-1

IL, interleukin; GM-CSF, granulocyte–macrophage colony-stimulating factor; ICAM, intercellular adhesion molecule; MCP, monocyte chemoattractant protein; MIP, macrophage inflammatory protein; NK, natural killer; SCF, stem-cell factor; TNF, tumour necrosis factor; VCAM, vascular cell adhesion molecule.

where methylprednisolone improved immunosuppressive efficacy with no increase in adverse effects other than suppression of endogenous cortisol production.

Pulse therapy has been used to treat a range of conditions, including transplant rejection, rapidly progressive glomerulonephritis, immune mediated diffuse alveolar haemorrhage, acute systemic lupus erythematosus (SLE) and myeloma. Common immunologically mediated diseases such as acute asthma and rheumatoid disease are treated with low to moderate dosage systemic glucocorticoids.

Radiation

Total body radiation has been used prior to stem cell transplantation and is profoundly immunosuppressive. It causes 80% of lymphocytes to undergo intermitotic death, including B cells and T-cell progenitors. Radiation also impairs cell homing. This technique has also been used for Hodgkin's disease, solid organ rejection and severe rheumatoid disease [61].

Small molecule drugs

Small molecule drugs encompass a variety of nonprotein agents that inhibit different parts of molecular processes that are required for full expression of immune recognition, activation, proliferation and effector mechanisms to cells that are recognized as non-self [61–63,68].

Antiproliferative and cytotoxic agents include cyclophosphamide, methotrexate, azathioprine and mycophenolate.

Cyclophosphamide

Cyclophosphamide is an alkylating agent that has been used for many years to reduce reliance on high dosages of corticosteroids for immunosuppression. It is used prior to stem cell transplantation and in the treatment of SLE and vasculitis. Unwanted effects include leucopenia, gonadal failure, haemorrhagic cystitis and significant risk of future malignancy. In SLE, the addition of cyclophosphamide to glucocorticoid regimens increased both short- and long-term adverse effects including mortality rates [63].

Methotrexate

Methotrexate, through its effects on folate metabolism, kills proliferating cells. It has been used in a variety of diseases including graft-versus-host disease, SLE, rheumatoid disease and psoriasis. Apart from expected haematological effects, monitoring to identify and prevent serious hepatic adverse effects is required. Unlike cyclophosphamide, methotrexate does not appear to be carcinogenic but it is teratogenic.

Azathioprine

Azathioprine is metabolized to 6-mercaptopurine, which is incorporated into DNA and results in killing of rapidly dividing cells such as lymphocytes and intestinal epithelium. Except in people with abnormal drug metabolism, standard doses cause immunosuppression without suppressing white cell counts. Nevertheless, its long-term use is associated with malignancies, bacterial and opportunistic infections.

Mycophenolate mofetil

Mycophenolate mofetil is an ester of mycophenolic acid that inhibits inosine monophosphate dehydrogenase. It inhibits the guanosine nucleotide synthetic pathway without incorporating into DNA. T and B lymphocytes are critically dependent on this pathway in contrast to other cell lines which can use other pathways. It also down-regulates adhesion molecule expression on endothelial cells. Its main adverse effects are gastrointestinal (diarrhoea), neutropenia and mild anaemia. Therapeutic drug monitoring is not required, but may be helpful given the variability of oral absorption and propensity for drug interactions.

Calcineurin inhibitors

Ciclosporin was a major advance in immunosuppressant therapeutics, allowing greater use of corticosteroid-sparing regimens and also making need for pretransplant blood transfusion immune modulation obsolete. Tacrolimus is a more potent calcineurin inhibitor that has been introduced to clinical practice recently. Both agents have limited and variable oral bioavailability, their elimination pathways are subject to induction and inhibition by other drugs and they have a narrow therapeutic window with significant adverse effects. The intravenous dosage of these calcineurin inhibitors is much less than the oral dosage and treatment for both agents is guided by therapeutic drug monitoring. Given similar efficacy, drug choice may be determined by individual patient risk factors. Ciclosporin causes nephrotoxicity, hypertension, hyperlipidaemia, post-transplant diabetes mellitus, neurotoxicity and aesthetic problems such as hirsutism and gum hyperplasia as well as haemolytic-uraemic syndrome. Tacrolimus is associated with a higher incidence of post-transplant diabetes mellitus and neurotoxicity but a lower incidence of the other ciclosporin-induced problems listed above.

Target of rapamycin (mTOR) inhibitors

Sirolimus, and its sister drug, everolimus, inhibits mTOR and prevents IL-2 driven T-cell proliferation. In addition to its primary use as an immunosuppressant, sirolimus is also used to prevent coronary restenosis after stenting [1]. As its primary target differs from the calcineurin inhibitors, it can be used to complement these agents although the combination of tacrolimus with sirolimus is more nephrotoxic than the combination of tacrolimus with mycophenolate. Its principal non-immune adverse effects include hyperlipidaemia, thrombocytopenia, delayed wound healing, mouth ulcers, pneumonitis and interstitial lung disease.

Other small molecule immunosuppressants

FTY720 is a derivative of myriocin, a fungal product that is an antagonist for sphingosine-1-phosphate receptors. It results in enhanced homing of lymphocytes to lymphoid tissues and prevents their egress, with resulting lymphopenia. It causes nausea, vomiting, diarrhoea, alterations of liver enzymes and first-dose bradycardia. It is currently undergoing phase III clinical trials.

Depleting antibodies

Depleting antibodies destroy T or B cells, or both, and the release of cytokines after administration can produce severe adverse effects. These include polyclonal antithymocyte globulin, muromonab-CD3, alemtuzumab and rituximab.

Antithymocyte globulin

Antithymocyte globulin, obtained from immunizing horses or rabbits, produces profound and long-lasting lymphopenia. This can leave the patient very vulnerable to immunodeficiency complications as well as thrombocytopenia, cytokine-release syndrome and hypersensitivity reactions such as serum sickness.

Muromonab-CD3

Muromonab-CD3 is a mouse antibody against CD3 and has been used for induction of immunosuppression in transplantation and to treat rejection episodes. Like antithymocyte globulin, it can cause a severe cytokine release syndrome and its use is associated with subsequent lymphoproliferative disorders including malignant lymphoma.

Alemtuzumab

Alemtuzumab is an anti-CD52 antibody and massively depletes lymphocytes, macrophages and NK cells. It is licensed for the treatment of chronic lymphocytic anaemia but has been used 'off-label' in transplantation.

Rituximab

Rituximab is an anti-CD20 antibody that depletes B cells and is licensed for use in B-cell lymphomas. Again it has been used 'off-label' as an adjunct to other immunosuppressives and because its target is more selective than some of the other depleting antibodies, the associated adverse effects appear less.

Non-depleting antibodies and fusion proteins

These are drugs that reduce responsiveness of cells without destroying lymphoid populations and include daclizumab, basiliximab and belatacept (LEA29Y). Daclizumab and basiliximab are anti-CD25 monoclonal antibodies that are used in transplantation as part of an induction regimen. They cause little depletion of T cells and, in combination with calcineurin inhibitors, reduce rejection episodes by approximately one-third. Belatacept is a fusion protein combined with IgG. It prevents co-stimulation of T cell CD28 molecules by B7 (CD80 and CD86) ligands on antigen presenting cells. Preventing this important co-stimulation offers the prospect of long-term use of non-depleting antibodies to reduce the need for small molecule immunosuppressants such as the calcineurin inhibitors [69]. Further study of this and other agents is required to confirm whether the considerable early promise of these approaches is effective and less toxic in the long term [70].

Intravenous immunoglobulin

Intravenous immunoglobulin (IVIG) is widely used as immune modulator in diseases such as Guillain–Barré syndrome, myasthenia gravis, Kawasaki's syndrome, ANCA-positive vasculitis, autoimmune uveitis and prevention of graft-versus-host disease in bone marrow transplantation, as well as a miscellany of other conditions [71]. The mode of action is complex, involving functions of Fc receptors, interference with activation of complement and cytokine networks, through anti-idiotypic antibodies and through modulation of activation, differentiation and effector functions of T cells. Adverse effects occur in less than 5% of patients, most often including chills, headache, nausea, fatigue, myalgia, arthralgia and hypertension. Aseptic meningitis and acute renal failure are also well documented.

Rhesus antigens and anti-D

Polyclonal human IgG solutions containing an enriched fraction of antibodies against the D blood group have been given to suppress immune responses of rhesus negative mothers with rhesus positive offspring [61]. This highly successful immunological management policy has prevented many cases of haemolytic anaemia of the newborn or erythroblastosis fetalis.

Infection and malignancy following transplantation

Infection and late malignancy are problems of major concern to clinicians and patients. Immunosuppression predisposes patients to infection, especially when combined with breakdown of natural barriers following surgery or pre-bone marrow transplant

'conditioning' with cytotoxic agents and subsequent mucositis. They include an increased incidence of infections found in non-immunocompromised hosts such as bacterial urinary tract infections, as well as those most often found in immunocompromised individuals. Patients are at risk both from new infections and reactivation of old or latent infections [72–74]. Some immunosuppressive regimens require prophylaxis against likely pathogens such as the herpes viruses or *Pneumocystis jerovecci* [75]. Infection is a major barrier to xenotransplantation in humans [76].

Malignancy is another long-term risk of immunosuppressed patients that has been extensively studied [77,78]. Immunosuppressed allograft patients have a three- to fourfold increased risk of developing tumours. With the exception of lip and cutaneous malignancies, particular types of malignancy are associated with immunosuppression: lymphomas, lymphoproliferative disorders, Kaposis's sarcoma, renal carcinoma, cervical carcinoma, hepatobiliary carcinomas, anogenital carcinomas and various other sarcomas [77]. Some of these tumours are associated with viruses such as Epstein–Barr virus, human herpes virus 8 and human papillomavirus [78]. Some tumours respond to reduction in immunosuppression although immunosuppression itself does not fully account for the causal link between immunosuppressives and cancer. Ciclosporin increases metastatic disease in laboratory animals devoid of an immune system and sirolimus can prevent tumours or cause them to regress in some circumstances [78]. Therapeutically, substitution of sirolimus for other immunosuppressive agents has been associated with remission of Kaposi's sarcoma and this together with new approaches to immunosuppression gives some hope that the risks of cancer in these patients can be reduced in addition to improved graft survival [70,78].

Conclusions

In summary, innate and adaptive immunity is essential for the survival of large multicellular organisms. These immune mechanisms may be subverted unintentionally by a variety of means during clinical practice and these may be important for host survival in some circumstances. Intentional immuno-suppression is required for those patients requiring allogeneic transplants or control of autoimmune diseases. The goal is to refine immunosuppressive regimens to maximize patient benefits while decreasing adverse effects and risks. Research and innovation continue.

References

1 Moliterno DJ. Healing Achilles: sirolimus versus paclit-axel. *N Engl J Med* 2005; **353**: 724–7.

2 Delves PJ, Roitt IM. The immune system (First and second of two parts). *N Engl J Med* 2000; **343**: 37–49; 108–17.

3 Medzhitov R, Janeway C. Innate immunity. *N Engl J Med* 2000; **343**: 338–44.

4 Tosi MF. Innate immune responses to infection. *J Allergy Clin Immunol* 2005; **116**: 241–9.

5 Lin MT, Albertson TE. Genomic polymorphisms in sepsis. *Crit Care Med* 2004; **32**: 569–79.

6 Sheeran P, Hall GM. Cytokines in anaesthesia. *Br J Anaesth* 1997; **78**: 201–19.

7 Janeway CA, Travers P, Walport M, Sclomchik MJ. *Immunobiology*, 6th edn. New York: Garland Science Publishing, 2005.

8 Kumar CR. Graying of the immune system: can nutrient supplements improve immunity in the elderly? *JAMA* 1997; **277**: 1398–9.

9 Tracey KJ. TNF and Mae West or: too much of a good thing. *Lancet* 1995; **345**: 75–6.

10 Cook JA. The toll of sepsis: altered innate immunity in polymicrobial sepsis. *Crit Care Med* 2003; **31**: 1860–2.

11 Sessler DI. Complications and treatment of mild hypothermia. *Anesthesiology* 2001; **95**: 531–43.

12 Polderman KH. Application of therapeutic hypothermia in the ICU: opportunities and pitfalls of a promising treatment modality. Part 1: Indications and evidence. *Intensive Care Med* 2004; **30**: 556–75.

13 Polderman KH. Application of therapeutic hypothermia in the ICU: opportunities and pitfalls of a promising treatment modality. Part 2: Practical aspects and side effects. *Intensive Care Med* 2004; **30**: 757–69.

14 Turina M, Fry DE, Polk HC. Acute hyperglycemia and the innate immune system: clinical, cellular and molecular aspects. *Crit Care Med* 2005; **33**: 1624–33.

15 Van den Berghe G, Wouters PM, Weekers F, *et al.* Intensive insulin therapy in critically ill patients. *N Engl J Med* 2001; **345**: 1359–67.

16 Allen DB, Maguire JJ, Mahdavian M, *et al.* Wound hypoxia and acidosis limit neutrophil bacterial killing mechanisms. *Arch Surg* 1997; **132**: 991–6.

17 Zuckerberg AL, Goldberg LI, Lederman HM. Effects of hypoxia on interleukin-2 mRNA expression by T lymphocytes. *Crit Care Med* 1994; **22**: 197–203.

18 Hopf HW, Hunt TK, West JM, *et al.* Wound tissue oxygen tension predicts the risk of wound infection in surgical patients. *Arch Surg* 1997; **132**: 997–1005.

19 Greif R, Akca O, Horn EP, Kurz A, Sessler DI. Supplemental perioperative oxygen to reduce the incidence of wound infection. *N Engl J Med* 2000; **342**: 161–7.

20 Gennari R, Alexander JW. Effects of hypoxia on bacterial translocation and mortality during gut-derived sepsis. *Arch Surg* 1996; **131**: 57–62.

21 West M, Li MH, Seatter SC, Bubrick MP. Pre-exposure to hypoxia or septic stimuli differentially regulates endotoxin release of tumour necrosis factor, interleukin-6, interleukin-1, prostaglandin E_2, nitric oxide, and superoxide by macrophages. *J Trauma* 1994; **37**: 82–90.

22 Bertges DJ, Fink MP, Delude RL. Hypoxic signal transduction in critical illness. *Crit Care Med* 2000; **28** (Suppl.): N78–86.

23 Jensen LS, Andersen AJ, Christiansen PM, *et al.* Postoperative infection and natural killer cell function following blood transfusion in patients undergoing elective colorectal surgery. *Br J Surg* 1982; **79**: 513–6.

24 Ross WB, Yap PL. Blood transfusion and organ transplantation. *Blood Rev* 1990; **4**: 252–8.

25 Raghavan M, Marik PE. Anemia, allogenic blood transfusion and immunomodulation in the critically ill. *Chest* 2005; **127**: 295–307.

26 Blajchman MA. Immunomodulation and blood transfusion. *Am J Ther* 2002; **9**: 389–96.

27 Silliman CC, Moore EE, Johnston JL, Gonzalez RJ, Biffle WL. Transfusion of the injured patient: proceed with caution. *Shock* 2004; **21**: 291–9.

28 Jensen LS, Puho E, Pedersen L, Mortensen FV, Sorenesen HT. Long-term survival after colorectal surgery associated with buffy-coat-poor and leucocyte depleted blood transfusions: a follow-up study. *Lancet* 2005; **365**: 681–2.

29 Van Hilten JA, van de Watering LMG, van Bockel JH, *et al.* Effects of transfusion with red cells filtered to remove leucocytes: randomised controlled trial in patients undergoing major surgery. *Br Med J* 2004; **328**: 1281–8.

30 Hebert PC, Wells G, Blajchman MA, *et al.* A multicenter randomized controlled clinical trial of transfusion requirements in critical care. *N Engl J Med* 1999; **340**: 409–17.

31 Angele MK, Faist E. Immunodepression in the surgical patient and increased susceptibility to infection. *Crit Care* 2002; **6**: 298–305.

32 Martin C. Immune responses after trauma and haemorrhagic shock. In: Galley HF, ed. *Critical Care Focus 11*. Oxford: Blackwell Publishing, 2005: 26–35.

33 Boddie DE, Currie DG, Eremin O, Heys SD. Immune suppression and isolated severe head injury: a significant clinical problem. *Br J Neurosurg* 2003; **17**: 405–17.

34 Christou NV, Meakins JL, Gordon J, *et al.* The delayed hypersensitivity response and host resistance in surgical patients: 20 years later. *Ann Surg* 1995; **222**: 534–46.

35 Faist E, Ertel W, Cohnert T, *et al.* Immunoprotective effects of cyclooxygenase inhibitors in patients with major surgical trauma. *J Trauma* 1990; **30**: 8–18.

36 Jarrar D, Kuebler JF, Wang P, Bland KI, Chaudry IH. DHEA: a novel adjunct for the treatment of male trauma patients. *Trends Mol Med* 2001; **7**: 81–5.

37 Windsor ACJ, Klava A, Somers SS, Guillou PJ, Reynolds JV. Manipulation of local and systemic host defence in the prevention of perioperative sepsis. *Br J Surg* 1995; **82**: 1460–7.

38 Hoeben D, Dosogne H, Heyneman R, Burvenich C. Effect of antibiotics on the phagocytic and respiratory burst activity of granulocytes. *Eur J Pharmacol* 1997; **332**: 289–97.

39 Van Vlem B, Vanholder R, dePaepe P, Vogelaers D, Ringoir S. Immunomodulating effects of antibiotics: literature review. *Infection* 1996; **24**: 275–91.

40 Nielsen HJ, Christiansen IJ, Moesgard F, Kehlet H and the Danish RANX05 Colorectal Cancer Study Group. Ranitidine as an adjuvant treatment in colorectal cancer. *Br J Surg* 2002; **89**: 1416–22.

41 Noble DW. Proton pump inhibitors and stress ulcer prophylaxis: pause for thought? *Crit Care Med* 2002; **30**: 1175–6.

42 Gregor JC. Acid suppression and pneumonia. *JAMA* 2004; **295**: 2012–3.

43 Loop T, Bross T, Humar M, *et al.* Dobutamine inhibits phorbo-myristate-acetate-induced activation of nuclear factor-κB in human T lymphocytes *in vitro*. *Anesth Analg* 2004; **99**: 1508–15.

44 Nomoto Y, Karasawa S, Uehara K. Effects of hydrocortisone and adrenaline on natural killer cell activity. *Br J Anaesth* 1994; **73**: 318–21.

45 Cuthbertson BH, Noble DW. Dopamine and oliguria. *Br Med J* 1997; **314**: 690–1.

46 Cunningham-Rundles S, McNeeley DF, Moon A. Mechanisms of nutrient modulation of the immune response. *J Allergy Clin Immunol* 2005; **115**: 1119–28.

47 Reichlin S. Neuroendocrine-immune interactions. *N Engl J Med* 1993; **329**: 1246–53.

48 Khansari DN, Murgo AJ, Faith RE. Effects of stress on the immune system. *Immunology Today* 1990; **11**: 170–5.

49 Agarwal SK, Marshall GD. Stress effects on immunity and its application to clinical immunology. *Clin Exp Allergy* 2001; **31**: 25–31.

50 Bruce DL, Wingard DW. Anesthesia and the immune response. *Anesthesiology* 1971; **34**: 271–82.

51 Duncan PG, Cullen BF. Anesthesia and immunology. *Anesthesiology* 1976; **45**: 522–38.

52 Walton B. Anaesthesia, surgery and immunology. *Anaesthesia* 1978; **33**: 322–48.

53 Walton B. Effects of anaesthesia and surgery on immune status. *Br J Anaesth* 1979; **51**: 37–43.

54 Stevenson GW, Hall SC, Rudnick S, Seleny FL, Stevenson HC. The effect of anaesthetic agents on the human immune response. *Anesthesiology* 1990; **72**: 542–52.

55 Salo M. Effects of anaesthesia and surgery in the immune response. *Acta Anesthesiol Scand* 1992: **36**: 201–20.

56 Galley HE, DiMatteo MA, Webster NR. Immunomodulation by anaesthetic agents: Does it matter? *Intensive Care Med* 2000; **26**: 267–74.

57 Moudgil GC, Singal DP. Halothane and isoflurane enhance melanoma tumour metastasis in mice. *Can J Anaesth* 1997; **44**: 90–4.

58 Melamed R, Bar-Yosef S, Shakhar G, Shakhar K, Ben-Eliyahu S. Suppression of natural killer cell activity and promotion of tumour metastasis by ketamine, thiopental and halothane but not by propofol: mediating mechanisms and prophylactic measures. *Anesth Anal* 2003; **97**: 1331–9.

59 Vallejo R, Hord ED, Barna SA, Santiago-Palma J, Ahmed S. Perioperative immunosuppression in cancer patients. *J Environ Pathol Toxicol Oncol* 2003; **22**: 139–46.

60 Moudgil GC. Anaesthesia and leucocyte locomotion. *Can J Anaesth* 1992; **39**: 899–904.

61 Nelson RP, Ballow M. Immunomodulation and immunotherapy: drugs, cytokines, cytokine receptors and antibodies. *J Allergy Clin Immunol* 2003; **111**: S720–32.

62 Halloran PF. Immunosuppressive drugs for kidney transplantation. *N Engl J Med* 2004; **351**: 2715–29.

63 Fine DM. Pharmacological therapy for lupus nephritis. *JAMA* 2005; **293**: 3053–60.

64 Czock D, Keller F, Rasche FM, Haussler U. Pharmacokinetics and pharmacodynamics of systemically administered glucocorticoids. *Clin Pharmacokinet* 2005; **44**: 61–98.

65 Barnes PJ, Adcock IM. How do corticosteroids work in asthma? *Ann Intern Med* 2003; **139**: 359–70.

66 Barnes PJ, Karin M. Nuclear factor-κB: a pivotal transcription factor in chronic inflammatory diseases. *N Engl J Med* 1997; **336**: 1066–71.

67 Hamrahian AH, Oseni TS, Arafah BM. Measurement of free cortisol in the critically ill. *N Engl J Med* 2004; **350**: 1629–38.

68 Kahan BD. Koch SM. Current immunosuppressant regimens: considerations for critical care. *Curr Opin Crit Care* 2001; **7**: 242–50.

69 Vicenti F, Larsen C, Durrbach A, *et al.* Costimulation blockade with belatacept in renal transplantation. *N Engl J Med* 2005; **353**: 770–81.

70 Ingelfinger JR, Schwartz RS. Immunosuppression: the promise of specificity. *N Engl J Med* 2005; **353**: 836–9.

71 Kazatchkine MD, Kaveri SV. Immunomodulation of autoimmune and inflammatory diseases with intravenous immune globulin. *N Engl J Med* 2001; **345**: 747–55.

72 Kang I, Park SH. Infectious complications in SLE after immunosuppressive therapies. *Curr Opin Rheumatol* 2003; **15**: 528–34.

73 Fishman JA, Rubin RH. Infection in organ-transplant recipients. *N Engl J Med* 1998; **338**: 1741–51.

74 Lionakis MS, Kontoylannis DP. Glucocorticoids and invasive fungal infections. *Lancet* 2003; **362**: 1828–38.

75 Thomas CF, Limper AH. *Pneumocystis* pneumonia. *N Engl J Med* 2004; **350**: 2487–98.

76 Webster NR. Animal tissues into humans. *Br J Anaesth* 1998; **80**: 281–2.

77 Penn I. Post-transplant malignancy: the role of immunosuppression. *Drug Saf* 2000; **23**: 101–13.

78 Dantal J, Soulillou J-P. Immunosuppressive drugs and the risk of cancer after organ transplantation. *N Engl J Med* 2005; **352**: 1371–3.

CHAPTER 9

Mechanisms of anaesthesia: a role for voltage-gated K channels?

Peter Århem, Kristoffer Sahlholm and Johanna Nilsson

Introduction

The mechanisms of how general anaesthetics induce unconsciousness are little known. This is surprising considering the fact that general anaesthesia was introduced more than 150 years ago, when Crawford Long performed the first surgical operation with ether anaesthesia [1].

The lack of knowledge concerning anaesthetic mechanisms pertains to all levels of brain organization. At the macroscopic level, we have knowledge about a number of brain structures that are affected by general anaesthetics but we have little detailed knowledge about which structures are critical for anaesthesia. Similarly, at the mesoscopic level, we know how anaesthetics modulate cellular processes in a number of systems but not which modifications are critical. At the microscopic level, we know how anaesthetics phenomenologically affect membrane proteins, but not by which molecular mechanisms and not which membrane proteins are critically affected. Consequently, we do not know how these interact to produce anaesthesia.

One of the problems complicating the determination of the anaesthetic mechanisms at all levels is the fact that anaesthetics form a very diverse chemical group. General anaesthetics comprise: chemically unrelated compounds such as nitrous oxide, diethyl ether, halogenated hydrocarbons, alcohols, barbiturates, and ketamine and propofol. Does this imply that anaesthesia is caused by many different mechanisms? It seems so, and consequently a unitary theory, once dominant, now appears obsolete.

The difficulty in solving the general anaesthesia problem is highlighted by its close connection to the consciousness problem, one of the greatest challenges to human rationality. We do not know which brain structures cause conscious processes, which cellular activity is associated with experiencing or which physical brain processes correlate critically with mental activity.

The main aim of this chapter is to summarize briefly some aspects of current knowledge about the function of general anaesthetics at different organization levels. In particular, we highlight the possible role of voltage-gated K channels as targets for anaesthetics.

Target brain structures — three principal theories

Which structures of the brain are critically affected by general anaesthetics? Which structures are critically associated with loss of consciousness? Three principal theories have come to dominate the field. They differ in locating the critical structure to cortex, thalamus or to the reticular activating system. They all aim to explain the characteristics of cortical activity at the different steps of general anaesthesia as reflected by electroencephalography (EEG): at the level of sedation, the paradoxical increase in power at all frequencies; at hypnosis, the occurrence of delta waves and the decrease in power at high frequencies; and at anaesthesia, the emergence of burst suppression (i.e. irregular activity at low power interrupted by periods of silence). The changes in cortical activity are paralleled by changes in the activity of thalamic intralaminar relay neurones; at sedation, tonic firing is transformed into burst activity, associated with increased Ca currents and induced Ca-activated K currents. The increased Ca current is assumed to be caused by a hyperpolarization of the relay neurones, resulting in a faster recovery from inactivation [2].

The changes in EEG during the time evolution of general anaesthesia are not uniform, with the anterior and posterior parts of the cortex showing separate modifications. John [3] summarizes the results from a long series of quantitative EEG studies of anaesthetic effects:

1 A general lowering of frequency over the whole cortex

2 A relative increase in the activity of anterior cortical regions compared with posterior

3 An increased coherence between low frequency activity in frontal areas and an uncoupling between activity in anterior and posterior regions.

Both increased and decreased activity, as well as increased and decreased coherence, thus characterizes anaesthetic-induced unconsciousness. From this we can conclude that neither simple suppression nor simple disruption of coherence explains general anaesthesia. Obviously, we have to search for more sophisticated theories.

Cortex theories assume that the observed effects are caused mainly by a direct effect on cortical neurones. This is supported by neocortical slice studies as well as simulation studies [4]. A major problem is that it has not been possible to record delta waves from isolated neocortical slices.

Thalamus theories assume that the observed effects are caused by direct effects on thalamic intralaminar relay neurones. This implies that general anaesthetics cause the observed tonic to bursting transition, in turn causing the observed cortical effects. How? Why are the relay neurones hyperpolarized? By direct activation of K channels in the relay neurones or by indirect inhibitory GABA activity? The thalamus theories are supported by the fact that experiments on neocortical slices including thalamic neurones show delta waves [2].

Reticular system theories assume direct effects on neurones in the reticular activating system, causing a switch-like transformation of the activity on both the thalamus and cortical level, much like sleep induction. This theory has little experimental support at present. Very little is known about direct effects on reticular activating system (RAS) neurones. These theories derive their support from the similarity between general anaesthesia and sleep processes.

This series of principal theories also displays a gradual transformation from process-specific theories to neurone-specific theories. In cortical theories, the general anaesthetics are often assumed to simultaneously attack a large dynamic network of cells, while in RAS theories they are assumed to attack a smaller and more specified neuronal target. Within the framework of all these theories, we find two competing ideas: one of direct suppression and the other of disrupting coherence [5]. Presumably, the final theory of general anaesthesia will make use of a combination of these ideas.

These questions reflect closely related problems in the discussion on the neuronal correlate of consciousness. Here we can also separate two sorts of theories. Either consciousness depends on activity in specific groups of neurones, or it depends on specific processes in unspecified neurones in a larger dynamic population. Roughly speaking, the view of Crick and Koch [6] can be classified as neurone-specific. They search for specific awareness neurones, possibly characterized by a tendency to fire bursts synchronously, and possibly distributed in cortex (the lower layers), thalamus and the limbic system. Equally roughly speaking, we can classify the attempts by Tononi and Edelman [7] as process-specific. These workers look for a specific form of activity in cortical neurones that forms a coherent but variable dynamic core as the correlate to consciousness. Similar ideas have been presented in terms of adaptive resonance, interneural synchrony, coherent oscillations and temporal coherence. Considering the different arguments used in the debate, we find the most likely solution to be a combination of the two main theories: consciousness depends on specific coherent activity in a specific population of cortical neurones. Similarly, we find the most likely explanation of anaesthesia to be an anaesthetic-induced modification of specific coherent activity in specific neurones; different neurones for different anaesthetics. Note, however, that the neurones directly involved in consciousness need not necessarily be the neurones directly affected by general anaesthetics.

Molecular effects — the dominant theories are focused on ion channels

We now consider the molecular mechanism of anaesthesia. Of the different organization level approaches to the problem of anaesthesia, the molecular level approach has probably been the most fertile so far. A number of investigations have described effects of general anaesthetics in molecular detail [8].

The first, more detailed molecular theory was advanced by Charles Ernest Overton in his classic *Studien über die Narkose* 1901. In this classic work he demonstrates the correlation between anaesthetic effect and lipid solubility, measured as distribution coefficient in water–alcohol. Over the years, however, the Overton lipid theory lost ground to theories assuming proteins to be the critical targets. Today, protein theories focus on ion channels [8].

Which anaesthetic-induced ion channel modifications are critical in causing anaesthesia? The dominant theories are focused on two ligand-gated channels: γ-aminobutyric acid (GABA) and *N*-methyl-D-aspartate (NMDA) channels. Voltage-activated channels have also been suggested as main targets. However, the problem is not to demonstrate that anaesthetics affect channels, but to demonstrate which effects are critical in causing anaesthesia.

At the centre of the debate is the ionotropic $GABA_A$ channel. In most scenarios, the anaesthetics are assumed to activate $GABA_A$ channels in thalamic neurones, which leads to hyperpolarization and decreased activity in postsynaptic cortical cells [9]. This is in accordance with the suppression idea. Mihic *et al.* [10] have, by clever use of chimeric constructs, localized the binding sites for volatile anaesthetics on the $GABA_A$ channel. But is this mechanism general-izable and does it also apply to other anaesthetics? Other than some investigations on alcohol effects, we have little further information.

Another influential theory calls attention to the NMDA channel as the critical target for general anaesthetics [11]. The NMDA channel has a unique position among channels in necessitating a dual action of both ligand (glutamate) and voltage to open. This means that NMDA channels can function as coincidence detectors and act in associative networks. In accordance with this view, ketamine acts as a specific NMDA channel blocker. But what about other general anaesthetics? Do they block NMDA channels specifically? Under all circumstances, Flohr [11] argues that ultimately all general anaesthetics directly or indirectly inhibit NMDA currents and thereby some aspects of neuronal activity, essential for consciousness.

Recently, a subfamily of K channels has come into focus as critical target for anaesthetic action. Both enhancement and block of certain two-pore loop K channels have been reported at relatively low concentrations of various volatile anaesthetics [2,12,13]. This might explain the remarkable anaesthetic-induced enhancement of leak current in specific neurones of the snail *Lymnea stagnalis*. Another case of anaesthetic-induced effects on a background channel is the block of flicker channels in myelinated axons at low concentrations of local anaesthetics [14]; but the picture is still fragmentary.

Kv channels — a novel target for general anaesthetics

Here we explore the role of yet another channel family in general anaesthesia, voltage-gated K channels (Kv). Most general anaesthetics have been shown also to block voltage-gated channels, but as a rule they have been assumed to act at higher concentrations than those blocking $GABA_A$ and NMDA channels [8]. However, a number of investigations have shown that both volatile and intravenous anaesthetics affect voltage-gated channels, including Kv channels, at clinically used concentrations, implying that they in some cases affect Kv channels at the same concentration as they affect GABA$_A$ channels [15–17]. That Kv channels are critically involved in anaesthesia has been clear long since; the Shaker channel is named after the *Drosophila* mutant, which under ether narcosis shows shaking movements [18]. The Shaker mutant was shown to lack the Shaker channel. The neural activity under ether narcosis evidently depends on the occurrence of Kv channels in neurones. But how channel specific are the effects? Can we find specific ultrasensitive voltage-gated channels? A growing number of studies suggest that this may be the case [19].

Voltage-gated channels and their close relatives form the third largest superfamily of signal-transduction proteins, only outnumbered by G-protein-coupled receptors and protein kinases, and comprise 143 members in the human genome [20]. Of these, K channels form a 88-member main body, including the classic voltage-gated (Kv) and the mentioned two-pore loop (K2p; 15 members in 15 subfamilies) channels [20].

The human Kv family has 40 members, classified into 12 subfamilies. The classic voltage-gated K channels belong to four subfamilies, Kv1–Kv4, comprising delayed rectifiers and inactivating channels (associated with A-type K current). These four subfamilies form the mammalian counterparts to the well-studied *Drosophila* K channels *Shaker, Shab, Shaw* and *Shal*. Kv5–Kv9 comprise subunits that form non-functional homotetramers, but function as regulators in Kv2 heterotetramers. Kv10–Kv12 are channels that are voltage-dependent but also regulated by cyclic nucleotides. Kv10–Kv12 are the mammalian counterparts to the *Drosophila ether-a-go-go* channels.

These channels regulate the resting potential and sculpture the firing patterns of activated neurones, two features essential in all molecular theories of anaesthesia. Assuming that disruption of coherence has a role in general anaesthesia, it is not surprising that K channels have come into focus as targets for general anaesthetics.

The molecular structure of Kv channels is better known than the structure of any other channel, and one bacterial Kv channel has recently been crystallized and partly structurally determined [21]. To understand the molecular mechanism of general an-

aesthetic action on Kv channels it is of some interest to review briefly the molecular structure of a Kv channel as we know it today. Kv channels are composed of four similar or identical subunits, symmetrically arranged around a central ion-conducting pore. These subunits consist of assemblies of six transmembrane α helices, S1–S6, where S1–S4 form a voltage-sensing domain, and S5 and S6 an ion-conducting pore domain (Fig. 9.1a). The outer portion of the pore domain forms a selectivity filter — a narrow pathway that determines which ion will pass. At the intracellular part of the pore, the four S6s form an inner vestibule, at the internal end limited by a narrow passage (a gate) that can open up when the channel is activated (Fig. 9.1b).

Role of Kv channels in normally functioning brain

Because of the diversity of the Kv channel family, the role of Kv channels in normally functioning brain is

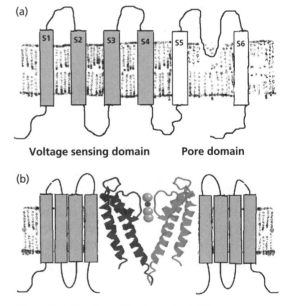

Figure 9.1 Structure of Kv channels. (a) The transmembrane topology of a subunit. The first four transmembrane segments (S1–S4) form the voltage sensing domain and the last two the pore domain. (b) Side view of a channel, comprising two subunits. The pore region (represented by KcsA [47]) shows the selectivity filter and the internal vestibule.

highly complex. The importance of a specific channel relates to its specific kinetics, its specific distribution in the brain and its specific distribution on the neuronal surface. Although our knowledge is still fragmentary, something of a consensus view is available both for the kinetics of Kv channels and for the distribution of Kv channels, at least in hippocampus neurones. We therefore summarize briefly what is known about the localization of Kv channels in hippocampal neurones and the expected functional relevance. For simplicity, we here focus on the four 'classic' types of Kv channels, the members of the Kv1–Kv4 subfamilies.

The Kv1 subfamily

The Kv1 subfamily is the most diverse of the Kv subfamilies, comprising eight members. Kv1 homotetramers are mainly delayed rectifiers; the Kv1.4 homotetramer being an exception in forming rapidly inactivating channels. Kv1.4 also confers its inactivation capacity to heterotetramers, as do several accessory β subunits. In hippocampus, the Kv channels are mainly heteromeric, forming two main groups: one consisting of Kv1.1–Kv1.4 channels and another of Kv1.1–Kv1.2 channels [22]. Kv1.1, 1.2 and 1.4 subunits are mainly located axonally, thus being in the position to regulate transmitter release [23]. Specifically, Kv1.4 has been assumed to be involved in synaptic frequency facilitation [24]. Kv1.1 knockout experiments suggest relatively small effects at the neuronal level [25]. In a study of the effects of truncating the Kv1.1 channel on neuronal activity, we found that the mutation induced increased firing frequencies in interneurones (mossy cells in the dentate gyrus) [26]. At the system level, the situation is more difficult to review. Knockout experiments show that eliminating Kv1.1 causes epilepsy, reflected as strong low-frequency oscillations of the electric field in cortex [25,26].

The Kv2 subfamily

The Kv2 subfamily is a small two-member subfamily, both members displaying slow delayed rectifier properties. Kv2.1 has been located to the soma and proximal dendrites in hippocampal principal neurones [27]. Antisense-knockdown experiments suggest that Kv2.1 expression is necessary for

action potential repolarization during high-frequency (1 Hz) stimulation, but not during low-frequency (0.2 Hz) stimulation in cultured CA1 pyramidal neurones. Additionally, Kv2.1 conductance has been shown to affect dendritic Ca^{2+} influx, suggesting a role for Kv2.1 in synaptic plasticity [28]. In summary, Kv2.1 seems to support high frequency firing at a cellular level. The implications of this at the system level are still unclear.

The Kv3 subfamily

The Kv3 subfamily comprises four members, Kv3.1 and Kv3.2 forming homotetrameric delayed rectifiers, and Kv3.3 and Kv3.4 forming inactivating homotetramers. Kv3.4 imparts its inactivation capacity to heterotetramers [29]. The steady-state activation–voltage curves of homomeric Kv3 channels, independent of expression system, are all shifted rightwards compared to those of other Kv channels, implying that Kv3 channels deactivate much faster than other Kv channels [30]. This capacity suggests that Kv3 has a role in fast-spiking neurones, a hypothesis supported by experimental evidence [27,31]. Kv3 channels are less restricted with reference to its localization than the other Kv channels, in hippocampus being located in proximal dendrites, soma, axons and terminals of preferentially interneurones [27,29]. At the system level, knockout experiments suggest that Kv3 channels paradoxically keep the frequency of electrical field fluctuations in cortex down. Kv3 knockout experiments with mice resulted in increased gamma and decreased delta frequencies on EEG [32].

The Kv4 subfamily

The Kv4 subfamily comprises three members, all forming rapidly inactivating channels. Kv4 channels activate already at subthreshold potentials, and recover very fast from inactivation upon repolarization [33]. Kv4.2 and Kv4.3 are expressed in dendrites of hippocampal principal neurones [23], and are presumed to regulate action potential back-propagation and Ca^{2+}-influx in dendrites, thus possibly having a role in associative long-term potentiation [34,35]. They favour low-frequency, regularly spiking activity; the subthreshold activation attenuating action potential initiation [27]. The role of Kv4 channels at the system level is much less studied, but it is not difficult to conceive the synaptic gatekeeper role as fundamental at higher organization levels.

In summary, the four major subfamilies of voltage-gated channels seem to serve several basic functions. At a cellular level, Kv2 and Kv3 channels seem involved in high-frequency firing, while Kv1 and Kv4 may have more of a dampening effect on neural activity. At a system level, the picture is less clear because of the highly non-linear relationship between individual cell firing and fluctuations in the cortical mean field. Elimination of Kv1 results in strong low-frequency field oscillations (i.e. epilepsy), while elimination of Kv3 results in increased high-frequency (gamma band) activity.

General anaesthetics affect different Kv channels differently

Against this background of growing knowledge about species-specific roles of Kv channels for cellular and system level function, we ask how general anaesthetics affect the different Kv channels. It is clear that the picture is complex. Reported effects of inhalational and intravenous anaesthetics on Kv channels include both activation and block, as well as modified voltage dependence, reflected in bidirectional shifts of activation and inactivation curves. Thus, halothane and chloroform in clinical doses decrease the open probability of Shaker channels, while isoflurane increases the open probability [15]. We have similarly described a barbiturate-induced increase in Kv currents, although only at high potentials [36]. However, there are few comparative studies on the sensitivity of different Kv channels. In a few cases, a specific Kv channel has been suggested to be especially sensitive, even being identified as the main target for general anaesthetics. Covarrubias and Rubin [37] argue that Shaw channels are much more sensitive to volatile anaesthetics than are Shaker, Shal, Kv1 and Kv3.4 channels.

To obtain information on Kv species sensitivity for general anaesthetics, we analysed effects of intravenous anaesthetics on Kv1, Kv2 and Kv3 channels, expressed in *Xenopus* oocytes. The results show that Kv2.1 channels are more sensitive to propofol and ketamine (three- to 10-fold) than are Kv1.2 and

Kv3.2 [38]. Furthermore, the mechanism of action on Kv2.1 differs between the anaesthetics. Ketamine seems to block all channels in an open-state dependent manner. This is reflected in a leftward shift of the steady-state activation curve. Propofol seems to block Kv2.1 preferentially in the closed state, reflected in the rightward shift of the activation curve. The binding seems to depend critically on the S5–S6 (ketamine) and the S4–S5 (propofol) linker, respectively [39]. Furthermore, the mechanism of action seems to differ for the different channels; propofol modifies the activation in a voltage-dependent way in Kv1.2, causing the channel to open at low voltages. Similar effects have been reported for local anaesthetics on dorsal root ganglion cells [40]. Other results have been found for other Kv channels [41,42].

A block of K channel activity is generally assumed to increase the excitability of the affected neurone, while an increase is assumed to cause the reverse effect. Assuming a general suppression theory as an explanation of general anaesthesia, we would therefore expect a facilitating effect of general anaesthetics on Kv channels. However, most reported effects are inhibitions. As shown below, this does not necessarily mean an increased excitability. The mechanism of blocking the channel is essential.

Summarizing the results of these and other studies, general anaesthetics show channel-specific and mechanism-specific effects on Kv channels. Our studies suggest that Kv2.1 channels are especially sensitive. Kv2.1 seems to confer fast spiking capacity to neurones, suggesting that general anaesthetic block of Kv2.1 might decrease the firing frequency in some neurones. What that means at the system level of neural activity is poorly understood. The finding that Kv3-like channels also seem highly sensitive, falls in a similar explanatory pattern [19].

Specific blocking of channels can cause a transition of firing patterns

One way to investigate the effects on neuroneal and neural activity of blocking specific channels is to use mathematical models. Figure 9.2 shows model simulations based on recordings from an interneurone in hippocampus [43]. This type of neurone shows several interesting features, such as graded action potentials and spontaneous activity induced by single channel openings [44]. Figure 9.2 shows the time evolution of the oscillatory behaviour at different stimulation intensities for a model neurone with normal Na and K channel densities (Fig. 9.2a) and with 75% of both channel types blocked (Fig. 9.2b). As seen, the block forces the oscillatory activity into damped responses at high stimulation levels without eliminating the excitability per se. The frequency increases continuously with increased stimulation intensity until it reaches a saturation value of approximately 100 Hz.

Using stability analysis [45] we can investigate the effect of blocking the Kv channels in further detail. Such an analysis shows that by continuously increasing the block of Kv, the firing of a certain model neurone passes through distinct patterns, described by different mathematical characteristics (Fig. 9.3): Hopf-bifurcations imply that the oscillations start immediately with non-zero frequency at the threshold, and saddle-node bifurcations implying that the oscillations start with very low frequency when stimulation reaches the threshold level [46]. The consequences of these subtle changes in firing patterns for the network activity are being explored at present.

General anaesthetics comprise compounds of great structural and functional diversity, including anaesthetics blocking voltage-gated channels selec-

tively. Thus, the discussed theoretical cases should be demonstrated experimentally. Furthermore, and as discussed below, the blocking mechanism per se (i.e. whether it is state-dependent or independent) can be shown to be of importance for modifying the dynamic behaviour of the cell.

Different blocking mechanisms modify the firing patterns differently

Blocking mechanisms have been studied extensively [18]. Since the recent structural breakthroughs [21,47], the block of Kv channels have come into focus. We have thus analysed effects of local anaesthetics in molecular [38] and atomic (using molecular dynamic) simulations [48]. Summarizing these and other studies, we can broadly classify the block of Kv channels in either open state dependent or state independent mechanisms.

Taking the kinetics of the Kv channel in the interneurone model described above as point of departure [43]:

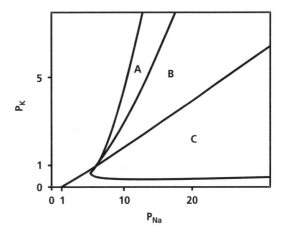

Figure 9.3 The channel-dependent oscillatory behaviour can be classified in three distinct types. The model neurone in Fig. 9.2 is capable of oscillatory activity in area A, B and C at some level of stimulation. Areas A and B represent an oscillatory activity that starts abruptly with relatively high frequency at threshold stimulation, while area C represents an activity that starts continuously with low frequencies. Mathematically, area B represents Hopf bifurcation behaviour and area C saddle-node bifurcation behaviour.

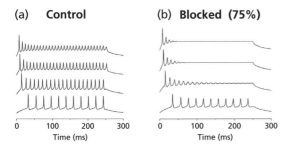

Figure 9.2 Blocking Na and K channels modifies the oscillatory behaviour. Simulation of the voltage response to constant stimulation levels (7, 11, 15, 19 and 23 pA) in a model neurone, described by Johansson and Århem [43]. (a) The control situation, assuming a 20-fold higher channel density than in the experimentally studied small-sized hippocampal interneurones. (b) The effect of blocking 75% of the channels.

$$C \leftrightarrow C \leftrightarrow O \qquad\qquad \text{Scheme 1}$$

an open state dependent block is described by:

$$C \leftrightarrow C \leftrightarrow O \qquad\qquad \text{Scheme 2}$$
$$\updownarrow$$
$$B$$

while the kinetics of a state independent block is described by:

$$C \leftrightarrow C \leftrightarrow O \qquad\qquad \text{Scheme 3}$$
$$\updownarrow \quad \updownarrow \quad \updownarrow$$
$$B \leftrightarrow B \leftrightarrow B$$

Figure 9.4 shows how the firing pattern of these two basic types of Kv channel block modifies the firing patterns differently, even assuming the same affinity. It shows simulations of the same model interneurone as in Figures 9. 2 and 9.3, with the K

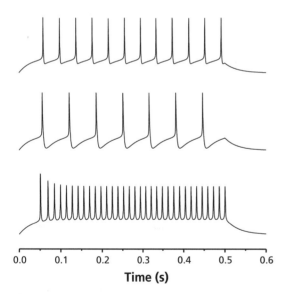

Figure 9.4 Different blocking mechanisms cause different modifications of oscillatory behaviour. Simulation of the same model neurone as in Fig. 9.2 at a stimulation level of 7 pA. Upper panel shows the control situation; the middle panel the effect of blocking 50% of the K channels state dependently (Scheme 2); and the lower panel the effect of blocking 50% of the K channels state independently (Scheme 3).

channels selectively blocked state dependently according to Scheme 2 (middle panel) and state independently according to Scheme 3 (lower panel). In both cases, a steady-state block of 50% was assumed. As seen, the state independent block increases and the state dependent block decreases the frequency of the oscillations. The reason for the differential result is that the state independent block shortens the recovery time and poises the membrane at a level close to threshold while the state dependent block induces a longer recovery time because of a 'foot-in-the-door' effect. The two types of mechanism thus theoretically disrupt oscillatory activity in different ways.

In summary, general anaesthetics act through a variety of mechanisms, including different forms of state independent and state dependent block. Considering the accumulating evidence for an essential role of voltage-gated channels in anaesthesia, the simulation data presented here may explain some aspects of the varying profiles of anaesthesia induced by different anaesthetics.

Conclusions

What conclusions can be drawn from these studies of general anaesthetic effects on Kv channels? A key problem that has first to be rectified is whether the reported effects occur at relevant concentrations. How should we understand the fact that many, but not all [15–17], IC_{50} values (concentration at which the current is reduced 50%) reported for Kv channels are higher than the clinical concentrations? There are several explanations. Many reports are based on effects on channels expressed in oocytes, a methodology known to require 100-fold higher concentrations than for the same channels expressed in other cells. Simulations with model neurones show that effects on the firing pattern are evident at up to 100-fold lower concentration than the IC_{50} values. Also, we should remember that there are an increasing number of investigations reporting effects on Kv channels at clinical concentrations (e.g. chloroform [15]). Taken together, this suggests that effects on Kv channels in many cases are expected to contribute to general anaesthesia. The degree of action probably depends on the specific general anaesthetic. Thus, it is not unreasonable to expect an increasing interest in K channel theories of anaesthesia in the near future.

Concerning the system level theories, the fragmentary data presented above suggest at least a thalamus dependent mechanism; general anaesthetics directly or indirectly hyperpolarize neurones in thalamo-cortical loops, and thereby disrupt coherent oscillatory activity in the cortex. However, the explanatory gaps are obvious. The importance of an integrated approach is forced upon us. The computational cases presented above are illustrative; subtle changes at the ion channel level cause drastic differences in the activity at the cellular level.

The problem of understanding the mechanisms of anaesthesia is closely related to the problem of determining the neural correlate of consciousness. Possibly, consciousness is a case of degeneracy, as discussed by Edelman and Gally [49]. Consciousness is, according to this view, caused by many interacting mechanisms, each in itself or in interaction with other mechanisms sufficient to create consciousness. Is it the degenerate character of the neural mechanisms causing consciousness that is the reason for the difficulties in defining its neuronal correlate?

The remarkable fact that such structurally different compounds cause anaesthesia suggests that anaesthesia can also be a case of degeneracy (i.e. that there are many interconnected ways for anaesthetics to cause unconsciousness) [50]. This could suggest that unconsciousness, possibly like sleep, is an evolutionary adaptive phenomenon. Populations of animals with brains that easily switch from conscious to unconscious states have survival advantages compared with populations with more robust brains that resist unconsciousness. Such a view opens up new approaches in understanding the anaesthesia problem (including constructing novel general anaesthetics), but also, perhaps, the classic problem of consciousness.

References

1 Friedman M, Friedland G. *Medicine's 10 greatest discoveries*. New Haven and London: Yale University Press, 1998.

2 Antkowiak B. *In vitro* networks: cortical mechanisms of anaesthetic action. *Br J Anaesth* 2002; **89**: 102–11.

3 John ER. A field theory of consciousness. *Conscious Cogn* 2001; **10**: 184–213.

4 Steyn-Ross ML, Steyn-Ross DA, Sleigh JW. Modelling general anaesthesia as a first-order phase transition in the cortex. *Prog Biophys Mol Biol* 2004; **85**: 369–85.

5 Cariani P. Anaesthesia, neural information processing, and conscious awareness. *Conscious Cogn* 2000; **9**: 387–95.

6 Crick F, Koch C. Towards a neurobiological theory of consciousness. *Semin Neurosci* 1990; **2**: 263–75.

7 Tononi G, Edelman G. Consciousness and complexity. *Science* 1998; **282**: 1846–51.

8 Franks NP, Lieb WR. Molecular and cellular mechanisms of general anaesthesia. *Nature* 1994; **367**: 607–14.

9 Alkire MT, Haier RJ, Fallon JH. Toward a unified theory of narcosis: brain imaging evidence for a thalamocortical switch as the neurophysiologic basis of anaesthetic-induced unconsciousness. *Conscious Cogn* 2000; **9**: 370–86.

10 Mihic SJ, Ye Q, Wick MJ. Sites of alcohol and volatile anaesthetic action on GABA(A) and glycine receptors. *Nature* 1997; **389**: 385–9.

11 Flohr H. Sensations and brain processes. *Behav Brain Res* 1995; **71**: 157–61.

12 Patel AJ, Honore E, Lesage F, *et al.* Inhalational anaesthetics activate two-pore-domain background K^+ channels. *Nat Neurosci* 1999; **2**: 422–6.

13 Rudolph U, Antkowiak B. Molecular and neuroneal substrates for general anaesthetics. *Nat Rev Neurosci* 2004; **5**: 709–20.

14 Bräu ME, Nau C, Hempelmann G, Vogel W. Local anaesthetics potently block a potential insensitive potassium channel in myelinated nerve. *J Gen Physiol* 1995; **105**: 485–505.

15 Correa AM. Gating kinetics of Shaker K^+ channels are differentially modified by general anaesthetics. *Am J Physiol* 1998; **275**: C1009–21.

16 Friederich P, Benzenberg D, Trellakis S, Urban BW. Interaction of volatile anaesthetics with human Kv channels in relation to clinical concentrations. *Anesthesiology* 2001; **95**: 954–8.

17 Lingamaneni R, Hemmings HC Jr. Differential interaction of anaesthetics and antiepileptic drugs with neuroneal Na^+ channels, Ca^{2+} channels, and GABA(A) receptors. *Br J Anaesth* 2003; **90**: 199–211.

18 Hille B. *Ionic Channels of Excitable Membranes*, 3rd edn. Sunderland: Sinauer Associates, 2001.

19 Harris T, Shahidullah M, Ellingson JS, Covarrubias M. General anaesthetic action at an internal protein site involving the S4–S5 cytoplasmic loop of a neuroneal K⁺ channel. *J Biol Chem* 2000; **275**: 4928–36.

20 Yu FH, Catterall WA. The VGL-chanome: a protein superfamily specialized for electrical signaling and ionic homeostasis. *Sci STKE* 2004; **253**: 15.

21 Jiang Y, Lee A, Chen J, *et al*. X-ray structure of a voltage-dependent K⁺ channel. *Nature* 2003; **423**: 33–41.

22 Monaghan MM, Trimmer JS, Rhodes KJ. Experimental localization of Kv1 family voltage-gated K⁺ channel alpha and beta subunits in rat hippocampal formation. *J Neurosci* 2001; **21**: 5973–83.

23 Trimmer JS, Rhodes KJ. Localization of voltage-gated ion channels in mammalian brain. *Annu Rev Physiol* 2004; **66**: 477–519.

24 Cooper EC, Milroy A, Jan YN, Jan LY, Lowenstein DH. Presynaptic localization of Kv1.4-containing A-type potassium channels near excitatory synapses in the hippocampus. *J Neurosci* 1998; **18**: 965–74.

25 Smart SL, Lopantsev V, Zhang CL, *et al*. Deletion of the K(V)1.1 potassium channel causes epilepsy in mice. *Neurone* 1998; **20**: 809–19.

26 Petersson S, Persson AS, Johansen JE, *et al*. Truncation of the Shaker-like voltage-gated potassium channel, Kv1.1, causes megencephaly. *Eur J Neurosci* 2003; **18**: 3231–40.

27 Martina M, Schultz JH, Ehmke H, Monyer H, Jonas P. Functional and molecular differences between voltage-gated K⁺ channels of fast-spiking interneuronees and pyramidal neuronees of rat hippocampus. *J Neurosci* 1998; **18**: 8111–25.

28 Du J, Haak LL, Phillips-Tansey E, Russell JT, McBain CJ. Frequency-dependent regulation of rat hippocampal somato-dendritic excitability by the K⁺ channel subunit Kv2.1. *J Physiol* 2000; **522**: 19–31.

29 Baranauskas G, Tkatch T, Nagata K, Yeh JZ, Surmeier DJ. Kv3.4 subunits enhance the repolarizing efficiency of Kv3.1 channels in fast-spiking neuronees. *Nat Neurosci* 2003; **6**: 258–66.

30 Rudy B, McBain CJ. Kv3 channels: voltage-gated K⁺ channels designed for high-frequency repetitive firing. *Trends Neurosci* 2001; **24**: 517–26.

31 Lien CC, Jonas P. Kv3 potassium conductance is necessary and kinetically optimized for high-frequency action potential generation in hippocampal interneurones. *J Neurosci* 2003; **23**: 2058–68.

32 Joho RH, Ho CS, Marks GA. Increased gamma- and decreased delta-oscillations in a mouse deficient for a potassium channel expressed in fast-spiking interneurones. *J Neurophysiol* 1999; **82**: 1855–64.

33 Serodio P, Rudy B. Differential expression of Kv4 K⁺ channel subunits mediating subthreshold transient K⁺ (A-type) currents in rat brain. *J Neurophysiol* 1998; **79**:1081–91.

34 Johnston D, Christie BR, Frick A, *et al*. Active dendrites, potassium channels and synaptic plasticity. *Phil Trans R Soc Lond B Biol Sci* 2003; **358**: 667–74.

35 Hoffman DA, Magee JC, Colbert CM, Johnston D. K⁺ channel regulation of signal propagation in dendrites of hippocampal pyramidal neurones. *Nature* 1997; **387**: 869–75.

36 Århem P, Kristbjarnarson H. On the mechanism of barbiturate action on potassium channels in the nerve membrane. *Acta Physiol Scand* 1985; **123**: 369–71.

37 Covarrubias M, Rubin E. Ethanol selectively blocks a noninactivating K⁺ current expressed in *Xenopus* oocytes. *Proc Natl Acad Sci U S A* 1993; **90**: 6957–60.

38 Nilsson J, Madeja M, Århem P. Local anaesthetic block of Kv channels: role of the S6 helix and the S5–S6 linker for bupivacaine action. *Mol Pharmacol* 2003; **63**: 1417–29.

39 Nilsson J, Madeja M, Arhem P. Selective block of Kv channels by general anaesthetics. *Biophys J* 2004; **86**: 539A.

40 Olschewski A, Wolff M, Brau ME, *et al*. Enhancement of delayed-rectifier potassium conductance by low concentrations of local anaesthetics in spinal sensory neurones. *Br J Pharmacol* 2002; **136**: 540–9.

41 Århem P, Rydqvist B. The mechanism of action of ketamine on the myelinated nerve membrane. *Eur J Pharmacol* 1986; **126**: 245–51.

42 Veintemilla F, Elinder F, Århem P. Mechanisms of propofol action on ion currents in the myelinated axon of *Xenopus laevis*. *Eur J Pharmacol* 1992; **218**: 59–68.

43 Johansson S, Århem P. Computed potential responses of small cultured rat hippocampal neurones. *J Physiol* 1992; **445**: 157–67.

44 Johansson S, Århem P. Single-channel currents trigger action potentials in small cultured hippocampal neurones. *Proc Natl Acad Sci U S A* 1994; **91**: 1761–5.

45 Århem P, Klement G, Blomberg C. Channel density regulation of firing patterns in a cortical neuron model. *Biophys J* 2006; **90**: 1–13.

46 Koch C. *The Quest for Consciousness*. Englewood: Roberts and Company, 2004.

47 Doyle DA, Morais Cabral J, Pfuetzner RA, *et al*. The structure of the potassium channel: molecular basis of K⁺ conduction and selectivity. *Science* 1998; **280**: 69–77.

48 Luzhkov VB, Nilsson J, Arhem P, Aqvist J. Computational modelling of the open-state Kv 1.5 ion channel block by bupivacaine. *Biochim Biophys Acta* 2003; **1652**: 35–51.

49 Edelman GM, Gally JA. Degeneracy and complexity in biological systems. *Proc Natl Acad Sci U S A* 2001; **98**: 13763–8.

50 Arhem P, Klement G, Nilsson J. Mechanisms of anaesthesia: towards integrating network, cellular, and molecular level modeling. *Neuropsychopharmacology* 2003; **28**: S40–7.

CHAPTER 10

Use and abuse of antibiotics

Jeremy Cohen and Jeffrey Lipman

Introduction

It is an unusual patient who stays for any length of time in an intensive care unit (ICU) without at least one course of broad-spectrum antibiotic treatment. While the clinical benefits of appropriate and timely antimicrobial therapy should not be underestimated, their widespread use has been associated with a number of adverse consequences, not the least of which is the propagation of highly resistant organisms. In this chapter we discuss important aspects of the evidence base for antibiotic prescribing practice in the critical care environment, in particular the issues of appropriate prescribing, duration of antibiotic therapy and the controversies surrounding dosing and spectrum of cover. At the same time we hope to discourage the inappropriate use of these drugs.

Epidemiology

The increasing use of antibiotics on ICUs is partly driven by an increase in the incidence and awareness of sepsis. In 1990, the Centers for Disease Control estimated the annual incidence of septicaemia in the USA at 450 000 and that the condition was responsible for more than 100 000 deaths [1]. While there have been a number of studies defining the incidence of severe sepsis in patients treated in ICUs, less is known about the population incidence of severe sepsis. Studies in ICUs suggest that 11–15% of patients admitted to ICUs have, or develop, severe sepsis [2–4], and recent studies suggest the mortality rate for patients with severe sepsis treated in ICUs varies between 30 and 60% [2–5]. Martin *et al.* [6], using ICD9-CM codes, found the incidence of sepsis increased from 0.83 cases per 1000 population in

1979 to 2.40 cases per 1000 population in 2000. In 1995–2000, 33.6% of patients with sepsis also had organ failure, suggesting an incidence of severe sepsis in 2000 of 0.81 per 1000 population. In contrast, Angus *et al.* [5] examined the incidence of severe sepsis using a database constructed from the 1995 hospital discharge databases of seven US states. They used different ICD9-CM codes to separately identify infection and organ dysfunction and estimated the incidence of severe sepsis at 3.0 cases per 1000 of population. The study further estimated that severe sepsis is responsible for 215 000 deaths per annum in the USA [5]. Thus, two recent studies using similar methodology have produced quite different estimates for the incidence of severe sepsis in the USA.

The Australian and New Zealand Intensive Care Society Clinical Trials Group (ANZICS CTG) investigated the epidemiology of sepsis in 2004. Examining 23 ICUs from 21 hospitals in Australia and New Zealand they were able to estimate a population incidence of 0.7 per 1000, and an ICU incidence of severe sepsis of 11.8 patients per 100 [7]. These data fall within the lower range of the estimates from the USA, but compares well with data from 99 Italian units suggesting a rate of 11.6 per 100 ICU admissions [4]. Data from the UK gives a higher rate of 27.1% of admissions fulfilling severe sepsis criteria [8].

Thus, severe sepsis continues to be a significant problem in intensive care, contributing heavily to mortality and prolonged hospital stays. The rapid development of highly resistant bacteria, coupled with the decrease in development of novel antibiotics means the threat of untreatable nosocomial infections is becoming more real. The remaining weapons

Table 10.1 Antibiotics commonly underdosed.

	Drug	Recommended i.v. dose
Quinolones	Ciprofloxacin	400 mg q. 8 h
	Levofloxacin	750 mg once a day
Aminoglycosides	Gentamicin/tobramycin	7 mg/kg once a day
	Amikacin	20 mg/kg once a day
Glycopeptides	Vancomycin	30 mg/kg/day or more in divided doses (q. 6 h or q. 12 h)
Carbapenems	Meropenem	3 g/day in divided doses (q. 6 h or q. 8 h)
Beta-lactams	Piperacillin/tazobactam	4.5 g q. 6 h
	Cefepime/cefpirome	2 g q. 8 h
	Ceftriaxone	2 g/day or more in divided doses (q. 8 h or q. 12 h)

Note: these doses are for an adult with normal renal function.

in our antibiotic arsenal must be used wisely (Table 10.1).

Early and appropriate use of antibiotics

There is now a significant body of evidence that suggests early, appropriate antibiotic use decreases mortality in critically ill patients.

Examining ventilator-associated pneumonia (VAP), Rello *et al.* [9] determined that inadequate initial therapy was associated with a related mortality of 37% versus 15.4% in patients receiving appropriate initial antibiotic cover ($P < 0.05$) [9]. In a study of 132 mechanically ventilated patients, Luna *et al.* [10] demonstrated that in patients who received inadequate treatment, as determined by bronchoalveolar lavage (BAL) fluid culture, mortality was 91%, compared with 38% in the adequately treated group. Late change to adequate therapy did not improve the mortality rate, suggesting that early treatment was a key factor. Similarly, a study from Spain demonstrated an attributable mortality of 24.7% in patients with VAP managed initially with inadequate antibiotics, compared with 16.2% in those whom the initial treatment was adequate [11].

Garnacho-Montero *et al.* [12] examined 406 patients who were admitted to ICU with a diagnosis of sepsis, and determined that the risk of death in medical patients receiving initial inadequate anti-

microbial cover was eight times higher than in those receiving adequate cover. Data from Kollef *et al.* [13] demonstrated a higher in-hospital mortality for ICU patients receiving initial adequate antimicrobial treatment (42% versus 17.7%). Examining patients with blood stream infections, adequate empirical antibiotic selection was found to be the most important factor for survival, reducing mortality to 51.7% from 79.4% in the first 48 hours [14]. Similar data from Ibrahim *et al.* [15] demonstrated a reduction in mortality from 62% to 28% in the hospital mortality rate of patients with documented bacteraemia.

MacArthur *et al.* [16] and Harbarth *et al.* [17] retrospectively looked at 'adequate' or 'inadequate' antibiotic therapy in two large (2614 and 900 patients, respectively) multicentred negative mediator trials. MacArthur *et al.* [16] showed a 10% absolute crude mortality difference between the two groups. Harbarth *et al.* [17] showed a 15% decrease in 28-day mortality.

These data are all highly suggestive that early correct antibiotic treatment may have a greater impact on mortality than therapies such as activated protein C (APC), low tidal volume ventilation or tight glucose control.

Accurate diagnosis of infection

Rational use of antibiotics is based upon accurate diagnosis of infection. Blood cultures may often be negative in septic patients, and distinguishing between an infecting organism and one that is simply colonizing can be difficult. The ubiquitous systemic inflammatory response syndrome (SIRS) response makes interpretation of clinical signs complex, and proof of bacterial growth does not equate to proof of infection. There is therefore intense interest in biochemical markers specific for sepsis.

Procalcitonin

Current interest has focused upon the use of procalcitonin (PCT), a 116 amino-acid precursor of calcitonin. It is probably produced primarily in liver and undergoes cleavage in thyroid, lung and pancreas [18,19]. The most potent inducer of PCT is the lipopolysaccharide of cell walls of Gram-negative bacteria. After a bacterial stimulus the levels of PCT start to increase at about the 3–4 hour mark, with a peak level reached at 6 hours. PCT is degraded by specific proteases and has a half-life of 25–30 hours [18,19]. A similar stimulus produces a later rise in C-reactive protein (CRP) at approximately 12–18 hours after the bacterial challenge [18,19]. Normal levels of PCT are <0.1 ng/mL and levels of >1000 ng/mL have been documented in some bacterial infections. To diagnose bacterial infections various cut-off levels have been quoted: anything between 0.2 and 5 ng/mL. However, while the most potent stimulus for PCT production may be Gram-negative sepsis, PCT is part of the innate immune response to many stimuli [19]. It is therefore not surprising that Carrol *et al.* [18] came to the conclusion that PCT is 'A tool that should complement thorough clinical assessment, good clinical acumen and judgment . . . and cannot and should not be used alone to determine appropriate treatment'. Still another recent analysis by Gattas and Cook [20] asked the question, 'Can PCT accurately distinguish sepsis in patients with systemic inflammatory response syndrome (SIRS) who have a suspected infection?' They too came to the conclusion that PCT could not. It has poor sensitivity and specificity for the diagnosis of bacterial infections, and there are no consistent cut-off levels. However, when PCT levels are very high there seems to be no doubt that there is a bacterial infection present, and falling levels over time seem to correlate with patient improvement.

Thus, while PCT is a better marker of sepsis than CRP, its specificity and sensitivity is less than ideal. The place of PCT in clinical practice is still debatable and its use to guide antibiotic therapy, either institution thereof or stoppage, while tempting, is presently still premature on the available data. Nevertheless, PCT is currently still our best hope for the future ability to differentiate sepsis from the non-specific inflammatory response of SIRS.

Soluble TREM-1

A recently described receptor and its soluble form have been evaluated in terms of predicting infection and as a guide to outcome. TREM-1 (triggering receptor expressed on myeloid cells 1) is known to be present on many cells and is part of the signalling pathway involving Toll-like receptors. However, a similar protein is also present in the plasma and is called soluble TREM-1 (sTREM-1). It lacks the transmembrane portion of the membrane-bound form. It has been shown that increased sTREM-1 is a very sensitive and specific marker of infection. In a study comparing concentrations of sTREM-1, PCT and CRP during sepsis, sTREM-1 concentrations were significantly lower at admission in non-survivors than in survivors, whereas PCT levels were higher among non-survivors. CRP levels did not differ between the two groups of patients. Plasma PCT and CRP decreased during the 14-day period of study in both survivors and non-survivors. Conversely, sTREM-1 plasma concentrations remained stable or even increased in non-surviving patients and decreased in survivors. An elevated baseline sTREM-1 level was found to be an independent protective factor, with an odds ratio of dying of 0.1.

In conclusion, a progressive decline of plasma sTREM-1 concentration indicates a favourable clinical evolution during the recovery phase of sepsis. In addition, baseline sTREM-1 level may prove useful in predicting outcome of septic patients [21].

Duration of treatment

Few data exist to rationally guide duration of antibiotic treatment in critically ill patients. However, increasing awareness of the risks of prolonged courses of broad-spectrum agents has led internationally to a trend towards shortening the length of treatment.

Most courses of antibiotics in the ICU are given for an empirical duration based upon site of infection and pathogen. Some data exist to modify durations based upon clinical response.

The Infectious Disease Society of America (IDSA) guidelines on management of community acquired pneumonia (CAP) in adults [22] suggests that length of treatment should be guided by clinical factors, such as response, severity and comorbidities. Specifically, they note that pneumonia caused by *Streptococcus pneumoniae* should be treated until the patient has been afebrile for at least 72 hours, and grade this as a C-III recommendation. Similar recommendations are made for management of neutropenic patients with cancer [23], based on duration of fever and neutrophil count.

Evidence-based data to guide duration of treatment are sparse. Singh *et al.* [24] examined the effect of a 3-day course of ciprofloxacin compared with standard antibiotic treatment for 10–21 days for ICU patients with pulmonary infiltrates, but who were thought to have a low risk of pneumonia. They documented no difference in mortality and a lower length of stay in the short duration group. Antimicrobial resistance and superinfection rates were higher in the group receiving standard treatment. A French study examined the effects of an 8-day antibiotic course compared with 15 days in the management of VAP [25]. A total of 401 patients were enrolled, and no difference in mortality, duration of mechanical ventilation or length of stay was noted. The authors did comment on a higher recurrence rate of pulmonary infections in patients with *Pseudomonas aeruginosa* managed with the shorter course; this was not associated with unfavourable outcomes. Denneson *et al.* [26] examined the resolution of infectious parameters in 27 patients with diagnosed VAP. They determined that maximum resolution occurs in the first 6 days of treatment, while acquired colonization with resistant pathogens appears primarily in the second week. Based on these data, the authors hypothesized that a 1-week course of antibiotics may be sufficient to treat VAP while decreasing the rate of emergence of resistant bacteria.

In summary, while there is little evidence to guide the clinician in deciding the optimal duration of treatment of infections in the critically ill, there is a move to decrease the duration of antibiotic therapy.

Increasing awareness of the emergence of multiresistant pathogens is leading to reluctance to engage in protracted courses of broad-spectrum antibiotics, and while this appears to be supported by the data, larger clinical trials are urgently required.

The use of 'double Gram-negative cover'

Although the use of combination therapy for Gram-negative infections is relatively common, the data supporting it are sparse. Synergy demonstrated *in vitro* is an oft quoted reason for its use, and supporting clinical data comes primarily from two trials. The EORTC group studied Gram-negative bacteraemias in neutropenic patients with cancer [27], and demonstrated a superiority in response for ceftazidime in combination with a full course of aminoglycoside. Hilf *et al.* [28] prospectively studied 200 patients with *Pseudomonas* bacteraemia and determined that combination therapy conferred a significant survival advantage. However, more recent work has failed to confirm these findings. Examining febrile neutropenic patients, a meta-analysis of 47 trials encompassing 7807 patients failed to demonstrate any outcome difference between single and combination therapy. Indeed, combination therapy was associated with a higher incidence of adverse events, especially renal failure [29]. Likewise, in non-neutropenic patients, a meta-analysis of 74 trials with 7586 patients demonstrated no difference in fatality and a higher rate of clinical failure and nephrotoxicity with combination therapy [30]. Given the high level of clinical concern regarding the development of drug resistance in certain organisms, the authors performed a subgroup analysis of general *Pseudomonas* infections; again, no difference was observed. However, in another meta-analysis by Safdar *et al.* [31], a subgroup analysis did suggest a 50% mortality reduction with the use of combination therapy, specifically in *Pseudomonas* bacteraemia, although again no overall benefit was shown.

Thus, the weight of evidence at present suggests that there is no requirement for double antibiotic cover in most Gram-negative infections. However, in the case of blood stream infection with *Pseudomonas*, combination therapy may be of benefit.

The problem of resistance

The widespread use of potent broad-spectrum anti-biotics has been paralleled by the development of re-sistance in bacteria, culminating in the prevalence of highly resistant bacteria in some ICUs.

Bacteria can be regarded as self-maintaining enti-ties with sophisticated survival strategies, participat-ing in a promiscuous type of global gene pool, often freely swapping material [32]. DNA transfer between bacteria is common and occurs via integrons, gene cassettes, transposons and/or plasmids. Flux within this gene pool is largely a product of selection pres-sure. The necessity to use appropriate first-line ther-apy for serious infections combines with the rising tide of resistance to drive increasing empiric use of broad-spectrum antibiotics in the critically ill. There is evidence that this selection pressure operates in clinically relevant ways. Inappropriate use of anti-biotics, for example in the colonized patient with SIRS, merely fuels this problem. Extreme selection pressure in certain scenarios may promote the devel-opment of highly adaptable populations of muta-tion-repair defective organisms. The archetype is *Pseudomonas aeruginosa* infection in the cystic fibrosis patient. In this scenario, there may be a significant population of organisms with mutations in their DNA mismatch-repair system [33,34].

These concepts help explain why the ability of bacteria to become resistant to our antibiotics is frightening. The intensive care community faces the realistic prospect of untreatable nosocomial infec-tions. As there has been no new class of antibiotic developed for Gram-negative sepsis since the 1980s when the carbapenems were released [35], it be-hoves us to use antibiotics appropriately and not abuse the ease of becoming a 'just in case' prescriber. Antibiotics will kill susceptible bacteria but, within any colony of organisms, resistant bacteria will still grow. Indiscriminate use just propagates the devel-opment of resistant organisms. Wise antibiotic use translates into using the correct antibiotic (not nec-essarily using dual Gram-negative cover), in the cor-rect dose, for the correct duration and only in sepsis, not using it for SIRS, etc. Inadequate dosing of any antibiotic, but especially for quinolones, leads to re-sistance [36,37]. Incorrect dosing of aminoglycosides

occurs unless extended interval dosing is used [38]. High creatinine clearance in some ICU patients leads to high drug clearances and hence potential under-dosing of antibiotics [39]. Antibiotics commonly un-derdosed, with their suggested doses, are shown in Table 10.1.

Selective digestive decontamination

The use of selective digestive decontamination (SDD) is probably the most controversial topic in the current ICU antibiotic literature [40,41] as well as, paradoxically, the one with the largest amount of experimental data.

Introduced into ICUs in the mid-1980s [42], SDD aims to eradicate pathogenic organisms from the gastrointestinal tract, while preserving the non-pathogenic normal anaerobic flora. Classically, SDD consists of four components: topical application of non-absorbable antibiotics to the oral cavity and gastrointestinal tract; systemic antibiotic admini-stration for the first few days of admission; regular surveillance cultures to monitor effectiveness; and optimal hygiene. In practice, SDD regimes vary widely, in choice and dose of antibiotics used, dura-tion and omission or inclusion of the systemic portion. There can be no doubting the evidence pointing to efficacy [43]. Numerous studies have demonstrated a decrease in VAP incidence using an SDD protocol, although the methodological quality of some of these studies has been called into ques-tion. What is less clear is the effect on mortality. However, two more recent studies have been able to demonstrate a survival benefit with SDD [44,45], al-though in both cases these were units with low en-demic rates of multiresistant organisms, raising questions as to how generally applicable these find-ings might be.

Despite encouraging data, SDD has yet to be accepted as a standard therapy in the general ICU community. Underpinning this reluctance is almost certainly the concern that widespread prophylactic use will dramatically increase selection pressure on multiresistant pathogens. Although emergence of multiresistant organisms has not yet been adequately demonstrated with the use of SDD, opponents point out the protocol has not been studied in environments with high levels of pre-existing resistant pathogens, notably methicillin-resistant *Staphylococcus aureus* (MRSA) [46]. In summary, while SDD appears to be a promising mechanism for reduction of infections, concerns regarding emergence of drug resistance have prevented its widespread acceptance. A large-scale trial of the sort recently carried out into fluid resuscitation [47] is likely the only way to help solve the controversy.

Conclusions

Broad-spectrum antibiotics form one of the primary therapeutic modalities of critical care, and when used early and appropriately, save more lives than many other more recent ICU interventions. The correct antibiotic, in the correct dose, for a limited duration is enlightened practice. However, the ability of microorganisms to develop resistance, coupled with the slowdown in development of new antibiotic classes, means that their effectiveness may become compromised. A number of strategies are available to combat this trend. The development of accurate biochemical markers of sepsis will help rationalize prescribing practice and lead to more stringent inclusion criteria in research studies. Stronger data on treatment duration may lead to shorter courses of antibiotics, and thus to a reduction in selection pressure. Awareness of the dosing vagaries in critically ill patients will allow for the correct dose selection. Work in all these areas as well as investigating other strategies (possibly SDD and antibiotic rotation) is required if we are to prevent the catastrophe of untreatable nosocomial infections arising in our ICUs.

References

1 Centers for Disease Control. Increase in National Hospital Discharge Survey rates for septicemia: United States, 1979–1987. *JAMA* 1990; **263**: 937–8.

2 Brun-Buisson C, Doyon F, Carlet J, *et al*. Incidence, risk factors, and outcome of severe sepsis and septic shock in adults: a multicenter prospective study in intensive care units. French ICU Group for Severe Sepsis. *JAMA* 1995; **274**: 968–74.

3 Pittet D, Rangel-Frausto S, Li N, *et al*. Systemic inflammatory response syndrome, sepsis, severe sepsis and septic shock: incidence, morbidities and outcomes in surgical ICU patients. *Intensive Care Med* 1995; **21**: 302–9.

4 Salvo I, de Cian W, Musicco M, *et al*. The Italian SEPSIS study: preliminary results on the incidence and evolution of SIRS, sepsis, severe sepsis and septic shock. *Intensive Care Med* 1995; **21**(Suppl 2): S244–9.

5 Angus DC, Linde-Zwirble WT, Lidicker J, *et al*. Epidemiology of severe sepsis in the United States: analysis of incidence, outcome, and associated costs of care. *Crit Care Med* 2001; **29**: 1303–10.

6 Martin GS, Mannino DM, Eaton S, Moss M. The epidemiology of sepsis in the United States from 1979 through 2000. *N Engl J Med* 2003; **348**: 1546–54.

7 Finfer S, Bellomo R, Lipman J, *et al*. Adult-population incidence of severe sepsis in Australian and New Zealand intensive care units. *Intensive Care Med* 2004; **30**: 589–96.

8 Padkin A, Goldfrad C, Brady AR, *et al*. Epidemiology of severe sepsis occurring in the first 24 hrs in intensive care units in England, Wales, and Northern Ireland. *Crit Care Med* 2003; **31**: 2332–8.

9 Rello J, Gallego M, Mariscal D, Sonora R, Valles J. The value of routine microbial investigation in ventilator-associated pneumonia. *Am J Respir Crit Care Med* 1997; **156**: 196–200.

10 Luna CM, Vujacich P, Niederman MS, *et al*. Impact of BAL data on the therapy and outcome of ventilator-associated pneumonia. *Chest* 1997; **111**: 676–85.

11 Alvarez-Lerma F. Modification of empiric antibiotic treatment in patients with pneumonia acquired in the intensive care unit. ICU-Acquired Pneumonia Study Group. *Intensive Care Med* 1996; **22**: 387–94.

12 Garnacho-Montero J, Garcia-Garmendia JL, Barrero-Almodovar A, *et al*. Impact of adequate empirical antibiotic therapy on the outcome of patients admitted to the intensive care unit with sepsis. *Crit Care Med* 2003; **31**: 2742–51.

13 Kollef MH, Sherman G, Ward S, Fraser VJ. Inadequate antimicrobial treatment of infections: a risk factor for hospital mortality among critically ill patients. *Chest* 1999; **115**: 462–74.

14 Valles J, Rello J, Ochagavia A, Garnacho J, Alcala MA. Community-acquired bloodstream infection in critically ill adult patients: impact of shock and inappropriate antibiotic therapy on survival. *Chest* 2003; **123**: 1615–24.

15 Ibrahim EH, Sherman G, Ward S, Fraser VJ, Kollef MH. The influence of inadequate antimicrobial treatment of

bloodstream infections on patient outcomes in the ICU setting. *Chest* 2000; **118**: 146–55.

16 MacArthur RD, Miller M, Albertson T, *et al.* Adequacy of early empiric antibiotic treatment and survival in severe sepsis: experience from the MONARCS trial. *Clin Infect Dis* 2004; **38**: 284–8.

17 Harbarth S, Garbino J, Pugin J, *et al.* Inappropriate initial antimicrobial therapy and its effect on survival in a clinical trial of immunomodulating therapy for severe sepsis. *Am J Med* 2003; **115**: 529–35.

18 Carrol ED, Thomson AP, Hart CA. Procalcitonin as a marker of sepsis. *Int J Antimicrob Agents* 2002; **20**: 1–9.

19 Becker KL, Nylen ES, White JC, Muller B, Snider RH Jr. Clinical review 167: procalcitonin and the calcitonin gene family of peptides in inflammation, infection, and sepsis — a journey from calcitonin back to its precursors. *J Clin Endocrinol Metab* 2004; **89**: 1512–25.

20 Gattas DJ, Cook DJ. Procalcitonin as a diagnostic test for sepsis: health technology assessment in the ICU. *J Crit Care* 2003; **18**: 52–8.

21 Gibot S, Cravoisy A, Kolopp-Sarda MN, *et al.* Time course of sTREM (soluble triggering receptor expressed on myeloid cells)-1, procalcitonin and C-reactive protein concentrations during sepsis. *Crit Care Med* 2005; **33**: 792–6.

22 Bartlett JG, Dowell SF, Mandell LA, *et al.* Practice guidelines for the management of community-acquired pneumonia in adults. Infectious Diseases Society of America. *Clin Infect Dis* 2000; **31**: 347–82.

23 Hughes WT, Armstrong D, Bodey GP, *et al.* 2002 Guidelines for the use of antimicrobial agents in neutropenic patients with cancer. *Clin Infect Dis* 2002; **34**: 730–51.

24 Singh N, Rogers P, Atwood CW, Wagener MM, Yu VL. Short-course empiric antibiotic therapy for patients with pulmonary infiltrates in the intensive care unit: a proposed solution for indiscriminate antibiotic prescription. *Am J Respir Crit Care Med* 2000; **162**: 505–11.

25 Chastre J, Wolff M, Fagon JY, *et al.* Comparison of 8 vs 15 days of antibiotic therapy for ventilator-associated pneumonia in adults: a randomized trial. *JAMA* 2003; **290**: 2588–98.

26 Dennesen PJ, van der Ven AJ, Kessels AG, Ramsay G, Bonten MJ. Resolution of infectious parameters after antimicrobial therapy in patients with ventilator-associated pneumonia. *Am J Respir Crit Care Med* 2001; **163**: 1371–5.

27 EORTC International Antimicrobial Therapy Cooperative Group. Ceftazidime combined with a short or long course of amikacin for empirical therapy of gram-negative bacteremia in cancer patients with granulocytopenia. *N Engl J Med* 1987; **317**: 1692–8.

28 Hilf M, Yu VL, Sharp J, *et al.* Antibiotic therapy for *Pseudomonas aeruginosa* bacteremia: outcome correlations in a prospective study of 200 patients. *Am J Med* 1989; **87**: 540–6.

29 Paul M, Soares-Weiser K, Leibovici L. Beta lactam monotherapy versus beta lactam-aminoglycoside combination therapy for fever with neutropenia: systematic review and meta-analysis. *Br Med J* 2003; **326**: 1111–5.

30 Paul M, Benuri-Silbiger I, Soares-Weiser K, Leibovici L. Beta lactam monotherapy versus beta lactam-aminoglycoside combination therapy for sepsis in immunocompetent patients: systematic review and meta-analysis of randomised trials. *Br Med J* 2004; **328**: 668–81.

31 Safdar N, Handelsman J, Maki DG. Does combination antimicrobial therapy reduce mortality in Gram-negative bacteraemia? A meta-analysis. *Lancet Infect Dis* 2004; **4**: 519–27.

32 Hendrix RW, Smith MC, Burns RN, Ford ME, Hatfull GF. Evolutionary relationships among diverse bacteriophages and prophages: all the world's a phage. *Proc Natl Acad Sci U S A* 1999; **96**: 2192–7.

33 Blazquez J. Hypermutation as a factor contributing to the acquisition of antimicrobial resistance. *Clin Infect Dis* 2003; **37**: 1201–9.

34 Oliver A, Canton R, Campo P, Baquero F, Blazquez J. High frequency of hypermutable *Pseudomonas aeruginosa* in cystic fibrosis lung infection. *Science* 2000; **288**: 1251–4.

35 Amyes SG. The rise in bacterial resistance is partly because there have been no new classes of antibiotics since the 1960s. *Br Med J* 2000; **320**: 199–200.

36 Fantin B, Farinotti R, Thabaut A, Carbon C. Conditions for the emergence of resistance to cefpirome and ceftazidime in experimental endocarditis due to *Pseudomonas aeruginosa*. *J Antimicrob Chemother* 1994; **33**: 563–9.

37 Zhou J, Dong Y, Zhao X, *et al.* Selection of antibiotic-resistant bacterial mutants: allelic diversity among fluoroquinolone-resistant mutations. *J Infect Dis* 2000; **182**: 517–25.

38 Pinder M, Bellomo R, Lipman J. Pharmacological principles of antibiotic prescription in the critically ill. *Anaesth Intensive Care* 2002; **30**: 134–44.

39 Lipman J, Wallis SC, Boots RJ. Cefepime versus cefpirome: the importance of creatinine clearance. *Anesth Analg* 2003; **97**: 1149–54.

40 van Saene HK, Petros AJ, Ramsay G, Baxby D. All great truths are iconoclastic: selective decontamination of the digestive tract moves from heresy to level 1 truth. *Intensive Care Med* 2003; **29**: 677–90.

41 Bonten MJ, Brun-Buisson C, Weinstein RA. Selective decontamination of the digestive tract: to stimulate or stifle? *Intensive Care Med* 2003; **29**: 672–6.

42 Stoutenbeek CP, van Saene HK, Miranda DR, Zandstra DF. The effect of selective decontamination of the digestive tract on colonisation and infection rate in multiple trauma patients. *Intensive Care Med* 1984; **10**: 185–92.

43 de Jonge E. Effects of selective decontamination of digestive tract on mortality and antibiotic resistance in the intensive-care unit. *Curr Opin Crit Care* 2005; **11**: 144–9.

44 Krueger WA, Lenhart FP, Neeser G, et al. Influence of combined intravenous and topical antibiotic prophylaxis on the incidence of infections, organ dysfunctions, and mortality in critically ill surgical patients: a prospective, stratified, randomized, double-blind, placebo-controlled clinical trial. *Am J Respir Crit Care Med* 2002; **166**: 1029–37.

45 de Jonge E, Schultz MJ, Spanjaard L, et al. Effects of selective decontamination of digestive tract on mortality and acquisition of resistant bacteria in intensive care: a randomised controlled trial. *Lancet* 2003; **362**: 1011–6.

46 Bonten MJ, Kullberg BJ, van Dalen R, et al. Selective digestive decontamination in patients in intensive care. The Dutch Working Group on Antibiotic Policy. *J Antimicrob Chemother* 2000; **46**: 351–62.

47 Finfer S, Bellomo R, Boyce N, et al. A comparison of albumin and saline for fluid resuscitation in the intensive care unit. *N Engl J Med* 2004; **350**: 2247–56.

PART 2

Physiology

CHAPTER 11
Inflammation and immunity

Helen F. Galley

Introduction

The immune system in humans is a very adaptable system that has evolved to provide protection against both invading pathogenic organisms and cancer cells. This extremely complex system is able to recognize and eliminate a huge variety of foreign cells and molecules. An immune response can be functionally divided into recognition and response. Immune recognition is extremely specific, enabling discrimination between the subtle chemical differences that distinguish foreign pathogens from each other. In addition, the immune system is able to recognize the body's own cells and proteins from foreign ones. Once a foreign molecule has been recognized — the recognition response — the immune system recruits the involvement of a number of other cells and molecules to elicit an appropriate response to enable the neutralization or elimination of the particular organism — the effector response. Exposure to the same organism again at a later date induces a memory response, with enhanced immune reactivity which eliminates the pathogen and prevents disease. This chapter describes basic mechanisms involved in innate and acquired immune responses and describes the particular relevance for sepsis. In addition, recent discoveries in signalling pathways for bacterial and viral agents and novel immunotherapeutic strategies are discussed.

Innate immunity

Immunity can be defined as the state of protection from infectious disease, and comprises both specific and non-specific components. Non-specific, or innate immunity, is the basic in-built resistance to disease that we have, regardless of there being no prior exposure to the antigen. Innate immunity comprises four defensive barriers, which offer protection through anatomical, physiological, phagocytic/endocytic and inflammatory strategies.

Anatomical barriers

Anatomical barriers are the body's first line of defence, preventing entry of pathogens and hence infection. These include the skin and mucous membranes.

The skin

Intact skin prevents the penetration of most pathogens. Skin consists of two layers: the thinner outer epidermis, and the thicker dermis. The epidermis is renewed every 2–4 weeks and does not contain blood vessels. The dermis is composed of connective tissue and contains blood vessels, hair follicles, sebaceous glands and sweat glands. The sebaceous glands produce the oily substance sebum, made up of lactic acid and fatty acids, which keeps the pH of the skin at around pH 4 to inhibit bacterial growth. Bacteria that metabolize sebum live on the skin and are responsible for a rare form of acne; acne treatments such as isotretotoin inhibit sebum formation. Breaks in the skin such as small cuts and insect bites are obvious routes of infection, and diseases such as malaria and Lyme disease are spread via insect bites.

Mucous membranes

The conjunctivae and the alimentary, respiratory and urogenital tracts are covered by mucous membranes instead of skin. Many pathogens enter the body by binding to and penetrating mucous membranes, but they are protected by saliva, tears and mucus, which wash away organisms and also contain antiviral and antibacterial substances. In the lower respiratory and gastrointestinal tracts, organisms trapped in mucus are propelled out of the body by ciliary action. Some organisms have evolved such that they can evade this defence mechanism. For example, the influenza virus has a surface molecule that enables it to attach to cells in the mucus membrane, preventing it being washed away through the action of cilia. The adherence of bacteria to mucous membranes is dependent on the interaction of protrusions on the bacteria and specific glycoproteins on some mucous membrane epithelial cells, which explains why only certain tissues are susceptible to bacterial invasion.

Physiological barriers

If an organism manages to breach the anatomical barriers, other innate defences come into play. Physiological barriers include temperature, pH and a variety of soluble factors, including lysozyme, interferons (IFNs) and complement. Many species are resistant to certain diseases because their body temperature inhibits pathogen growth. Hens, for example, have a high body temperature which inhibits the growth of anthrax. Gastric acidity prevents the growth of many organisms, and newborn infants are more prone to some diseases because their stomach contents are less acidic. Lysozyme, found in mucus, is an enzyme that cleaves the peptidoglycan layer of bacterial cell walls. Interferons are produced by virus-infected cells and bind to nearby cells, causing a generalized antiviral state (see below). Complement is a group of serum proteins that circulate in an inactive state. They can be activated by non-specific immune mechanisms that convert the inactive pro-enzymes to active enzymes through an enzyme cascade, which results in membrane damaging reactions, destroying pathogenic organisms and facilitating their clearance.

Complement

The complement system is activated via a sequential enzymatic cascade and has an important role in antigen clearance. There are two pathways of complement activation. The classic pathway involves activation by specific immunoglobulin molecules, and the alternative pathway is activated by a variety of microorganisms and immune complexes. Each pathway results in the activation of different complement proteins but the endpoint is the same — the generation of a membrane attack complex which is how complement is able to lyse foreign cells. This complex displaces phospholipids within cell membranes, making large holes, disrupting the membrane and resulting in cell lysis. Complement components also amplify reactions between antigens and antibodies, attract phagocytic cells to sites of infection and promote phagocytosis, and activate B lymphocytes. The complement system is non-specific and will, in theory, attack its own body cells as well as foreign cells. To prevent host cell damage there are regulatory mechanisms that restrict complement reactions to specific targets. This is achieved by spontaneous breakdown of active complement components and the release of inactivating proteins.

Endocytosis and phagocytosis

Another important innate defence mechanism is the ingestion of extracellular macromolecules and particles by the processes of endocytosis and phagocytosis, respectively. In endocytosis, macromolecules in extracellular fluid are internalized by invagination of the plasma membrane to form endocytic vesicles. Endocytosis can take place through two mechanisms: pinocytosis and receptor-mediated endocytosis. Pinocytosis occurs through non-specific membrane invagination, whereas in receptor-mediated endocytosis macromolecules are selectively engulfed after binding to specific membrane receptors. The ingested material is degraded by enzymes of the endocytic processing pathway.

Phagocytosis involves ingestion of particles, including whole microorganisms, via expansion of the plasma membrane to form phagosomes. Virtually all cells are able to endocytose but phagocytosis occurs in only a few specialized cells. Professional phagocytes are the polymorphonuclear neutrophils, mast cells and macrophages, and non-professional phagocytes include endothelial cells and hepatocytes. Cells infected with viruses and parasites are killed by large granular lymphocytes, termed natural killer (NK) cells, and eosinophils. Once particles are ingested into phagosomes, the phagosomes fuse with lysosomes and the contents are digested in a similar way to endocytosis.

The inflammatory response

The inflammatory response to tissue damage or invasion by pathogenic organisms results in vasodilatation, increased capillary permeability and influx of phagocytic cells. Vasodilatation occurs as the vessels constrict, resulting in engorgement of the capillary network, causing tissue redness or erythema, and increased tissue temperature, while increased capillary permeability enables an influx of fluid and cells from the capillaries into the tissue. The accumulating fluid — exudate — has a high protein content and its accumulation contributes to the tissue swelling, or oedema. The increased capillary permeability also helps the migration of leucocytes into the tissues, particularly phagocytes. Movement of phagocytic cells involves a complex series of events including margination or adherence of cells to the endothelial cell wall, extravasation or movement of the cells between the capillary cell walls into the tissue, and chemotaxis, the migration of the cells through the tissue to the site of inflammation. The process of leucocyte margination is a carefully regulated process involving adhesion molecules. These comprise three structurally dissimilar groups of molecules which are located on the extracellular portion of the cell membrane of both endothelial cells and leucocytes. Examples include E-selectin, intercellular adhesion molecule (ICAM) and vascular cell adhesion molecule (VCAM). These molecules cause circulating white cells initially to slow down and then roll along the endothelium so that firm adherence and transmigration can occur.

The inflammatory response is initiated by a series of interactions that involve several chemical mediators, produced from the invading organisms, from damaged cells, from cells of the immune system and from plasma enzyme systems. Among the chemical mediators released as a result of tissue damage are the acute phase proteins. The circulating levels of these increase considerably during tissue damaging infections. C-reactive protein is a major acute phase protein produced by the liver and which binds to the C polysaccharide component found on many bacteria and fungi. This binding activates the complement system, resulting in both complement-mediated lysis and increased phagocytosis. Histamine is a chemical released from mast cells, basophils and platelets in response to tissue injury, which binds to receptors on capillaries and venules, leading to increased vascular permeability and vasodilatation. Kinins are small peptides that cause vasodilatation and increased capillary permeability and are also important mediators of the inflammatory response to injury. In addition, bradykinin also stimulates pain receptors in the skin.

Regulation of the inflammatory response

Severe infection with Gram-negative organisms leads to the appearance of endotoxin or lipopolysaccharide (LPS) in the blood stream which interacts with LPS-binding protein (LBP) and binds to CD14 receptors, transducing signals via Toll-like receptors, which culminate in the activation of the transcription factor nuclear factor κB (NF-κB) [1–3]. Toll-like receptors (TLRs) are pathogen-associated molecular pattern (PAMP) receptors for a variety of diverse molecules derived from bacteria, viruses and fungi [4]. Engagement of TLRs by PAMPs on cells, such as macrophages and neutrophils, drives innate immune effector function, while activation of TLRs expressed on antigen-presenting cells (most notably dendritic cells) leads to the initiation of adaptive immunity through induction of interleukin-12 (IL-12) and T-cell activation. Recruitment of the adaptor protein, MyD88 to TLR complexes ultimately leads to the activation of NF-κB. MyD88 is involved in NF-κB activation by every TLR tested so far except TLR3.

NF-κB regulates, in part, gene expression of many cytokines, growth factors, adhesion molecules and enzymes involved in the inflammatory response (see below) [2]. It is maintained in a non-activated state in the cytoplasm by association with an inhibitor subunit, IκB. Proteolysis of IκB in response to activation stimuli, including LPS and cytokines, reveals a previously hidden nuclear recognition site (Fig. 11.1). This then prompts the NF-κB to move into the nucleus where it binds onto target DNA and results in mRNA expression. NF-κB activation leads to increased gene expression of several important mediators involved in the inflammatory response, including chemokines, cytokines and adhesion molecules. Although some cells (e.g. endothelial cells) do not themselves express CD14, LPS can activate

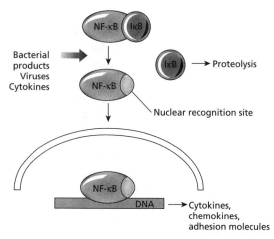

Figure 11.1 Activation of nuclear factor κB (NF-κB). Reproduced with permission from Galley and Webster [32].

these cells via interaction with soluble CD14 and LBP circulating in the blood stream.

Interferons are the body's first line of antiviral defence. By inducing the expression of hundreds of IFN-stimulated genes, which have antiviral functions, IFNs can block virus replication. Viruses are able to counteract the antiviral response through mechanisms that control IFN signalling and block the actions of IFN-stimulated gene products. Studies of influenza, hepatitis C, herpes simplex and vaccinia viruses have revealed the importance of IFNs for the control of virus replication and pathogenesis. Various viral proteins are able to either activate TLRs or to block TLR function, demonstrating the interplay between detection of viruses by the innate immune system, and evasion of the TLR system for the viruses' own purposes. Some viruses may even need cellular activation via TLRs to enable entry into the cell or replication. The discovery that viruses activate TLRs and activate NF-κB leading to production of IFNs, is providing a crucial 'missing' link in the understanding of exactly how viral infection leads to the IFN response [5].

To date, 10 TLR family members have been identified [4]. TLR2 is crucial for the propagation of the inflammatory response to components of Gram-positive and Gram-negative bacteria and mycobacteria such as LPS, peptidoglycan, lipoteichoic acid,

bacterial lipoproteins, lipopeptides, and lipoarabinomannan. TLR2 is predominantly expressed in the cells involved in innate immunity, including monocytes, macrophages, dendritic cells and neutrophils, but endothelial cells also express TLR2. TLR4 has been identified as the receptor for LPS and lipoteichoic acid. Double-stranded RNA is a molecular pattern produced by many viruses, and so is considered a viral PAMP. It has recently been shown that TLR3 can mediate cellular responses to viral infection [6]. TLR3 localization varies in different types of cells; it is expressed on the cell surface of fibroblasts but intracellularly in dendritic cells [7].

Another receptor that is important for host responses to infection has recently been described, triggering receptor expressed on myeloid cells (TREM-1) [8]. It is expressed on neutrophils and a subset of monocytes. *In vitro* studies have shown that TREM-1 is up-regulated in response to Gram-positive and Gram-negative bacteria, mycobacteria and bacterial cell wall components, including both LPS and lipoteichoic acid. Triggering of the TREM-1 receptor induces the secretion of IL-8, tumour necrosis factor α (TNF-α), IL-1β and monocyte chemotactic protein (MCP-1) and release of the enzyme myeloperoxidase [9]. TREM-1 is one of several pathways with a role in signalling in the innate immune response (Fig. 11.2) and has been shown to have a role in sepsis [10].

There are several human primary immunodeficiencies caused by germ line mutations in genes encoding molecules involved in cell signalling downstream from TLRs [11]. These patients have defects in TLR/NF-κB signalling and increased bacterial infection rates in childhood, but despite the infectious phenotype, defects are restricted and this suggests that TLRs are largely redundant in protective immunity *in vivo*. Indeed, other cell-surface receptors are also involved in LPS-mediated immune responses, including the type A macrophage-scavenger receptor [12], β2 integrin (CD11b/CD18) [13] and a voltage-dependent K^+ channel [14]. Nod1 and Nod2 proteins are also involved in responses to LPS in some cells [15].

Apoptosis

Cells that are damaged by injury, such as by mechan-

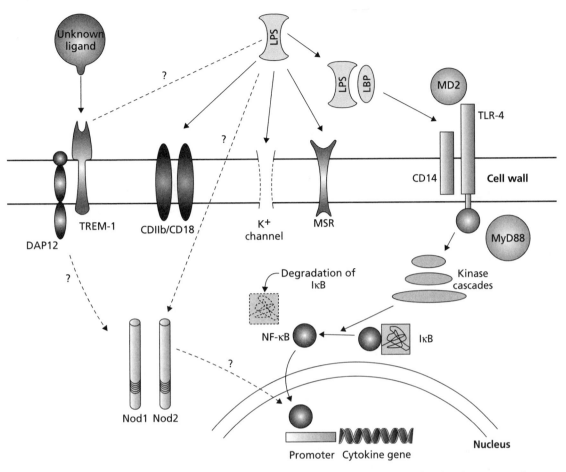

Figure 11.2 Outline of TREM-1 and cytokines in inflammatory response to bacteria. Reproduced with permission from Cohen [8]. IκB, inhibitor of κB; LPS, lipopolysaccharide; MSR, macrophage-scavenger receptor; MyD88, myeloid differentiation factor 88.

ical damage or exposure to toxic chemicals, undergo swelling caused by disruption of the ability of the plasma membrane to control the passage of ions and water, with consequent leakage of cell contents, leading to inflammation of surrounding tissues. This process is called necrosis.

Apoptosis, or programmed cell death, is a crucial process for normal development and maintenance of tissue homoeostasis via removal of damaged, infected or otherwise harmful cells such as tumour cells. Cells that are induced to 'commit suicide' by apoptosis, in contrast to necrosis, shrink and the mitochondrial membrane becomes breached. Phagocytic cells such as macrophages engulf the cell

fragments, leading to a 'quiet' and orderly removal of dead cells [16].

Deregulation of apoptosis has a role in various diseases such as cancer, autoimmune diseases, neurodegenerative disorders and AIDS. Apoptosis is an active and tightly regulated process. It is induced by activation of effector protease enzymes called caspases which cleave specific substrates, resulting in the events leading to cellular disassembly. Because of the orderly way in which apoptosis takes place, release of inflammatory mediators in the extracellular environment is prevented. Hence, apoptosis clearly differs from necrosis, which causes an inflammatory reaction.

The cascade of events leading to apoptosis takes place as a result of either the withdrawal of positive signals (i.e. signals needed for continued survival) or the initiation of negative signals (i.e. those that instigate cell death). Signals can arise within the cell or from so-called 'death activators' binding to receptors at the cell surface. Caspases initially exist as immature pro-caspases (zymogens) and require processing to be activated, in a similar way to the proteins of the clotting or complement cascades.

Apoptosis pathways

Like complement activation, the process of apoptosis can be activated by two pathways: one dependent on mitochondria and the other independent of mitochondria. The mitochondria-dependent or intrinsic apoptotic pathway is triggered by various stress signals, including DNA damage (e.g. that induced by radiation or chemotherapeutic agents), stress molecules (e.g. reactive oxygen species and reactive nitrogen species) or growth factor withdrawal. These stress signals can trigger the release of pro-apoptotic proteins from the mitochondrial intermembrane space into the cytosol. Important apoptosis regulators of the mitochondrial pathway are the BCL2 protein family, in which members are either death antagonists or death agonists. The ratio of pro-apoptotic to anti-apoptotic BCL2 family proteins controls the cell's sensitivity to apoptotic signals via the mitochondrial pathway.

The extrinsic apoptotic pathway is initiated by activation of so-called death receptors on the cell membrane. Several of the human death receptors belong to the TNF receptor superfamily. Apoptosis triggered by death receptor activation also triggers the mitochondrial apoptotic pathway. Apoptosis can be inhibited at several stages in the pathway.

Proteasome

The proteasome is the term given to an enzyme complex found in both the nucleus and the cytoplasm of cells that effectively functions as a protein shredder. The function of the proteasome is to degrade or process intracellular proteins, some of which are mediators of cell-cycle progression and apoptosis, such as the caspases, BCL2 and NF-κB. It therefore has an important role in the regulation of intracellular pro-

tein degradation and as such regulates apoptosis and inflammatory response processes. Malignant cells are more susceptible to certain proteasome inhibitors, which might be explained, in part, by the reversal or bypass of some of the effects of the mutations in cell-cycle and apoptotic checkpoints that have led to tumorigenesis. Inhibition of the activity of the proteasome has been proposed as an anticancer therapeutic target [17].

Acquired immunity

Acquired (specific) immunity inactivates microorganisms that are not destroyed by the innate immune system. Specificity, diversity, memory and the ability to discriminate self from non-self are key features of the acquired immune system. The acquired immune system has four distinct phases: recognition of antigen, activation of lymphocytes, effector phase of antigen elimination and return to homoeostasis and antigenic memory. Acquired immunity is intricately involved with the innate immune response. Phagocytic cells for example, activate specific immune responses and stimulate the release of soluble mediators that control and regulate the inflammatory response and the interplay involved in the elimination of a foreign organism. The specificity of the immune system is such that even a single amino acid substitution can mean that an antigen escapes recognition and hence elimination.

The acquired immune response can also be classified into humoral (from body fluid) and cell-mediated immunity. The humoral component involves interaction of B cells with antigen and their proliferation and differentiation into plasma cells, the antibody secreting cells. Antibody is the effector of the humoral response due to its binding to the antigen, neutralizing and facilitating its removal. This process also activates the complement system. Unlike B cells, where membrane bound antibody enables direct recognition of antigen, T cells can only recognize antigen in the presence of cell membrane proteins called the major histocompatibility complex (MHC) molecules. Effector T cells generated in response to antigen associated with MHC are responsible for cell-mediated immunity. There are two main types of T cells: T helper (Th) cells and T cytotoxic (Tc) cells. Th cells secrete cytokines, which are low molecular weight proteins, and which activate various phagocytic cells, B cells, Tc cells, macrophages and other cells. Under the influence of cytokines secreted by Th cells, Tc cells that recognize antigen–MHC molecule complex are able to eliminate cells displaying antigen — that is, altered self cells, such as virus infected cells, foreign tissue grafts and tumour cells.

Major histocompatibility complex

The MHC is a tightly linked cluster of genes located on chromosome 6 that encodes proteins required for antigen recognition. MHC also have major roles in the acceptance of self (histocompatible) or non-self (histoincompatible). The MHC proteins have an important role in antigen recognition by T cells, and determine the response of an individual to infectious antigens and hence susceptibility to disease. Human MHC molecules are called human leucocyte antigens (HLA). The MHC genes are organized into those encoding three classes of molecules: classes I–III. Class I genes encode glycoproteins expressed on the surface of most nucleated cells and present antigens for the activation of specific T cells. Class II genes encode glycoproteins expressed mainly on antigen presenting cells, including macrophages and B cells, where they present antigen to other defined T-cell populations. Class III genes encode several different immune products, including complement system components, enzymes and TNF-α, and have no role in antigen presentation. Class I molecules are expressed on all nucleated cells, whereas class II molecules are mainly expressed on specialized antigen presenting cells such as dendritic cells, macrophages and B lymphocytes. MHC molecule expression is enhanced by cytokines such as IFN-γ.

Cell-mediated immunity

Leucocytes develop from a common pluripotent stem cell during haematopoiesis, and proliferate and differentiate into the different cells in response to haematopoietic growth factors, balanced by programmed cell death or apoptosis. The lymphocyte, the only cell to possess specificity, diversity, memory and recognition of self/non-self, is the central line of the immune system. Monocytes, macrophages and

neutrophils are accessory immune cells that phagocytose, facilitated by complement and antibody, which increase attachment of antigen to the membrane of the phagocyte. Macrophages also are important in antigen processing and presentation in association with a class II MHC molecule, and secretion of the cytokine, IL-1. Lymphocytes constantly recirculate via interaction between cell adhesion molecules on the vascular endothelium and receptors for the adhesion molecules on the circulating cells.

Different maturational stages of lymphocytes can be distinguished by their expression of specific molecules on the cell membranes, which are called cluster of differentiation (CD) antigens.

Lymphocytes

Antibodies activate the complement system, stimulate phagocytic cells and specifically inactivate microorganisms. Lymphocytes, the basis of the acquired immune defence system, consist of antibody producing plasma cells derived from B lymphocytes, and T lymphocytes which control intracellular infections. Binding of microorganisms to antibodies on the cell surface of B cells leads to preferential selection of these antibody producing cells. This is termed priming, and subsequent responses are faster and amplified, and provide the basis of vaccination. T cells exploit two main strategies to combat intracellular infections: secretion of soluble mediators that activate other cells to enhance microbial defence mechanisms, and production of cytotoxic T lymphocytes that kill the target organism. NK cells have an important role in tumour cell destruction. They are large granular lymphocytes that do not exhibit immunological memory and are non-specific in their recognition of tumour cells.

Control of adaptive T-cell selection

Regulation of MHC gene expression (e.g. by cytokines) has a fundamental role in the immune system, because alterations of cell surface expression of class I or II molecules can affect the efficiency of antigen presentation. T helper (Th) cells are CD4$^+$ and recognize class II MHC molecules which produce IFN-γ and other macrophage activating factors. Cytotoxic or killer T cells (Tc) are CD8$^+$ and recognize both specific antigens and class I MHC molecules on the surface of infected cells.

T helper cells

Circulating Th cells are capable of unrestricted cytokine expression and are prompted into a more restricted and focused pattern of cytokine production, depending on signals received at the outset of infection (Fig. 11.3). The cells can be classified according to the pattern of cytokines they produce. Th1 category cells secrete a characteristic set of cytokines that push the system towards cellular immunity (cellular cytotoxicity). Th2 cells are associated with humoral or antibody mediated immunity. Typically, Th1 cells secrete IL-2, IFN-γ, TNF-β and transforming growth factor β (TGF-β) whereas Th2 cells secrete IL-4, IL-5, IL-6, IL-9, IL-10 and IL-13 and also help B-cell antibody production. Both cell types produce

IL-3, TNF-α and granulocyte macrophage colony stimulating factor (GM-CSF).

Polarization of Th cells toward either a Th1 or Th2 response can significantly influence host immunity to pathogens. IFN-γ and IL-4 are the signature cytokines of Th1 and Th2 cells, respectively. At an early stage of development, Th1 and Th2 populations are heterogeneous with a reversible cytokine profile, suggesting that a number of molecular changes are needed for committed profiles of cytokine gene expression. The control of Th cell differentiation is a function of a number of factors; the most important of which is cytokine environment. There appear to be two 'master switches' that control Th cytokine commitment. IL-4 is the principal cytokine driving naïve T cells (Th0) to Th2 differentiation. IL-4 is synthesized by differentiating Th2 cells and by fully differentiated Th2 cells. The human

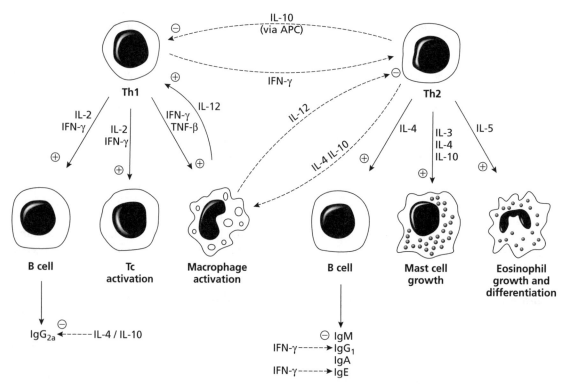

Figure 11.3 Cross-regulation by cytokines secreted from T helper 1 (Th1) and Th2 subsets. Solid arrows indicate stimulatory effects; dashed arrows indicate inhibitory effects. IFN, interferon; Ig, immunoglobulin; IL, interleukin. Reproduced with permission from Webster and Galley [33].

IL-4 promoter consists of multiple DNA binding motifs, which bind several classes of transcription factor. The GATA-binding protein 3 (GATA-3) is a Th2-specific regulatory factor necessary to direct Th cells to Th2 differentiation [18]. The key cytokine for promoting Th1 differentiation is IFN-γ. A number of transcription factors have an important role in regulation of IFN-γ. However, control of Th1 lineage commitment and IFN-γ expression seems to be controlled by the Th1-restricted transcription factor protein, T-bet, which is able to initiate Th1 differentiation while repressing Th2 differentiation [19].

Serious injury results in predominance of the Th2 phenotype as opposed to the Th1 phenotype, rather than generalized Th suppression [20,21]. Th1 predominance is associated with cell mediated responses that are generally considered to be most beneficial to recovery. A shift to Th2 dominated phenotypes increases the risk for infection (e.g. after burn injury) [21]. The Th1:Th2 ratio is reduced in patients with sepsis caused by both a decrease in Th1 cells and an increase in Th2 cells [22].

Processing and presentation of antigens

Antigens are substances including proteins, carbohydrates and glycoproteins, that are capable of interacting with the products of a specific immune response. An antigen that is capable of eliciting a specific immune response by itself is called an immunogen. Foreign protein antigens must be degraded into small peptides and complexed with class I or II MHC molecules in order to be recognized by a T cell. This is called antigen processing. Complexing with class I or II MHC molecules seems to be determined by the way in which the antigen enters the cell.

Mature immunocompetent animals possess large numbers of antigen reactive T and B cells and long before any contact with an antigen, each T and B lymphocyte already possesses specificity to antigens. This is achieved by random gene rearrangements in the bone marrow during maturation of lymphocytes. When antigen interacts with, and activates, mature, antigenically committed T and B cells it causes the expansion of the particular population of cells with that antigenic specificity. This is called clonal selec-

tion and expansion. This process explains both specificity and memory attributes. Specificity is implicit because only those lymphocytes possessing appropriate receptors will be clonally expanded. Memory occurs because there is a larger number of antigen reactive lymphocytes present after clonal selection and many of these lymphocytes have a longer lifespan — these are called memory cells. The initial encounter of antigen-specific lymphocytes with an antigen induces a primary response, and later encounters are more rapid and heightened secondary response (Fig. 11.4). Self/non-self recognition is achieved by elimination of lymphocytes that bear receptors identifying them as self.

Antibody structure

The protein molecules that combine specifically with antigens are called antibodies or immunoglobulins. Antibody molecules consist of two identical light

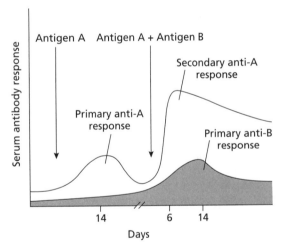

Figure 11.4 Differences in the primary and secondary response to injected antigen (humoral response) reflect the phenomenon of immunological memory. When an animal is injected with an antigen, it produces a primary serum antibody response of low magnitude and relatively short duration, peaking at approximately 10–17 days. A second immunization with the same antigen results in a secondary response that is greater in magnitude, peaks in 2–7 days and lasts longer (months to years) than the primary response. Reproduced with permission from Webster and Galley [33].

chains and two identical heavy chains joined by disulphide bonds. Each heavy and light chain has a
variable amino acid sequence region and a constant
region. The unique heavy chain constant region sequences determine the five classes or isotypes of antibody: IgM, IgG, IgD, IgA and IgE (Table 11.1). These
isotypes vary in their effector function, serum concentration and half-life. IgG is the most common isotype and the only immunoglobulin to cross the
placenta. IgM exists as a pentamer and is most effective in viral neutralization, bacterial agglutination
and complement activation. IgA is the predominant
isotype in external secretions including breast milk
and mucus. IgD and IgE are the least abundant isotypes; IgD and IgM are the major isotype on mature B
cells and IgE mediates mast cell degranulation.

Monoclonal antibodies are antibodies with the
same antigenic specificity. These antibodies are produced by a hybridoma, which is a group of identical
cells called a clone. These clones are manufactured
by fusing normal lymphocytes with myeloma cells;
the clone keeps its normal antibody functions and
receptors of lymphocytes but has the immortal
growth characteristics of myeloma cells. Monoclonal
antibodies provide an indefinite supply of antibody
with a highly defined antigenic specificity.

Cytokines

Orchestration of immune and inflammatory responses depends upon communication between
cells by soluble molecules given the generic term cytokines, including chemokines, interleukins, growth
factors and IFNs. They are involved in both innate
and acquired immune responses. Cytokines are low
molecular weight secreted proteins that regulate
both the amplitude and duration of immune responses and have the properties of redundancy, plei-
otrophy, synergism and antagonism. They have a
transient and tightly regulated action. Cytokines are
highly active at very low concentrations, combining
with small numbers of high affinity cell surface receptors and producing changes in the patterns of
RNA and protein synthesis. They have multiple effects on growth and differentiation in a variety of cell
types with considerable overlap and redundancy between them, partially accounted for by the induction
of synthesis of common proteins. Interaction may
occur in a sort of network in which one cytokine induces another, through modulation of the receptor
of another cytokine and through either synergism or
antagonism of two cytokines acting on the same cell.
Cytokines should not be considered as having
identifying labels for being growth stimulators or

Table 11.1 Characteristics of immunoglobulin isotypes.

Antibody isotype (half-life in serum)	Specific effector function	Other information
IgG (23 days)	Neutralization of bacteria Facilitation of phagocytosis Complement activation (classic pathway) ADCC mediated by NK cells Inhibits B-cell activation	Crosses placenta: provides neonatal passive immunity
IgM (5 days)	Antigen receptor for naïve B cells Complement activation (classic pathway)	Membrane bound
IgD (3 days)	Antigen receptor for naïve B cells	Membrane bound, no secreted form
IgA (6 days)	Provides mucosal immunity	Secreted into gut lumen, respiratory tract and breast milk
IgE (2 days)	ADCC mediated by eosinophils Mast cell degranulation	Provides immunity against helminths Involved in hypersensitivity reactions

ADCC, antibody-dependent cellular cytotoxicity; Ig, immunoglobulin; NK, natural killer.

inhibitors and pro- or anti-inflammatory actions; their specific action depends on the stimulus, the cell type and the presence of other mediators and receptors.

Chemokines are small chemoattractant molecules characterized by four conserved cysteine residues. The α chemokines have two pairs of cysteine residues separated by a variable amino acid (C-X-C) and chemoattract neutrophils (e.g. IL-8, platelet basic protein, epithelial neutrophil activating peptide), whereas β chemokines have two adjacent pairs of cysteine groups (C-C) and are chemotactic for monocytes/macrophages (e.g. platelet factor 4, monocyte chemotactic protein 1, macrophage inflammatory protein 1) and T cells (e.g. RANTES). Chemokines have been said to have more restricted actions than cytokines, but this is more likely to be a result of differential expression of receptors.

Interferons (IFN-α, IFN-β, IFN-γ) are a family of broad-spectrum antiviral agents that also modulate the activity of other cells, particularly IL-8 and platelet activating factor (PAF) production, antibody production by B cells and activation of cytotoxic macrophages. Growth factors regulate the differentiation, proliferation, activity and function of specific cell types. The best known are colony-stimulating factors which cause colony formation by haematogenic progenitor cells (e.g. granulocyte–macrophage colony-stimulating factor, GM-CSF). Other examples include factors that regulate the growth of nerve cells, fibroblasts, epidermis and hepatocytes.

In addition to the low molecular weight protein mediators, there are also lipid mediators of inflammation which include PAF and arachidonic acid metabolites. PAF is a labile alkyl phospholipid released from a variety of cells in the presence of antigen and leucocytes in response to immune complexes. In addition to its actions on platelets, the effects of PAF include the priming of macrophages to other inflammatory mediators and alterations of microvascular permeability. Arachidonic acid metabolites include the prostaglandins and leukotrienes, which have profound inflammatory and vascular actions, and may regulate and be regulated by other cytokines.

TNF-α and TNF-β have a vast range of similar effects and are usually referred to as pro-inflammatory cytokines. They have a central role in initiating the cascade/network of other cytokines and factors that make up the immune response to infection. The wide variety of effects can be explained by the wide distribution of their receptors, their ability to activate multiple signal transduction pathways and their ability to induce or suppress many genes including those for growth factors, cytokines, transcription factors, receptors and acute phase proteins. Although both TNFs have similar biological activities, regulation of the expression and processing of the two is quite different.

Receptors and antagonists

The biological activities of cytokines are regulated by specific cellular receptors. Often these receptors comprise multiple subunits providing phased stages of activation and biological action. For example the IL-2 receptor (IL-2R) complex consists of three subunits: IL-2Rα, IL-2Rβ and IL-2Rγ. Although the IL-2Rα/β combination can bind IL-2, IL-2Rγ is also required for high affinity binding, ligand internalization and signalling, which are all required for maximal effect. Other cellular receptors are present in more than one type which act alone but have different binding affinities for different forms of a cytokine protein (e.g. IL-1 receptor type I binds IL-1α better than IL-1β, and IL-1 receptor type II has more affinity for IL-1β). Binding of a cytokine to one type of receptor may result in interactions with another receptor; the two receptors for TNF, for example, use ligand passing in which TNF binds transiently to receptor type I, with full signal transduction, but may then move onto the type II receptor with activation of another signal for apoptosis or programmed cell killing.

Soluble cytokine receptors have been identified that compete with membrane-bound receptors, thus regulating cytokine signals. Exceptions to this are soluble receptors for IL-6 and ciliary neurotrophic factor, which act as agonists rather than antagonists. Such soluble receptors may be membrane-bound receptors that are shed into the circulation either intact or as truncated forms (e.g. soluble TNF receptors, sTNF-R), or may begin as related precursor molecules that are enzymatically cleaved (e.g. IL-1R). Soluble receptors may appear in response to stimuli as part of a naturally occurring independent regulatory process to limit the harmful effects of a mediator (e.g. sTNF-R), but some soluble receptors have little binding activity and may represent superficial and unimportant losses of cellular receptors (e.g. the soluble form of IL-2Rα). Soluble cytokine receptors not only mediate biological activity but control desensitization to ligands by reduced availability, decreased signalling and by stimulating cellular mechanisms that can result in lack of activity.

The biological actions of some cytokines are also regulated by receptor antagonists. The receptor antagonist for IL-1 (IL-1ra) competes with cell receptors for IL-1, but when bound does not induce signalling. IL-1ra binds to cell receptors much more avidly than to soluble receptors, such that soluble receptors will have little effect of the inhibitory action of the receptor antagonist. The soluble receptor also inhibits activation of the pro-IL-1β precursor. The appearance of IL-1ra is independently regulated by other cytokines as part of the inflammatory process.

Hypersensitivity reactions

A localized inflammatory reaction, delayed type hypersensitivity (DTH), can occur when some subpopulations of activated Th cells encounter certain antigens. Tissue damage is usually limited and DTH has an important role in defence against intracellular pathogens and contact antigens. Development of a DTH response requires a sensitization episode beforehand, when Th cells are activated and clonally expanded by antigen presented along with the required class II MHC molecule. A second exposure to the antigen induces an effector response, where T cells produce a variety of cytokines leading to recruitment and activation of macrophages and other non-specific inflammatory cells. The activated T cells are generally Th1 subtype. A DTH response becomes apparent after approximately 24 hours following secondary antigen contact, peaking after approximately 48–72 hours. The delay is caused by the time taken for cytokines to activate and recruit macrophages. A complex and amplified interaction of many non-specific cells then occurs, but only approximately 5% of the participating cells are antigen specific. The macrophage is the primary effector cell of DTH responses and the influx and activation of these cells

provides an effective host response against intracellular pathogens. Generally, the pathogen is cleared with little tissue damage, but prolonged DTH responses can themselves be damaging, ultimately leading to tissue necrosis in extreme cases.

Immediate hypersensitivity reactions occur within 8 hours of secondary allergen exposure and are not cell-mediated but humoral in nature, resulting in generation of antibody-secreting plasma cells and memory cells. The hypersensitivity reactions can be classified into type I (IgE dependent), type II (antibody-mediated cytotoxicity), type III (immune complex-mediated hypersensitivity) and type IV (delayed type hypersensitivity) and are shown in Table 11.2. Type I reactions are mediated by IgE antibodies which bind to receptors on mast cells or basophils, leading to degranulation and release of mediators. The principal effects are smooth muscle contraction and vasodilatation, and can result in serious life-threatening systemic anaphylaxis, asthma, hay fever and eczema.

Type II hypersensitivity reactions occur when antibody reacts with antigenic markers on the cell surface leading to cell death through complement-mediated lysis or antibody-dependent cytotoxicity. Type II reactions include haemolytic disease of the newborn and autoimmune diseases such as Goodpasture's syndrome and myasthenia gravis.

Type III reactions are mediated by formation of antigen–antibody or immune complexes and subsequent complement activation. Deposition of immune complexes near the site of antigen entry can cause the release of lytic enzymes by accumulated neutrophils and results in localized tissue damage. The formation of circulating immune complexes is involved in a number of conditions including allergies to penicillin, infectious diseases including hepatitis, and autoimmune diseases such as rheumatoid arthritis.

The characteristics of hypersensitivity reactions are given in Table 11.2 and common antigens are listed in Table 11.3.

Lymphoid tissue

Although the immune system operates throughout the body, there are certain sites where the cells of the

Table 11.2 Hypersensitivity reactions.

Type of reaction	Immune mechanism	Effector mechanism	Example
Type I Immediate	Th2 cells IgE Mast cells Eosinophils	Mast cell-derived mediators Cytokine-mediated inflammation	Systemic and local anaphylaxis (see Table 11.3)
Type II Antibody-mediated	IgM, IgG	Complement-mediated recruitment/activation of neutrophils/macrophages Phagocytosis Abnormal cell function	Blood transfusion reactions Autoimmune haemolytic anaemia
Type III Immune complex- mediated	Immune complexes deposited in vascular basement membrane	Complement-mediated recuitment and activation of neutrophils/macrophages	Systemic lupus erythematosus Rheumatoid arthritis Glomerular nephritis
Type IV T-cell-mediated Delayed	CD4+ T cells CD8+ cytoxic T cells	Macrophage activation Direct target cell lysis Cytokine-mediated inflammation	Contact dermatitis Graft rejection

Table 11.3 Common antigens associated with type I hypersensitivity.

Proteins	Foods	Plant pollens	Insect venom	Drugs	Mould spores	Animal hair and dander
Foreign serum	Nuts	Rye grass	Bee	Penicillin	*Aspergillus*	Dogs
Vaccines	Seafood	Ragweed	Wasp	Sulphonamides		Cats
Latex	Eggs	Timothy grass	Ant	Local anaesthetics		Horses
	Peas, beans	Birch trees		Salicylates		

immune system are organized into specific structures. These are classified as central lymphoid tissue (bone marrow, thymus) and peripheral lymphoid tissue (lymph nodes, spleen, mucosa-associated lymphoid tissue).

Bone marrow

All the cells of the immune system are derived from stem cells in the bone marrow. The bone marrow is the site of origin of red blood cells, white cells (including lymphocytes and macrophages) and platelets.

Thymus

In the thymus gland, lymphoid cells undergo a process of maturation prior to release into the circulation. This process allows T cells to develop self-tolerance. The thymus comprises an outer cortex and an inner medulla. Immature lymphoid cells enter the cortex, proliferate, mature and pass on to the medulla. From the medulla, mature T lymphocytes enter the circulation.

Lymph nodes

Lymph nodes are small bean-shaped structures lying

along the course of lymphatics. Within lymph nodes, phagocytic cells act as filters for particulate matter and microorganisms and antigen is presented to the cells of the immune system. Lymph passes into the node through the afferent lymphatic into the marginal sinus, through the cortical sinuses, to reach the medullary sinuses before leaving via the efferent lymphatic.

Spleen

The spleen has two main functions: acting as part of the immune system and as a filter. There are two distinct components of the spleen: the red pulp and the white pulp. The red pulp consists of large numbers of sinuses and sinusoids filled with blood and is responsible for the filtration function of the spleen. The white pulp consists of aggregates of lymphoid tissue and is responsible for the immunological function of the spleen as it contains T and B cells and antigen presenting dendritic cells.

Mucosa-associated lymphoid tissue

In addition to the lymphoid tissue concentrated within the lymph nodes and spleen, lymphoid tissue is also found at other sites, most notably the gastrointestinal, respiratory and urogenital tracts. B-cell precursors and memory cells are stimulated by antigen in Peyer's patches, which are aggregates of lymphoid tissue found in the small intestine.

Lymphocyte recirculation

Lymphocytes and macrophages can recirculate between lymphoid and non-lymphoid tissues, facilitating the distribution of effector cells to the sites where they are needed. The recirculation is a complex process, depending on interactions between the immune cells and other cell types such as endothelial cells. The complex patterns of recirculation depend on the state of activation of the lymphocytes, the adhesion molecules expressed by endothelial cells and the presence of chemotactic molecules which selectively attract particular populations of lymphocytes or macrophages.

Transplantation immunology

Transplantation is the transfer of cells, tissues or or-

gans from one site to another. Tissues that are antigenically similar or histocompatible do not induce rejection, and the opposite is called histoincompatible. Graft rejection is an immunological response involving cell-mediated responses, specifically T lymphocytes. The immune response is mounted against tissue antigens on the transplanted tissue that differ from those of the host. However, even with identical HLA antigens, differences in minor histocompatibility loci outside the MHC can contribute to graft rejection.

Graft rejection can be divided into sensitization and effector stages. During sensitization, leucocytes derived from the donor migrate from the donor tissue into lymph nodes where they are recognized as foreign by Th cells, stimulating Th cell proliferation. This is followed by migration of the effector Th cells into the graft and rejection follows. Graft rejection can be suppressed by specific and non-specific immunosuppressive agents. Non-specific agents include purine analogues, corticosteroids, cyclosporin, total lymphoid X-irradiation and antilymphocyte serum. Specific approaches such as blocking the proliferation of activated T cells using monoclonal antibodies to the IL-2 receptor, or depletion of T-cell populations with anti-CD3 or CD4 antibodies, have also been used.

Blood transfusion and postoperative immunocompetence

It is well recognized that blood transfusion suppresses some aspects of the immune response, giving rise to depressed delayed hypersensitivity reactions, decreased NK cell activity, decreased Th cells and decreased IL-2 production [23]. Although there are several theories to explain these effects, the explanation is still not clear and nor is it known for certain which of the components of the blood transfusion are responsible for the changes. However, it appears that the donor leucocytes carrying foreign antigens are most likely to be responsible for the immunosuppression.

In the patient undergoing surgery, the immunosuppressive effects of transfusion are compounded by the effects of anaesthesia and the stress response of the surgery itself. Three areas of concern have been highlighted: tumour recurrence rate, postoperative infection rate and the clinical course of pre-existing inflammatory disorders such as Crohn's disease.

Cancer immunology

Tumour cells display surface structures that are recognized as antigenic and that promote an immune response. Macrophages mediate tumour destruction by lytic enzymes and production of TNF-α; NK cells recognize tumour cells by an unknown mechanism and either bind to antibody coated tumour cells — antibody-dependent cell-mediated cytotoxicity — or by secretion of a cytotoxic factor that is apparently only cytotoxic for tumour cells. Tumour cell antigens can often elicit the generation of specific serum antibodies, which activate the complement system, producing the membrane attack complex. However, some tumours are able to endocytose the hole in the cell membrane produced by the membrane attack complex pore and repair the cell membrane before lysis occurs. Complement products can also induce chemotaxis of macrophages and neutrophils and release of toxic mediators. Ironically, antibodies to tumour cells may also enhance tumour growth, possibly by masking tumour antigens and preventing recognition by NK cells.

Cancer immunotherapy

A number of experimental immunotherapy regimens have been used in the treatment of cancer. Injections of cytokines including IFNs and TNF-α have been shown to be beneficial in some cancers. However, cytokine therapy may also result in unwanted side-effects including fever, hypotension and decreased leucocyte counts. Chronic lymphocytic leukaemia is characterized by the accumulation of leukaemic B cells and depressed immune responses. In particular, the T-cell abnormalities in these patients lead to increased risk of infection and hamper recognition and elimination of leukaemic cells by the immune system. *In vitro* expansion and activation of patients' T-cell populations has been tested as a potential therapy, and results in decreased numbers of leukaemic B cells, through increased apoptosis [24]. Most cancer immunotherapy strategies work by enhancing apoptosis of tumour cells and genetic ap-

proaches are now being tested [25]. Specifically, trials in patients with IFN-β resistant tumours such as glioma or melanoma, in whom the IFN-β gene is delivered in liposomes, have had some success [26].

HIV and AIDS

Human immunodeficiency virus (HIV) is the causative agent for acquired immunodeficiency syndrome (AIDS). The virus infects host cells by binding to CD4 molecules on the cell membranes of T lymphocytes. When the virus enters the cell, it copies its RNA into DNA and the DNA can then integrate into the host DNA, forming a pro-virus that can remain in a dormant state for varying lengths of time. Activation of an HIV-infected Th cell also triggers activation of the pro-virus, leading to destruction of the host cell and severe immune system depression. Because only approximately 0.01% of the Th cells are infected by the virus in an HIV-infected individual, the extensive depletion of the Th cell population implies that uninfected Th cells are also destroyed. Several mechanisms have been proposed for this, including complement-mediated lysis, apoptosis or antibody-mediated cytotoxicity. Early immunological changes include loss of *in vitro* proliferative responses of Th cells; reduced IgM synthesis; increased cytokine synthesis and reduced DTH responses. Later abnormalities include loss of germinal centres in lymph nodes; marked decreases in Th cell numbers and functional activity; lack of proliferation of HIV-specific B cells and lack of anti-HIV antibodies; shift in cytokine production from Th1 to Th2 subsets; and complete absence of DTH responses.

Treatment of HIV infection is via highly active antiretroviral therapy, usually in combinations of several drugs. Current therapeutic options and previously unexploited viral and cellular targets have been recently reviewed by Barbaro *et al.* [27].

Sepsis, SIRS and multiorgan failure

Severe infection leads triggering of the innate immune responses such as activation of phagocytic cells and activation of the alternative complement cascade, leading to the production of TNF-α and IL-1β. Secondary mediators including other cytokines, prostaglandins and PAF are then released, with further activation of complement and the acute phase response, expression of adhesion molecules, T-cell selection, antibody production and release of oxygen-derived free radicals. Other toxins and cellular debris must also trigger such a systemic inflammatory response, because this process also occurs in the absence of LPS release — resulting in the systemic inflammatory response syndrome (SIRS).

Local effects of the inflammatory response are essential for the control of infection. Prolonged systemic exposure to high concentrations of cytokines and other components of the immuno-inflammatory cascade may contribute to the development of multiorgan dysfunction syndrome. Damage and activation of the endothelium, which plays a pivotal role in the regulation of haemostasis, vascular tone and fibrinolysis, has profound consequences. The endothelium produces several substances that regulate inflammation and regional perfusion, including nitric oxide, vasoactive arachidonic acid metabolites and cytokines. Changes in the balance of concentrations of these substances may contribute to the pathogenesis of multiorgan failure. Phagocytic cells are in constant contact with the endothelium and disturbance of the relationship between these two cell types may result in direct tissue damage as a result of local production of oxygen-derived free radicals, hypochlorous acid and proteolytic enzymes. Another hypothesis to explain the observed tissue damage and organ dysfunction is that of local tissue ischaemia and hypoxia as a result of microthrombi formed by a coagulopathy or platelet or white cell aggregates. There is evidence for all of these mechanisms and it is probable that the pathogenesis of multiorgan dysfunction syndrome and failure is diverse and complex and is unlikely to be attributable to a single mechanism.

Immunotherapy in sepsis

Mortality from sepsis associated with metabolic acidosis, oliguria, hypoxaemia or shock, has remained high, even with intensive medical care, including treatment of the source of infection, intravenous fluids, nutrition, mechanical ventilation for respiratory failure, all of which are recognized standard treatments of sepsis. During the initial response to infection, tissue macrophages generate inflammatory cytokines, including TNF-α, IL-1 and IL-8 in response to bacterial cell wall products. Although cytokines play an important part in host defence by attracting activated neutrophils to the site of infection, inappropriate and excessive release into the systemic circulation may lead to widespread microvascular injury and multiorgan failure. All clinical series (with one exception) have shown that tested immunotherapies aimed at modulating the excessive expression of key cytokines, such as interleukins and TNF-α, designed to reduce the mortality rate associated with sepsis, have been either equivalent or inferior to placebo [28].

Both soluble receptors and monoclonal antibodies directed against receptors can be used to block the interaction of a cytokine with its receptor. This then prevents transduction of the appropriate biological signal in the target cell. The cloning of genes encoding cytokine receptor chains and the characterization of their soluble forms has resulted in new approaches to anticytokine therapy. Injection of a recombinant soluble receptor might prevent the deleterious effect of excessive cytokine production. In addition to soluble receptors, monoclonal antibodies that block cellular cytokine receptors can be used as anticytokine therapy. However, these small molecules have short half-lives and therefore derivatized molecules with longer half-lives and higher affinity have now been developed. However, it has been shown that cytokine complexed to such binding proteins is still available for receptor binding. It is possible that these complexes can still act as agonists *in vivo*, depending on concentrations of other mediators and relative receptor expression. Another approach to minimizing the deleterious effects of the uncontrolled inflammatory process is to blunt the final common pathways of damage (i.e. using either agents that decrease free radical production or antioxidants that inactivate free radicals as they are produced).

Blockade of any single or combined inflammatory mediator may not be successful for a number of reasons [28]. First, the inflammatory process is a normal response to infection and is essential not only for the resolution of infection but also for the initiation of other adaptive stress responses required for host survival. Secondly, the profound redundancy of action of many cytokines means that there are many overlapping pathways for cellular activation and further mediator release. In addition, the synergism of actions and effects of cytokines suggests that imbalance in the process of the immune response may be adversely affected by inhibition of a single agent. Exogenously administered anticytokine therapy may have unrecognized effects because of interaction with naturally occurring immunomodulators or their receptors. Finally, the timing of any potential anticytokine therapy is clearly crucial.

Activated protein C

The inflammatory and pro-coagulant host responses to infection are intricately linked. Infectious agents, endotoxin and inflammatory cytokines such as TNF-α and IL-1β activate coagulation by stimulating the release of tissue factor from monocytes and endothelial cells. Up-regulation of tissue factor leads to the formation of thrombin and a fibrin clot. While inflammatory cytokines are capable of activating coagulation and inhibiting fibrinolysis, thrombin is capable of stimulating several inflammatory pathways. The end result may be widespread injury to the vascular endothelium, multiorgan dysfunction and ultimately death. Protein C is an endogenous protein, a vitamin K dependent serine protease, that promotes fibrinolysis, while inhibiting thrombosis and inflammatory responses. It is therefore an important modulator of the coagulation and inflammatory pathways seen in severe sepsis.

Activated protein C can intervene at multiple points during the systemic response to infection. It exerts an antithrombotic effect by inactivating factors Va and VIIIa, limiting the generation of thrombin. As a result of decreased thrombin levels, the thrombin-mediated inflammatory, pro-coagulant and antifibrinolytic response is attenuated. *In vitro* data indicate that activated protein C exerts an anti-inflammatory effect by inhibiting the production of TNF-α, IL-1β and IL-6 by monocytes, and limiting monocyte and neutrophil adhesion to the endothelium [29]. Reduced levels of protein C are found in the majority of patients with sepsis and are associated with an increased risk of death. A multicentre trial revealed that administration of human recombinant activated protein C in patients with severe sepsis reduced mortality, such that one additional life would be saved for every 16 patients treated with activated protein C [30].

Immunosuppression in sepsis and SIRS: CARS

Depressed immune status including decreased blood cell counts, low expression of surface markers (e.g. MHC class II antigen), altered NK cell activity, diminished cellular cytotoxicity and reduced antigen presentation, poor proliferation in response to mitogens and depressed cytokine production have been described in some patients with sepsis and SIRS [31]. This is termed compensatory anti-inflammatory response syndrome (CARS). It has been suggested that when the SIRS response predominates, it is associated with organ dysfunction and cardiovascular compromise leading to shock; in contrast, when CARS predominates, it is characterized by anti-inflammatory responses associated with a suppression of the immune system — immunoparalysis. Although alterations in immune response are probably associated with an enhanced sensitivity to nosocomial infections, there is no clear demonstration that they are directly responsible for poor outcome in sepsis.

References

1 Aderem A, Ulevitch RJ. Toll-like receptors in the induction of the innate immune response. *Nature* 2000; 406: 782–7.
2 Delhalle S, Blasius R, Dicato M, Diederich M. A beginner's guide to NF-κB signaling pathways. *Ann N Y Acad Sci* 2004; **1030**: 1–13.
3 Xiao C, Ghosh S. NF-κB, an evolutionarily conserved mediator of immune and inflammatory responses. *Adv Exp Med Biol* 2005; **560**: 41–5.
4 Takeda K, Kaisho T, Akira S. Toll-like receptors. *Annu Rev Immunol* 2003; **21**: 335–76.
5 Rassa JC, Ross SR. Viruses and Toll-like receptors. *Microbes Infect* 2003; **5**: 961–96.
6 Tabeta K, Georgel P, Janssen E, *et al.* Toll-like receptors 9 and 3 as essential components of innate immune defense against mouse cytomegalovirus infection. *Proc Natl Acad Sci U S A* 2004; **101**: 3516–21.
7 Matsumoto M, Funami K, Tanabe M, *et al.* Subcellular localization of Toll-like receptor 3 in human dendritic cells. *J Immunol* 2003; 171: 3154–62.
8 Cohen J. TREM-1 in sepsis. *Lancet* 2001; **358**: 776–8.

9 Bouchon A, Dietrich J, Colonna M. Inflammatory responses can be triggered by TREM-1, a novel receptor expressed on neutrophils and monocytes. *J Immunol* 2000; **164**: 4991–5.

10 Bouchon A, Facchetti F, Weigand MA, Colonna M. TREM-1 amplifies inflammation and is a crucial mediator of septic shock. *Nature* 2001; **410**: 1103–7.

11 Ku CL, Yang K, Bustamante J, et al. Inherited disorders of human Toll-like receptor signaling: immunological implications. *Immunol Rev* 2005; **203**: 10–20.

12 Haworth R, Platt N, Keshav S, et al. The macrophage scavenger receptor type A is expressed by activated macrophages and protects the host against lethal endotoxic shock. *J Exp Med* 1997; **186**: 1431–9.

13 Perera PY, Mayadas TN, Takeuchi O, et al. CD11b/CD18 acts in concert with CD14 and Toll-like receptor (TLR) 4 to elicit full lipopolysaccharide and taxol-inducible gene expression. *J Immunol* 2001; **166**: 574–81.

14 Blunck R, Scheel O, Muller M, et al. New insights into endotoxin-induced activation of macrophages: involvement of a K+ channel in transmembrane signaling. *J Immunol* 2001; **166**: 1009–15.

15 Inohara N, Ogura Y, Chen FF, Muto A, Nunez G. Human Nod1 confers responsiveness to bacterial lipopolysaccharides. *J Biol Chem* 2001; **276**: 2551–4.

16 Green D. Apoptotic pathways: ten minutes to dead. *Cell* 2005; **121**: 671–4.

17 Adams J. The proteasome: a suitable antineoplastic target. *Nat Rev Cancer* 2004; **4**: 349–60.

18 Zheng W, Flavell RA. The transcription factor GATA-3 is necessary and sufficient for Th2 cytokine gene expression in CD4 T cells. *Cell* 1997; **89**, 587–96.

19 Szabo SJ, Kim ST, Costa GL, et al. A novel transcription factor, T-bet, directs Th1 lineage commitment. *Cell* 2000; **100**: 655–69.

20 O'Sullivan ST, Lederer JA, Horgan A, et al. Major injury leads to predominance of the T helper-2 lymphocyte phenotype and diminished interleukin-12 production associated with decreased resistance to infection. *Ann Surg* 1995; **222**: 482–90.

21 Guo Z, Kavanagh E, Zang Y, et al. Burn injury promotes antigen-driven Th2-type responses *in vivo*. *J Immunol* 2003; **15**: 3983–90.

22 Ferguson NR, Galley HF, Webster NR. T helper cell subset ratios in patients with severe sepsis. *Intensive Care Med* 1999; **25**: 106–9.

23 Wheatley T, Veitch PS. Effect of blood transfusion on postoperative immunocompetence. *Br J Anaesth* 1997; **78**: 489–92.

24 Bonyhadi M, Frohlich M, Rasmussen A, et al. In vitro engagement of CD3 and CD28 corrects T cell defects in chronic lymphocytic leukemia. *J Immunol* 2005; **174**: 2366–75.

25 Hougardy B, Maduro J, van der Zee A, et al. Clinical potential of inhibitors of survival pathways and activators of apoptotic pathways in treatment of cervical cancer: changing the apoptotic balance. *Lancet Oncol* 2005; **6**: 589–98.

26 Yoshida J, Mizuno M, Wakabayashi T. Interferon-beta gene therapy for cancer: basic research to clinical application. *Cancer Sci* 2004; **95**: 858–65.

27 Barbaro G, Scozzafava A, Mastrolorenzo A, Supuran CT. Highly active antiretroviral therapy: current state of the art, new agents and their pharmacological interactions useful for improving therapeutic outcome. *Curr Pharm Des* 2005; **11**: 1805–43.

28 Nasraway SA. The problems and challenges of immunotherapy in sepsis. *Chest* 2003; **123** (Suppl): 451S–9S.

29 White B, Schmidt M, Murphy C, et al. Activated protein C inhibits lipopolysaccharide-induced nuclear translocation of nuclear factor kappa B (NF-κB) and tumour necrosis factor α (TNF-α) production in the THP-1 monocytic cell line. *Br J Haematol* 2000; **110**: 130–4.

30 Bernard GR, Vincent J-L, Laterre P-F, et al. for the Recombinant Human Activated Protein C Worldwide Evaluation in Severe Sepsis (PROWESS) Study Group. Efficacy and safety of recombinant human activated protein C for severe sepsis. *N Engl J Med* 2001; **344**: 699–709.

31 Cavaillon J-M, Galley HF. Immunoparalysis. In: Galley HF, ed. *Critical Care Focus 10: Inflammation and Immunity*. London: BMJ Books, 2003: 1–17.

32 Galley HF, Webster NR. The immune system. In: Hemmings HC Jr, Hopkins PM, eds. *Foundations of Anesthesia*, 2nd edn. Philadelphia: Mosby Elsevier, 2006: 647–57.

33 Webster NR, Galley HF. Immunology and body defences. In: Aitkenhead AR, Rowbotham DJ, Smith G, eds. *Textbook of Anaesthesia*, 4th edn. London: Churchill Livingstone, 2001: 270–7.

Further reading

Galley HF, ed. *Critical Care Focus 10: Inflammation and Immunity*. London: BMJ Books, 2003.

Abbas AK, Lichtman AH, eds. *Cellular and Molecular Immunology*, 4th edn. Philadelphia, Saunders: 2000.

Abbas AK, Lichtman AH, eds. *Basic Immunology*, 2nd edn. Philadelphia, Saunders: 2004.

CHAPTER 12

Shock: pathogenesis and pathophysiology

Anand Kumar

Introduction

The inability of cells to obtain or utilize oxygen in sufficient quantity to optimally meet their metabolic requirements has classically been considered to be the pathophysiological basis of all forms of shock. In the first half of the 20th century, the study of shock focused on the relatively distinct haemodynamic physiology that characterizes the different forms of shock. Since then, evidence has accumulated that the various types of clinical shock have significant overlap in their haemodynamic characteristics. In parallel, shock of most aetiologies has been shown to involve similar biochemical and metabolic pathways. In this chapter, the pathophysiology and pathogenesis of shock is reviewed from the haemodynamic to the molecular level.

Haemodynamic basis of shock

From a haemodynamic perspective, shock is the failure of cardiovascular adaptation to systemic dyshomoeostasis induced by trauma, infection or other insult such that cardiac output or blood pressure are compromised. This failure is manifested by inadequate organ and tissue perfusion. Although effective perfusion is also dependent upon microcirculatory and intracellular factors (Table 12.1), the haemodynamic aspects of shock can be described, in part, by the contributions of cardiac and arterial vascular function to blood pressure and cardiac output.

Arterial pressure

Although cardiac output may be expressed as a function of mean arterial pressure (MAP) and systemic vascular resistance (SVR), $[CO = (MAP - CVP)/SVR]$, cardiac output (CO) is not directly dependent on MAP in most physiological states. Instead, blood pressure is typically dependent on cardiac output and vascular resistance. However, blood pressure provides a mechanism to indirectly sense cardiac output and global perfusion perturbations for autoregulatory purposes.

The ability of vascular beds in all organs to support normal blood flow is dependent on maintenance of blood pressure within the defined range for that organ (Fig. 12.1) [1]. Vital organs, the brain and heart in particular, are able to autoregulate blood flow over a wide range of blood pressure. Failure to maintain the minimal MAP and perfusion pressure required for autoregulation during hypodynamic circulatory shock indicates a severe reduction in cardiac output. Pharmacological support of blood pressure in such situations (with α-adrenergic agonists) usually results in decreased total systemic perfusion as sensitive vascular beds constrict and overall vascular resistance increases. However, because of their strong autoregulatory capacity, vital organs will maintain increased perfusion under these conditions.

In addition to sufficient cardiac output, effective perfusion requires appropriate distribution of blood flow. Failure to maintain blood pressure within the autoregulatory range results in distribution of blood flow that is strictly dependent on the passive mechanical properties of the vasculature [2]. This may result in inappropriate distribution of perfusion between and within tissues and organs. Late

Table 12.1 Determinants of effective tissue perfusion in shock.

1 Cardiovascular performance (total systemic perfusion/cardiac output)

Cardiac function
Preload
Afterload
Contractility
Heart rate

Venous return
Right atrial pressure (dependent on cardiac function)
Mean circulatory pressure
Stressed vascular volume
Mean vascular compliance
Venous vascular resistance

Distribution of blood flow

2 Distribution of cardiac output
Intrinsic regulatory systems (local tissue factors)
Extrinsic regulatory systems (sympathetic/adrenal activity)
Anatomic vascular disease
Exogenous vasoactive agents (inotropes, vasopressors, vasodilators)

3 Microvascular function
Pre- and postcapillary sphincter function
Capillary endothelial integrity
Microvascular obstruction (fibrin, platelets, WBC, RBC)

4 Local oxygen unloading and diffusion
Oxyhaemoglobin affinity
Red blood cell 2,3-DPG
Blood pH
Temperature

5 Cellular energy generation/utilization capability
Citric acid (Kreb's) cycle
Oxidative phosphorylation pathway
Other energy metabolism pathways (e.g. ATP utilization)

ATP, adenosine triphosphate; 2,3-DPG, 2,3-diphosphoglycerate; RBC, red blood cells; WBC, white blood cells.

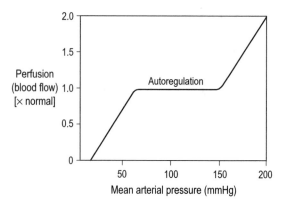

Figure 12.1 Idealized representation of blood flow autoregulation. Outside the range of autoregulation, perfusion becomes dependent on mean arterial pressure.

haemorrhagic shock is characterized by abnormal microvascular flow with dilatation of precapillary sphincters [3].

Cardiac output

The fact that total systemic perfusion is defined by cardiac output underlies its importance in shock. The product of heart rate (HR) and stroke volume (SV) determines cardiac output [CO = HR × SV]. Stroke volume (a measure of myocardial performance) is dependent on preload, afterload and contractility.

Preload represents the extent of precontraction myocardial fibre (or sarcomere) stretch. *In vivo*, preload is the end-diastolic ventricular volume. Because measurement of such volumes in the clinical context is difficult, intracardiac pressures, which can be determined more easily, are frequently substituted. There are difficulties with this approach. The relationship of ventricular end-diastolic volume (preload) to end-diastolic pressure is non-linear. Further, alterations of myocardial compliance render CVP and pulmonary wedge pressure (PWP) unreliable as estimates of preload in critically ill patients [4].

Preload is dependent on circulating volume, venous tone, atrial contraction and intrathoracic pressure among other factors [1,5]. Atrial contraction is particularly important in those with impaired ventricular function. Although accounting for only 5–10% of cardiac output in healthy humans, synchronized atrial contraction contributes as much as 40–50% of the cardiac output in patients with severe left ventricular dysfunction [5]. Increased intrathoracic pressure or increased venous capacitance affect preload by reducing venous return [1,6]. Nitrovasodilators such as nitroglycerin may decrease cardiac output despite arteriolar vasodilatation as a result of their venodilatory (decreased preload) effects. Conversely, the earliest increases in cardiac output seen with sympathetic stimulation and exogenous catecholamine infusion are related to venoconstriction-induced increases of venous return and preload [7]. Cardiogenic and some forms of obstructive shock are typically characterized by increased preload. Pre-resuscitation distributive shock and hypovolaemic shock are uniformly associated with decreased preload.

Afterload refers to the total resistance to ejection of blood from the ventricle during contraction. Increasing afterload results in decreased extent and velocity of myocardial contraction. Excessive afterload (aortic dissection, pulmonary embolus) causes some forms of obstructive shock. *Ex vivo*, afterload can be easily defined as a resistive force applied to an isolated papillary muscle. Because the heart does not displace a fixed mass, but rather rhythmically moves a viscous non-Newtonian fluid through branching viscoelastic conduits, the definition of afterload *in vivo* is difficult.

Afterload has been suggested to be equivalent to systolic myocardial wall stress. This definition suggests that afterload is substantially dependent on intrinsic cardiac mechanical and functional properties [8]. An alternative approach equates left ventricular afterload with the mechanical properties of the arterial side of the circulatory system. Aortic input impedance, which represents the total resistance to flow from outside the left ventricle, is determined by the inertial and viscous properties of blood, and the resistive and viscoelastic properties of the arterial system. The term is inclusive of SVR, heart rate effects and pulse wave reflections in the arterial tree [8]. While an accurate measure of afterload in pulsatile systems, assessment of impedance is technically difficult, requiring continuous harmonic analysis of rhythmic variations of aortic pressure and flow. SVR is a limited approximation of aortic input impedance based on a model that assumes non-pulsatile flow. At a heart rate of 0, SVR and aortic input impedance are equivalent. From a clinical point of view, SVR is the most practical way of assessing afterload.

Afterload is increased in pathological conditions such as aortic stenosis, systemic embolism and hypertension. Vasopressors including α-agonists (e.g.

phenylephrine, noradrenaline) and vasopressin also increase afterload while nitrates and other vasodilator agents decrease it. Increased intrathoracic pressure, resulting from mechanical ventilation and positive end-expiratory pressure (PEEP), decreases left ventricular afterload while increasing right ventricular afterload. Hypodynamic and hyperdynamic shock are usually characterized by increased and decreased afterload, respectively.

Contractility refers to the intrinsic ability of myocardial fibres to shorten under given loading conditions. Under normal conditions, determinants of contractility include myocardial mass and sympathoadrenal activation state. In pathological states (e.g. shock), hypoperfusion/ischaemia, myocardial cell injury (e.g. reperfusion injury, myocarditis), acidosis and circulating myocardial depressant substances (such as seen in sepsis) depress cardiac contractility.

As with preload and afterload, the *ex vivo* and *in vitro* assessments of contractility are straightforward. Assessment of *in vivo* contractility (even in experimental animals) is substantially more difficult because of intrinsic lability of preload and afterload. Relatively load-independent variables such as peak systolic pressure : end-systolic volume ratio may be the most clinically useful measures of contractility [9]. Many of these variables can be obtained echocardiographically.

Microvascular function in shock

Preserved microvascular function (vessels of less than 100–150 μmol diameter) is a critical determinant of appropriate tissue perfusion during shock. Although adequate cardiac output at sufficient blood pressure is required for appropriate global perfusion and systemic haemodynamics, effective tissue perfusion also requires intact local and systemic microvascular function.

Distribution of cardiac output is a complicated process involving local intrinsic autoregulation and extrinsic regulation mediated by autonomic tone and humoral factors. Blood flow to individual organs may be affected by systemwide changes in micro-arteriolar tone or by local alterations in metabolic activity. Blood flow within organs also requires microvascular regulation to match blood flow to areas of highest metabolic activity.

Autoregulation

Intrinsic control (autoregulation) of blood flow is thought to occur through two mechanisms. Rapid alterations of microvascular tone are mediated through endothelial stretch receptors so that sudden changes in perfusion pressure can be compensated by opposing changes in vascular resistance in order to maintain perfusion [10]. Increases in metabolic activity within tissues and organs are thought to cause local elevation of various metabolites (e.g. CO_2, H^+), resulting in vasodilatation and increased perfusion to match substrate demand [10].

Extrinsic control

Extrinsic control of vascular tone is primarily exerted through the autonomic nervous system. Parasympathetic release of acetylcholine to blood vessels results in nitric oxide and cyclic guanosine 3′,5′-monophosphate (GMP) generation in endothelial cells and vascular smooth muscle leading to vascular relaxation. Increases of sympathetic tone cause local noradrenaline (norepinephrine) release, activation of vascular α-adrenoreceptors and increased vascular tone. Under stress, adrenaline and noradrenaline can be systemically released by sympathetic stimulation of the adrenal medulla. Basal control of blood pressure and flow resides in the activity of the renin–angiotensin system.

Alterations in microvascular function are effected through pre- and postcapillary sphincters that are sensitive to both intrinsic and extrinsic control mechanisms. Because exchange of carbon dioxide, oxygen and other substrates and metabolites, and compartmental regulation of fluids occurs at the capillary level, alteration of tone of either sphincter can have varying effects. Opening of either non-nutrient capillary sphincters (microanatomic shunts) [11] or increased flow to hypometabolic tissues (functional shunts) [12] will result in suboptimal distribution of substrate supply with increased mixed venous oxygen saturation (MVO_2). Failure to dilate sphincters supplying metabolically active tissues may result in ischaemia and anaerobic metabolism with lactate production. Increased precapillary tone as seen with

sympathetic stimulation results in increased blood pressure systemically and decreased hydrostatic pressure locally. This decreased hydrostatic pressure will favour redistribution of volume from the interstitium to the circulation. Increased postcapillary tone (relative to precapillary) results in vascular pooling of blood and loss of fluid to interstitium (because of increased hydrostatic pressure).

Blood flow

Organ blood flow changes are well characterized in shock states. Autoregulation of blood flow is dependent on maintenance of blood pressure within a defined range which varies between organs. The autoregulatory capacity of various organs can be determined by mechanically altering blood pressure in the organ vascular bed. With isolated local hypotension, the brain exhibits dominant autoregulatory capability with the ability to maintain blood flow over a wide range of pressures (30–200 mmHg in dogs) [2]. Coronary perfusion is also substantially autoregulated at 40–100 mmHg. In contrast, mesenteric and renal blood flow becomes pressure dependent below approximately 60 mmHg, while the vascular bed of skeletal muscle behaves in a passive manner at pressures outside 50–100 mmHg. Human data suggest that overall, good autoregulation of blood flow exists in humans between pressures of 60–100 mmHg [2]. In the context of normal physiology, blood flow is not effectively autoregulated outside this range. Without local adaptation, this would result in mismatching of blood flow and metabolic demands producing organ failure and the metabolic correlates of shock. However, extrinsic adaptive mechanisms to protect the most vital organs come into play.

Hypovolaemia

During hypovolaemia and other hypodynamic forms of shock, extrinsic blood flow regulatory mechanisms overwhelm the autoregulatory response of most vascular beds. Blood flow to the heart and brain are well preserved because of dominant local autoregulation of flow. Blood flow to other organs is reduced relative to the decrease in total cardiac output, as organ vascular resistance increases to maintain blood pressure [13]. This effect is mediated in part by both sympathetic neural activity and adrenal release of catecholamines [2,13]. This adaptive mechanism maintains perfusion to vital organs at mild to moderate levels of reduced cardiac output. If the insult is sufficiently severe or prolonged, organ ischaemia and subsequent organ failure may develop. Even if resuscitation restores systemic circulatory haemodynamics, microvascular perfusion abnormalities persist for days [14]. Experimental data suggest that perfusion of brain, kidneys, liver and other splanchnic organs remains impaired following resuscitation from haemorrhagic shock [14]. Persistence of inadequate matching of tissue substrate demand and delivery after resuscitation of shock can lead to continued ischaemia or hypoxia of some tissues. This may explain why haemorrhagic shock-related tissue injury can be irreversible if the duration and severity is excessive. Animal models suggest this irreversible phase of severe haemorrhagic shock is characterized by vasodilatation of precapillary sphincters [3].

Sepsis

During sepsis and septic shock, organ blood flow is disturbed at higher mean arterial pressures, suggesting a primary defect of microvascular function. Cerebral blood flow to the brain in humans has been shown to be depressed even before the onset of septic shock in patients with systemic inflammatory response syndrome [15]. This pathological vasoconstriction (apparently a unique response of the cerebral circulation to sepsis) does not appear to be the cause of septic encephalopathy. Cerebral autoregulation remains intact during sepsis [16]. The greater decrease in coronary than systemic vascular resistance during human septic shock may suggest that myocardial autoregulation also remains intact despite the fact that, in contrast to the brain, myocardial perfusion is often increased during septic shock [17,18].

Animal models demonstrate that all other vascular beds (splanchnic, renal, skeletal, cutaneous) exhibit decreased vascular resistance, with flow in these beds becoming increasingly dependent on cardiac output. This suggests both an active vasodilatory process and failure of extrinsic control of blood flow [2]. Inappropriate levels of splanchnic and skeletal muscle perfusion are also observed in humans during sepsis [19]. Other experimental data suggest that

sepsis and septic shock are also associated with aberrant distribution of flow within organs [12]. In sepsis, vasodilatation and autoregulatory failure of the microvasculature may be responsible for mismatches of oxygen delivery and demand, resulting in anaerobic glycolysis with lactate production despite increased mixed venous oxygen saturation.

During both irreversible haemorrhagic shock and septic shock, peripheral vascular failure results in worsened matching of tissue demand and substrate supply, leading to failure of all organs and death. Among the potential responsible mechanisms are:

1 Tissue acidosis [20]

2 Catecholamine depletion and mediator-related vascular resistance to catecholamines [21]

3 Release of vasodilating and vasoconstricting arachidonic acid metabolites [22]

4 Decreased sympathetic tone resulting from altered central nervous system (CNS) perfusion [23]

5 Pathologic generation of nitric oxide by vascular smooth muscle cells [24,25].

In addition to vasomotor dysfunction, shock is associated with other microvascular pathologies. Prime among these is disruption of endothelial cell barrier integrity. The endothelial layer is responsible for maintaining oncotic proteins (mostly albumin) within the circulatory space. During shock, capillary permeability is increased resulting in loss of plasma proteins into the interstitium. Endothelial injury, through the action of neutrophil-generated free radicals [26] and nitric oxide generation [27] may account for this phenomenon. Release of vasoactive intermediaries such as histamine, bradykinin, platelet activating factor (PAF), leukotrienes and tumour necrosis factor α (TNF-α) appear to drive this pathological process. Injury is initiated by leucocyte–endothelial cell interactions via adhesion molecules (integrins, selectins) which allow emigration of neutrophils to the tissues. Blockade of such activity or depletion of neutrophils attenuates tissue injury in animal models of shock [28]. With the loss of plasma proteins, the plasma oncotic pressure drops, interstitial oedema develops and circulating volume falls.

There is also evidence of intravascular haemagglutination of red cells, white cells and platelets in almost all shock syndromes [12,29]. This may be because of primary microvascular clotting leading to microthrombi. Alternately, clotting may occur as a consequence of primary endothelial damage resulting from circulating cytokines, free radicals produced by reperfusion and neutrophils or complement activation. In any case, the result may be further endothelial cell injury, microvascular abnormalities and inadequate distribution of perfusion within tissues. Decreased deformability of erythrocytes resulting from membrane free radical injury may also have a role in microcirculatory alterations in haemorrhagic and septic shock [30].

Mechanisms of cellular injury in shock

Shock of all forms involves common cellular metabolic processes that typically end in cell injury, organ failure and death. The pathogenesis of cellular dysfunction and organ failure as a consequence of shock appears to involve multiple inter-related factors including cellular ischaemia, circulating or local inflammatory mediators and free radical injury.

Cellular ischaemia

Cellular ischaemia clearly has a major role in cellular injury in most forms of shock. During early hypovolaemia, physiological adaptive mechanisms appear to compensate for decreased preload so that tissue perfusion is unaffected. Once cardiac output cannot be maintained and tissue perfusion of nonvital, followed by vital, organs are compromised, increasing dependence on anaerobic glycolysis for cellular energy requirements becomes manifest. Intracellular lactate rises and pH falls. During circulatory shock, such adaptation is absent and progressive defects of mitochondrial metabolism and adenosine triphosphate (ATP) generation occur. Essential ATP-dependent intracellular metabolic processes that may be adversely affected include maintenance of transmembrane electrical potential (sodium and potassium transport) [31], mitochondrial function [32], carbohydrate metabolism [33] and energy-dependent enzyme reactions. Some vital organs, such as the liver and kidney, are particularly sensitive and ATP-dependent processes are rapidly impaired [31,34–37]. Eventually, other organs

including skeletal muscle become involved. Ultrastructural deterioration of mitochondria becomes apparent [38]. Worsening of shock, organ failure and death ensue.

In sepsis, tissue ATP levels may initially remain normal and mitochondrial function unaffected. This may suggest that ischaemia does not contribute to early septic organ dysfunction [39,40]. Overall normal levels of ATP, however, do not rule out the possibility of patchy focal deficits within tissues, related to inadequately distributed perfusion. Inflammatory microthrombi in the microvasculature may mechanically obstruct microcirculatory flow. This could result in cellular dysfunction resulting from persistent focal ischaemic areas. Evidence to support ischaemia as a contributor to cell dysfunction in sepsis includes evidence of oxygen supply-dependent oxygen consumption, washout of organic acids (from ischaemic tissues) into the circulation in patients with sepsis and multiorgan dysfunction syndrome (MODS) after treatment with vasodilators, and elevated ATP degradation products with decreased acetoacetate:hydroxybutyrate ratio (suggestive of altered hepatic mitochondrial redox potential). Based on the totality of evidence, however, the question of whether ischaemia has a role in sepsis pathophysiology remains an open question.

Inflammatory mediators

Inflammatory mediator effects on cellular metabolism are of prime importance in organ dysfunction resulting from sepsis and septic shock. Circulating inflammatory mediators may also have a substantial role in other forms of shock, including haemorrhagic shock associated with extensive tissue trauma [41,42]. Both sepsis and trauma are associated with generalized systemic activation of the inflammatory response. Resulting cell injury and hypermetabolism may culminate in organ failure. A number of triggers can result in activation of the inflammatory cascade. The best studied is endotoxin from Gram-negative bacteria but other bacterial antigens and cell injury itself can also initiate the cascade. Macrophage production of cytokines such as TNF-α and interleukin 1β (IL-1β) appears to be central.

TNF-α is a 51-kDa trimeric peptide produced by macrophages in response to a variety of inflammatory stimuli including bacterial antigens and other cytokines. Circulating levels of TNF-α are transiently elevated soon after the onset of shock (particularly septic shock) [43]. Administration of TNF to animals or humans results in a hyperdynamic circulatory state (with or without a dose-dependent hypotension) similar to untreated sepsis and septic shock [44]. Although clinical trials to date have yielded disappointing results, anti-TNF strategies protect animals from experimental endotoxic and septic shock [45]. Among the many effects of TNF are release of IL-1, IL-6, IL-8, PAF, leukotrienes, thromboxanes and prostaglandins; stimulation of production and activity of polymorphonuclear leucocytes; promotion of immune cell adhesion to endothelium; activation of coagulation and complement systems; direct endothelial cell cytotoxicity; depression of myocardial contractility; and fever production by the hypothalamus [44,46]. Notably, TNF causes alterations of skeletal transmembrane electrical potential similar to those described in haemorrhagic and septic shock [47]. These membrane effects precede haemodynamic alterations suggesting that TNF exerts a primary effect on cell metabolism independent of perfusion alterations. While TNF appears to be of central importance in the pathogenesis of septic shock, it is also known to be elevated in congestive heart failure [48] and haemorrhagic shock [41].

There are other substances involved in the inflammatory process:

• *The interleukins.* IL-1β, which can potentiate the *in vivo* effects of TNF; IL-2, which can cause haemodynamic abnormalities in humans; IL-6, which is involved in the acute phase response; and IL-10, which is an anti-inflammatory cytokine that limits macrophage generation of pro-inflammatory cytokines.

• *γ-Interferon* (IFN-γ) promotes the release of other cytokines and enhances adhesion of immune cells and promotes macrophage activation.

• *Transforming growth factor* β (TGF-β) is an anti-inflammatory cytokine that, in addition to limiting macrophage pro-inflammatory responses, also blocks the effects of pro-inflammatory cytokines on target cells.

• *Endothelin-1* strongly promotes vasoconstriction, particularly in the renal vascular bed, possibly result-

ing in renal hypoperfusion and decreased glomerular filtration rate.

• *Platelet activating factor* (PAF) stimulates TNF, thromboxane and leukotriene release, stimulates free radical formation and alters microvascular permeability.

• *Leukotrienes* can release other arachidonic acid metabolites, alter vascular endothelial permeability and may mediate vascular and myocardial depression in shock.

• *Thromboxanes* contribute to altered microvascular vasomotor and permeability function.

• *Prostaglandins* produce fever, induce vasodilatation and inhibit thrombus formation.

• *Complement fragments C3a and C5a* constrict vascular smooth muscle, release histamine and promote chemotaxis [46].

In recent years, several newly recognized mediators have been shown to have important roles in shock, particularly septic shock. These include most notably, macrophage migration inhibitory factor (MIF) and high mobility group 1 protein (HMG-1). MIF has been shown to be produced by monocytes and macrophages following exposure to bacterial toxins including endotoxin, toxic shock syndrome toxin 1, streptococcal pyrogenic toxin A and to pro-inflammatory cytokines including TNF-α and IFN-γ [49]. MIF results in expression of other pro-inflammatory mediators by monocytes and/or macrophages and activation of T cells. Increased MIF concentrations have been shown in the blood of mice subjected to peritonitis and in humans with septic shock [50]. Injection of MIF during experimental murine *Escherichia coli* peritonitis increases mortality [50]. HMG-1 also appears to have a key role in the pathogenesis of Gram-negative sepsis [51]. Mice show increased levels of HMG-1 in serum 8–32 hours after endotoxin administration. Patients succumbing to septic shock also demonstrate increased serum HMG-1 levels [51]. Administration of HMG-1 to control and endotoxin-resistant mice induces dose-dependent mortality with signs consistent with endotoxic shock [51].

A circulating myocardial depressant substance is present in the blood of patients with septic shock who exhibit myocardial depression with biventricular dilatation and reduced ventricular ejection fractions [52]. Similar substances have been shown to be present in animal models of haemorrhagic shock [53]. Other data suggest canine myocardial infarction [54] and human cardiogenic shock [55] may also be associated with circulating myocardial depressant substances. Serum from appropriate septic patients or animal models depresses myocardial tissue *in vitro* [52,56]. Myocardial depressant substances from both septic and haemorrhagic shock appear to be dependent on calcium [57]. The substance implicated in human sepsis appears to represent a synergistic combination of TNF and IL-1 that can produce depression by inducing myocardial nitric oxide production [52,58,59]. TNF and IL-1 are both elevated in shock and cause similar depression of myocardial tissue [58,60].

Nitric oxide

Another important mediator, nitric oxide, has a vital role in normal intracellular signal transduction [61]. Of particular importance to shock, nitric oxide is the mediator through which endothelial cells normally cause relaxation of adjacent smooth muscle [61]. Endothelial cells, through a constitutive nitric oxide synthase, produce picomolar quantities of nitric oxide in response to a number of vasodilatory mediators such as acetylcholine and bradykinin. This nitric oxide diffuses to adjacent smooth muscle and activates guanylate cyclase to produce cyclic GMP which causes vascular relaxation. Nitrovasodilators bypass nitric oxide synthase to relax smooth muscle directly through the guanylate cyclase pathway. During septic shock, an inducible nitric oxide synthase capable of producing nanomolar quantities of nitric oxide is generated in vascular smooth muscle [25,61]. Studies have also implicated nitric oxide in late vascular dysfunction seen in haemorrhagic shock [24]. Nitric oxide-mediated generation of cyclic GMP may explain the profound loss of arterial vascular tone and venodilatation seen in septic shock [25,26] and may, in part, explain irreversible vascular collapse seen late in haemorrhagic shock [24]. A potential role for nitric oxide in inflammation-associated oedema and third-spacing during shock has also been suggested [27,62]. The *in vitro* myocardial depressant effects of TNF, IL-1 and serum

from septic humans may be mediated by a similar nitric oxide and cyclic GMP dependent pathway [44,58].

Finally, as part of the release of inflammatory mediators, immune cells including macrophages, polymorphonuclear leucocytes and lymphocytes may be activated in some forms of hypodynamic shock (e.g. haemorrhagic shock) resulting in a self-perpetuating systemic inflammatory response (similar to that seen in sepsis). This response can contribute to vascular and parenchymal injury and culminate in MODS.

Free radicals

Free radical injury induced by reperfusion or neutrophil activity is a mechanism of organ injury during haemorrhagic and septic shock as well as burns and myocardial infarction [63]. During tissue ischaemia, oxygen deficiency leads to accumulation of ATP degradation products including adenosine, inosine and hypoxanthine [64]. With resuscitation and reperfusion of ischaemic areas, oxygen drives the generation of superoxide ($O_2^{-\bullet}$), the most common precursor of reactive oxidants, by xanthine oxidase, in endothelial cells. Most of the superoxide is converted, either spontaneously or through superoxide dismutase, to hydrogen peroxide (H_2O_2). This further reacts to produce tissue damaging hydroxyl radicals (or other highly reactive free radicals) [63]. These radicals interact with critical cell targets such as the plasma membrane, lipid membranes of organelles and various enzymes resulting in cell lysis and tissue injury. Oxidant activity, directly and through endothelial damage, attracts and activates neutrophils resulting in amplification of superoxide generation by a neutrophil nicotinamide adenine dinucleotide phosphate (NADPH)-oxidase and in further tissue damage resulting from neutrophil protease release [63]. Injured tissue may release xanthine oxidase into the circulation resulting in systemic microvascular injury [65].

A parallel process occurs during reperfusion of ischaemic myocardium following myocardial infarction [66]. Thrombolytic therapy or balloon angioplasty results in sudden delivery of oxygen to ischaemic myocardium. Although substantial salvage of myocardial function results, free oxygen radical mediated reperfusion injury can contribute to myocardial 'stunning' [67]. Cardiogenic shock during this phase may resolve as the reperfusion injury settles. Free radical damage likely also has a role in tissue damage during sepsis and septic shock. Following activation by inflammatory mediators and during phagocytosis, polymorphonuclear leucocytes undergo a respiratory burst during which they consume oxygen and generate both superoxide and hydrogen peroxide through a membrane-associated NADPH-oxidase [63]. Macrophages similarly produce oxygen radicals upon activation. Activation also enhances adhesion and tissue migration of leucocytes so that both vascular endothelial and parenchymal tissue damage may result. Free radical injury may have an important role in the development of organ failure following shock [68].

Cellular membrane function

One of the most notable results of cellular injury in shock involves cellular membrane function. Movement of most solutes through cells is partially dependent on active transport through the plasma cell membrane. During both haemorrhagic and septic shock, marked changes of plasma membrane function occur. Normal gradients of sodium, chloride, potassium and calcium are not maintained. Changes of intracellular electrolytes and pH may affect sensitive intracellular enzyme systems and further impair cell metabolism. Impairment of membrane function is reflected by reversible changes in transmembrane electrical potential in skeletal muscle and liver. Because maintenance of membrane transport functions and electrochemical gradient is an energy-dependent process, decreased production of ATP during shock has been proposed as the cause of this defect [35]. However, alterations of liver and skeletal muscle transmembrane potential occur early in shock prior to the decrease in levels of high-energy phosphates and onset of hypotension. Further, the membrane defect is not prevented by administration of membrane-permeable forms of high-energy phosphates such as ATP-MgCl$_2$ [69].

Gene expression

Variations in stress response genes between individuals and alteration of gene expression in immune, endothelial, muscle and organ parenchymal cells is another important aspect of cellular dysfunction and injury in circulatory shock. Although shock can be present immediately after injury (massive trauma, haemorrhage or endotoxin infusion) prior to the onset of substantial alterations of gene expression, its evolution is dependent on a combination of the ongoing nature of the insult, the genetically passive compensatory physiological and metabolic response, the underlying genotype with respect to stress response elements, and stress-related modulation of gene expression in a variety of cells.

The clinical presentation of shock, progression of the syndrome and final outcome may be substantially controlled by genetic factors [70]. Genetic factors have been best studied in septic shock. Studies have demonstrated that the human TNF promoter polymorphism, TNF2, imparts an increased susceptibility to and mortality from septic shock [71]. Other studies suggest increased TNF generation, severity of sepsis and mortality with another human TNF gene polymorphism [72]. A specific locus on chromosome 12 in mice has been shown to be associated with resistance to mortality resulting from TNF-induced shock [73]. Recently, a human IL-1 receptor antagonist gene polymorphism has been linked to increased susceptibility to sepsis [74]. Several additional linked polymorphisms have been described in recent years [75]. It appears likely that gene polymorphisms may also have similar roles in other forms of shock.

Beyond the role of gene alleles in the development and clinical response to shock, the progression of irreversible circulatory shock and MODS may have its basis in genetically driven vascular or parenchymal responses. Production of cytokines by macrophages during shock requires acute expression of the genes coding for TNF, IL-1 and other pro-inflammatory cytokines. The production of adhesion molecules by endothelial cells and inducible nitric oxide synthase by vascular smooth muscle during shock requires active up-regulation of gene expression. Both events are thought to be key to the development of MODS following shock in humans. In addition, human and animal research indicate that apoptosis, a genetically programmed process of cell autolysis, occurs in a variety of organs during shock and subsequent organ failure [76,77]. Further research should elucidate the important link between irreversible and refractory shock and shock-associated MODS and genetically programmed cell responses to inflammatory stimulation and/or injury.

Whatever the initiating event or events, progressive cell metabolic failure occurs. Mitochondrial activity continues to deteriorate, subcellular organelles are damaged and intracellular (and possibly systemic) release of lysosome hydrolytic enzymes occurs, accelerating cell death and organ failure.

Oxygen supply dependency in shock

Reduced oxygen consumption relative to requirements has a pivotal role in all hypodynamic shock states and may also have a significant role in hyperdynamic shock associated with hypermetabolism. Without a sufficient supply of oxygen, mitochondrial oxidation of pyruvate (the citric acid cycle) is inhibited. This blocks aerobic energy production with resulting anaerobic production of ATP through the cytoplasmic pyruvate–lactate shunt pathway. Anaerobic metabolism yields just 5% of the energy of the aerobic pathway and results in accumulation of lactate (Fig. 12.2). Acidosis results as ATP is hydrolysed. The deficiency of energy production can lead to manifestations of organ failure due to shock. The

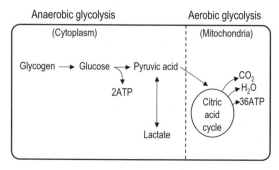

Figure 12.2 Aerobic and anaerobic glucose metabolism. Under anaerobic conditions, pyruvic acid cannot enter the citric acid cycle in the mitochondria to support aerobic production of adenosine triphosphate (ATP). Shunting to the lactate pathway within the cytoplasm produces less high-energy phosphates per mole of glucose metabolized. Intracellular acidosis results when hydrolysis of ATP molecules results in production of H^+ ions which cannot be cleared via anaerobic metabolism. After Mizock and Falk [121] with permission.

relationship of systemic oxygen delivery to oxygen consumption in shock and related states has been the subject of substantial research over the last two decades. Newer trends in therapy of shock and related states are predicated on concepts developed through this work [78].

Systemic oxygen delivery (Do_2) is the amount of oxygen delivered to the body per unit time and is the product of cardiac output or systemic perfusion (Q) and total oxygen content of arterial blood (Cao_2). Systemic oxygen consumption (Vo_2) can be defined by the difference between the oxygen content of arterial and venous blood (or the difference between systemic oxygen delivery and return) so that $Vo_2 = Q \times (Cao_2 - Cvo_2)$ where Cvo_2 equals the oxygen content of venous blood. The oxygen extraction ratio, a measure of the proportional amount of oxygen utilized for the amount of oxygen delivered, is represented by Vo_2/Do_2 or more simply by $Sao_2 - Svo_2/Sao_2$. Normal extraction ratio in humans at rest is 0.25–0.33 [79] reflecting a mixed venous oxygen saturation of 65–70%. Under conditions of reduced cardiac output, mixed venous oxygen saturation can fall to 25–30%, indicating extraction ratios of approximately 0.7 [79].

Humans and other large vertebrates share the ability to maintain a constant Vo_2 over a wide range of oxygen deliveries (Fig. 12.3). As oxygen delivery is lowered, however, a critical oxygen delivery point (Do_2crit) is reached below which Vo_2 becomes a linear function of Do_2. This critical oxygen delivery appears to be constant (for a given metabolic rate) and is independent of the method by which oxygen delivery is reduced (decreased perfusion, haemoglobin concentration or arterial oxygen saturation). Above this critical delivery, oxygen extraction ratio varies to maintain a constant Vo_2. At the Do_2crit extraction ratio is maximal and further decreases in oxygen delivery cannot be supported while maintaining Vo_2. Below this point, tissue hypoxia ensues and anaerobic metabolism is thought to support limited ATP generation resulting in lactate production. Constant Vo_2 while Do_2 increases have been used to infer that Vo_2 is equivalent to basal oxygen demand when Do_2 is not a limiting factor. A similar biphasic oxygen consumption response is seen in isolated tissues and organs and available evidence suggests that organ

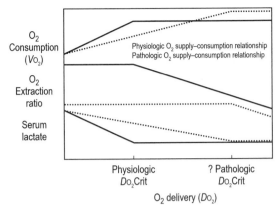

Figure 12.3 Oxygen supply dependent oxygen consumption in shock. Physiological supply dependent oxygen consumption is characterized by a biphasic relationship between oxygen delivery (Do2) and oxygen consumption (Vo2). The inflection point defines the physiologic critical oxygen delivery (Do2crit). Below this Do2crit, Vo2 is linearly dependent on Do2, the oxygen extraction ratio is maximal and lactate (indicating anaerobic metabolism) is produced. Above the physiological Do2crit, Vo2 is independent of Do2, the oxygen extraction ratio varies to maintain a constant Vo2 and lactate is not produced. Pathological oxygen supply dependency exists when oxygen consumption is dependent on oxygen delivery over a much wider range of oxygen delivery values. The Do2 is shifted to the right, the oxygen extraction ratio varies throughout a wide range of Do2 values and lactate is produced with higher than normal oxygen delivery. This condition has been thought to be associated with hyperdynamic shock states, particularly septic shock.

Do_2crit *in vivo* is similar to whole body Do_2crit [80]. In anaesthetized humans, the critical point appears to be 8–10 mL/min/kg [81]. A number of difficulties preclude obtaining a similar definitive value for the critically ill (primarily that the metabolic rate of critically ill patients is not at all stable within or between patients). In those studies in which a critical value was found, it ranged widely, from 7 to 15 mL/kg/min [81]. This phenomenon of a biphasic relationship between Do_2 and Vo_2 with Vo_2 being independent of Do_2 at higher delivery levels and linearly dependent on Do_2 below a critical delivery value is termed physiologic oxygen supply dependency.

Because hypoxaemia and anaemia can be acutely compensated by increased cardiac output, physiological oxygen supply dependency in humans is primarily seen during low output circulatory shock (hypovolaemic, cardiogenic and obstructive) associated with increased lactate levels. Evidence supporting oxygen supply dependency in other conditions such as congestive heart failure, sleep apnoea, pulmonary hypertension and chronic obstructive lung disease is less certain. During hypovolaemic, cardiogenic and obstructive shock, the extraction ratio is maximal but Do_2 is reduced below the critical point.

Experimental animal and clinical human data have suggested that during septic shock, sepsis, trauma and related hypermetabolic conditions with elevated lactate levels (such as Acute Respiratory Distress Syndrome [ARDS] and MODS), a pathological oxygen supply dependency may exist [82]. Pathological supply dependency is defined by an increased critical oxygen delivery and decreased maximal oxygen extraction ratio so that oxygen supply dependency appears to exist over a wide range of oxygen delivery values. In the hypermetabolic conditions postulated to be associated with this phenomenon, oxygen demand and delivery are typically elevated, extraction ratio is reduced and the Do_2crit is shifted far to the right such that oxygen supply dependency may be observed throughout normal or even elevated cardiac outputs [83].

The reasons for the defect of oxygen extraction in septic conditions may have to do with the microvascular and cellular metabolic alterations that characterize sepsis and other states of systemic inflammatory activation: microvascular thrombi, altered vasomotor regulation, endothelial cell injury and, later, cellular metabolic dysfunction.

Most available evidence suggests that pathological oxygen supply dependency seen in septic conditions remains associated with tissue ischaemia and anaerobic glycolysis (for ATP generation) because lactic acidosis is usually present. In addition, increases in Vo_2 with increasing Do_2 (through fluid loading or inotrope administration) appear to be dependent on the presence of elevated lactate.

The methodology of studies that support the existence of pathological oxygen supply dependency in hypermetabolic states such as sepsis has been questioned. Most have utilized the Fick principle by calculating oxygen consumption as the difference between arterial oxygen transport from the heart and venous oxygen delivery back to the heart. Because both Vo_2 and Do_2 are derived from shared variables (particularly cardiac output), the possibility exists that covariation of the two may be a result of mathematical coupling. In addition, other supportive studies have involved augmentation of cardiac output with catecholamines. However, catecholamines are associated with dose-dependent increases of oxygen consumption (as well as oxygen delivery) in normal volunteers that could mimic 'pathologic' oxygen supply dependency [84]. Studies using differences of inspired and expired oxygen content to determine Vo_2 have tended to suggest that pathologic supply dependency is not present in either sepsis or ARDS associated with normal or increased serum lactate [85,86]. These studies suggest that the Do_2crit is similar in both septic and nonseptic critically ill patients and may be as low as 4–5 mL/kg/min [87]. Nuclear magnetic spectroscopy studies, by demonstrating normal high-energy phosphate generation in septic tissues, are consistent with the view that pathological oxygen supply dependency does not exist in septic states [39].

For low output forms of shock, standard resuscitation to normal stressed cardiac output and blood pressure generally results in oxygen delivery above the relatively unchanged Do_2 crit. Evidence of hypoperfusion (whether clinical examination, blood pressure or mixed venous oxygen saturation) indicating that oxygen delivery may be deficient necessitates continued resuscitation. Bland et al. [88] have demonstrated that high-risk survivors of surgical procedures have higher values of cardiac index, Do_2 and Vo_2 (median 4.5 L/min/m², 600 mL/min/m² and 170 mL/min/m², respectively) than do non-survivors. In several prospective randomized trials, an improved survival rate was found in hyperdynamic resuscitation protocol surgical patients compared with controls resuscitated to standard parameters [89,90].

The haemodynamic approach (after standard resuscitation) to sepsis, septic shock and related conditions is more controversial. Augmentation of cardiac index or oxygen delivery values using inotropes has been suggested to potentially improve mortality. Shoemaker et al. [91] suggested target values for car-

diac index, Do_2 and Vo_2 of 5.5 L/min/m², 1000 mL/min/m² and 190 mL/min/m², respectively, based on median values of a series of survivors. While evidence continues to suggest increased cardiac index and Do_2 are associated with improved survival in septic shock, no studies have been able to demonstrate a conclusive causal relationship. Several well-designed randomized studies of sepsis and septic shock in medical patients have suggested mortality may be increased when inotropes are routinely utilized to achieve supranormal oxygen delivery targets [92,93]. Similarly, increased cardiac index, oxygen delivery or oxygen consumption characterizes survivors of trauma (another hypermetabolic condition) [94] but clear data to demonstrate that survival can be improved by augmenting oxygen transport to supranormal values are not entirely convincing [89,95]. The efficacy of this approach in high-risk septic surgical patients also remains an open question [90]. A recent randomized controlled trial has suggested efficacy when early goals directed therapy of septic shock is implemented in a protocolized manner [78].

Compensatory responses to shock

Shock is usually not a discrete condition occurring abruptly after injury or infection. With the onset of haemodynamic stress, homoeostatic compensatory mechanisms engage to maintain effective tissue perfusion. At this time, subtle clinical evidence of haemodynamic stress may be apparent (tachycardia, decreased urine output) but overt evidence of shock (hypotension, altered sensorium, metabolic acidosis) may not. Therapeutic interventions have a high probability of preventing ischaemic tissue injury and initiation of systemic inflammatory cascades during this early compensated stage. Adaptive compensatory mechanisms fail and organ injury ensues if the injury that initiates the shock is too extensive or progresses despite therapy. As the duration of established shock increases, therapy is less likely to be effective in preventing organ failure and death.

Various sensing mechanisms involved in physiological compensatory responses exist to recognize haemodynamic and metabolic dyshomoeostasis. Low-pressure right atrial and pulmonary artery stretch receptors sense volume changes. A decrease in circulating volume (or increase of venous capacitance) results in an increase in sympathetic discharge from the medullary vasomotor centre [1,96,97]. Aortic arch, carotid and splanchnic high-pressure baroreceptors sense early blood pressure changes close to the physiologic range [1,96,97]. An increase of sympathetic discharge from the medullary vasomotor centre results from a small to moderate decrease in blood pressure associated with early shock. However, once mean arterial pressure falls below approximately 80–90 mmHg, aortic baroreceptor activity is absent. Subsequently, carotid baroreceptor response is eliminated as mean pressure falls below 60 mmHg. As blood pressure falls further, carotid and aortic chemoreceptors, sensitive to decreased Po_2, increased Pco_2 and increased hydrogen ion concentrations (decreased pH), dominate the response. These receptor complexes, active only when mean blood pressure is less than approximately 80 mmHg, are of minimal relevance during physiological states [1]. During shock, they make a substantial contribution to increases of sympathetic tone.

During severe shock, the most powerful stimulus to sympathetic tone is the CNS ischaemic response [1]. The lower medullary chemoreceptors for this response (thought to be sensitive to increased CO_2 associated with decreased cerebral perfusion) become active when mean blood pressure falls below 60 mmHg. Sympathetic stimulation provided by these receptors peaks at mean pressures of 15–20 mmHg and results in maximal stimulation of the cardiovascular system [1]. The Cushing response to increased intracranial pressure is an example of activation of this reflex under different circumstances.

Other mechanisms also have a role in the compensatory response to shock. Vasopressin release is regulated by alterations of serum osmolality. During effective hypovolaemia resulting from intravascular volume loss or increased vascular capacitance, low pressure, right atrial stretch receptors can override osmolar control of vasopressin response to effect retention of body water [1,98]. Similarly, during hypovolaemia and shock, the juxtaglomerular apparatus in the kidneys respond to decreased perfusion pressure by renin release [1].

All compensatory responses to shock, whether haemodynamic, metabolic or biochemical, support oxygen delivery to vital organs. These responses are similar (to varying extents) for different classes of shock and can be broken down into four components:

1 Maintenance of mean circulatory pressure (a measure of venous pressure) by either maintaining total intravascular volume, or increasing stressed volume (i.e. increasing venous tone)
2 Optimizing cardiac performance
3 Redistributing perfusion to vital organs
4 Optimizing unloading of oxygen at the tissue (Table 12.2; Fig. 12.4).

Mean circulatory pressure and venous return are sustained in early shock by a number of mechanisms.

Table 12.2 Cardiovascular/metabolic compensatory responses to shock.

---

1 Maintain mean circulatory pressure (venous pressure)
Volume
Fluid redistribution to vascular space
    from interstitium (Starling effect)
    from intracellular space (osmotic)
Decreased renal fluid losses
    glomerular filtration rate
    aldosterone
    vasopressin

Pressure
Decreased venous capacitance
    sympathetic activity
    circulating (adrenal) adrenaline
    angiotensin
    vasopressin

2 Maximize cardiac performance
Increase contractility
Sympathetic stimulation
Adrenal stimulation

3 Redistribute perfusion
Extrinsic regulation of systemic arterial tone
Dominant autoregulation of vital organs (heart, brain)

4 Optimize oxygen unloading
Red cell 2,3-DPG
Tissue acidosis
Pyrexia
Tissue Po_2

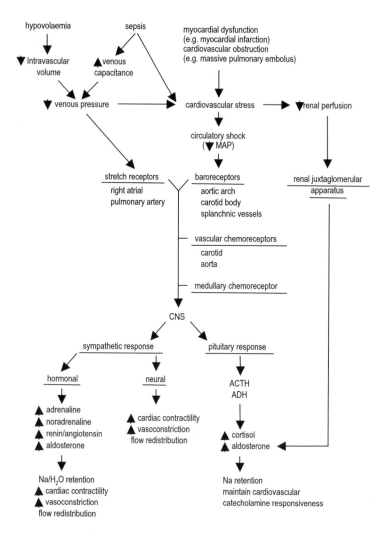

Figure 12.4 Neurohormonal response to shock. During early cardiovascular stress, the neurohormonal response may involve increased activity of the juxtaglomerular apparatus and stimulation of right atrial and pulmonary artery low pressure mechanoreceptors. With progressive hypotension, high pressure vascular baroreceptors, vascular chemoreceptors and the medullary chemoreceptor are sequentially stimulated resulting in augmented neurohormonal activity.

Increased pituitary hormone (adrenocorticotrophic hormone [ACTH] and antidiuretic hormone [ADH]) release and increased sympathetic outflow from the central nervous system result. Volume retention, increased venous tone, increased cardiac contractility and blood flow redistribution to vital organs occur as a consequence.

Acutely, total intravascular volume is supported by alterations of capillary hydrostatic pressure as described by Starling [99]. Sympathetic activation results in precapillary vasoconstriction. In combination with initial hypotension, this results in decreased capillary hydrostatic pressure [99]. A decrease in capillary hydrostatic pressure enhances intravascular fluid shift due to maintained plasma oncotic pressures. Transcapillary fluid influx following removal of 500–1000 mL blood volumes in humans can be as high as 2 mL/min with full correction of intravascular volume by 24–48 hours [100]. The intravascular volume may also be supported by the osmotic activity of glucose generated by glycogenolysis. Increased

extracellular osmolarity results in fluid redistribution from the intracellular to the extracellular space.

Intravascular volume is also conserved by decreasing renal fluid losses. Renal compensatory mechanisms are of limited value in acute shock but can have more impact in the subacute phase. Decreased renal perfusion associated with reduced cardiac output and afferent arteriolar constriction results in a fall in glomerular filtration rate and urine output. In addition, decreased renal perfusion pressure, sympathetic stimulation and compositional changes in tubular fluid [1] result in renin release from the juxtaglomerular apparatus. Renin release leads to adrenal cortical release of aldosterone (via antiotensin II) which increases sodium reabsorption in the distal tubules of the kidney in exchange for potassium or hydrogen ion [1]. Angiotensin II also exerts a powerful direct vasoconstricting effect (particularly on mesenteric vessels) while increasing sympathetic outflow and adrenal adrenaline release. Vasopressin (antidiuretic hormone) release occurs through activation of right atrial low pressure. Angiotensin II augments this release by increasing sympathetic outflow. The release of vasopressin from the posterior pituitary results in water retention at the expense of osmolarity. Hyponatraemia can result. Vasopressin, like angiotensin II, also results in vasoconstriction, particularly of the splanchnic circulation.

Finally, increased sympathetic activity and release of adrenal adrenaline results in systemic venoconstriction, particularly of the venous capacitance vessels of the splanchnic circulation. This supports mean circulatory pressure and venous return by increasing stressed volume.

Increased sympathetic nervous system activity accounts for most of the enhancement of cardiac performance during shock. Local release of noradrenaline by sympathetic nerves and systemic release of adrenaline result in stimulation of cardiac α- and β-adrenergic receptors resulting in increases of heart rate and contractility that optimize cardiac output and support blood pressure. Angiotensin II may also exert direct as well as indirect (sympathetic stimulation) inotropic effects on myocardium. Improved cardiac function also results in decreased right atrial pressure which tends to increase venous return.

Redistribution of blood flow during shock has already been discussed. Increased sympathetic vasoconstrictor tone, systemic release of adrenaline from the adrenals, vasopressin, endothelin and angiotensin II cause vasoconstriction in all sensitive vascular beds including skin, skeletal muscle, kidneys and splanchnic organs [2]. Dominant autoregulatory control of blood flow spares brain and heart bloodwork from these effects. Redistribution of flow to these vital organs is the effective result.

The effects of decreased delivery of oxygen to the tissues during shock can be attenuated by local adaptive responses. Hypoperfusion and tissue ischaemia will result in local acidosis because of decreased clearance of CO_2 and anaerobic metabolism. Local acidosis results in decreased affinity between oxygen and haemoglobin at the capillary level [1]. The resultant rightward shift of the oxyhaemoglobin dissociation curve allows greater unloading of oxygen from haemoglobin for a given Po_2. Tissue ischaemia is also accompanied by decreased tissue Po_2 (relative to normal) which will further augment unloading of oxygen. Pyrexia associated with sepsis may also contribute to a rightward shift of the oxyhaemoglobin dissociation curve while hypothermia is associated with a leftward shift. For that reason, maintenance of normothermia during resuscitation from shock is helpful in optimizing oxygen unloading.

Organ system dysfunction resulting from shock (Table 12.3)

Central nervous system

Central nervous system neurones are extremely sensitive to ischaemia. Fortunately, the CNS vascular supply is highly resistant to extrinsic regulatory mechanisms. Although cerebral perfusion is clearly impaired in shock, flow remains relatively well preserved until the later stages [101,102]. Absent primary cerebrovascular impairment, cerebral function is well supported until mean arterial pressure falls below approximately 50–60 mmHg [103]. Eventually, irreversible ischaemic injury may occur to the most sensitive areas of the brain (cerebral cortex). Before this fixed injury, an altered level of consciousness, varying from confusion to unconsciousness, may be seen depending on the degree of perfusion deficit. Disturbances of serum pH and electrolytes may also contribute. Electroencephalographic (EEG) recordings demonstrate non-specific changes compatible with encephalopathy. Sepsis-related encephalopathy may occur at higher blood pressures (caused in part by the effects of circulating inflammatory mediators) and is associated with increased mortality [104].

Heart

The major clinically apparent manifestations of shock on the heart are a result of sympatho-adrenal stimulation. Increased heart rate, in the absence of disturbances of cardiac conduction, is almost universally present. Vagally mediated paradoxical bradycardia may be seen on occasion in severe haemorrhage

Table 12.3 Organ system dysfunction in shock.

Central nervous system
Encephalopathy (ischaemic or septic)
Cortical necrosis

Heart
Tachycardia, bradycardia
Supraventricular tachycardia
Ventricular ectopy
Myocardial ischaemia
Myocardial depression

Pulmonary
Acute respiratory failure
Acute respiratory distress syndrome

Kidney
Prerenal failure
Acute tubular necrosis

Gastrointestinal
Ileus
Errosive gastritis
Pancreatitis
Acalculous cholecystitis
Colonic submucosal haemorrhage
Transluminal translocation of bacteria/antigens

Liver
Ischaemic hepatitis
'Shock' liver
Intrahepatic cholestasis

Haematology
Disseminated intravascular coagulation
Dilutional thrombocytopenia

Metabolic
Hyperglycaemia
Glycogenolysis
Gluconeogenesis
Hypoglycaemia (late)
Hypertriglyceridaemia

Immune
Gut barrier function depression
Cellular immune depression
Humoral immune depression

[105]. In patients predisposed to myocardial ischaemia or irritability, catecholamine driven supraventricular tachycardias and ventricular ectopy with ischaemic ECG changes are not common. Like the brain, the blood supply to the heart is autoregulated. This, in combination with the resilient nature of myocardial tissue, renders it resistant to sympathetically driven vasoconstriction and shock-related hypoperfusion injury. Overt necrosis does not typically occur although evidence of cellular injury may be present.

Most forms of shock are associated with increased contractility of healthy myocardium. Despite this, shock has substantial impact on myocardial contractility and compliance. Hypotension during cardiogenic (and other forms of shock) is associated with decreased coronary artery perfusion pressure. In patients with coronary artery disease or increased filling pressures, decreased coronary artery perfusion pressure may lead to overt ischaemia. Further, circulating myocardial depressant substances contribute to myocardial depression in septic [52] and haemorrhagic [53] shock. This has been linked to decreased β-adrenoreceptor affinity and density as well as potential defects of intracellular signal transduction involving nitric oxide, G-proteins, cyclic adenosine monophosphate (AMP) and cyclic GMP [44]. Circulating depressant substances may also be present during cardiogenic shock [55].

Respiratory system

Early alterations of pulmonary function seen during acute circulatory shock are primarily related to changes in central drive or muscle fatigue. Increased minute volume occurs as a result of augmented respiratory drive because of peripheral stimulation of pulmonary J receptors and carotid body chemoreceptors as well as hypoperfusion of the medullary respiratory centre. This results in hypocapnia and primary respiratory alkalosis [1,106]. With increased minute volume and decreased cardiac output, the ventilation–perfusion (V/Q) ratio is increased. Unless arterial hypoxaemia complicates shock, pulmonary resistance is initially unchanged or minimally increased. Coupled with an increased workload, respiratory and diaphragmatic muscle impairment resulting from hypoperfusion (manifested by decreased transmembrane electrical potential) may lead to early respiratory failure [107]. ARDS may develop as a late cause of respiratory failure from inflammatory or free radical injury to the alveocapillary cell layers following established shock.

Kidney

Acute renal failure is a major complication of circulatory shock with associated mortality rates of 35–80% [108]. Although initial injury manifested by decreased urine output occurs, other clinical manifestations of renal dysfunction (increased creatinine, urea and potassium) may not be noted for 1–3 days. Once haemodynamic stabilization has been achieved, it becomes apparent that urine output does not immediately improve and both serum creatinine and urea continue to rise. The single most common cause of acute renal failure is renal hypoperfusion resulting in acute tubular necrosis (ATN). The most frequent cause of renal hypoperfusion is haemodynamic compromise from septic shock, haemorrhage, hypovolaemia, trauma and major operative procedures. ATN that occurs in the setting of circulatory shock is associated with a higher mortality than in other situations.

Part of the reason for the kidney's sensitivity to hypoperfusion has to do with the nature of its vascular supply. The renal vascular bed is moderately autoregulated. Increases of efferent arteriolar tone can initially maintain glomerular perfusion despite compromise of renal flow [109]. Renal hypoperfusion does not become critical until relatively late in shock when maximal vasoconstriction of renal preglomerular arterioles [109] results in cortical, then medullary, ischaemic injury.

Decreased urine output in shock can pose a diagnostic dilemma because it can be associated with both oliguric ATN and hypoperfusion-related prerenal failure without ATN. Indices suggestive of the latter include: a benign urine sediment; urine sodium concentration <20 mmol/L; fractional urine sodium excretion <1%; urine osmolality >450 mOsm/L; and urine : plasma creatinine ratio >40. Useful markers of acute renal failure resulting from ATN include: haematuria and haeme granular casts; urine sodium concentration to >40 mmol/L; fractional excretion of urine sodium to >2%; urine osmolarity <350 mOsm/L; and urine : plasma creatinine ratio <20 [110]. Of note, ATN caused by circulatory shock may be associated with urine sodium <20 mmol/L and fractional excretion <1% if the acute renal injury is superimposed upon chronic effective volume depletion as may be seen with cirrhosis and congestive heart failure [111].

Gastrointestinal

The gut is relatively sensitive to circulatory failure. The splanchnic vasculature is highly responsive to sympathetic vasoconstriction. Typical clinical gut manifestations of hypoperfusion, sympathetic stimulation and inflammatory injury associated with shock include ileus, errosive gastritis, pancreatitis, acalculous cholecystitis and colonic submucosal haemorrhage. Enteric ischaemia produced by circulatory shock and free radical injury with resuscitation may breach gut barrier integrity with translocation of enteric bacteria and antigens (notably endotoxin) from the gut lumen to the systemic circulation resulting in propagation and amplification of shock and MODS [112,113].

Liver

Like the gut, the liver is highly sensitive to hypotension and hypoperfusion injury. 'Shock liver' associated with massive ischaemic necrosis and major elevation of transaminases is atypical in the absence of extensive hepatocellular disease on very severe insult [114]. Centrilobular injury with mild increases of transaminases and lactate dehydrogenase is more typical. Transaminases usually peak within 1–3 days of the insult and resolve over 3–10 days. In either case, early increases in bilirubin and alkaline phosphatase are modest. Despite the production of acute phase reactants in early circulatory shock, synthetic functions may be impaired with decreased generation of prealbumin, albumin and hepatic coagulation factors. After haemodynamic resolution of shock, evidence of biliary stasis with increased bilirubin and alkaline phosphatase can develop even though the patient is otherwise improving. Post-shock MODS involves similar hepatic pathology.

Haematology

Haematological   manifestations   of   circulatory

shock tend to be dependent on the nature of shock. Disseminated intravascular coagulation (DIC), characterized by microangiopathic haemolysis, consumptive thrombocytopenia, consumptive coagulopathy and microthrombi with tissue injury, is most commonly seen in association with septic shock. Because it is caused by simultaneous systemic activation of coagulation and fibrinolysis cascades, it can be differentiated from the coagulopathy of liver failure by determination of endothelial cell-produced factor 8 (normal or increased with hepatic dysfunction). In the absence of extensive tissue injury or trauma, haemorrhagic shock is rarely associated with DIC [115]. Dilutional thrombocytopenia is the most common cause of coagulation deficits after resuscitation for haemorrhage [116].

Metabolism

Metabolic alterations associated with shock occur in a predictable pattern. Early in shock, when haemodynamic instability triggers compensatory responses, sympatho-adrenal activity is enhanced. Increased release of adrenocorticotrophic hormone (ACTH), glucocorticoids and glucagon, and decreased release of insulin results in glycogenolysis, gluconeogenesis and hyperglycaemia [98,117]. Increased release of adrenaline results in skeletal muscle insulin resistance, sparing glucose for use by glucose-dependent organs (heart and brain). Late in shock, hypoglycaemia may develop, possibly resulting from glycogen depletion or failure of hepatic glucose synthesis. Fatty acids are increased early in shock but fall later as hypoperfusion of adipose-containing peripheral tissue progresses. Hypertriglyceridaemia is often seen during shock as a consequence of catecholamine stimulation and reduced lipoprotein lipase expression induced by circulating TNF [117]. Increased catecholamines, glucocorticoids and glucagon also increase protein catabolism resulting in a negative nitrogen balance [117].

Immune system

Immune dysfunction, frequent during and after circulatory shock and trauma, rarely has immediate adverse effects but likely contributes to late mortality. Underlying mechanisms of immune dysfunction include ischaemic injury to barrier mucosa (particul-

arly of the gut) leading to anatomical breaches (colonic ulceration) and potential mucosal translocation of bacteria and bacterial products; parenchymal tissue injury because of associated trauma, inflammation, ischaemia or free radical injury; and direct ischaemic or mediator (immunosuppressant cytokines, corticosteroids, prostaglandins, catecholamines, endorphins) induced dysfunction of cellular and humoral immune system [118,119]. In particular, macrophage function is adversely affected during trauma and circulatory shock. A decrease in antigen presenting ability impairs the activation of T and B lymphocytes. Associated with this defect are a decrease in Ia antigen expression, decrease in membrane IL-1 receptors, and the presence of suppressor macrophages. Phagocytic activity of the reticuloendothelial system is also compromised, partially because of an acute decrease in fibronectin levels. Suppression of T-lymphocyte immune function is manifested by decreased responsiveness to antigenic stimulation, and a decreased helper:suppressor ratio. Decreased production of IgG and IgM suggests B-cell suppression. Non-specific immunosuppression is expressed as decreased neutrophil bactericidal function, chemotaxis, opsonization and phagocytosis.

Resuscitation agents used in shock may also substantially depress immune function. Dopamine, used for haemodynamic support in shock, has been shown to suppress pituitary production of prolactin (required for optimal immune function) resulting in suppression of T-cell proliferative responses [120]. Thus, dopamine may contribute, along with stress-induced increases in immunosuppressive glucocorticoids, to T-cell anergy seen in critically ill patients.

All of these factors may contribute to the propensity of critically ill patients to develop ongoing organ system dysfunction as well as a variety of infections during the post-shock phase. It is notable that one-third to half of patients with shock die late in their course following resolution of the acute shock phase.

Conclusions

The pathogenesis and pathophysiology of shock has undergone tremendous advances in recent decades.

From studies of the clinical cardiovascular physiology of shock just 30 years ago, we have advanced to molecular analysis of subcellular signalling mechanisms and transcriptional regulation, and *in vivo* imaging of metabolic pathways. In the future, more detailed examination of shock pathophysiology may involve a variety of techniques including gene array and proteonomic technology. Advances derived from such future studies can be expected to appear as startling to us as current advances appear to our predecessors.

References

1 Guyton AC. *Textbook of Medical Physiology*, 8th edn. Philadelphia: W.B. Saunders, 1991.

2 Bond RF. Peripheral macro- and microcirculation. In: Schlag G, Redl H, eds. *Pathophysiology of Shock, Sepsis and Organ Failure*. Berlin: Springer-Verlag, 1993: 893–907.

3 Bond RF, Johnson GI. Vascular adrenergic interactions during haemorrhagic shock. *Fed Proc* 1985; **44**: 281–9.

4 Calvin JE, Driedger AA, Sibbald WJ. Does the pulmonary wedge pressure predict left ventricular preload in critically ill patients? *Crit Care Med* 1981; **9**: 437–43.

5 Braunwald E, Frahm CJ. Studies on Starling's law of the heart. IV. Observations on haemodynamic functions of the left atrium in man. *Circulation* 1961; **24**: 633–42.

6 Sylvester JT, Goldberg HS, Permutt S. The role of the vasculature in the regulation of cardiac output. *Clin Chest Med* 1983; **4**: 111–26.

7 Bressack MA, Raffin TA. Importance of venous return, venous resistance, and mean circulatory pressure in the physiology and management of shock. *Chest* 1987; **92**: 906–12.

8 Milnor WR. Arterial impedance as ventricular afterload. *Circ Res* 1975; **36**: 565–70.

9 Carabello BA, Spann JF. The uses and limitations of end-systolic indices of left ventricular function. *Circulation* 1984; **69**: 1058–64.

10 Johnson PC. Autoregulation of blood flow. *Circ Res* 1986; **59**: 483–95.

11 Cohn JD, Greenspan M, Goldstein CR, *et al.* Arteriovenous shunting in high cardiac output shock syndromes. *Surg Gynecol Obstet* 1968; **127**: 282–8.

12 Thijs LG, Groenveld ABJ. Peripheral circulation in septic shock. *Appl Cardiopulmon Pathol* 1988; **2**: 203–14.

13 Gutteriez G, Brown SD. Response of the macrocirculation. In: Schlag R, Redl H, eds. *Pathophysiology of Shock, Sepsis and Organ Failure*. Berlin: Springer-Verlag, 1993: 215–29.

14 Wang P, Hauptman JG, Chaudry IH. Hemorrhage produces depression in microvascular blood flow which persists despite fluid resuscitation. *Circ Shock* 1990; **32**: 307–18.

15 Bowton DL, Bertels NH, Prough DS, Stump DA. Cerebral blood flow is rduced in patients with sepsis syndrome. *Crit Care Med* 1989; **17**: 399–403.

16 Ekstrom-Jodal B, Haggendal E, Larsson LE. Cerebral blood flow and oxygen uptake in endotoxic shock: an experimental study in dogs. *Acta Anaesthesiol Scand* 1982; **26**: 163–70.

17 Cunnion RE, Schaer GL, Parker MM, *et al.* The coronary circulation in human septic shock. *Circulation* 1986; **73**: 637–44.

18 Dhainaut JF, Huyghebaert MF, Monsallier JF, *et al.* Coronary haemodynamics and myocardial metabolism of lactate, free fatty acids, glucose, and ketones in patients with septic shock. *Circulation* 1987; **75**: 533–41.

19 Finley RJ, Duff JH, Holliday RL, *et al.* Capillary muscle blood flow in human sepsis. *Surgery* 1975; **78**: 87–94.

20 Cryer HM, Kaebrick H, Harris PD, Flint LM. Effect of tissue acidosis on skeletal muscle microcirculatory responses to haemorrhagic shock in unanesthetized rats. *J Surg Res* 1985; **39**: 59–67.

21 Coleman B, Glaviano VV. Tissue levels of norepinephrine in haemorrhagic shock. *Science* 1963; **139**: 54.

22 Chernow B, Roth BL. Pharmacologic manipulation of the peripheral vasculature in shock: clinical and experimental approaches. *Circ Shock* 1986; **18**: 141–55.

23 Koyama S, Aibiki M, Kanai K, *et al.* Role of the central nervous system in renal nerve activity during prolonged haemorrhagic shock in dogs. *Am J Physiol* 1988; **254**: R761–9.

24 Thiemermann C, Szabö C, Mitchell JA, Vane JR. Vascular hyporeactivity to vasoconstrictor agents and haemodynamic decompensation in haemorrhagic shock is mediated by nitric oxide. *Proc Natl Acad Sci U S A* 1993; **90**: 267–71.

25 Lorente JA, Landin L, Renes E, *et al.* Role of nitric oxide in the haemodynamic changes of sepsis. *Crit Care Med* 1993; **21**:759–67.

26 Carden DI, Smith JK, Zimmerman BJ, *et al.* Reperfusion injury following circulatory collapse: the role of

reactive oxygen metabolites. *J Crit Care* 1989; **4**: 294–300.

27 Kubes P. Nitric oxide modulates microvascular permeability. *Am J Physiol* 1992; **262**: H611–5.

28 Redl H, Schlag G, Kneidinger R, *et al.* Activation/adherence phenomena of leucocytes and endothelial cells in trauma and sepsis. In: Redl H, Schlag G, eds. *Pathophysiology of Shock, Sepsis and Organ Failure.* Berlin: Springer-Verlag, 1993: 549–63.

29 Shah DM, Dutton RE, Newell JC, Powers SR. Vascular autoregulatory failure following trauma and shock. *Surg Forum* 1977; **28**: 11–3.

30 Hurd TC, Dasmahapatra KS, Rush BF Jr, *et al.* Red blood cell deformability in human and experimental sepsis. *Arch Surg* 1988; **123**: 217–20.

31 Van Rossum GD. The relation of sodium and potassium ion transport to respiration and adenine nucleotide content of liver slices treated with inhibitors of respiration. *Biochem J* 1972; **129**: 427–38.

32 Vogt MT, Fraber E. The effects of ethionine treatment on the metabolism of liver mitochondria. *Arch Biochem Biophys* 1970; **141**: 162–73.

33 Chaudry IH. Cellular mechanisms in shock and ischaemia and their correction. *Am J Physiol* 1983; **245**: R117–34.

34 Horpacsy G, Schnells G. Metabolism of adenine nucleotides in the kidney during haemorrhagic hypotension and after recovery. *J Surg Res* 1980; **29**: 11–7.

35 Chaudry IH, Sayeed MM, Baue AE. Alteration in high-energy phosphates in haemorrhagic shock as related to tissue and organ function. *Surgery* 1976; **79**: 666–8.

36 Chaudry IH, Sayeed MM, Baue AE. Effect of adenosine triphosphate-magnesium chloride administration in shock. *Surgery* 1974; **75**: 220–7.

37 Chaudry IH, Sayeed MM, Baue AE. Effect of haemorrhagic shock on tissue adenine nucleotides in conscious rats. *Can J Physio Pharmacol* 1974; **52**: 131–7.

38 Chaudry IH, Ohkawa M, Clemens MG, Baue AE. Alterations in electron transport and cellular metabolism with shock and trauma. *Prog Clin Biol Res* 1983; **111**: 67–88.

39 Solomon MA, Correa R, Alexander HR, *et al.* Myocardial energy metabolism and morphology in a canine model of sepsis. *Am J Physiol* 1994; **266**: H757–68.

40 Chaudry IH, Wichterman KA, Baue AE. Effect of sepsis on tissue adenine nucleotide levels. *Surgery* 1979; **85**: 205–11.

41 Ayala A, Perrin MM, Meldrum DR, *et al.* Hemorrhage induces an increase in serum TNF which is not associated with elevated levels of endotoxin. *Cytokine* 1990; **2**: 170–4.

42 Calandra T, Baumgartner J, Grau GE, *et al.* Prognostic values of tumor necrosis factor/cachectin, interleukin-1, and interferon-γ in the serum of patients with septic shock. *J Infect Dis* 1990; **161**: 982–7.

43 Girardin E, Grau GE, Dayer JM, *et al.* Plasma tumor necrosis factor and interleukin-1 in the serum of children with severe infectious purpura. *N Engl J Med* 1989; **319**: 397–400.

44 Kumar A, Krieger A, Symeoneides S, *et al.* Myocardial dysfunction in septic shock, Part II: Role of cytokines and nitric oxide. *J Cardiovasc Thoracic Anesth* 2001; **15**: 485–511.

45 Zanotti S, Kumar A, Kumar A. Cytokine modulation in sepsis and septic shock. *Expert Opin Investig Drugs* 2002; **11**: 1061–75.

46 Bone RC. The pathogenesis of sepsis. *Ann Intern Med* 1991; **115**: 457–69.

47 Tracey KJ, Lowry SF, Beutler B, *et al.* Cachectin/tumor necrosis factor mediates changes of skeletal muscle plasma membrane potential. *J Exp Med* 1986; **164**: 1368–73.

48 Levine B, Kalman J, Mayer L, *et al.* Elevated circulating levels of tumor necrosis factor in severe chronic heart failure. *N Engl J Med* 1990; **323**: 236–41.

49 Calandra T, Echtenacher B, Roy DL, *et al.* Protection from septic shock by neutralization of macrophage migration inhibitory factor. *Nat Med* 2000; **6**: 164–70.

50 Calandra T, Glauser MP. Immunocompromised animal models for the study of antibiotic combinations. *Am J Med* 1986; **80**: 45–52.

51 Wang H, Yang H, Czura CJ, *et al.* HMGB1 as a late mediator of lethal systemic inflammation. *Am J Respir Crit Care Med* 2001; **164**: 1768–73.

52 Parrillo JE, Burch C, Shelhamer JH, *et al.* A circulating myocardial depressant substance in humans with septic shock. Septic shock patients with a reduced ejection fraction have a circulating factor that depresses *in vitro* myocardial cell performance. *J Clin Invest* 1985; **76**: 1539–53.

53 Hallstrom S, Vogl C, Redl H, Schlag G. Net inotropic plasma activity in canine hypovolemic traumatic shock: low molecular weight plasma fraction after prolonged hypotension depresses cardiac muscle performance *in vitro*. *Circ Shock* 1990; **30**: 129–44.

54 Brar R, Kumar A, Schaer GL, *et al.* Myocardial infarction and reperfusion produces soluble myocardial depressant activity that correlates with infarct size. *Crit Care Med* 1996; **24**: A30.

55 Coraim F, Trubel W, Ebermann R, Werner T. Isolation of low molecular weight peptides in hemofiltrated patients with cardiogenic shock: a new aspect of myocar-

dial depressant substances. *Contrib Nephrol* 1991; **93**: 237–40.

56 Shoemaker WC, Appel PL, Kram HB. Measurement of tissue perfusion by oxygen transport patterns in experimental shock and in high-risk surgical patients. *Intensive Care Med* 1990; **16**(Suppl 2): S135–44.

57 Hallstrom S, Koidl B, Muller U, *et al*. A cardiodepressant factor isolated from blood blocks Ca^{2+} current in cardiomyocytes. *Am J Physiol* 1991; **260**: H869–76.

58 Kumar A, Thota V, Dee L, *et al*. Tumor necrosis factor-alpha and interleukin-1 beta are responsible for depression of *in vitro* myocardial cell contractility induced by serum from humans with septic shock. *J Exp Med* 1996; **183**: 949–58.

59 Kumar A, Brar R, Wang P, *et al*. The role of nitric oxide and cyclic GMP in human septic serum-induced depression of cardiac myocyte contractility. *Am J Physiol* 1999; **276**: R265–76.

60 Cain BS, Meldrum DR, Dinarello CA, *et al*. Tumor necrosis factor-α and interleukin-1β synergistically depress human myocardial function. *Crit Care Med* 1999; **27**: 1309–18.

61 Nathan C. Nitric oxide as a secretory product of mammalian cells. *FASEB J* 1992; **6**: 3051–64.

62 Kilbourn RG, Gross SS, Jubran A, *et al*. N-methyl-L-arginine inhibits tumor necrosis factor-induced hypotension: implications for the involvement of nitric oxide. *Proc Natl Acad Sci U S A* 1990; **87**: 3629–33.

63 McCord JM. Oxygen-derived free radicals. *New Horizons* 1993; **1**: 70–6.

64 Saugstad OD, Ostrem T. Hypoxanthine and urate levels of plasma during and after haemorrhagic hypotension in dogs. *Eur Surg Res* 1977; **9**: 48–56.

65 Yokoyama Y, Parks DA. Circulating xanthine oxidase: release of xanthine oxidase from isolated rat liver. *Gastroenterology* 1988; **94**: 607–11.

66 Jolly SR, Kane WJ, Bailie MB, *et al*. Canine myocardial reperfusion injury: its reduction by the combined administration of superoxide dismutase and catalase. *Circ Res* 1984; **54**: 277–85.

67 Przyklenk K, Kloner RA. Superoxide dismutase plus catalase improve contractile function in the canine model of the 'stunned myocardium'. *Circ Res* 1986; **58**: 148–56.

68 Granger DN, Rutili G, McCord JM. Superoxide radicals in feline intestinal ischaemia. *Gastroenterology* 1981; **81**: 22–9.

69 Peitzman AB, Shires GTI, Illner H, Shires GT. Effect of intravenous ATP-MgCl$_2$ on cellular function in liver and muscle in haemorrhagic shock. *Curr Surg* 1981; **38**: 300.

70 Murphy K, Haudek SB, Thompson M, Giroir BP. Molecular biology of septic shock. *New Horizons* 1998; **6**: 181–93.

71 Mira J, Cariou A, Grall F, *et al*. Susceptibility to and mortality of septic shock are associated with TNF2, a TNF-alpha promotor polymorphism: a multicenter study. *JAMA* 1999; **282**: 561–8.

72 Stuber F, Petersen M, Bokelmann F, Schade U. A genomic polymorphism within the tumor necrosis factor locus influences plasma tumor necrosis factor-alpha concentrations and outcome of patients with severe sepsis. *Crit Care Med* 1996; **24**: 381–4.

73 Libert C, Wielockx B, Hammond GL, *et al*. Identification of a locus on distal mouse chromosome 12 that controls resistance to tumor necrosis factor-induced lethal shock. *Genomics* 1999; **55**: 284–9.

74 Fang XM, Schroder S, Hoeft A, Stuber F. Comparison of two polymorphisms of the interleukin-1 gene family: interleukin-1 receptor antagonist polymorphism contributes to susceptibility to severe sepsis. *Crit Care Med* 1999; **27**: 1330–4.

75 Holmes CL, Russell JA, Walley KR. Genetic polymorphisms in sepsis and septic shock: role in prognosis and potential for therapy. *Chest* 2003; **124**: 1103–15.

76 Lightfoot EJ, Horton JW, Maass DL, *et al*. Major burn trauma in rats promotes cardiac and gastrointestinal apoptosis. *Shock* 1999; **11**: 29–34.

77 Xu YX, Wichmann MW, Ayala A, *et al*. Trauma-hemorrhage induces increased thymic apoptosis while decreasing IL-3 release and increasing GM-CSF. *J Surg Res* 1997; **68**: 24–30.

78 Rivers E, Nguyen B, Havstad S, *et al*. Early goal-directed therapy in the treatment of severe sepsis and septic shock. *N Engl J Med* 2001; **345**: 1368–77.

79 Finch CA, Lenfant C. Oxygen transport in man. *N Engl J Med* 1972; **286**: 407–15.

80 Nelson DP, Samsel RW, Wood LD, *et al*. Pathological supply dependency of systemic and intestinal O$_2$ uptake during endotoxemia. *J Appl Physiol* 1988; **64**: 2410–9.

81 Shibutani K, Komatsu T, Kubal K, *et al*. Critical level of oxygen delivery in anesthetized man. *Crit Care Med* 1983; **11**: 640–3.

82 Rackow EC, Astiz ME, Weil MH. Cellular oxygen metabolism during sepsis and shock: the relationship of oxygen consumption to oxygen delivery. *JAMA* 1988; **259**: 1989–93.

83 Gutierrez G, Pohil RJ. Oxygen consumption is linearly related to oxygen supply in critically ill patients. *J Crit Care* 1986; **1**: 45–53.

84 Ensinger H, Weichel T, Lindner KH, *et al*. Effects of norepinephrine, epinephrine, and dopamine on oxygen consumption in volunteers. *Crit Care Med* 1993; **21**: 1502–8.

85 Ronco JJ, Phang PT, Walley KR, *et al*. Oxygen consumption is independent of changes in oxygen delivery in severe adult respiratory distress syndrome. *Am Rev Respir Dis* 1991; **143**: 1267–73.

86 Ronco JJ, Fenwick JC, Wiggs BR, *et al*. Oxygen consumption is independent of increases in oxygen delivery by dobutamine in septic patients who have normal or increased plasma lactate. *Am Rev Respir Dis* 1993; **147**: 25–31.

87 Ronco JJ, Fenwick JC, Tweeddale MG, *et al*. Identification of the critical oxygen delivery for anaerobic metabolism in critically ill and nonseptic humans. *JAMA* 1993; **270**: 1724–30.

88 Bland RD, Shoemaker WC, Abraham E, Cobo JC. Haemodynamic and oxygen transport patterns in surviving and nonsurviving postoperative patients. *Crit Care Med* 1985; **13**: 85–90.

89 Fleming A, Bishop M, Shoemaker W, *et al*. Prospective trial of supranormal values as goals of resuscitation in severe trauma. *Arch Surg* 1992; **127**: 1175–81.

90 Boyd O, Grounds M, Bennett ED. A randomized clinical trial of the effect of deliberate perioperative increase of oxygen delivery on mortality in high-risk surgical patients. *JAMA* 1993; **270**: 2699–707.

91 Shoemaker WC, Appel PL, Kram HB, *et al*. Haemodynamic and oxygen transport monitoring to titrate therapy in septic shock. *New Horizons* 1993; **1**: 145–59.

92 Hayes MA, Timmins AC, Yau EHS, *et al*. Elevation of systemic oxygen delivery in the treatment of critically ill patients. *N Engl J Med* 1994; **330**: 1717–22.

93 Gattinoni L, SVO2 Collaborative Group. A trial of goal-oriented haemodynamic therapy in critically ill patients. *N Engl J Med* 1995; **333**: 1025–32.

94 Bishop MH, Shoemaker WC, Appel PL, *et al*. Relationship between supranormal circulatory values, time delays, and outcome in severely traumatized patients. *Crit Care Med* 1993; **21**: 56–63.

95 Bishop MH, Shoemaker WC, Appel PL, *et al*. Prospective, randomized trial of survivor values of cardiac index, oxygen delivery, and oxygen consumption as resuscitation endpoints in severe trauma. *J Trauma* 1995; **38**: 780–7.

96 Chien S. Role of the sympathetic nervous system in hemorrhage. *Physiol Rev* 1967; **47**: 214–88.

97 Bond RF, Green HD. Cardiac output redistribution during bilateral common carotid artery occlusion. *Am J Physiol* 1969; **216**: 393–403.

98 Woolf PD. Endocrinology of shock. *Ann Emerg Med* 1986; **15**: 1401–5.

99 Haupt MT. The use of crystalloidal and colloidal solution for volume replacement in hypovolemic shock. *Crit Rev Clin Lab Sci* 1989; **27**: 1–23.

100 Skillman JJ, Awwad HK, Moore FD. Plasma protein kinetics of the early transcapillary refill after hemorrhage in man. *Surg Gynecol Obstet* 1967; **125**: 983–96.

101 Forsyth RP, Hoffbrand BI, Melmon KL. Redistribution of cardiac output during hemorrhage in the unanesthetized monkey. *Circ Res* 1970; **27**: 311–20.

102 Kaihara S, Rutherford RB, Schwentker EP, Wagner HN. Distribution of cardiac output in experimental haemorrhagic shock in dogs. *J Appl Physiol* 1969; **27**: 218–22.

103 Harper AM. Autoregulation of cerebral blood flow: Influence of the arterial blood pressure on the blood flow though the cerebral cortex. *J Neurol Neurosurg Psychiatry* 1966; **29**: 398–403.

104 Sprung CL, Peduzzi PN, Shatney CH, *et al*. Impact of encephalopathy on mortality in the sepsis syndrome. The Veterans Administration Systemic Sepsis Cooperative Study Group. *Crit Care Med* 1990; **18**: 801–6.

105 Sander-Jensen K, Secher NH, Bie P, *et al*. Vagal slowing of the heart during hemorrhage: observations from twenty consecutive hypotensive patients. *Br Med J* 1986; **295**: 364–6.

106 Douglas ME, Downs JB, Dannemiller FB, *et al*. Acute respiratory failure and intravascular coagulation. *Surg Gynecol Obstet* 1976; **143**: 555–60.

107 Roussos C, Macklem PT. The respiratory muscles. *N Engl J Med* 1982; **307**: 786–97.

108 Hou SH, Bushinsky DA, Wish JB, *et al*. Hospital acquired renal insufficiency: a prospective study. *Am J Med* 1983; **74**: 243–8.

109 Myer B, Moran S. Haemodynamically mediated acute renal failure. *N Engl J Med* 1986; **314**: 97–105.

110 Rose BD. *Meaning and Application of Urine Chemistries: Clinical Physiology of Acid–Base and Electrolyte Disorders.* New York: McGraw-Hill, 1984: 271–8.

111 Diamond JR, Yoburn DC. Nonoliguric acute renal failure associated with a low fractional excretion of sodium. *Ann Intern Med* 1982; **96**: 597–600.

112 Mainous MR, Deitch EA. Bacterial translocation. In: Schlag G, Redl H, eds. *Pathophysiology of Shock, Sepsis and Organ Failure.* Berlin: Springer-Verlag, 1993: 265–78.

113 Lillehei RC, MacLean LD. The intestinal factor in irreversible endotoxin shock. *Ann Surg* 1958; **148**: 513–9.

114 Champion HR, Jones RT, Trump BF, *et al*. A clinicopathologic study of hepatic dysfunction following shock. *Surg Gynecol Obstet* 1976; **142**: 657–63.

115 Garcia-Barreno P, Balibrea JL, Aparicio P. Blood coagulation changes in shock. *Surg Gynecol Obstet* 1978; **147**: 6–12.

116 Counts HB, Haisch C, Simon TL, *et al.* Hemostasis in massively transfused trauma patients. *Ann Surg* 1979; **190**: 91–9.

117 Arnold J, Leinhardt D, Little RA. Metabolic response to trauma. In: Schlag G, Redl H, eds. *Pathophysiology of Shock, Sepsis and Organ Failure*. Berlin: Springer-Verlag, 1993: 145–60.

118 Hoyt DB, Junger WG, Ozkan AN. Humoral mechanisms. In: Schlag G, Redl H, eds. *Pathophysiology of Shock, Sepsis and Organ Failure*. Berlin: Springer-Verlag, 1993: 111–30.

119 Stephan R, Ayala A, Chaudry IH. Monocyte and lymphocyte responses following trauma. In: Schlag G, Redl H, eds. *Pathophysiology of Shock, Sepsis and Organ Failure*. Berlin: Springer-Verlag, 1993: 131–44.

120 Devins SS, Miller A, Herndon BL, *et al.* The effects of dopamine on T-cell proliferative response and serum prolactin in critically ill patients. *Crit Care Med* 1992; **20**: 1644–9.

CHAPTER 13
Cellular physiology

Nigel R. Webster

Introduction

This chapter aims to bridge the gap between basic biochemistry and molecular and cell biology on the one hand, and organ and systems physiology on the other. These topics are all well covered in a range of major textbooks which are used in undergraduate and postgraduate training. However, cellular physiology is often less well appreciated and detailed in these textbooks.

In essence, all cells require energy and nutrients to fulfil three functions:

1 Ion transport
2 Locomotion
3 Multiplication/reproduction.

Humans are free-living animals who can move about and survive in vastly diverse environments — deserts, altitude and extreme cold. However, individual cells can only survive and function within a narrow range of physical and chemical conditions. The body can therefore only survive extreme conditions by maintaining the environment around cells within narrow limits — called homoeostasis. Achieving homoeostasis requires various component physiological systems to function in a coordinated fashion. For example, to maintain electrolyte homoeostasis for potassium and sodium, the cells of the gut, central nervous system, kidney and endocrine system must cooperate.

The organization of the body can be viewed hierarchically (Fig. 13.1) as being made up of functionally distinct entities or compartments that act together as physiological systems. This compartmentalization can continue further down in scale to include individual cells and indeed individual organelles within cells. Each compartment can have its own special local environment maintained to permit optimal performance. Each cell is separated from the extracellular environment by the cell membrane, and each of the organelles within cells is separated from the cytoplasm of the cell by membranes. Each of the membranes is especially adapted to allow different functions to be carried out under optimal conditions — examples include protein synthesis in the endoplasmic reticulum and oxidative metabolism in the mitochondria.

Cell and subcellular membranes are lipid bilayers made up largely of phospholipids. These have hydrophilic or polar heads (and contain phosphates) attached to hydrophobic or non-polar tails made up of fatty acids. The phospholipids assemble into sheets, with the polar heads packed together. Two sheets combine at their hydrophobic surfaces to form a bilayer with the two hydrophilic surfaces exposed to the aqueous environment within and outside the cell. The individual lipid molecules within the membrane are free to move, and the membrane therefore behaves like a two-dimensional fluid. Two other lipids are also found within membranes, cholesterol and sphingolipids, and also proteins. Many of these proteins are transmembrane in that they penetrate both sheets of the membrane and mediate transport of water and electrolytes through ion channels and in other cases larger molecules such as proteins or hormones (as seen with receptors) (Fig. 13.2).

Transport mechanisms are central to homoeostasis. Furthermore, for coordinated regulation of physiological functions, communication must occur between compartments and this must involve the transmission, receiving and translation of signals. This often involves second and third messengers (such as inositol triphosphate, cyclic adenosine monophosphate [AMP] and cyclic guanosine monophosphate [GMP]) and may also involve the internalization of the protein components of the cell membrane (as in corticosteroid signalling).

It is therefore clear that homoeostasis and its regulation is crucial for the survival of the cell and

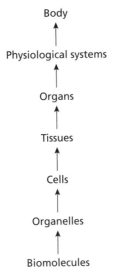

Body

↑

Physiological systems

↑

Organs

↑

Tissues

↑

Cells

↑

Organelles

↑

Biomolecules

Figure 13.1 The hierarchy of the organization of the body.

the body. This process depends on the normal functioning of membranes and their signalling functions. This chapter is therefore primarily concerned with the membrane-mediated processes that are essential to physiology. Other chapters cover specifics of receptors, second and third messengers, and aspects of systems physiology.

Diffusion and permeability

The distribution of electrolytes in the compartments of the body varies radically and the intracellular fluid can also vary between individual cells, depending on the nature and function of the cell. It is apparent that the electrolyte concentrations differ markedly in the various compartments; for example, the low content of protein anions in the interstitial fluid and the fact that Na^+ and Cl^- are largely extracellular whereas most of the K^+ is intracellular. The differences in composition are caused in large part by the nature of the barriers separating the compartments. The cell membrane separates the intracellular fluid from the interstitial fluid and the capillary wall separates the

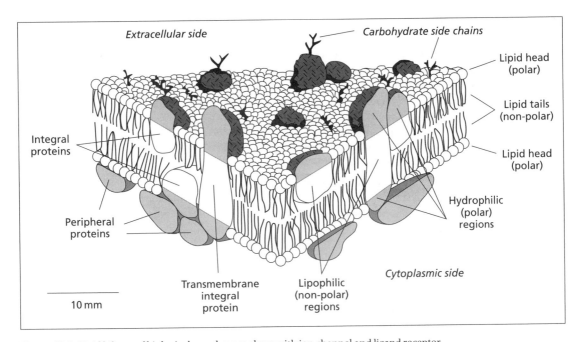

Figure 13.2 Lipid bilayer of biological membranes along with ion channel and ligand receptor.

plasma from the interstitial fluid. The primary forces producing movement of water, electrolytes and other molecules around the system are diffusion, osmosis, active transport and exocytosis and endocytosis.

Diffusion is the process by which molecules in solution (including a gas) expand to fill all the available volume. This process depends on the motion of the particles and is an entirely random process. An individual particle is equally likely to move into or out of an area in which it is in high concentration. However, because there are more particles in areas of high concentration, the total number of particles moving to areas of lower concentration is greater — there is a net flux (J) of particles from areas of high to those of lower concentration. Flux is the amount of material passing through a certain cross-sectional area in a given time. Flux is proportional to the concentration gradient — $\Delta C / \Delta x$ — where ΔC is the change of concentration with distance Δx.

$$J \, \alpha \, \Delta C / \Delta x$$

or

$$J = -D \, (\Delta C / \Delta x)$$

where the proportionality constant, D, is known as the diffusion coefficient. The minus sign denotes the fact that the diffusion is occurring down the concentration gradient. This latter equation is Fick's first law of diffusion and has the dimensions of cm^2/s.

The time required for equilibrium to occur by diffusion is proportional to the square of the distance for diffusion. This effectively means that displacement of particles does not increase linearly with time — in fact it increases with the square root of time. This results in a very inefficient way to move molecules around over large distances.

We can now introduce membranes into the system and apply Fick's law:

$$J = -D \, [(Ci - Co) / \Delta x]$$

where Ci and Co are the concentrations inside and outside the membrane and Δx is the thickness of the membrane as biological membranes are hydrophobic, while the aqueous solution on either side is highly polar, solutes show differing solubilities in the

membrane relative to the aqueous solution and the partition coefficient (β) becomes important:

$$\beta = C_{mem} / C_{aq}$$

where C_{aq} is the solute concentration in aqueous solution and C_{mem} is the solute concentration inside the membrane.

When $\beta < 1$ (solute dissolves better in aqueous solution than in the membrane), the concentration gradient in the membrane is reduced and flux is decreased. When $\beta > 1$ (solute dissolves better in the membrane than in aqueous solution), the concentration gradient is increased and flux is enhanced. Should $\beta = 0$, then flux would be zero and the membrane would be completely impermeable to that substance. This now leads to the concept of membrane permeability (P):

$$P = D\beta / \Delta x$$

and the units of permeability are cm/s or velocity.

Membrane permeability coefficients for a variety of biologically important molecules are given in Table 13.1. In general, small neutral molecules such as water, oxygen and carbon dioxide can permeate membranes readily. Larger and more hydrophilic molecules permeate more slowly. However, inorganic ions (Na^+, K^+, Cl^- and Ca^{2+}) are essentially impermeable. Also shown in Table 13.1 are the various time constants (τ) for diffusion which more graphically illustrate this concept in a given cell of 20 μm diameter. It is readily apparent that, with the exception of small neutral molecules, almost everything that is

Table 13.1 Permeability of lipid bilayer membrane to solutes calculated on the basis of a spherical cell of diameter 20 μm.

Solute	P (cm/s)	τ
Water	10^{-4}–10^{-3}	0.5–5 s
Urea	10^{-6}	8 min
Glucose	10^{-7}	14 hours
Cl$^-$	10^{-11}	1.6 year
Na$^+$	10^{-13}	160 years

biochemically important and biologically relevant cannot pass through a lipid bilayer membrane simply by diffusion. Biological membranes have therefore evolved with special mechanisms to transport molecules across membranes — ion pumps, carrier proteins for substances like glucose and amino acids, and endocytosis and exocytosis for larger molecules such as proteins.

Osmosis and water movement

Diffusion is the net movement of molecules down concentration gradients and has the effect of abolishing concentration differences — diffusion causes mixing. However, if two solutions are separated and solute is prevented from moving down a concentration gradient because the membrane is not permeable to that particular solute, then the concentration difference could persist. However, this does not occur when the membrane is permeable to the solute. Here, the converse of the concentration gradient for solute can be considered to exist — the more concentrated solution (side of the membrane) has fewer solvent molecules than in the less concentrated solution. As before, solvent molecules are free to diffuse across the membrane and this has the same ultimate effect of equalizing concentrations across the semipermeable membrane. However, when the process is complete, there will be a net movement of solvent molecules from the less concentrated solution to the more concentrated solution, with the end result being an increase in volume of the initially more concentrated solution. In a closed environment, this increase in volume has the effect of increasing pressure. The pressure arising from unequal solute concentrations across a semi-permeable membrane is termed osmotic pressure. The larger the concentration difference then the greater is the osmotic pressure.

Osmotic pressure, like vapour pressure lowering, or freezing-point depression, depends on the number rather than the type of particles in solution. In an ideal solution, osmotic pressure (P) is related to temperature and volume in the same way as the pressure of a gas:

$$P = n\text{RT/V}$$

where n is the number of particles, R is the gas constant, T is the absolute temperature and V is the volume. It is therefore clear that if T is constant, osmotic pressure is proportional to the number of particles per unit volume of solution. With non-ionizing solutes such as glucose, the osmotic pressure is a function of the number of glucose molecules present. If the solute ionizes, each ion is osmotically active. For example, NaCl dissociates into Na^+ and Cl^- ions, so that each mole in solution would supply two moles of osmotically active particles (2 osm). Clearly, although a homogeneous solution may have within it osmotically active particles, it can only exert an osmotic pressure when in contact with another solution across a membrane permeable to the solvent but not the solute. The total solute concentration in the fluids of the body are approximately 300 mmol and the osmotic pressure resulting from this solute concentration at 37°C is approximately 7.5 atm.

However, membranes are never completely impermeable to solute and this requires us to consider a parameter called the reflection coefficient (σ):

$$\sigma = 1 - (P_{solute}/P_{water})$$

If the membrane permeability to solute is 0, the reflection coefficient is 1 and in this case all solute molecules are 'reflected' by the membrane. Under these circumstances, the full osmotic effect is achieved. If the membrane allows completely free passage to the solute, $\sigma = 0$ and the osmotic pressure should also be zero.

The reflection coefficient can now be incorporated into the osmotic pressure equation:

$$\Delta\pi = \sigma RT\Delta C_{solute}$$

where $\Delta\pi$ is the effective osmotic pressure difference across the membrane.

We can now describe the forces that govern water movement across membranes — the Starling equation. As far as water is concerned, both hydrostatic and osmotic pressures can act similarly — both can drive water through a membrane.

$$\text{Fluid movement} = Kf\left[(Pc + \pi I) - (Pi + \pi c)\right]$$

where Kf is the filtration coefficient. It is apparent from the equation that the direction and volume of water flow across the membrane is determined by the balance of the hydrostatic and osmotic pressures. Figure 13.3 shows a schematic representation of the pressure and osmotic forces across a capillary joining an arteriole and a venule. Arrows indicate the magnitude and direction of the fluid movement at various sites along the capillary. Over the length of the capillary there is a slight excess of filtration over absorption with a net flow of a small amount of fluid into the interstitium. This excess fluid is collected by the lymphatics and is eventually returned into the circulation. Knowledge of the various factors and forces governing fluid movement across the capillary explain the various processes that can result in the appearance of oedema.

Because impermeable solutes remain trapped within cells, when a cell is exposed to changing external osmotic conditions the only changes that can occur rapidly to the cell are volume changes produced by gain or loss of water. It is for this reason that

the amount of impermeable intracellular solutes ultimately determine cell volume.

Ion gradients

At any membrane in a living cell, biologically active ions are distributed asymmetrically on either side of the membrane — concentrations of Na^+, K^+ and Cl^- are different (Table 13.2). This asymmetrical distribution obviously results in a concentration gradient, but what may not be so obvious is that there is also an electrical gradient. In practice, the maintenance of normal cell volume depends on sodium and potassium pumping. In the absence of such pumping, chloride and sodium ions would enter the cells down their concentration gradients and water would follow along the osmotic gradient thus created, causing the cells to swell until the pressure inside balanced the influx.

Ions will move across membranes in the direction of their concentration gradients. However, if the membrane is selectively permeable to some ions, there will be a resultant charge to the cell. For example, the intracellular potassium concentration is higher than that of the extracellular fluid so potassium ions tend to leave the cell. This results in an excess of positive charges to the outside of the cell because chloride ions do not automatically follow. An electrical potential difference develops as the cell interior becomes progressively more negative. Eventually, the developing electrical field opposes further migration of potassium ions: the negative interior attracts K^+ while the positive exterior repels K^+. Eventually, an electrochemical equilibrium is reached

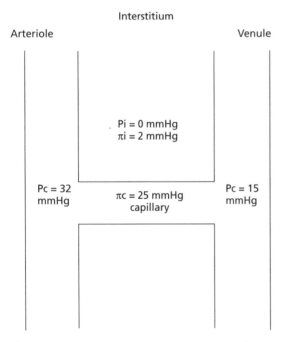

Figure 13.3 Schematic diagram of the pressure gradients across a capillary with examples given at either end of the capillary. In this example the pressure differential at the arteriolar end of the capillary is $[(32 + 2) − (0 + 25)] =$ 9 mmHg outward and at the opposite end is $[(15 + 2) − (0 + 25) = 8$ mmHg inwards.

Table 13.2 Concentrations of monovalent ions for a typical mammalian cell.

	Concentration (mmol/L)		Equilibrium potential (mV)
Ion	Inside cell	Outside cell	
Na^+	15.0	150.0	+60
K^+	150.0	5.0	−90
Cl^-	9.0	110.0	−70

and this potential difference where there is no net movement of an individual ion is termed the equilibrium potential. Each ion will have its own equilibrium potential which can be determined from the Nernst equation:

$$E_{eq} = RT/FZ \ln [C_{out}/C_{in}]$$

Where E_{eq} is the equilibrium potential, R is the universal gas constant, T is the absolute temperature, F is Faraday's constant, Z is the electrical valency of the ion (e.g. +1 for K^+ and −1 for Cl^-) and C_{out} and C_{in} are the extracellular and intracellular concentrations of the ion.

The magnitude of the membrane potential at any given time depends upon the distribution of Na^+, K^+ and Cl^- and the permeability of the membrane to each of these ions. The Goldman constant field equation describes this relationship and is the same as the Nernst equation, but is the sum of the concentration ratios with, in each case, a permeability factor for the three ions. Clearly, a cell can alter its membrane potential merely by manipulating the relative permeabilities of the major ions — as occurs in nerve cells for example.

Two transport proteins are primarily responsible for the resting membrane potential: a K^+ leak channel that permits potassium to diffuse out of the cell and the Na^+, K^+ ATPase pump.

Ion channels

The permeability of phospholipid bilayer membranes to ions is very small and consequently ions cross membranes by either binding to a carrier molecule or through an aqueous pore. However, transport by carrier molecule, although facilitating movement, would still be too slow to allow neuronal signalling. Ion channels are large protein structures which often comprise several subunits. They extend across the lipid bilayer and are in contact with the aqueous environment on both sides of the membrane. This channel allows ions to cross by diffusion and is considerably faster. The pore of the ion channel is not necessarily open all of the time and they may open or close spontaneously and in response to external stimuli, acting like a gate. Voltage-gated ion channels open depending on the membrane potential, while ligand-gated channels open in response to binding of another molecule (e.g. neurotransmitter) to a receptor located on the channel.

An understanding of the function of channels is important for much of the physiology of excitable tissues and also pharmacology. The topic of ion channels is covered in other chapters within this book.

Transport processes

To mediate and regulate the transfer of water and polar solutes, membranes contain integral proteins known as channels, carriers and pumps.

Channels in biological membranes are proteins with central pores that are open to both the extracellular fluid and cytoplasm at the same time. They usually have a narrowing within them, the selectivity filter, which determines which substances can pass through. Aquaporins are selectively permeable to water and similar channels are highly selective for Na^+, K^+ and Ca^{2+}, whereas others are less selective and may be permeable to both Na^+ and K^+.

Permeability through channels depends to an extent on the density of the channels in the particular membrane. For example, the relative permeability to water depends on the number of channels present per unit area and hormones can vary this (e.g. vasopressin and the renal collecting ducts). In diabetes insipidus, aquaporin-2 insertion into the membranes of the epithelial cells of the collecting ducts is deficient, causing an intrinsically low water permeability in these ducts which prevents water reabsorption.

Another mechanism of controlling channel permeability is by gating, as discussed previously. Examples of gating include voltage or ligand gating with either Ca^{2+} or ATP.

In contrast to channels, carriers are integral membrane proteins that open to only one side of the membrane at a time. A solute binds to the carrier at one side of the membrane, then, as a result of a conformational change, the gate on the opposite side of the membrane is opened and the solute dissociates from the carrier. In the simplest case, carriers move substances down their concentration gradients but at a much faster rate than would otherwise be the case — facilitated diffusion. A good example is the simple glucose carrier or glucose transporter,

GLUT-1. Transport by carriers exhibits kinetic properties similar to those of enzymes and it follows Michaelis–Menten kinetics. This means that they can be saturated if the solute concentration rises sufficiently to exceed the limited number of carrier molecules. Carrier-mediated transport exhibits specificity for substrates and, like other receptors, is subject to competitive and non-competitive inhibition. Carrier-mediated transport can also be regulated; for example, another glucose transporter, GLUT-4, is regulated by insulin because it increases the density of GLUT-4 molecules in the membrane and thus enhances glucose uptake. β-Adrenergic agents appear to inhibit GLUT-4 activity because glucose uptake is reduced; however, this occurs because of enhanced glycogenolysis which increases the intracellular glucose concentration and thereby results in a relatively unfavourable concentration gradient.

Co-transport occurs when the transport of one solute is coupled to that of another. If both solutes move in the same direction the process is called symport and if two coupled solutes move in opposite directions then it is called countertransport or antiport or exchange. Sodium is co-transported with a variety of solutes including proton ions such as K^+, glucose and amino acids.

Active transport converts the chemical energy from ATP into electrochemical potential energy stored in solute gradients. For example, the Na^+ pump uses the energy from ATP to build up and maintain the sodium electrochemical gradient which is then used to drive the secondary transport of another solute. The sodium pump is an integral membrane protein that hydrolyses one ATP molecule to ADP while transporting three Na^+ ions out of the cell and two K^+ ions into the cell. Because more positive charges leave the cell than enter with each turn of the cycle, there is a net flow of charge resulting in an actual resting membrane potential that is slightly more negative than that predicted from the Goldman equation.

Molecular motors

Cell motility is an essential feature of many biological processes; for example, the beating of cilia, cell movement, cell division and development and mainte-

nance of cell architecture, as well as the more obvious muscle contraction. Moreover, the normal function of cells requires the directional transport within the cell of numerous substances and subcellular organelles such as vesicles, mitochondria and chromosomes. All types of cellular motility are driven by *molecular motors*. These motors produce unidirectional movement along structural elements in the cell — filaments of *actin* and *microtubules* made of the protein tubulin. Three distinct motors have been described: *myosin*, *kinesin* and *dynein*. All molecular motors convert chemical energy (ATP) into kinetic energy (movement).

Myosin is an actin-based motor that moves along actin filaments and produces muscle contraction. Kinesin and dynein transport organelles along microtubules with kinesins being involved in mitotic and meiotic spindle formation, chromosome separation and protein transport, while dyneins are associated with the beating of cilia and vesicular transport.

The first kinesin-based motor to be discovered is called 'conventional' kinesin — it transports vesicular cargo packages along microtubule tracks. It comprises two heavy peptide chains and two light chains (Fig. 13.4). At the N-terminus of the heavy chains is the motor domain that contains the site for microtubule binding and ATP hydrolysis. The neck linker domain is critical in determining the direction of the motor domains along the microtubule. The light chains are involved in cargo binding. The kinesin moves along the microtubule with the two motor domains alternately stepping from one tubulin subunit to another. When kinesin is bound to a microtubule with the leading head free of nucleotide and the trailing head bound to ADP, both of the neck linkers are mobile. When ATP binds to the leading head, the neck linker becomes docked on to the leading head which throws the trailing head forward towards the next tubulin binding site.

Conclusions

Knowledge of cellular and molecular physiological processes is fundamental to understanding organ function and how tissues fail in various pathological processes. The maintenance of homoeostasis is crucial for normal cell and organ function. The crucial

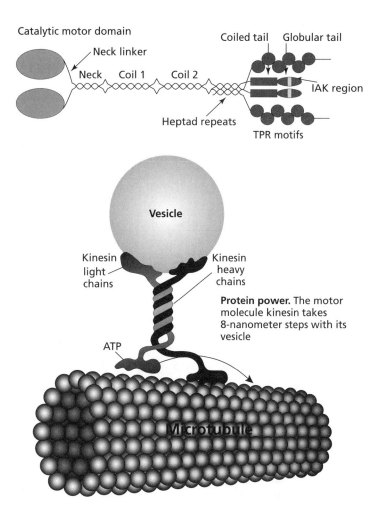

Figure 13.4 Conventional kinesin structure and movement.

role of the membrane in this homoeostasis has been highlighted. In addition, the need for specialized areas within the membrane that facilitate the transfer of molecules and ions from one side of the membrane to the other has been detailed. Specialized cells have individual and specifically tailored receptors and ion channels and these permit nerve conduction and muscle contraction. Further discussion of the pharmacokinetics and pharmacodynamics of these units are presented elsewhere in this book.

Further reading

Blaustein MP, Lederer WJ. Sodium/calcium exchange: its physiological implications. *Physiol Rev* 1999; **79**: 763–854.

Catterall WA. Structure and function of voltage-gated ion channels. *Annu Rev Biochem* 1995; **64**: 493–531.

Catterall WA. Structure and regulation of voltage-gated Ca^{2+} channels. *Annu Rev Cell Dev Biol* 2000; **16**: 521–55.

Gennis RB. *Biomembranes: Molecular Structure and Function.* New York: Springer-Verlag, 1989.

Joost HG, Thorens B. The extended GLUT-family of sugar/polyol transport facilitators: nomenclature, sequence characteristics, and potential function of its novel members. *Mol Membr Biol* 2001; **18**: 247–56.

MacLennan DH, Green NM. Structural biology: pumping ions. *Nature* 2000; **405**: 633–4.

Vale RD, Milligan RA. The way things move: looking under the hood of molecular motor proteins. *Science* 2000; **288**: 88–95.

Verhey KJ, Rapoport TA. Kinesin carries the signal. *Trends Biochem Sci* 2001; **26**: 545–50.

CHAPTER 14

Acid–base balance: albumin and strong ions

John A. Kellum

Introduction

Regulation of blood pH is an essential component of homoeostasis. In health, the pH of the arterial blood is maintained between 7.35 and 7.45 by a precise balance of alveolar ventilation and carbon dioxide (CO_2) production matched to non-volatile acid production and elimination. This non-volatile or 'fixed' component of acid–base balance is traditionally referred to as 'metabolic'. However, because CO_2 is generated by metabolism and because most non-volatile acids are not, the term 'metabolic' is misleading at best. This chapter focuses on the non-volatile components of acid–base balance, which can be divided into weak acids and strong ions. Recent advances in the understanding of the regulation and interaction of weak acids and strong ions, along with the application of basic physical and chemical principles, permit a simpler, yet more comprehensive treatment of acid–base balance. At the same time, this 'new' approach is grounded in the same basic principles as more traditional approaches (and is, in fact, entirely consistent with them). What is different with this new approach is a more careful consideration of the independent determinants of blood pH. Consideration of the independent variables is important not only for understanding mechanism but also for planning treatment.

The pH of blood

In order to understand acid–base physiology, it is first necessary to agree on how to describe and measure it. Since Sörensen first introduced the pH notation, the pH scale has been used to quantify acid–base bal-ance. The pH scale has tremendous advantages because it lends itself to colorimetric and electrometric techniques. There is also some physiological relevance to the logarithmic pH scale [1]. However, pH is a confusing variable. It is a non-linear transformation of H^+ concentration — the logarithm of its reciprocal. Strictly speaking, pH can only be thought of as a dimensionless representation of H^+ concentration and is not, itself, a concentration. Indeed, pH is actually the logarithmic measure of the volume required to contain 1 Eq of H^+. In blood plasma at pH 7.4, this volume is roughly 25 million litres [2].

Since Hasselbalch adapted the Henderson equation to the pH notation of Sörensen, the following equation has been used to understand the relationship between volatile and non-volatile acid–base variables:

$$pH = pK \times \log [HCO_3^-/(0.03 \times pCO_2)]$$

This is the Henderson–Hasselbalch (HH) equation and it is important to realize what this equation tells us. An increase in pCO_2 results in a decrease in pH and an increase in HCO_3^- concentration. Thus, a patient found to have a low blood pH, a condition known as acidaemia, will either have an increased pCO_2 or a pCO_2 that is 'not increased'. In the former circumstance, the disorder is classified as a 'respiratory acidosis'. The term 'acidosis' is used to describe the process resulting in acidaemia, and 'respiratory' because the apparent cause is an increased pCO_2. This is logical because carbonic acid results when CO_2 is added to water (or blood) and the resultant decrease in pH is entirely expected. In the latter condition, pCO_2 is not increased and thus there cannot be a respiratory acidosis. This condition is referred to as 'metabolic' because some non-volatile acid must be the cause of the acidaemia. The above logic can be reversed and used to easily classify simple conditions of alkalaemia as either resulting from respiratory or metabolic alkaloses. Thus, the HH equation allows us to classify disorders as to the primary type of acid being increased or decreased.

Over time, physiology superimposes its effects on simple chemistry and the relationship between pCO_2 and HCO_3^- is altered in order to reduce the alterations in pH. However, by carefully examining the changes that occur in pCO_2 and HCO_3^- in relationship to each, one can discern highly conserved patterns. In this way rules can be established to allow one to discover mixed disorders and to separate chronic from acute respiratory derangements. For example, one such rule is the convenient formula [3] for predicting the expected pCO_2 in the setting of a metabolic acidosis: $pCO_2 = (1.5 \times HCO_3^-) + 8 \pm 5$. This rule tells what the pCO_2 should be secondary to the increase in alveolar ventilation that accompanies a metabolic acidosis. If pCO_2 does not change enough or changes too much, the condition is classified as a 'mixed' disorder, with either a respiratory acidosis if the pCO_2 is still too high, or a respiratory alkalosis if the change is too great.

It is equally, important to understand what the HH equation does not tell us. First, it does not allow us to discern the severity (quantity) of the metabolic derangement in a manner analogous to the respiratory component. For example, when there is a respiratory acidosis, the increase in the pCO_2 quantifies the derangement even when there is a mixed disorder. However, the metabolic component can only be approximated by the change in HCO_3^-.

Secondly, the HH equation does not tell us about any other acids other than carbonic acid. The relationship between CO_2 and HCO_3^- provides a useful clinical 'road map' to guide the clinician in uncovering the aetiology of an acid–base disorder. However, the total CO_2 concentration, and hence the HCO_3^- concentration, is determined by the pCO_2, which is in turn determined by the balance between alveolar ventilation and CO_2 production. HCO_3^- cannot be regulated independently of pCO_2. The HCO_3^- concentration in the plasma will always increase as the pCO_2 increases, yet this is not an alkalosis. To understand how the pH and HCO_3^- concentration are altered independently of pCO_2, it is necessary to look beyond the HH equation.

Determinants of blood pH

Almost all biological solutions share two important characteristics. First, virtually all are aqueous (composed of water) and, secondly, most are alkaline (OH^- concentration > H^+ concentration). Because these characteristics are so universal in human physiology, they are often ignored in reviews of physiology, especially for clinical medicine, yet they are extremely important. Aqueous solutions contain a virtually inexhaustible source of H^+. Although pure water dissociates only slightly into H^+ and OH^-, electrolytes and CO_2 produce powerful electrochemical forces that influence water dissociation. Similarly, aqueous solutions that are alkaline behave very differently compared with acidic solutions in terms of the extent to which changes in their composition influence changes in pH (Fig. 14.1). Importantly, this property of alkaline solutions is often overlooked and what has often been attributed to the power of buffering systems is merely a physicochemical property of alkaline solutions.

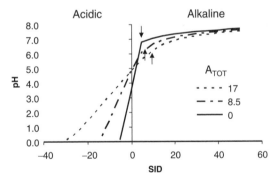

Figure 14.1 Plot of pH versus strong ion difference (SID). For this plot, pCO_2 was held constant at 40 mmHg. The three curves correspond to three different concentrations of A_{TOT} (normal, 50% of normal and zero). The plots assume a water dissociation constant for blood of 4.4×10^{-14} (Eq/L). The arrows refer to the point of neutrality ($OH^- = H^+$). To the right of these points, $OH^- > H^+$ and the solutions are alkaline. To the left of these points, $H^+ > OH^-$ and the solutions are acidic. Note how different the slopes of these lines are when the solutions are acidic versus alkaline.

Thus, for aqueous solutions, water is the primary source of H^+ and the determinants of pH are the determinants of water dissociation. Fortunately, even for an aqueous solution as complex as blood plasma, there are but three independent variables that determine pH:

1 pCO_2
2 Strong ion difference (SID)
3 Total weak acid concentration (A_{TOT}).

The last two compose the non-volatile acids and are the focus of this review.

Strong ions

Blood plasma contains numerous ions. These ions can be classified both by charge: positive 'cations' and negative 'anions', as well as by their tendency to dissociate in aqueous solutions. Some ions are completely dissociated in water; for example, Na^+, K^+, Ca^{2+}, Mg^{2+} and Cl^-. These ions are called 'strong ions' to distinguish them from 'weak ions' (e.g. albumin, phosphate and HCO_3^-), which can exist both as charged (dissociated) and uncharged forms. Certain ions, such as lactate, are so nearly completely dissociated that they may be considered strong ions under physiological conditions. In a neutral salt solution containing only water and NaCl, the sum of strong cations (Na^+) minus the sum of strong anions (Cl^-) is zero (i.e. $Na^+=Cl^-$). However, in blood plasma, strong cations (mainly Na^+) outnumber strong anions (mainly Cl^-). The difference between the sum of all strong cations and all strong anions is known as SID. SID has a powerful electrochemical effect on water dissociation and hence on blood pH. As SID becomes more positive the pH increases in order to maintain electrical neutrality (Fig. 14.1).

In healthy humans, the plasma SID is 40–42 mEq/L, although it is often quite different in critically ill patients. According to the principle of electrical neutrality, blood plasma cannot be charged, so the remaining negative charges balancing the SID come from CO_2 and the weak acids (A^-) and, to very small extent, from OH^-. At physiological pH, the contribution of OH^- is so small (nEq range) that it can be ignored. A_{TOT} (mainly albumin and phosphate) can be considered together and where $AH + A^- = A_{TOT}$. The SID of a blood sample can be estimated from the value of the remaining negative charge because SID $- (CO_2 + A^-) = 0$. This estimate of SID has been termed the effective SID (SIDe) [4] but it is really no different from the term 'buffer base', first described over a half century ago [5]. Thus, SID and buffer base are mirror images of each other. Furthermore, because the base excess (BE) is the change in buffer base required to return a blood sample to a pH of 7.4 where $pCO_2 = 40$ mmHg [6], the BE therefore defines the change in SID from this equilibrium point.

An alternative estimate of SID is $(Na^+ + K^+ + Ca^{2+} + Mg^{2+}) - (Cl^- + lactate^-)$. This is referred to as the 'apparent' SID (SIDa) because some 'unmeasured' ions might also be present [4]. Neither SIDe nor SIDa are perfect estimates of the true SID. Blood samples from patients may contain unmeasured strong ions (e.g. sulphate, ketones) making the SIDa an inaccurate estimate of SID. Similarly, these patients may have abnormal weak ions (e.g. proteins) that will make the SIDe inaccurate. However, in healthy humans, SIDa and SIDe are nearly identical and are thus valid estimates of SID [4]. Furthermore, when SIDa and SIDe are not equal, a condition referred to as the strong ion gap (SIG), where SIDa – SIDe = SIG, abnormal strong and/or weak ions must be present [7]. The SIG is positive when unmeasured anions > unmeasured cations and negative when unmeasured cations > unmeasured anions. Unexplained anions, and in some cases cations, have been found in the circulation of patients with a variety of diseases [7–10] and in animals under experimental conditions [11].

Mechanisms regulating strong ions

In order to alter the SID, the body must affect a change in the relative concentrations of strong cations and strong anions. The kidney is the primary organ that affects this change. However, the kidney can only excrete a very small amount of strong ion into the urine each minute and several minutes to hours are therefore required to impact significantly on the SID. The handling of strong ions by the kidney is extremely important because every Cl^- filtered but not reabsorbed decreases the SID. Because most of the human diet contains similar ratios of strong cations to strong anions, there is usually sufficient Cl^- available for this to be the primary regulating mechanism. This is particularly apparent when one considers that renal Na^+ and K^+ handling are influenced by other priorities (e.g. intravascular volume and plasma K^+ homoeostasis). Accordingly, 'acid handling' by the kidney is generally mediated through Cl^- balance. How the kidney handles Cl^- is obviously very important. Traditional approaches to this problem have focused on H^+ excretion and emphasized the importance of NH_3 and its conjugate acid NH_4^+. However, H^+ excretion per se is irrelevant as water provides an essentially infinite source of H^+. Indeed, the kidney does not excrete H^+ any more as NH_4^+ than it does as H_2O. The purpose of renal ammoniagenesis is to allow the excretion of Cl^- without Na^+ or K^+. This is achieved by supplying a weak cation (NH_4^+) to excrete with Cl^-.

Thus, NH_4^+ is important to systemic acid–base balance, not because of its carriage of H^+ or because of its direct action in the plasma (normal plasma NH_4^+ concentration is <0.01 mEq/L), but because of its 'co-excretion' with Cl^-. Of course, NH_4^+ is not only produced in the kidney; hepatic ammoniagenesis (and also glutaminogenesis) is important for systemic acid–base balance and, as expected, it is tightly controlled by mechanisms sensitive to plasma pH [12]. Indeed, this reinterpretation of the role of NH_4^+ in acid–base balance is supported by the evidence that hepatic glutaminogenesis is stimulated by acidosis [13]. Amino acid degradation by the liver can result in the production of urea, glutamine or NH_4^+. Normally, the liver does not release more than a very small amount of NH_4^+, but rather incorporates this nitrogen into either urea or glutamine. Hepatocytes have enzymes to enable them to produce either of these end products, and both allow for the regulation of plasma NH_4^+ at suitably low levels. However, the production of urea or glutamine has significantly different effects at the level of the kidney. This is because glutamine is used by the kidney to generate NH_4^+ and facilitate the excretion of Cl^-. Thus, the production of glutamine can be seen as having an alkalinizing effect on plasma pH because of the way in which the kidney utilizes it.

Further support for this scenario comes from the recent discovery of an anatomical organization of hepatocytes according to their enzymatic content [14]. Hepatocytes with a propensity to produce urea are positioned closer to the portal venule and thus have the first opportunity to metabolize NH_4^+ delivered from the splanchnic circulation. However, acidosis inhibits ureagenesis and under these conditions more NH_4^+ is available for the downstream hepatocytes which are predisposed to produce glutamine. Thus, the leftover NH_4^+ is 'packaged' as glutamine for export to the kidney where it is used to facilitate Cl^- excretion and hence increases the SID.

The gastrointestinal tract also has important effects on the SID. Along its length, the gastrointestinal tract handles strong ions quite differently. In the stomach, Cl^- is pumped out of the plasma and into the lumen, reducing the SID of the gastric juice and thus reducing the pH. On the plasma side, SID is increased by the loss of Cl^- and the pH is increased producing the so-called 'alkaline tide' which occurs at the beginning of a meal when gastric acid secretion is maximal [15]. In the duodenum, Cl^- is reabsorbed and the plasma pH is restored. Normally, only slight changes in plasma pH are evident because Cl^- is returned to the circulation almost as soon as it is removed. However, if gastric secretions are removed from the patient, either by suction catheter or vomiting, Cl^- will be progressively lost and the SID will steadily increase. It is important to realize that it is the Cl^- loss not the H^+ that is the determinant of plasma pH. Although H^+ is 'lost' as HCl, it is also lost with every molecule of water removed from the body. When Cl^- (a strong anion) is lost without loss of a strong cation, the SID is increased and therefore the plasma H^+ concentration is decreased. When H^+ is 'lost' as water rather than HCl, there is no change in the SID and hence no change in the plasma H^+ concentration.

In contrast to the stomach, the pancreas secretes fluid into the small intestine which has a SID much higher than plasma and is very low in Cl^-. Thus, the plasma perfusing the pancreas has its SID decreased, a phenomenon that peaks about an hour after a meal and helps counteract the alkaline tide. If large amounts of pancreatic fluid are lost (e.g. from surgical drainage), an acidosis will result as a consequence of the decreased plasma SID. In the large intestine, fluid also has a high SID because most of the Cl^- has been removed in the small intestine and the remaining electrolytes are mostly Na^+ and K^+. The body normally reabsorbs much of the water and electrolytes from this fluid but when severe diarrhoea exists, large amounts of cations can be lost. If this loss is persistent, the plasma SID will decrease and acidosis will result. Finally, whether the gastrointestinal tract is capable of regulating strong ion uptake in a compensatory fashion has not been well studied. There is some evidence that the gut may modulate systemic acidosis in experimental endotoxaemia by removing anions from the plasma [6]. However, the full capacity of this organ to affect acid–base balance is unknown.

Pathophysiology of strong ion imbalance

Metabolic acidoses and alkaloses are categorized according to the ions that are responsible. Thus, there is lactic acidosis and chloride-responsive alkalosis, etc. It is important to recognize that metabolic acidosis is produced by a decrease in the SID which produces an electrochemical force that results in a decrease in blood pH. A decrease in SID may be brought about by the generation of organic anions (e.g. lactate, ketones), the loss of cations (e.g. diarrhoea), the mishandling of ions (e.g. renal tubular acidosis) or the addition of exogenous anions (e.g. iatrogenic acidosis, poisonings). By contrast, metabolic alkaloses occur as a result of an inappropriately large SID, although the SID need not be greater than the 'normal' 40–42 mEq/L. This may be brought about by the loss of anions in excess of cations (e.g. vomiting, diuretics), or rarely by administration of strong cations in excess of strong anions (e.g. transfusion of large volumes of banked blood).

In the acute setting, acidosis is usually more of a problem than alkalosis, and in the critically ill the most common sources of metabolic acidosis are disorders of:

1 chloride homoeostasis
2 lactate
3 other anions.

Hyperchloraemic metabolic acidosis occurs either as a result of chloride administration or secondary to abnormalities in chloride handling or related to movements of chloride from one compartment to another. The effect of chloride administration on the development of metabolic acidosis has been known for many years [16,17]. Recently, new attention has been paid to this area in light of better understanding of the mechanisms responsible for this effect [18–22]. It has now been shown in animal models of sepsis [18] and in patients undergoing surgery [19,20,22] that saline causes metabolic acidosis not by 'diluting' HCO_3^-, but rather by its chloride content. From a physical chemical prospective this is completely expected. HCO_3^- is a dependent variable and cannot be the *cause* of the acidosis. Instead, Cl^- administration decreases the SID (an independent variable) and produces an increase in water dissociation and hence H^+ concentration. The reason this occurs with saline administration is that although saline contains equal amounts of both Na^+ and Cl^-, the plasma does not. When large amounts of salt are added, the Cl^- concentration increases much more than the sodium concentration. For example, 0.9% ('normal') saline contains 154 mEq/L of Na^+ and Cl^-. Administration of large volumes of this fluid will have a proportionally greater effect on total body Cl^- than on total body Na^+. Of note, it is the total body concentrations of these strong ions that must be considered and although the true volume of distribution of Cl^- is less, like Na^+, the effective volume of distribution (after some time of equilibration) is equal to total body water [18].

There are other important causes of hyperchloraemia (e.g. renal tubular acidosis, diarrhoea) and in addition, this form of metabolic acidosis is common in critical illness, especially sepsis. Although saline resuscitation undoubtedly has a role, there appears to be unexplained sources of Cl^-, at least in animal models of sepsis [18]. One possible explanation is that this Cl^- is coming from intracellular and interstitial compartments as a result of the partial loss of Donnan equilibrium resulting from albumin exiting the intravascular space [18]. However, this hypothesis is yet unproven.

Albumin and the weak acids

The second, non-volatile determinant of blood pH is the total weak acid concentration (A_{TOT}). The weak acids are mostly proteins (predominantly albumin) and phosphates, and they contribute the remaining charges to satisfy electroneutrality such that SID − $(CO_2 + A^-) = 0$. However, A^- is not an independent variable because it changes with alterations in SID and pCO_2. Rather, A_{TOT} (AH + A^-) is the independent variable because its value is not determined by any other. The identification of A_{TOT} as the third independent acid–base variable has led some authors to suggest that a third 'kind' of acid–base disorder exists [23]. Thus, along with respiratory and metabolic, there would also be acidosis and alkalosis caused by abnormalities in A_{TOT}. However, mathematical and therefore chemical independence does not necessarily imply physiological independence. Although the loss of weak acid (A_{TOT}) from the plasma space is an alkalinizing process [21], there is no evidence that the body regulates A_{TOT} to maintain acid–base balance. Furthermore, there is no evidence that clinicians should treat hypoalbuminaemia as an acid–base disorder. Indeed, a recent 7000 patient trial comparing albumin-based fluid resuscitation with saline found no difference in 28-day survival [24].

Critically ill patients frequently have hypoalbuminaemia and as such their A_{TOT} is reduced. However, these patients are not often alkalaemic and their SID is also reduced [25]. When these patients have a normal pH and a normal BE and HCO_3^- concentration, it would seem most appropriate to consider this to be physiological compensation for a decreased A_{TOT} [26] rather than classifying this condition as a complex acid–base disorder with a mixed metabolic acidosis/hypoalbuminaemic alkalosis. Thus, it seems far more likely that this 'disorder' is in fact the normal physiological response to a decreased A_{TOT}. Furthermore, because changes in A_{TOT} generally occur slowly, the development of alkalaemia would require the kidney to continue to excrete Cl^- despite an evolving alkalosis. Most authorities would consider such a scenario to be renal-mediated hypochloraemic metabolic alkalosis, the treatment for which would include fluids and/or chloride depending on the clinical conditions. Stewart's designation of a 'normal' SID of ~40 mEq/L was based on a 'normal' CO_2 and A_{TOT}. The 'normal' SID for a patient with an albumin of 2 g/dL would be much lower (e.g. ~32 mEq/L).

Unmeasured anions

Unmeasured anions can be quantified by the SIG, or less reliably by the anion gap (AG). The AG is calculated from the abundant strong ions and HCO_3^- without regard to weak acids ($AG = [Na^+ + K^+] - [Cl^- +$ $HCO_3^-]$). Normally, the SIG is near zero, while the AG is 8–12 mEq/L. The AG is an estimate of the sum of ($SIG + A^-$). Thus, subtracting A^- from the AG approximates the SIG. A convenient and reasonably accurate way to estimate A^- is to use the following formula [27]:

2 (albumin g/dL) + 0.5 (phosphate mg/dL)

or, for international units:

0.2 (albumin g/L) + 1.5 (phosphate mmol/L)

Note that the 'normal' AG for a person with no unmeasured anions or cations in their plasma is equal to A^- such that $AG - A^- = SIG = 0$. This technique allows one to 'calibrate' the AG for patients with abnormal albumin and/or phosphate concentrations.

In addition to the 'measured anions' (e.g. Cl^-, lactate), several other anions may be present in the blood of critically ill patients. Ketones are perhaps the most important of these, but sulphates and certain poisons (e.g. methanol, salicylate) are important in the appropriate clinical conditions. In addition, unmeasured anions have been shown to be present in the blood of many critically ill patients [7–10]. It is important to emphasize that both strong and weak ions will alter the SIG (and the anion gap for that matter). Thus, the exact chemical make-up of the SIG may vary significantly from patient to patient. Healthy humans and laboratory animals appear to have very little if any unmeasured anions and so their SIG is near zero. In one study, citing a previously published laboratory dataset calculated the total unmeasured anions in the blood of exercising humans at 0.3 ± 0.6 mEq/L [7].

However, unlike healthy exercising subjects or normal laboratory animals [11,18], critically ill patients seem to have much higher SIG values [28–33]. Recently, there has been controversy as to what constitutes a 'normal' SIG and whether an abnormal SIG is associated with adverse clinical outcomes. Reports from the USA [28,29,33] and from Holland [30] have found that the SIG was close to 5 mEq/L in critically ill patients, while studies from England and Australia [31,32] have found much higher values. The use of resuscitation fluids containing unmeasured anions (e.g. gelatins) could be the explanation but this has not been established. If exogenous anions are administered, the SIG will be a mixture of endogenous and exogenous anions and, quite possibly, of different prognostic significance. Interestingly, these two studies involving patients receiving gelatins [31,32] have failed to find a correlation between SIG and mortality, while a positive correlation between SIG and hospital mortality has been found in studies in patients not receiving gelatins [28,29,34]. Indeed, one recent study reported that pre-resuscitation SIG predicts mortality in injured patients better than blood lactate, pH or injury severity scores [29]. Dondorp *et al.* [34] had similar results with pre-resuscitation SIG as a strong mortality predictor in patients with severe malaria.

Interestingly, in none of these studies have the anions responsible for the SIG been identified. Given that individual patients may have SIG values of more than 10–15 mEq/L, it seems unlikely that any strong ion could be present in the plasma at these concentrations and be unknown to us. Yet, it seems stranger still for weak acids such as proteins to be the cause given that they are, in fact, weak. In healthy subjects, the total charge concentration of plasma albumin is only approximately 10–12 mEq/L. For a similarly charged protein to affect a SIG of 15 mEq/L, it would need to be present in very large quantities indeed. The answer, probably, is that the identity of the SIG in these patients is multifactorial. Endogenous strong ions such as ketones and sulphate are added to exogenous ones such as acetate and citrate. Reduced metabolism of these and other ions owing to liver [11] and kidney [35] dysfunction likely exacerbates this situation. The release of myriad of acute phase proteins, principally from the liver, in a setting of critical illness and injury is likely to add to the SIG. Furthermore, the systemic inflammatory response is associated with the release of a substantial quantity of proteins including cytokines and chemokines, some of which, like high-mobility group B1, have been linked to mortality [36].

The cumulative effect of all of these factors may well be a reflection of both organ injury and dysfunction. It is perhaps not surprising that there is a correlation between SIG and mortality. Indeed, whatever the source of SIG, it appears that its presence in the circulation, especially early in the course of illness or injury, portends a poor prognosis. While the prognostic significance of SIG is reduced (or abolished) when exogenous unmeasured anions are administered (e.g. gelatins), a SIG acidosis seems to be far worse than a similar amount of hyperchloraemic acidosis and more like lactic acidosis in terms of significance [37]. Although it is possible that saline-based resuscitation fluids contaminate the prognostic value of hyperchloraemia the same way gelatins appear to confound SIG, there remains strong evidence that not all metabolic acidoses are the same.

Clinical applications

While most cases of metabolic acidosis and alkalosis are mild and self-limiting, there are certain circumstances in which acid–base derangements are quite dangerous. Such is the case when the disorders are extreme (e.g. pH <7.0 or >7.7); especially when the acid–base derangement develops quickly. Such severe abnormalities can be the direct cause of organ dysfunction. Clinical manifestations can include cerebral oedema, seizures, decreased myocardial contractility, pulmonary vasoconstriction and systemic vasodilatation to name but a few. Furthermore, even less extreme derangements may produce harm because of the patient's response to the abnormality. For example, a spontaneously breathing patient with metabolic acidosis will attempt to compensate by increasing minute ventilation. The workload imposed by increasing minute ventilation can lead to respiratory muscle fatigue with respiratory failure or diversion of blood flow from vital organs to the respiratory muscles, resulting in organ injury. Acidaemia is associated with increased adrenergic tone and, on this basis, can promote the development of cardiac dysrrhythmias in critically ill patients, or increase myocardial oxygen demand in patients with myocardial ischaemia. In such cases, it may be prudent not only to treat the underlying disorder but also to provide symptomatic treatment for the acid–base disorder itself. Accordingly, it is important to understand both the causes of acid–base disorders and the limitations of various treatment strategies.

An extremely common cause of non-volatile acid–base derangements is fluid resuscitation. When intravenous solutions are administered to patients, the effect on the plasma pH is the result of changes in the independent variables determining it (i.e. pCO_2, A_{TOT} and SID). Commonly used fluids such as 0.9% ('normal') saline contain no weak acids and equal concentrations of strong ions (Na^+ and Cl^-) so that the SID of this solution is 0. When this solution is added to the plasma, the effect is to reduce the SID (an acidifying effect) (Fig. 14.2) while simultaneously reducing the albumin concentration (an alkalinizing effect). Because strong ions have more effect on the pH than weak acids, the addition of saline to the plasma will have a slight acidifying effect. Using *ex vivo* haemodilution of normal whole blood, Morgan *et al.* [21] have demonstrated that for crystalloids, the equilibrium point for these two opposing effects occurs at a SID of 24 mEq/L. When crystalloids with a SID <24 mEq/L are administered, acidosis will occur, while crystalloids with a SID >24 mEq/L result in alkalosis. When large volumes of saline (SID = 0) are used, the acidosis can be of sufficient magnitude to produce clinically important acidosis. Furthermore, if one fails to understand the reason for this acidosis, diagnostic and therapeutic mistakes may occur.

Finally, emerging evidence suggests that changes in acid–base variables influence immune effector cell function [38,39]. Thus, avoiding acid–base derangements may prove important in the management of critically ill patients for their own sake and the sake of standardizing study protocols that attempt to manipulate immunological responses (e.g. anticytokine therapies).

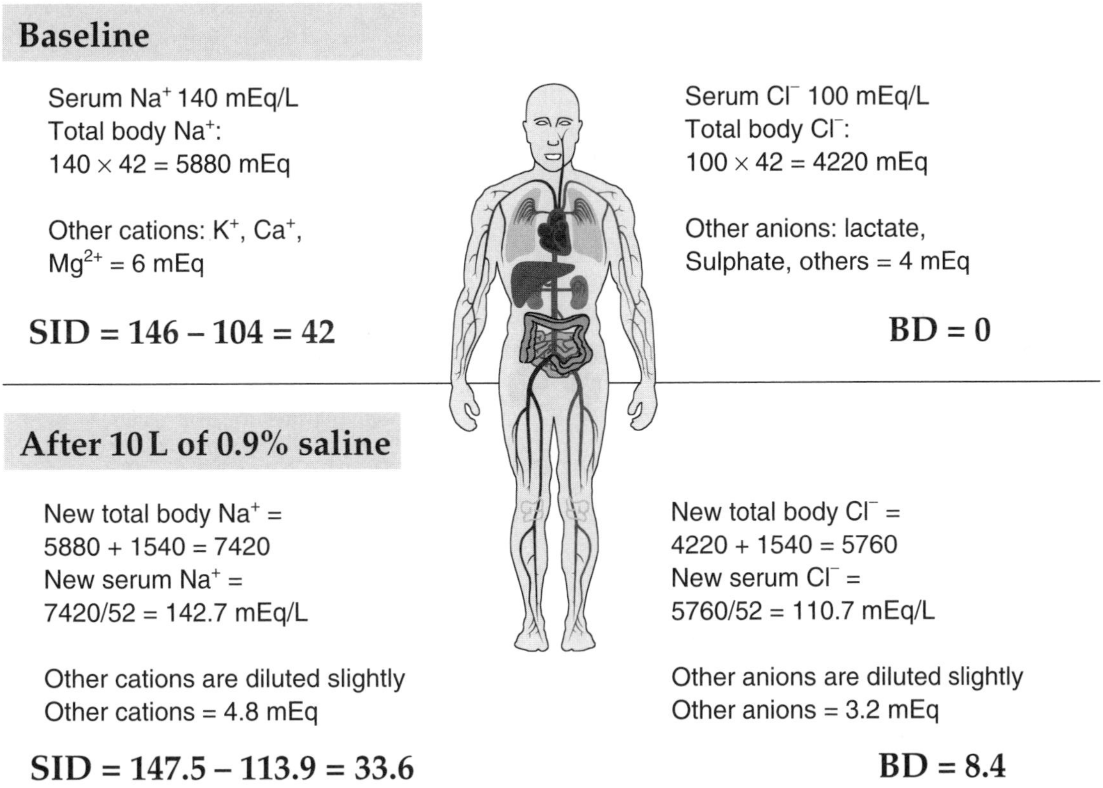

Baseline

Serum Na^+ 140 mEq/L
Total body Na^+:
$140 \times 42 = 5880$ mEq

Other cations: K^+, Ca^+,
$Mg^{2+} = 6$ mEq

$$SID = 146 - 104 = 42$$

Serum Cl^- 100 mEq/L
Total body Cl^-:
$100 \times 42 = 4220$ mEq

Other anions: lactate,
Sulphate, others = 4 mEq

$$BD = 0$$

After 10 L of 0.9% saline

New total body Na^+ =
$5880 + 1540 = 7420$
New serum Na^+ =
$7420/52 = 142.7$ mEq/L

Other cations are diluted slightly
Other cations = 4.8 mEq

$$SID = 147.5 - 113.9 = 33.6$$

New total body Cl^- =
$4220 + 1540 = 5760$
New serum Cl^- =
$5760/52 = 110.7$ mEq/L

Other anions are diluted slightly
Other anions = 3.2 mEq

$$BD = 8.4$$

Figure 14.2 The effects of a 10-L saline load in a 70-kg man with normal baseline acid–base status. The effects assume no fluid or electrolyte losses (no urine output) and sufficient time for equilibration (approximately 2–3 hours). Note that the change in strong ion difference (SID) is caused primarily by a greater relative increase in serum Cl^- compared with serum Na^+. Similar changes have been demonstrated experimentally [18]. The base deficit (BD) increases in direct proportion to the decrease in SID [40].

Conclusions

Unlike many other areas in clinical medicine, the approach to acid–base physiology has not often distinguished cause from effect. Although it is perfectly reasonable to describe an alteration in acid–base status by the observed changes in H^+ and HCO_3^-, this does not itself imply causation. The essence of the Stewart approach is the understanding that only three variables are important in determining blood pH: pCO_2, SID and A_{TOT}. Neither H^+ nor HCO_3^- can change unless one or more of these three variables change. Strong ions cannot be created or destroyed to satisfy electroneutrality but H^+ ions are generated or consumed by changes in water dissociation. Hence, in order to understand how the body regulates pH one need only ask how it regulates these three independent variables. Other approaches to acid–base physiology have ignored the distinction between independent and dependent variables, and while it is possible to describe an acid–base disorder in terms of H^+ or HCO_3^- concentrations or base excess, it is incorrect to analyse the pathology and potentially dangerous to plan treatment on the basis of altering these variables.

References

1 Severinghaus JW. More RipH. *JAMA* 1992; **267**: 2035–6.

2 Stewart PA. *How to Understand Acid–Base: A Quantitative Acid–Base Primer for Biology and Medicine*, 1st edn. New York: Elsevier, 1981.

3 Albert M, Dell R, Winters R. Quantitative displacement of acid–base equilibrium in metabolic acidosis. *Ann Intern Med* 1967; **66**: 312–5.

4 Figge J, Mydosh T, Fencl V. Serum proteins and acid–base equilibria: a follow-up. *J Lab Clin Med* 1992; **120**: 713–9.

5 Singer RB, Hastings AB. An improved clinical method for the estimation of disturbances of the acid–base balance of human blood. *Medicine (Baltimore)* 1948; **27**: 223–42.

6 Kellum JA, Bellomo R, Kramer DJ, Pinsky MR. Fixed acid uptake by visceral organs during early endotoxemia. *Adv Exp Med Biol* 1997; **411**: 275–9.

7 Kellum JA, Kramer DJ, Pinsky MR. Strong ion gap: a methodology for exploring unexplained anions. *J Crit Care* 1995; **10**: 51–5.

8 Gilfix BM, Bique M, Magder S. A physical chemical approach to the analysis of acid–base balance in the clinical setting. *J Crit Care* 1993; **8**: 187–97.

9 Mecher C, Rackow EC, Astiz ME, Weil MH. Unaccounted for anion in metabolic acidosis during severe sepsis in humans. *Crit Care Med* 1991; **19**: 705–11.

10 Kirschbaum B. Increased anion gap after liver transplantation. *Am J Med Sci* 1997; **313**: 107–10.

11 Kellum JA, Bellomo R, Kramer DJ, Pinsky MR. Hepatic anion flux during acute endotoxemia. *J Appl Physiol* 1995; **78**: 2212–7.

12 Bourke E, Haussinger D. pH homeostasis: the conceptual change. *Contrib Nephrol* 1992; **100**: 58–88.

13 Oliver J, Bourke E. Adaptations in urea and ammonium excretion in metabolic acidosis in the rat: a reinterpretation. *Clin Sci Mol Med* 1975; **48**: 515–20.

14 Atkinson DE, Bourke E. pH Homeostasis in terrestrial vertebrates: ammonium ion as a proton source. In: Heisler N, ed. *Comparative and Environmental Physiology. Mechanisms of Systemic Regulation, Acid–Base Regulation, Ion Transfer and Metabolism*. Berlin: Springer, 1995: 1–26.

15 Moore EW. The alkaline tide. *Gastroenterology* 1967; **52**: 1052–4.

16 Cushing H. Concerning the poisonous effect of pure sodium chloride solutions upon the nerve muscle preparation. *Am J Physiol* 1902; **6**: 77.

17 Shires GT, Tolman J. Dilutional acidosis. *Ann Intern Med* 1948; **28**: 557–9.

18 Kellum JA, Bellomo R, Kramer DJ, Pinsky MR. Aetiology of metabolic acidosis during saline resuscitation in endotoxemia. *Shock* 1998; **9**: 364–8.

19 Scheingraber S, Rehm M, Sehmisch C, Finsterer U. Rapid saline infusion produces hyperchloremic acidosis in patients undergoing gynecologic surgery. *Anesthesiology* 1999; **90**: 1265–70.

20 Waters JH, Bernstein CA. Dilutional acidosis following hetastarch or albumin in healthy volunteers. *Anesthesiology* 2000; **93**: 1184–7.

21 Morgan TJ, Venkatesh B, Hall J. Crystalloid strong ion difference determines metabolic acid–base change during *in vitro* hemodilution. *Crit Care Med* 2002; **30**: 157–60.

22 Waters JH, Miller LR, Clack S, Kim JV. Cause of metabolic acidosis in prolonged surgery. *Crit Care Med* 1999; **27**: 2142–6.

23 Fencl V, Jabor A, Kazda A, Figge J. Diagnosis of metabolic acid–base disturbances in critically ill patients. *Am J Respir Crit Care Med* 2000; **162**: 2246–51.

24 Finfer S, Bellomo R, Boyce N, *et al.* A comparison of albumin and saline for fluid resuscitation in the intensive care unit. *N Engl J Med* 2004; **350**: 2247–56.

25 Kellum JA. Recent advances in acid–base physiology applied to critical care. In: Vincent JL, ed. *Yearbook of Intensive Care and Emergency Medicine.* Heidelberg: Springer-Verlag, 1998: 579–87.

26 Wilkes P. Hypoproteinemia, SID, and acid–base status in critically ill patients. *J Appl Physiol* 1998; **84:** 1740–8.

27 Kellum JA. Determinants of blood pH in health and disease. *Crit Care* 2000; **4:** 6–14.

28 Balasubramanyan N, Havens PL, Hoffman GM. Unmeasured anions identified by the Fencl–Stewart method predict mortality better than base excess, anion gap, and lactate in patients in the pediatric intensive care unit. *Crit Care Med* 1999; **27:** 1577–81.

29 Kaplan L, Kellum JA. Initial pH, base deficit, lactate, anion gap, strong ion difference, and strong ion gap predict outcome from major vascular injury. *Crit Care Med* 2004; **32:** 1120–4.

30 Moviat M, van Haren F, van der Hoeven H. Conventional or physicochemical approach in intensive care unit patients with metabolic acidosis. *Crit Care* 2003; **7:** R41–5.

31 Cusack RJ, Rhodes A, Lochhead P, *et al.* The strong ion gap does not have prognostic value in critically ill patients in a mixed medical/surgical adult ICU. *Intensive Care Med* 2002; **28:** 864–9.

32 Rocktaschel J, Morimatsu H, Uchino S, Bellomo R. Unmeasured anions in critically ill patients: can they predict mortality? *Crit Care Med* 2003; **31:** 2131–6.

33 Gunnerson KJ, Roberts G, Kellum JA. What is normal strong ion gap (SIG) in healthy subjects and critically ill patients without acid–base abnormalities. *Crit Care Med* 2003; **31**(Suppl): A111.

34 Dondorp AM, Chau TT, Phu NH, *et al.* Unidentified acids of strong prognostic significance in severe malaria. *Crit Care Med* 2004; **32:** 1683–8.

35 Rocktaschel J, Morimatsu H, Uchino S, *et al.* Acid–base status of critically ill patients with acute renal failure: analysis based on Stewart–Figge methodology. *Crit Care* 2003; **7:** R60–6.

36 Wang H, Bloom O, Zhang M, *et al.* HMG-1 as a late mediator of endotoxin lethality in mice. *Science* 1999; **285:** 248–51.

37 Gunnerson KJ, Saul M, Kellum JA. Lactic versus non-lactate metabolic acidosis: a retrospective outcome evaluation of critically ill patients. *Crit Care* 2006; **10:** R22–7.

38 Kellum JA, Song M, Li J. Lactic, and hydrochloric acids induce different patterns of inflammatory response in LPS-stimulated RAW 264.7 cells. *Am J Physiol Regul Integr Comp Phsyiol* 2004; **286:** R686–92.

39 Kellum JA, Song M, Venkataraman R. Effects of hyperchloremic acidosis on arterial pressure and circulating inflammatory molecules in experimental sepsis. *Chest* 2004; **125:** 243–8.

40 Kellum JA, Bellomo R, Kramer DJ, Pinsky MR. Splanchnic buffering of metabolic acid during early endotoxemia. *J Crit Care* 1997; **12:** 7–12.

CHAPTER 15
Fluids and electrolytes

Martin Kuper and Neil Soni

History

Although the importance of fluids was acknowledged in the ancient world we have only recently had the ability to give fluids other than by the oral route. From an historical perspective the obvious fluid to give patients was blood and this was first attempted by Jean Baptiste Denis in 1667, who used lamb's blood to good effect initially although the next two patients died. Until recently, a common adage was 'if they have lost blood, give blood' and there is still interest in blood from sources other than humans. Human blood was first used successfully at St Thomas' Hospital, London in 1818 and was being used increasingly by the end of the 19th century.

There was growing interest in other fluids, with saline being tried in 1891 and other fluids such as Hartmann's following. Other aspects of the use of fluids developed concurrently and while haemodynamics were the domain of the physiologist, others were interested in maintaining haemodynamic stability. There was no equipment for giving fluids and improvization and innovation of administration methods were probably as important as the attempts to produce fluids and helped translate their use from the laboratory to the hospital. The advent of the First World War contributed significantly. The first plasma substitutes appeared in 1919 and were produced from gum acacia. The Second World War boosted the development of plasma substitutes. Initially polvinyl pyrrolidone (in the 1940s) and later an ever-increasing range of new colloids such as gelatins, dextrans and starches were produced, although human plasma remains important even today. More recently, new crystalloids such as hypertonic saline are being investigated.

Physiology

Physiology is the foundation of fluid management and for mammals this essentially comprises the maintenance of a fluid milieu in a fluid-deprived environment. Under normal temperate circumstances, an average adult might require in the order of 2.5 L fluid per day. Although largely taken as food and drink, there is also a contribution from metabolism. The actual amount required is determined by the quantity lost in urine, faeces and sweat. In pathological circumstances, losses depend on the disease and include everything from sweat to bowel losses or just bleeding. In these circumstances, the ability to maintain homoeostasis may be challenged and support is often necessary. In general terms, fluid management is based on seeking to maintain equilibrium by determining the ongoing requirements, with the addition of any untoward losses. This applies to both the intra- and extracellular spaces although it is the extravascular space that we can measure and manipulate. It is also this space, including the circulation, that is important in the distribution of substrates such as oxygen on which organ function depends.

Equilibrium can be considered in terms of normovolaemia. Although this baseline is hard to determine, it may be considered clinically as when the patient is haemodynamically stable as indicated by a normal (for them) blood pressure and a normal pulse rate, well perfused, with the adequacy of perfusion confirmed by clear indications of organ function such as urine output, cerebration or other endpoints. Homoeostasis is a dynamic process. In a single day in a 70 kg man, glomerular filtration is in the order of 200 L, carrying up to 30 000 mmol sodium. In the gut, over 10 L fluid and 1500 mmol sodium are secreted. Of this, 99% is reabsorbed and the fluid and sodium balances are kept within very tight constraints.

When things go wrong it becomes obvious reasonably rapidly, despite robust compensatory mechanisms for fluid deprivation or loss. With rapid fluid loss from the intravascular compartment, haemodynamic stability is maintained by compensatory means until 15–25% loss of intravascular volume, after which decompensation occurs with obvious alterations in haemodynamics and then organ function. The critical quantity of blood or fluid loss is determined by many factors in each individual but the ability of young mammals to compensate is always impressive. These mechanisms are far less impressive in the elderly or infirm.

The clinical signs of dehydration are more insidious with slower onset. They reflect total body losses despite fully employed compensatory mechanisms. Signs appear at 6% loss and 10% constitutes severe dehydration.

It is important to put fluid and electrolyte management into context. The human body, even when damaged, is an immensely complex but also robust and resilient 'machine'. The protective mechanisms that conserve fluid and electrolyte balance have evolved in mammals over the millennia and are sophisticated and relatively precise. In contrast, our best efforts are rather crude and unsophisticated. Fortunately, if we provide the basic components, the innate physiology usually effectively deals with the finer detail. The guiding principle in interacting with human physiology should therefore be 'keep it simple, keep it safe'.

A rule of thumb

The hourly 'maintenance' water requirement may be estimated as:

4 mL/kg for the first 10 kg, plus 2 mL/kg for the next 10 kg, plus 1 mL/kg for each subsequent kg of body weight

The predicted daily requirement for a 75-kg man is therefore:

$(10 \times 4\,mL) + (10 \times 2\,mL) + (55 \times 1\,mL) = 85\,mL/$ hour $= 2040\,mL/day$

Electrolytes

The specific composition of bodily fluids is of importance because cells require the correct milieu for their metabolic electrophysiological functions. Of necessity, this chapter does not cover the raison d'etre of the electrolyte components of compartments, which is available in any physiology text, but looks at the situation from the viewpoint of fluid management.

Sodium

Total body sodium is in the order of 3000 mmol in a 70-kg man, with a reasonably high daily turnover, so that a normal requirement in an adult is in the order of 100 mmol/day (1–1.5 mmol/kg). Serum sodium is usually around 140 mmol/L in the plasma compartment, with a similar value in the interstitial space, but a much lower intracellular concentration, where potassium is the dominant ion.

Consider the body as three compartments: the intravascular, interstitial and intracellular compartments (Fig. 15.1). Sodium is predominantly distributed across the intravascular and interstitial compartments and is in dynamic equilibrium between these compartments. The concentrations are not identical, but are essentially very similar. Distribution across the 'compartment barriers', which are permeable to sodium, results in equilibrium. As these compartments constitute the main location of sodium, the plasma sodium provides a reasonable indicator of total body sodium when taken in context with hydration. Sodium and fluid are linked closely and so are the control mechanisms. Control is mediated via both volume and osmoreceptors. Reduction in volume or in osmotic pressure result in sodium and water retention. Both high and low sodium concentrations occur in pathological states and are clinically relevant.

Potassium

A 70 kg man has approximately 3200 mmol potassium with a turnover of 40–120 mmol/day. The serum value is in the range 3.5–5 mmol/L. The majority of potassium is intracellular and varies in concentration between cells from 135 to 150 mmol/L. Only 2% of all potassium is in the intravascular compartment.

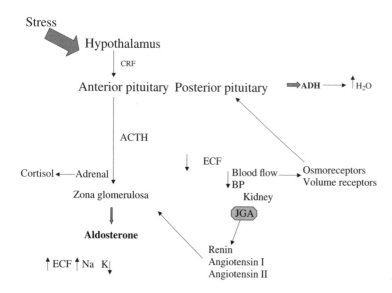

Figure 15.1 Diagram of the three-compartment model. ACTH, adrenocorticotrophic hormone; ADH, antidiuretic hormone; CRF, corticotrophin releasing factor; ECF, extracellular fluid; JGA, juxtaglomerular apparatus.

Unlike sodium, serum potassium represents only a tiny fraction of body potassium and is not necessarily representative of total body potassium. Potassium loss occurs from the gastrointestinal tract and in the urine. The quantity lost with diarrhoea can be very large. Efforts to conserve potassium may then result in hydrogen ion loss in preference to potassium, which can produce alkalosis. This may provide some indication of the degree of potassium depletion.

Chloride

Nature requires electrochemical neutrality and so anions are also important. Chloride will be retained by the kidneys if the bicarbonate is unusually low and reabsorbed sodium cannot be balanced by other anions such as phosphate, urate or acetoacetate. This produces hyperchloraemic acidosis, because chloride, unlike bicarbonate or phosphate, is unable to act as a buffer as it cannot accept hydrogen ions at physiological pH. This occurs in renal tubular acidosis and following transplantation of the ureters into the colon. Iatrogenic causes include carbonic anhydrase inhibition and the administration of large quantities of chloride as saline. The excess chloride is a strong ion and in excess, therefore, generates an acidosis. This is because the chloride ion seeks a cation to provide electrochemical neutrality. Chloride depletion occurs when chloride is lost without sodium (e.g. in pyloric stenosis). Normally, renal sodium is reabsorbed with chloride, but if chloride is absent then more bicarbonate is reabsorbed, producing an acid urine and a metabolic alkalosis. This illustrates that the anions and cations are closely interrelated with acid–base balance.

The response to injury

Significant stress, whether surgery trauma or infection, results in a predictable series of physiological responses that are protective in nature. Teleologically, these aim to conserve fluid and to maintain homoeostasis. There is increased secretion of adrenocortical hormones and, in particular, of antidiuretic hormone. The result is salt and water retention, which may last for several days after the event. The sodium conservation may increase potassium loss, which is often maximal at 24 hours but may be sustained. In the immediate postoperative or post-injury phase, these physiological responses should be considered when assessing the choice of fluid replacement as indeed should any ongoing losses (Table 15.1).

Distribution of fluids

The easiest way to look at fluid management is by using the three-compartment model whereby the body is simplistically divided into the intracellular,

Table 15.1 Electrolyte content of some body fluids.

	Na (mmol/L)	K (mmol/L)	Cl (mmol/L)
Stomach	60	9	84
Small intestine	111	4	104
Bile	148	5	100
Pancreatic juice	140	5	76
Ileostomy new	130	11	116
Ileostomy est.	46	3	21
Caecostomy	52	8	42

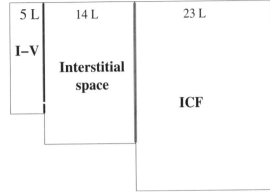

Figure 15.2 Simplified stress response. Salt and water conservation. ICF, intracellular fluid; IV, intravenous.

interstitial and intravascular compartments. Simple rules can be applied to the behaviour of these compartments which eases understanding. Like all models, its limitations need to be understood; this is a very limited model in various pathophysiological states, nevertheless it is a good starting point (Fig. 15.2).

1 Water constitutes 60–70% of total bodyweight and is distributed through all three compartments: the intravascular, extracellular and intracellular spaces.

2 Sodium distributes across the intravascular and interstitial spaces.

The intravascular space is small, accessible and is characterized by a high sodium and low potassium concentration. It equilibrates with the interstitial space, which has similar composition because both sodium and water can move freely. Other molecules also equilibrate, although there is resistance to the movement of larger molecules, and very large molecules and cells are retained in the intravascular space. The interstitial space is drained by lymphatics and can be considered an extension of the intravascular compartment.

In contrast to these two spaces, the intracellular compartment is protected by a cell membrane. Only water and dissolved gases such as oxygen can move freely across this membrane. Neither sodium nor potassium can move across this membrane easily with-

out using channels. Other ions such as calcium and magnesium are also limited in movement. Most larger molecules can only move into or out of the cell by active transport processes.

The interior of the cell has a large concentration of potassium and low sodium. The distribution of these ions, an active energy requiring process, results in a membrane potential and provides the electrophysiological properties of the cell. So, in simple terms sodium and water can move between interstitial and intravascular spaces while only water can move freely across all three compartments.

The concept of equilibration determines the amount of movement and the driving forces are predictable. Hydrostatic and osmotic gradients work across all three compartments to some degree. Oncotic pressure, largely determined by the pressure invoked by large immobile molecules, is seen to act between intravascular and interstitial spaces but its role at a cellular level is uncertain. Clearly, an active synthetic cell may well develop oncotic gradients and may influence water movement, but this is conjecture and is neither measurable nor can it be manipulated. Electrochemical gradients may also influence movement.

Other factors affecting movement are molecular shape, molecular charge and active transport mechanisms. The main determinants of movement are the pressure gradients whether hydrostatic, osmotic, oncotic or electrochemical, but it is helpful to appreciate that it is the gradient and not the absolute pressure that is important.

To illustrate this latter point let us consider a capillary. The hydrostatic pressure in the capillary will tends to drive fluid out into the low pressure interstitium. As fluid moves out, the concentration of molecules in the capillary will increase and this generates an oncotic gradient, pulling fluid back. Simultaneously, lymph drainage will reduce the hydrostatic pressure in the interstitium which otherwise would begin to impede movement as the gradient would decrease. Starling's equations relating to the movement of fluids and electrolytes in the capillary describes this very well (Fig. 15.3).

This is also a good example of how models need to be limited. The oncotic gradient eloquently described in Starling's equation depends on the integrity of the endothelial barrier. In normal circumstances this is accurately described in the equation, but in pathophysiological situations the 'integrity of the membrane' may fail (this is otherwise called permeability, but the exact nature of this change is unknown). When it fails, larger molecules can try to equilibrate as well by moving into the interstitium. Initially, their plasma concentration will fall, as will the gradient but, as the molecules disperse in the interstitium and are also diluted by the fluid they oncotically drag with them, a new gradient may establish itself which may be very similar to the old. The plasma concentration will be lower, but the gradient is not necessarily altered. Knowledge of the concentration of a protein on one side of the membrane will not necessarily inform on the gradient. This demonstrates a major flaw in extrapolating the model too far.

The mechanism by which fluid crosses the endothelium is also ill defined. Active transport that is driven by the Na/K pumps may be involved. Observations in animals, and in humans, show that there is active clearance of liquid from the alveoli across the alveolar membrane [1–5]. Failure of this mechanism would significantly influence the balance of forces in the Starling equation. It raises issues about the role of such mechanisms in the formation of pulmonary oedema, and of the role of hypoxia.

Fluid distribution

The only space we can measure and have access to is the intravascular compartment. Measurements can be made in a wide range of ways and then fluids can be given into that compartment and the effects on that space can be measured.

The interstitial space can be assessed clinically but not numerically, although some new devices such as PiCCO® (Pulsion, Munich, DE) suggest that some measure of extravascular lung water can be made. These tend to be indirect measurements and do require some assumptions. Clinically, loss of tissue turgor, or alternatively oedema, can be assessed.

The intracellular compartment is a mystery as it cannot be measured and even clinical assessment is

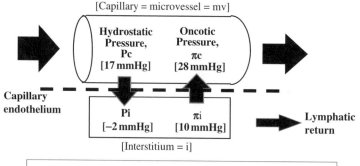

Figure 15.3 Schema of the Starling–Landis equation. This is a capillary with blood flowing through. Pc, hydrostatic pressure in the capillary; πc, the oncotic pressure in the capillary; Pi, the hydrostatic pressure in the interstitium; πi, interstitial oncotic pressure; Jv, net flux; Kfc, filtration coefficient; σ reflection coefficient (measure of permeability to proteins or large molecules — when it is 0 it is completely permeable).

Net fluid flux, $Jv = Kfc$. Net filtration pressure

$$Jv = Kfc\,[(Pc - Pi) - \sigma\,(\pi c - \pi i)]$$

difficult. This should be remembered when there is discussion about repleting the intracellular space.

Crystalloids

It is helpful to define common terms. Crystalloid, in colloidal chemistry, is an ionic or molecular substance with some or all the properties of a crystal, or a substance such as salt or sugar. In clinical practice this is loosely used to describe fluids that contain sugars or salts. Osmosis is the movement of water by diffusion from a region of high water concentration (low solute concentration) to low water concentration (high solute concentration). Molality is the number of particles dissolved in a mass of fluid (mmol/kg). Osmolality is usually expressed in terms of mOsm/kg. Molarity is the number of particles of a particular substance in a volume of fluid (e.g. mmol/L). Osmolarity depends on the number of osmotically active particles in a volume of solution and is expressed as mOsm/L.

The osmolarity of plasma is given approximately by the formula:

Osmolarity = 2 ([Na] + [K]) + [urea]
  + [glucose] mmol/L

The plasma osmolarity is normally 280–290 mOsm/L. The osmolar gap is the difference between measured and calculated osmolarity and is usually less than 10 mOsm/L.

There are two main considerations:

1 Salt solutions will equilibrate across the intravascular and interstitial compartments with distribution proportional to the volume of each compartment.

2 Water will distribute across all three compartments again proportional to the volume of each compartment.

For example, if 1 L half normal saline is added to 1 L saline the total volume will be 2 L but the concentration will have fallen to 0.75 normal saline. The 1 L half normal saline could be considered as 500 mL normal saline and 500 mL water (sometimes termed free water). The 2 L would consist of 1.5 L saline and 500 mL water. This simple concept allows identification of 'free water' (i.e. water that is not committed to sodium).

This concept aids working out fluid distribution. Administered fluid consists of the quantity that is iso-osmotic with the intravascular compartment and which will distribute through the extracellular space (intravascular and interstitial) and the free water which will distribute to extra- and intracellular spaces (i.e. all three compartments).

We can use these concepts to predict the behaviour of any solution, provided we know its composition. If we assume that normal saline is iso-osmotic, it has the same ionic concentration as the plasma and it will freely and quite rapidly distribute across the intravascular and interstitial spaces, which will behave as one space. If the intravascular space is 5 L and the interstitial space is 10 L then after 20 minutes or so, approximately 33% of the administered fluid will be intravascular and 66% will be interstitial. Proteins and other osmotically and oncotically active molecules will alter the distribution to a minor extent, but the predominant distribution will be in proportion to the size of the two spaces.

One litre of 5% dextrose is isotonic. Unlike salt, glucose is taken up by cells and metabolized, leaving 'free water'. Therefore dextrose solutions can be considered as free water in terms of distribution — unless they have added salt — because after administration the glucose will be metabolized and the remainder is water. This can freely cross all barriers and will distribute to all three spaces according to the relative volume of each space. If the intravascular volume is 5 L, interstitial 10 L and intracellular 15 L, the fluid will distribute in the ratio 5 : 10 : 15. The litre of fluid will split: 17% will remain intravascular, 33% interstitial and 50% intracellular.

Dextrose saline (4% dextrose and 1/5 normal saline) provides a means of illustrating this concept. In a litre bottle there is 1/5 L normal saline and 4/5 L water. The saline will distribute to the intravascular and interstitial spaces, the water to all three spaces.

This again is a simple model but it can be applied in practice to a limited degree. If intravascular filling is required, then any fluid will instantaneously fill the space, but its distribution will determine how long it stays there. Iso-osmotic salt-based fluid is more efficient than dextrose, which rapidly becomes water and therefore hypotonic. Conversely, if a patient is dehydrated and water-depleted then a solution that gets to all spaces is better, although on a practical level intravascular repletion should take precedence.

Put simply, a salt solution tends to fill the intravascular and interstitial space dependent on its tonicity. Dextrose solutions approximate rapidly to water and can be used to fill all spaces including the intracellular space.

It is important to remember that this is a model and that the ability to genuinely put fluid where it is required is very limited. This model tends to be thought of as a static model while it is clear in theory and in practice it is dynamic. If crystalloids are ad-

ministered rapidly, as occurs in resuscitation, the following phases could occur in the lungs (Fig. 15.4) [a–c].

1 The crystalloid will instantaneously dilute the intravascular compartment and reduce the oncotic pressure while increasing the hydrostatic pressure. This reduces the oncotic pressure holding the fluid in the compartment, while increasing the hydrostatic pressure tending to push the fluid out.

2 As the fluid distributes out into the interstitium it dilutes the interstitium, reducing the interstitial oncotic pressure and increasing the hydrostatic

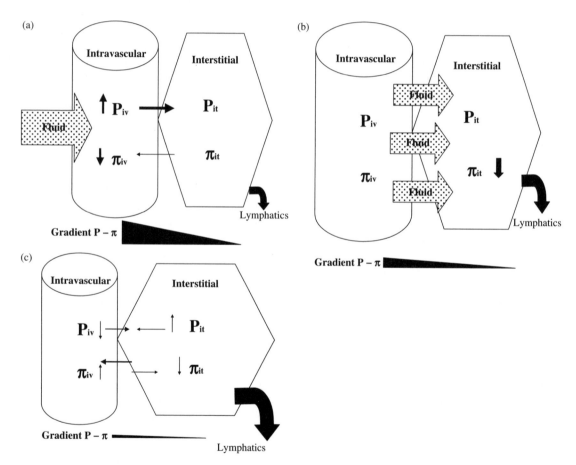

Figure 15.4 (a) Giving intravascular fluid increases intravascular pressure (Piv) and reduces intravascular oncotic pressure πiv. There is increased hydrostatic gradient and reduced oncotic gradient. P–π increases fluid moves into the interstitium. (b) Fluid moves out of the intravascular space. Interstitial hydrostatic pressure Pit rises, interstitial oncotic pressure πit falls. The resultant gradient is P–π. (c) As fluid moves out the Piv falls, πiv rises while Pit is increased and πit is still low. The gradient P–π is very low and fluid flux falls. Lymphatic flow, from the raised interstitial pressures, rises.

pressure in the interstitium. This will begin to resist further fluid inflow.

3 Simultaneously, the fluid leaving the intravascular space will tend to increase the intravascular oncotic pressure, and as fluid leaves the intravascular hydrostatic pressure will tend to fall. There is less force moving fluid out and equilibration occurs.

4 Even as this is happening, excessive fluid accumulation in the interstitium is prevented by alterations in lymph flow draining that compartment (flow can increase 10-fold).

Colloids and distribution

The discussion has focused on fluids with small molecules that can readily move out of the intravascular space. If the molecules are large they may be impeded in their movement. In normal plasma, the plasma proteins are the major colloids. The plasma protein concentration is approximately 0.9 mOsm/L which would give a predicted oncotic pressure of $0.9 \times 19.3\,\text{mmHg} = 17.4\,\text{mmHg}$. The actual plasma oncotic pressure measured with a colloid osmometer is usually higher, at approximately 25 mmHg, for two main reasons:

1 The negative charge of plasma proteins cause retention of positively charged sodium ions in the plasma, a Gibbs–Donnan equilibrium that increases the plasma osmolality.

2 Plasma proteins occupy significant volume, which is lost from the calculation introducing a significant error.

In a simple physical system with a known pore size it would be possible to predict which molecules would be unable to move. Reality is different. Size is a constraint on movement but this may vary between organs and certainly in different disease states. This will be considered again later. Nevertheless, the simple model of a fisherman's net with a known mesh size assumes that molecules of a certain size cannot move out of the intravascular space. Colloids are of a certain size and are less likely to move out. The larger the molecule the longer it will remain in the intravascular compartment. In situations where there is acute blood loss and the intention is to keep the circulating volume adequate for perfusion to occur, a fluid that stays in that space has obvious benefits. In theory, less will be required and it will not fill up the interstitial space.

Unfortunately, the model is not particularly good [6]. Colloids do move and the classic example is albumin. Albumin is able to move between the intravascular and interstitial space at a reasonable rate and indeed there is a reasonably large turnover on a daily basis. This is not surprising as the intravascular volume is, above all else, a transport system and the substrates it carries and the immunological defences such as white cells need to be able to get to the site of action, which may be the interstitium or even the cell itself. The mechanisms by which large molecules move are unclear. Certainly gaps or pores between endothelial cells may be a mechanism that alters in some conditions, while active transport may also be important (Fig. 15.5). Factors that are involved in the likelihood of movement include molecular size, shape, polarity, charge and disease states (there may be radically increased efflux of colloids in illness such as fulminant sepsis). However, it is true to say that colloids do tend to remain in the intravascular compartment longer than crystalloids.

A secondary problem that should be considered is what happens to these molecules once they are in the interstitium. Salt solutions are readily drained by the lymphatics and are passed back into the circulation and then excreted. Similarly, the gelatins probably find their way back into the circulation via the lymphatics and hence are passed in the urine. Molecules such as the starches may be taken up and trapped by the reticuloendothelial system or some

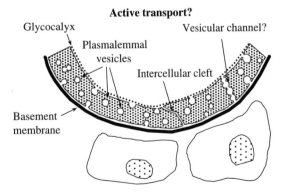

Figure 15.5 Some structures in a capillary wall. Where is the leak?

may be metabolized. The rate of clearance of these molecules may be slow. There has been discussion as to the clinical implications of retained colloids in the interstitium. In particular, there has been debate about whether late lung injury could be in part due to trapped colloid in the lung interstitium. To date this is purely conjecture.

In conclusion, colloids usually stay in the intravascular compartment longer and this is in part molecular size dependent. They are a more efficient way of filling the intravascular space and therefore result in less fluid administration and usually less clinical evidence of interstitial oedema. Whether this is clinically beneficial remains a source of contention. Furthermore, the model that colloids are trapped in the intravascular compartment is a useful idea, but needs considerable modification in practice. In severe sepsis, when everything is leaking, it is likely that even with colloids, the intravascular and interstitial space act effectively as one compartment, with relatively free fluid distribution from one to the other. The body then behaves as a two- rather than three-compartment model (Fig. 15.6).

The concept of 'leak'

In the critically ill it is readily observed that large amounts of fluid may be needed to sustain the circulation and that with time the patient appears oedematous. This is because of distribution of fluid and

expansion of the interstitial space. Several mechanisms are involved. The increase in fluid movement out of the intravascular space is called 'leak' and is caused by changes in 'permeability' (Fig. 15.5). Again, this is an easy concept that belies the actual mechanisms. The endothelial layer becomes permeable but the exact mechanism is unclear. It could be pore size, gaps between cells, membrane changes or other mechanisms, but the term permeability is useful to cover all possibilities, while the real nature of the leak is unknown. It is also likely that the efficacy of lymphatic drainage may play a part so that it may be partly drainage failure that makes the leak appear larger than it is.

Hypertonic solutions

There is resurgent interest in the use of hypertonic solutions. Using the same model this involves administering a hypertonic solution into the intravascular volume. This draws fluid from the interstitium and from the cells. The extra fluid is therefore endogenously derived. It is a short-term measure that appears to work. It cannot be used repeatedly as there are limited fluid reserves; it introduces a massive salt and hypertonic load that must be removed eventually. The advantage is reduced fluid administration and various niches are being sought for its application.

Fluid administration — therapeutics

Fluids are used in two main therapeutic manoeuvres.

Maintenance of normal homoeostasis and replacement of fluids that will replenish daily requirements of water and electrolytes

To do this, an assessment needs to be made of daily requirements to which is added measured or estimated losses. This includes situations where there are large losses from disease states such as diarrhoea or vomiting. An assessment should be made of the normal requirements to which any other losses are added. Due consideration should be made of the types of losses. Upper gastrointestinal losses may be rich in electrolytes and both the volume and content

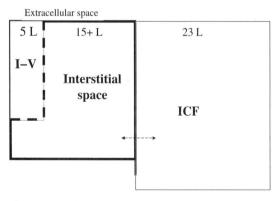

Figure 15.6 The two-compartment model. In leaky state, the intravascular and interstitial space act as a single compartment so fluid put intravascularly equilibrates rapidly. This expands the interstitial space which will increase in size, hence 15 + L. ICF, intracellular fluid.

need to be considered. In some conditions such as in diabetes insipidus or glycosuria, large volumes of water are lost and will need replacement.

Maintenance and replacement of losses can be easily managed with standard electrolyte solutions. The human body is extremely sophisticated and can usually fine-tune the distribution of fluids and electrolytes appropriately, provided approximately the correct amounts are being provided. Most situations can be managed using normal saline to provide salt and water and with dextrose solutions to provide 'free water'. Normal saline has more sodium than plasma and may be slightly hypertonic. It also provides an unnaturally large chloride load. Hence there is a tendency to use more balanced solutions such as Hartmann's or Ringer's lactate.

Care must be taken that the dextrose is being absorbed. In a diabetic patient, the dextrose could result in hyperglycaemia and this would produce an osmotic diuresis where more water would be lost. Dextrose may still be given but there should be adequate glucose control.

In most situations, extra potassium may be needed to supplement any requirements. Management of fluids mandates the needs to monitor the patient. Clinically, signs of dehydration such as thirst, altered haemodynamics and passing urine are helpful. This should be supplemented with electrolyte measurement and correction of any deficits. The frequency of monitoring should be dictated by the stability of the patient. In normal life outside of hospital most people avoid dehydration and overhydration using their intrinsic homoeostasis without even being aware of it. Usually, most of these mechanisms are still working in the conscious sick and should not be ignored. Thirst is the classic symptom that has an important message. Clearly, in the unconscious it is more difficult but other homoeostatic mechanisms will still be functioning.

Bedside monitoring involves regular clinical assessment. The haemodynamic state including peripheral perfusion pulse and blood pressure give an indication of the intravascular space. Assessment of peripheral oedema and pulmonary oedema give an idea of the state of the interstitium. The intracellular space is only accessible in severe dehydration where the loss of all interstitial fluid and tissue turgor imply depletion. Peripheral oedema alone does not indicate the state of the intravascular compartment but is a feature of sequestration.

Fluid balance charts are helpful and should list all input and output. Again this needs to be assessed in the context of the clinical situation. For routine ward management the chart should indicate not only unusual losses, but also the cumulative total of fluid input, which with antibiotics and other fluids may be far greater than expected. Invisible and unrecorded volumes, such as sweat or faeces, should be routinely assessed and can indicate fluid accumulation. In maintaining homoeostasis the message is 'keep it simple, keep it safe'.

Resuscitation: rapid re-establishment of an adequate circulating intravascular volume

When there is a significant loss of circulating blood volume, the intravascular volume may become inadequate to deliver substrates, especially oxygen, to the tissues, despite the best efforts of compensatory mechanisms. This may be a 20% fluid loss but it will depend on speed of loss, compensation and the general health of the patient. Physiological mechanisms will compensate for this fluid loss by:

1 Vasoconstriction, which effectively reduces the capacitance of the system and diverts any available intravascular volume to critical sites

2 Increased cardiac output to utilize the available delivery fluid more effectively

3 Distribution of fluid from other compartments into the intravascular space

4 Acidosis developing from tissue hypoxia shifts the Bohr equation and helps oxygen delivery to critical areas.

Two main principles should be employed: stop the fluid loss if possible and restore a functioning circulation as rapidly as possible.

It is mandatory that vital organs are adequately perfused. The fluid used is immaterial initially as anything is better than nothing. In more ideal circumstances, the choice may be either crystalloid or colloid and both have their proponents. If there is blood loss to the point at which oxygen carriage is threatened or where it is likely the situation is ongoing and therefore oxygen delivery will be threatened, then blood may need to be given. Transfusion thresholds are now much lower but need to take account of the circumstances, the comorbidity of the patient and the degree of control of the bleeding that exists. A margin of safety should be present if possible. Some authorities suggest a haemoglobin concentration of 7 g/dL is reasonable but in real life with active bleeding it is sensible to have a slightly higher threshold. If blood is not necessary then the choice of fluids becomes contentious. Any fluid will do in a crisis but where choice is involved it becomes difficult. The choice is crystalloid or colloid and having decided which to use, then which crystalloid or which colloid.

Crystalloids will achieve the goal and most authorities recommend starting with crystalloid. Saline, Hartmann's and Ringer's lactate are all preferable to the dextrose solutions (see above). When compared with colloid it is clear that crystalloids distribute more rapidly and so the benefit is not sustained and more fluid has to be given [7]. The volume of crystalloid may be up to five times the volume of blood lost. There is debate as to whether crystalloid is better or worse for microvascular perfusion [8–10]. The entire subject is confused by apparently paradoxical data such as the observation that while more extravascular lung water and more tissue oedema are found using crystalloid, no alteration in systemic or regional (i.e. mesenteric) oxygen uptake or greater ileal tissue acidosis are seen [11].

Dextrose solutions are poor for resuscitation as they distribute so rapidly and so are relatively ineffective unless very large volumes are used [12]. They also provide a potentially problematic glucose load and excessive volumes of free water in a patient who will retain both salt and water. The situation then prevails where hyponatraemia and osmotic dysequilibrium are likely. This can be used to illustrate a common iatrogenic problem. In the management of the postoperative elderly patient, fear of cardiac failure leads to avoidance of salt and therefore the irrational use of dextrose or dextrose saline, which is in effect, water. The operative stress response appropriately retains the fluid but as it is water, hyponatraemia ensues [13]. The stress response is appropriate but the iatrogenic water administration is not. The condition of inappropriate antidiuretic hormone se-

cretion presents similarly but without the entirely appropriate stress response [14–17].

In theory, colloids stay in the intravascular space and sustain intravascular volume. As there is no distribution, less fluid is needed and less ends up in the interstitium. Certainly, in volunteers and in most non-pathological situations such as minor and intermediate surgery, most colloids have a pronounced and sustained effect on the intravascular space. In situations where there is a significant inflammatory response such as trauma, major surgery and sepsis, there appears to be increased 'permeability' as seen by more rapid egress of the molecules from the intravascular space [18]. A less well-sustained clinical effect is seen.

Despite this reduction in efficacy under these circumstances, some clinicians prefer using colloids for resuscitation. Controversy has been intense for over three decades, with little hard evidence to show either benefit or detriment for either. This lends considerable weight to the argument that personal choice dictates what is used. There is intrinsic safety in routine and so changing practice for no clear reason may be hazardous. The Cochrane collaboration raised the spectre of danger in using colloids and in particular albumin. The safety issue has been refuted by the SAFE study that showed no mortality difference between albumin and saline in the critically ill [19–22]. The real outcome from both the Cochrane and the SAFE study was a clear demonstration on how little genuinely useful information is available on the relative merits of these commonly used therapies.

Given these basic principles, it should be possible to decide which fluids to use when their individual properties are known (Table 15.2).

Fluids available

Although fluids are often classified as either crystalloids or colloids, a more functional classification is:

1 *Isotonic crystalloids:* these distribute through the extracellular fluid

2 *Hypertonic crystalloids and colloids:* these distribute initially through the intravascular space only

3 *Dextrose solutions:* after metabolism of dextrose these solutions become hypotonic (i.e. water), and

Table 15.2 The composition of some standard intravenous fluids.

	Na (mmol/L)	K (mmol/L)	Cl (mmol/L)	Lactate (mmol/L)	Glucose (g/L)	Osmolality (mOsm/kg)
Hartmann's	130	4	110	28	–	275
Ringers lactate	131	4–5	109	28	–	273
5% Dextrose	–	–	–	–	50	252
Dextrose saline	31	–	31	–	40	262
Normal saline	153	0	153	0	–	306
Compare with extracellular fluid	140	5	103	<1		275–295

distribute through the intravascular interstitial and intracellular spaces.

Isotonic crystalloids

The isotonic crystalloids contain sodium in similar concentration to the extracellular fluid. 'Maintenance' fluid must meet daily requirements of both electrolytes and water. Stress such as surgery, infection, hypovolaemia and pain elicits an *appropriate* antidiuretic hormone (ADH) response. There is retention of water over and above sodium. Salt and water is better than water alone.

Normal saline 0.9% NaCl
Constitution: Na$^+$ 154 mmol/L, Cl$^-$ 154 mmol/L; calculated osmolality 300 mOsm/L as a result of incomplete dissociation of sodium and chloride ions.

Distribution: Peak plasma volume expansion of approximately 20% of administered volume in healthy volunteers.

Advantages: No anaphylactoid reactions. Volume effect is sustained at 6 hours compared with Hartmann's solution. Cheap [23].

Disadvantages: Distribution means that larger volumes given to sustain intravascular volume will potentially result in more interstitial fluid and more

oedema. Large volumes of saline can cause metabolic acidosis because of the accumulation of the strong anion chloride [24–27]. Whether this arises from the strong ion effect of hyperchloraemia or due to dilution of bicarbonate is debated [28]. It is uncertain as to whether there are clinical consequences. Rapid haemodilution by 20–30% causes a procoagulant state through unclear mechanisms [29,30].

Role: Still the mainstay of intravenous fluid administration. Although recent research has emphasized that normal saline is not 'normal' because it is hypertonic and hyperchloraemic compared with plasma, the clinical significance is disputed.

Balanced salt solutions
Constitution: Hartmann's solution Na$^+$ 131 mmol/L, K$^+$ 5 mmol/L, Ca^{2+} 2 mmol/L, Cl$^-$ 111 mmol/L, lactate 29 mmol/L. Calculated osmolality 276 mOsm/kg.

Distribution: Similar to saline, marginally less osmotically active particles and hence distributes faster [23–31]. Following rapid administration, half of the increase of plasma volume is gone by 6 hours in healthy volunteers. This poor intravascular retention of Hartmann's solution compared with normal saline may be because of mild hypotonicity causing inhibition of ADH secretion [32,33].

Metabolism: Lactate is metabolized. It is converted to pyruvate and further metabolized, either to glucose (gluconeogenesis), mainly in the liver but also in the kidneys, or through the Kreb's cycle to carbon dioxide and water (oxidation), which also occurs in cardiac and skeletal muscle. One litre provides 9 kcal. Both routes consume hydrogen ions so tend to cause alkalinization.

Advantages: No anaphylactoid reactions. Alkalinization tends to counter the mild metabolic acidosis that commonly occurs in illness. It is lower in chloride and avoids hyperchloraemic metabolic acidosis.

Disadvantages: Hartmann's solution has a dilutional procoagulant effect like normal saline. The tendency to alkalinize will be lost if lactate metabolism is impaired (e.g. in sepsis). In Hartmann's solution the amount of lactate is relatively small. The presence of lactate has been of considerable interest in the use of lactate buffers in dialysis in patients unable to clear lactate, but the volumes involved are far larger [34,35].

Role: Commonly used perioperatively. No clinical outcome benefit demonstrated compared with normal saline.

Colloids and hypertonic saline

With the exception of albumin none of the synthetic colloids are physiological in nature and even albumin in its treated form is different from the natural molecule. It might be expected that while they produce a volumetric effect, they have little in the way of other physiological roles. Physically they could dilute blood components such as coagulation factors. A threshold of blood volume to colloid ratio of 10:4 is where coagulation defects using thromboelastography are seen [36,37]. There is ongoing debate as to whether they have any advantage over crystalloids [38].

The ideal colloid is stable on the shelf at room temperature for a long time; can be stored in plastic so that it is easy to transport; is sterile, toxin free, antigen free and preferably not derived from human or animal products; is devoid of active ingredients; has an adequate colloid oncotic pressure; has a long half-

life in the circulation; is easily cleared from the interstitium (e.g. lymph drainage); is easily metabolized with no toxic metabolites or excreted; has no effect on the immune system; has no effects on coagulation and is cheap.

Albumin
Constitution: 4.5% (45 g/dL), 20% (200 g/dL). Both forms of albumin are rendered iso-osmotic by addition of sodium chloride. 4.5% Human albumin solution is also iso-oncotic. 20% Human albumin solution is hyperoncotic although iso-osmotic.

Distribution: In health, albumin is distributed approximately 40% in the intravascular compartment and 60% in the interstitial compartment [39]. Administered albumin is confined to the intravascular compartment so has a volume of distribution of approximately 3.5 L. Less than 10% of an administered dose leaves the plasma in 3 hours, and the plasma half-life is 16 hours with an elimination half-life of 19 days. Elimination is through intracellular metabolism by lysosomal proteases. In sepsis or burns, capillary leak may result in a greatly reduced reflection coefficient, such that less than half an administered dose of albumin remains in the intravascular compartment at 4 hours [18].

Advantages: Albumin is a larger molecule than gelatins so it persists in the longer intravascular space. Both forms of albumin will initially draw fluid into the intravascular volume. Albumin is a transport molecule, it can bind other molecules and toxins, it is a free radical scavenger and it has a role as a buffer in acid base [40]. Although theoretically ideal, few of these features, if any, have proven benefit. Anaphylactoid reactions are very rare (0.01%) [41].

Disadvantages: Expensive, each unit is derived from plasma pooled from as many as 65 000 donors. Although now sourced from America and treated to minimize risk, the possibility of infection with new variant Creutzfeldt–Jakob disease (nvCJD) in particular cannot be discounted.

Role: Utilization decreased dramatically after increased mortality with albumin administration in critical illness was suggested by meta-analysis [42] although a recent large Australasian randomized controlled trial (the SAFE study) found no difference in outcome compared with saline [21]. Administration of albumin with furosemide was reported to speed resolution of acute lung injury, but the subjects were young fit trauma patients resuscitated with large volumes of crystalloid, so relevance to the septic acute lung injury more commonly seen in the UK is unclear [43]. 20% or 'salt poor' albumin requires less sodium chloride administration for a given increase in oncotic pressure so is traditionally preferred where total body fluid volumes are increased, for instance in the treatment of liver failure with ascites [44,45]. There is a recent suggestion that it might be of use in hepatic encephalopathy induced by diuretic dehydration [46].

Gelatins

Constitution: 4% Succinylated gelatine, derived from bovine collagen. The osmolality is 279 mOsm. The average molecular weight is 30 kDa. However, this average emphasizes the contribution of heavier molecules. In terms of osmotic effects, the number of molecules is critical, so the number average molecular weight (arithmetic mean; i.e. the total weight divided by the number of particles) is probably more relevant and is only 22 600 kDa. The plasma half-life of gelofusin is enhanced beyond that expected on basis of size, because its negative charge repels the endothelium.

Distribution: The initial distribution is intravascular with a plasma half-life of approximately 2 hours. There is some minor metabolism in the liver but much is eliminated in the urine and elimination is complete. There are very few documented problems with coagulation. The finding of gelatin in the urine led to the myth of oncotic diuresis as a clinical entity. While gelatin is found in the urine there is no evidence that it causes a significant diuresis beyond that expected from volume expansion.

Advantages: It is an effective colloid [47,48], is cleared through the kidneys [49,50] and is cheap.

Disadvantages: Anaphylactoid reactions occur in approximately 1 in 1600. Although the collagen is sourced from 'BSE-free' cows, a theoretical risk of nvCJD transmission remains.

Role: It is the first line colloid in the UK. It has relatively poor intravascular persistence, but aside from anaphylactoid reactions has a good side-effect profile.

Dextrans

Constitution: Dextrans are glucose polymers produced by bacteria grown in sucrose. Dextran 70 has an average molecular weight of 67 000 kDa but a more relevant average molecular weight of 38 000 kDa and is supplied in either 5% dextrose or 0.9% sodium chloride solution. Dextran 70 has a colloid osmotic pressure of 350 mOsm/L. Dextran 40 has a higher oncotic pressure and will help 'pull' fluid from the intracellular space.

Maximum dose: 1.5 mL/kg/day.

Distribution: The distribution is relatively prolonged, with a plasma half-life of approximately 6 hours (Dextran 70) or 4 hours (Dextran 40).

Metabolism: There is no intravascular metabolism and smaller molecules below 55 kDa are filtered by the kidneys. Larger molecules are hydrolysed by tissue dextran-1,6-glucosidase.

Advantages: There is good intravascular persistence [51]. Dextran 40 has been used extensively to reduce blood viscosity and also increase the time to red cell aggregation through an effect on rouleaux formation. There is a recent suggestion that these agents may also influence leucocyte adherence. This may be of interest in ischaemia-reperfusion injury [52–54].

Disadvantages: Dextrans cause coagulopathy because of reduced formation of factors VII and VIII and inhibition of platelet aggregation and fibrin clot formation. The effects are very similar to von Willebrand disease and may be reversed in part with desmopressin [55]. Dextrans are intermediate between gelatins and starches in relation to serious anaphylactoid reactions, with an incidence of 1 in 2500 [41].

Dextrans can cause erythrocyte aggregation with rouleaux formation and can interfere with blood cross-matching. Acute renal failure has been reported resulting from increased urine viscosity caused by rapid clearance of low molecular weight molecules, particularly in dehydrated patients.

Role: Before the widespread use of low molecular weight heparins, dextrans were sometimes given to reduce occurrence of deep venous thrombosis following orthopaedic surgery, because of their associated coagulopathic effects [36,56,57] but are now largely discarded because of coagulopathic effects.

Starches

Constitution: Starch in 0.9% sodium chloride. Osmolarity 308 mOsm. Starches are described by the mean molecular weight/degree of substitution of glucose side chains with hydroxyethyl groups. Hydroxyethylation is usually at C2 but can be at C3 or C6. A high degree of substitution increases resistance to metabolism by amylase but is also associated with coagulopathy. One way of describing these agents is to consider their in vivo molecular weight which is determined by the original molecular weight and the C2 : C6 ratio which determines breakdown.

They are described therefore in three ways: by concentration, usually 3%, 6% or 10%; by average molecular weight: low 70 000 Da, medium 130–270 000 Da or high greater than 450 000 Da; degree of substitution (low is to 0.5 and high is 0.6 and above) (Table 15.3). Pentastarch is described as 264/0.5 making it a medium-range starch [58,59].

Currently available starches include: HES 130/0.4 (Voluven, Fresenius), maximum dose 33 mL/kg/day; HES 200/0.5 (Haes-steril, Fresenius), maximum dose 20 mL/kg/day [60,61].

Distribution: Distribution of starches is initially confined to the plasma, with a plasma half-life of approximately 6 hours. Small molecules are filtered by the kidney and large molecules are digested by amylase. The middle range starches such as HES 200/0.62 are very effective in the maintenance of plasma volume expansion over 24 hours in routine surgical patients [62]. These agents bind water with a capacity of 20–30 mL/kg. They have good volume expansion properties [63,64].

A rapid amylase-dependent breakdown occurs, with urinary excretion of approximately 40% of the dose in 48 hours. A high degree of hydroxyethylation inhibits breakdown and some accumulate in the reticuloendothelial system. In routine surgical patients there is minimal hydrolysis in 24 hours [65,66].

Advantages: Starches have the lowest risk of serious anaphylactoid reaction of any of the synthetic colloids at approximately 0.06%. There is a more persistent volume effect than gelatins. Some studies have suggested that starches may have beneficial effects in major surgery. Gelatins and Elohes were compared in patients undergoing aortic repair. Interleukin 6 (IL-6) and C-reactive protein (CRP) were both lower with starches [67,68]. Clinically, renal function appears to be better, with lower

Table 15.3 Description of a range of starches.

Concentration	MW (kDa)	Degree of substitution	Examples
6%	450	0.7	HES 450, 0.7, Hetastarch
6%	200	0.5	Pentastarch, HAES-steril 6%
6%	200	0.62	Elohes
6%	130	0.42	Venofundin
6%	130	0.4	Voluven
10%	200	0.5	HAES-steril 10%
6%	200	0.5	Hypertonic Hyper-HAES in 7.2% saline

MW, molecular weight.

creatinine values in the postoperative phase. An influence on the inflammatory reaction has also been suggested. A study reported that the use of starch seemed to reduce urinary albumin excretion, which was taken as a surrogate for capillary permeability [69,70]. 3% Hetastarch has been used in plasma exchange with no obvious ill effect [71].

Disadvantages: Starches can reduce factor VIII and fibrin polymerization and increase the activated partial prothrombin time (APTT). These effects are probably concentration related, and may be caused by von Willbrand factor and factor VI binding to starch [72]. The effect is worse with a high degree of substitution; 450/0.7 induces intracranial bleeding and is contraindicated in neurosurgery. Starches can also impair primary haemostasis through a reduction in von Willebrand factor activity [73–76]. Hydroxyethyl starch increases blood viscosity, decreases erythrocyte deformability and increases erythrocyte aggregation when compared with saline [77]. If thromboelastography is used to assess the effects of colloids on coagulation, the dilution ratio of blood volume to colloid solution volume appears to be critical. At a dilution of >10:4 problems may be seen [78–83]. Low molecular weight starches have less effect on coagulation. Those with a molecular weight less than 70 kDa are associated with barely detectable alterations in function [79,84]. Another issue is that hyperamylasaemia complicates the diagnosis of pancreatitis [85].

Starches result in persistent reticuloendothelial system storage, which probably causes the persistent itch reported in 13% of recipients [86,87]. Voluven has lower reticuloendothelial storage although it is not yet known if this will translate into a lower incidence of itching.

There is conflicting evidence about the effects on renal function. It has been suggested that low molecular weight starches in high concentration might impair renal function [67], but in renal allografts starches had no obvious effect on renal function [68,88].

Role: Starches are often used as a second line to gelofusine, as a result of the disadvantages mentioned,

despite better intravascular persistence and lower risk of anaphylactoid reaction.

Dose limitation: There are recommendations in place for the maximum dose per day of starch that can be used. For the third generation starches, 6% 130/0.4 the dose recommendation is 50 mL/kg, although higher doses have been used without documented ill effect and these limits are fairly arbitrary [83,89].

Hypertonic solutions

The notion of using hypertonic solutions is not new but is currently enjoying considerable interest. The concept is that in an acute situation with sudden volume loss from the intravascular space, the patient's own fluid reserves can be mobilized from the intracellular space and other spaces by the use of osmotically active agents. A wide range of hyperosmotic solutions have been used, from 1.8% saline to 7.2% saline in starch solutions [90–92]. The two most commonly used are 7.5% saline and 7.5% saline in Dextran 70 (HSD 70) [90,93–99]. The volume expansion is reputed to be in the order of 3–10 times the infused volume of fluid [100–102] and this expansion occurs almost immediately. In the immediate care this has the advantage of using much smaller resuscitation volumes.

Advantages: Hypertonic solutions have been evaluated in hypovolaemia and are effective [103–105]. There is a significant literature in burns patients and such solutions may have a role in the first 8 hours [95,106–108]. Use of hypertonic solutions in head trauma have shown favourable results in terms of reduced volumes required, and potentially less intracranial pressure changes [109–111]. However, this was not translated into outcome benefit in a clinical study [92]. Other benefits may include improved microcirculation, increased myocardial contractility and vasodilatation of the splanchnic circulation [112–114]. There is also a marked reduction in lymph production [115].

Disadvantages: There are potential problems with sodium excess and a lack of any free water. Plasma sodium increases and remains above baseline. In a study in dogs, high doses of hypertonic solution resulted in high plasma osmotic pressure (340.5–352.8 mOsm) and hyponatraemia (161.4–174.5 mmol/L) 10–90 minutes after fluid infusion [116]. This has also been reported in cardiac surgery [117]. Hypotensive episodes, sudden increases in pulmonary capillary wedge pressure and ventricular arrhythmias have all been reported. Other side-effects include electrolyte abnormalities, cardiac failure, bleeding diathesis and phlebitis. There is also a theoretical risk of central pontine myelinolysis and rebound intracranial hypertension [118].

Role: Many of the reported studies have been in animal models. A dose of 4–11.5 mL/kg of HSD has been recommended but in the bleeding patient the situation is confused. Animal studies suggest that 4 mL/kg will increase bleeding while 1 mL/kg will not [119]. Whether this can be extrapolated to provide an indication of what happens in resuscitation and increased pressure is uncertain. With hypertonic saline, a roadside dose of 250 mL along with other fluid has been used but specific dosage recommendations are hard to identify [120]. However, it is recommended that the serum sodium should not exceed 160 mmol/L and that this management is restricted to the first few hours. In burns, a suggested regimen is to use hypertonic solutions at a rate of 4 mL/kg percent burn area in the first 8 hours, to administer it as any other fluid and to modify administration against clinical effect.

Physiological colloid
The idea of placing a colloid in a more physiological medium has been explored. Using balanced solutions results in less metabolic acidosis than with saline, and in animal studies, better survival [26]. Hextend is 6% hetastarch (550/0.7) in a balanced solution with a lactate buffer and physiological levels of glucose. It is as effective as 6% hetastarch in saline for the treatment of hypovolaemia but has a more favourable side-effect profile in volumes of up to 5 L, compared with 6% hetastarch in saline. Using thromboelastography there appears to be less coagulopathy than with standard HES but more than with the newer lower molecular weight starches [63,121].

Acetyl starch has also been used and has the advantage of rapid and nearly complete enzymatic degradation [122].

Dextrose solutions
Dextrose is rapidly metabolized, leaving water or a hypotonic solution of sodium chloride. It distributes across all compartments rapidly so is ineffective for resuscitation. Insulin resistance is common in illness; it develops after burns, trauma, sepsis and elective surgery, in proportion to the insult [123]. Consequently, even slow administration of dextrose-containing solutions may cause hyperglycaemia, which indicates a corresponding intracellular hypoglycaemia resulting from impaired glucose uptake; hence the characterization of diabetes as 'starvation in the midst of plenty'.

5% Dextrose
Constitution: 5% Dextrose = 50 g/L in water. Molecular weight = 180 kDa. Osmolarity 253 mOsm/L. 5% Dextrose provides 170 kcal/L.

Distribution and metabolism: Because the blood volume comprises 7% of the total body water, only 70 mL of an administered 1 L will remain in the intravascular space after redistribution. In normal volunteers, rapid administration of 2 L 5% dextrose produced a similar expansion of plasma volume as normal saline at 1 hour, but by 2 hours the plasma volume had returned to baseline, and the entire administered volume had been passed as urine because of osmotic diuresis and inhibition of ADH secretion [31].

Advantages: The main role is to supply water, which cannot be given intravenously because the hypotonicity would cause haemolysis. 5% Dextrose should be given for fluid loss from the total body water; for example, resulting from fever. The requirement for water over and above saline is suggested by a supra-normal serum sodium concentration.

Disadvantages: 5% Dextran produces no sustained plasma volume expansion, so these solutions have no role in resuscitation. Rapid intravenous infusion causes hyperglycaemia, glycosuria and osmotic diuresis.

10% Dextrose
10% Dextrose = 100 g/L. 1 L provides 340 kcal.

Advantages: 10% Dextrose provides more calories than 5% dextrose.

Disadvantages: Initially hypertonic with an osmolality of 505 mOsm/L so can cause thrombophlebitis and requires a large free flowing vein. Hyperglycaemia also occurs.

Role: Often used in diabetics because it provides more calories than 5% dextrose.

50% Dextrose
50% Dextrose = 500 g/L. 1 L provides 1700 kcal.

Advantages: Is concentrated sugar so is very effective for raising blood sugar. It has little free water so is a means of giving sugar and calories without water.

Disadvantages: Initially 50% dextrose is strongly hypertonic, with an osmolality of 2525 mOsm/L, so prolonged administration requires central venous access to avoid phlebitis. Hyperglycaemia also occurs.

Role: Used for rapid treatment of hypoglycaemia in a dose of 20–50 mL. Also useful for administration in addition to isotonic crystalloid maintenance, provided central venous access is available, in order to provide energy without causing hyponatraemia; for example, 20 mL/hour of 50% dextrose provides 34 kcal/hour.

4% Dextrose
'Dextrose saline' 4% dextrose = 40 g/L. 0.18% sodium chloride Na = 30 mOsm, K = 30 mOsm, osmolality = 286 mOsm. 1 L provides 136 kcal.

Advantages: This solution provides a small amount of saline, 20% by volume and a larger amount of free water. It has no specific role.

Disadvantages: It gives an impression of giving some sodium but not too much. It is actually a water load. Inappropriate use can result in water overload with profound hyponatraemia.

Role: It can be used as part of a maintenance regimen as long as there is clear awareness of its relative salt and water components.

Potassium

Part of the regulation of fluids and electrolytes is the maintenance of 'reasonable' potassium levels. While serum potassium is poorly representative of whole body potassium, a value below 4 mmol/L representing part of the membrane gradient, greatly increases the occurrence of arrhythmias. Potassium is essential for the function of the sodium-potassium ATPase.

Factors affecting serum potassium
Acidosis and α-adrenergic agents promote potassium movement out of the cell. Alkalosis, β_2-adrenergic agents and insulin increase cellular uptake (hyperkalaemia increases insulin secretion). Aldosterone increases renal potassium loss.

Correction of hypokalaemia
Oral potassium is effective but slow, and many dietary components contain potassium. If rapid correction is required then intravenous administration is appropriate. The rate should not exceed 40 mmol/hour and it should be monitored. As potassium is irritant it should be given either very diluted or into a central vein. Rapid infusion is extremely hazardous.

Conclusions

Fluid management is simple. For maintenance, replace daily requirements, assess other losses and replace appropriate amounts of electrolytes and water. Assess the patient clinically as frequently as clinical conditions warrant. Keep an accurate fluid balance chart. Measure what is happening in the plasma. Keep the solutions simple and allow the patient to do the fine-tuning themselves. For resuscitation, fill the space. Determine from the illness, the patient and the situation which fluid is most appropriate for the case and use it to sustain intravascular volume.

References

1 Basset G, Crone C, Saumon G. Fluid absorption by rat lung *in situ*: pathways for sodium entry in the luminal membrane of alveolar epithelium. *J Physiol* 1987; **384**: 325–45.

2 Verghese GM, Ware LB, Matthay BA, Matthay MA. Alveolar epithelial fluid transport and the resolution of clinically severe hydrostatic pulmonary edema. *J Appl Physiol* 1999; **87**: 1301–12.

3 Suzuki S, Noda M, Sugita M, *et al*. Impairment of transalveolar fluid transport and lung Na(+)-K(+)-ATPase function by hypoxia in rats. *J Appl Physiol* 1999; **87**: 962–8.

4 Suzuki S, Noda M, Sugita M, *et al*. Role of Na(+)-glucose cotransport in fluid absorption across alveolar epithelium in isolated rat lungs. *Nihon Kyobu Shikkan Gakkai Zasshi* 1996; **34**: 1109–14.

5 Matthay MA, Wiener-Kronish JP. Intact epithelial barrier function is critical for the resolution of alveolar edema in humans. *Am Rev Respir Dis* 1990; **142**: 1250–7.

6 Lamke LO, Liljedahl SO. Plasma volume changes after infusion of various plasma expanders. *Resuscitation* 1976; **5**: 93–102.

7 Adams HA, Piepenbrock S, Hempelmann G. Volume replacement solutions: pharmacology and clinical use. *Anasthesiol Intensivmed Notfallmed Schmerzther* 1998; **33**: 2–17.

8 Funk W, Baldinger V. Microcirculatory perfusion during volume therapy: a comparative study using crystalloid or colloid in awake animals. *Anesthesiology* 1995; **82**: 975–82.

9 Cervera AL, Moss G. Crystalloid distribution following hemorrhage and hemodilution: mathematical model and prediction of optimum volumes for equilibration at normovolemia. *J Trauma* 1974; **14**: 506–20.

10 Wang P, Hauptman JG, Chaudry IH. Hemorrhage produces depression in microvascular blood flow which persists despite fluid resuscitation. *Circ Shock* 1990; **32**: 307–18.

11 Baum TD, Wang H, Rothschild HR, Gang DL, Fink MP. Mesenteric oxygen metabolism, ileal mucosal hydrogen ion concentration, and tissue edema after crystalloid or colloid resuscitation in porcine endotoxic

shock: comparison of Ringer's lactate and 6% hetastarch. *Circ Shock* 1990; **30**: 385–97.

12 Twigley AJ, Hillman KM. The end of the crystalloid era? A new approach to peri-operative fluid administration. *Anaesthesia* 1985; **40**: 860–71.

13 Amede FJ, James KA, Michelis MF, Gleim GW. Changes in serum sodium, sodium balance, water balance, and plasma hormone levels as the result of pelvic surgery in women. *Int Urol Nephrol* 2002; **34**: 545–50.

14 Tambe AA, Hill R, Livesley PJ. Post-operative hyponatraemia in orthopaedic injury. *Injury* 2003; **34**: 253–5.

15 Crook MA, Velauthar U, Moran L, Griffiths W. Review of investigation and management of severe hyponatraemia in a hospital population. *Ann Clin Biochem* 1999; **36**: 158–62.

16 McPherson E, Dunsmuir RA. Hyponatraemia in hip fracture patients. *Scott Med J* 2002; **47**: 115–6.

17 Baylis PH. The syndrome of inappropriate antidiuretic hormone secretion. *Int J Biochem Cell Biol* 2003; **35**: 1495–9.

18 Margarson MP, Soni NC. Changes in serum albumin concentration and volume expanding effects following a bolus of albumin 20% in septic patients. *Br J Anaesth* 2004; **92**: 821–6.

19 Schierhout G, Roberts I. Fluid resuscitation with colloid or crystalloid solutions in critically ill patients: a systematic review of randomised trials. *Br Med J* 1998; **316**: 961–4.

20 Roberts I. Human albumin administration in critically ill patients: systematic review of randomised controlled trials. *Br Med J* 1998; **317**: 235–40.

21 Finfer S, Bellomo R, Boyce N, *et al*. A comparison of albumin and saline for fluid resuscitation in the intensive care unit. *N Engl J Med* 2004; **350**: 2247–56.

22 Bunn F, Alderson P, Hawkins V. Colloid solutions for fluid resuscitation. *Cochrane Database Syst Rev* 2000; **2**: CD001319.

23 Reid F, Lobo DN, Williams RN, Rowlands BJ, Allison SP. (Ab)normal saline and physiological Hartmann's solution: a randomized double-blind crossover study. *Clin Sci (Lond)* 2003; **104**: 17–24.

24 Blanloeil Y, Roze B, Rigal JC, Baron JF. [Hyperchloremic acidosis druing plasma volume replacement]. *Ann Fr Anesth Reanim* 2002; **21**: 211–20.

25 Alfaro VP, J. Palacios, L. Acid–base disturbance during hemorrhage in rats: significant role of strong inorganic ions. *J Appl Physiol* 1999; **86**: 1617–25.

26 Kellum JA. Fluid resuscitation and hyperchloremic acidosis in experimental sepsis: improved short-term

survival and acid–base balance with Hextend compared with saline. *Crit Care Med* 2002; **30**: 300–5.

27 Waters JH, Bernstein CA. Dilutional acidosis following hetastarch or albumin in healthy volunteers. *Anesthesiology* 2000; **93**: 1617–25.

28 Wilkes NJ, Woolf R, Mutch M, *et al.* The effects of balanced versus saline-based hetastarch and crystalloid solutions on acid–base and electrolyte status and gastric mucosal perfusion in elderly surgical patients. *Anesth Analg* 2001; **93**: 811–6.

29 Ruttmann TG. Haemodilution enhances coagulation. *Br J Anaesth* 2002; **88**: 470–2.

30 Ruttmann TG, James MF, Finlayson J. Effects on coagulation of intravenous crystalloid or colloid in patients undergoing peripheral vascular surgery. *Br J Anaesth* 2002; **89**: 226–30.

31 Lobo DN, Stanga Z, Simpson JA, *et al.* Dilution and redistribution effects of rapid 2-litre infusions of 0.9% (w/v) saline and 5% (w/v) dextrose on haematological parameters and serum biochemistry in normal subjects: a double-blind crossover study. *Clin Sci (Lond)* 2001; **101**: 173–9.

32 Wilkes NJ. Hartmann's solution and Ringer's lactate: targeting the fourth space. *Clin Sci (Lond)* 2003; **104**: 25–6.

33 Kramer GC, Svensen CH, Prough DS. To bolus or not to bolus: is that the question? *Clin Sci (Lond)* 2001; **101**: 181–3.

34 Kierdorf HP, Leue C, Arns S. Lactate- or bicarbonate-buffered solutions in continuous extracorporeal renal replacement therapies. *Kidney Int* 1999; **56**(Suppl 72): S32–6.

35 Thongboonkerd V, Lumlertgul D, Supajatura V. Better correction of metabolic acidosis, blood pressure control, and phagocytosis with bicarbonate compared to lactate solution in acute peritoneal dialysis. *Artif Organs* 2001; **25**: 99–108.

36 Petroianu GA, Liu J, Maleck WH, Mattinger C, Bergler WF. The effect of *in vitro* hemodilution with gelatin, dextran, hydroxyethyl starch, or Ringer's solution on Thrombelastograph. *Anesth Analg* 2000; **90**: 795–800.

37 Salmon JB, Mythen MG. Pharmacology and physiology of colloids. *Blood Rev* 1993; **7**: 114–20.

38 Alderson P, Schierhout G, Roberts I, Bunn F. Colloids versus crystalloids for fluid resuscitation in critically ill patients. *Cochrane Database Syst Rev* 2000; **2**: CD000567.

39 Fleck A, Raines G, Hawker F, *et al.* Increased vascular permeability: a major cause of hypoalbuminaemia in disease and injury. *Lancet* 1985; **i**: 781–4.

40 Quinlan GJ, Margarson MP, Mumby S, Evans TW, Gutteridge JM. Administration of albumin to patients with sepsis syndrome: a possible beneficial role in plasma thiol repletion. *Clin Sci (Colch)* 1998; **95**: 459–65.

41 Laxenaire MC, Charpentier C, Feldman L. Anaphylactoid reactions to colloid plasma substitutes: incidence, risk factors, mechanisms: a French multicenter prospective study. *Ann Fr Anesth Reanim* 1994; **13**: 301–10.

42 Cochrane Injuries Group Albumin Reviewers. Human albumin administration in critically ill patients: systematic review of randomised controlled trials. *Br Med J* 1998; **317**: 235–40.

43 Martin GS, Mangialardi RJ, Wheeler AP, *et al.* Albumin and furosemide therapy in hypoproteinemic patients with acute lung injury. *Crit Care Med* 2002; **30**: 2175–82.

44 Moreau R, Valla D. Indications and role of albumin, plasma volume expansion excluded, in the preoperative or postoperative management of portal hypertension. *Ann Fr Anesth Reanim* 1996; **15**: 514–24.

45 Sort P, Navasa M, Arroyo V, *et al.* Effect of intravenous albumin on renal impairment and mortality in patients with cirrhosis and spontaneous bacterial peritonitis. *N Engl J Med* 1999; **341**: 403–9.

46 Jalan R, Kapoor D. Reversal of diuretic-induced hepatic encephalopathy with infusion of albumin but not colloid. *Clin Sci (Lond)* 2004; **106**: 467–74.

47 Beards SC, Watt T, Edwards JD, Nightingale P, Farragher EB. Comparison of the hemodynamic and oxygen transport responses to modified fluid gelatin and hetastarch in critically ill patients: a prospective, randomized trial. *Crit Care Med* 1994; **22**: 600–5.

48 Beyer R, Harmening U, Rittmeyer O, *et al.* Use of modified fluid gelatin and hydroxyethyl starch for colloidal volume replacement in major orthopaedic surgery. *Br J Anaesth* 1997; **78**: 44–50.

49 Schortgen F, Lacherade JC, Bruneel F, *et al.* Effects of hydroxyethylstarch and gelatin on renal function in severe sepsis: a multicentre randomised study. *Lancet* 2001; **i**: 911–6.

50 Ragaller MJ, Theilen H, Koch T. Volume replacement in critically ill patients with acute renal failure. *J Am Soc Nephrol* 2001; **12**(Suppl 17): S33–9.

51 Haljamae H. Volume substitution in shock. *Acta Anaesthesiol Scand Suppl* 1993; **98**: 25–8.

52 Dewachter P, Laxenaire MC, Donner M, Kurtz M, Stoltz JF. *In vivo* rheologic studies of plasma substitutes. *Ann Fr Anesth Reanim* 1992; **11**: 516–25.

53 Steinbauer M, Harris AG, Leiderer R, Abels C, Messmer K. Impact of dextran on microvascular disturbances and tissue injury following ischemia/reperfusion in striated muscle. *Shock* 1998; **9**: 345–51.

54 Harris AG, Steinbauer M, Leiderer R, Messmer K. Role of leukocyte plugging and edema in skeletal muscle ischemia-reperfusion injury. *Am J Physiol* 1997; **273**: H989–96.

55 Aberg M, Hedner U, Bergentz SE. Effect of Dextran 70 on factor VIII and platelet function in von Willebrand's disease. *Thromb Res* 1978; **12**: 629–34.

56 Coats TJ, Heron M. The effect of hypertonic saline dextran on whole blood coagulation. *Resuscitation* 2004; **60**: 101–4.

57 Inoue M, Hirose Y, Gamou M, Goto M. Effect of hemodilution with dextran and albumin on activated clotting time (ACT). *Masui* 1997; **46**: 809–12.

58 Wisselink W, Patetsios P, Panetta TF, *et al.* Medium molecular weight pentastarch reduces reperfusion injury by decreasing capillary leak in an animal model of spinal cord ischemia. *J Vasc Surg* 1998; **27**: 109–16.

59 Webb AR, Tighe D, Moss RF, *et al.* Advantages of a narrow-range, medium molecular weight hydroxyethyl starch for volume maintenance in a porcine model of fecal peritonitis. *Crit Care Med* 1991; **19**: 409–16.

60 James MF, Latoo MY, Mythen MG, *et al.* Plasma volume changes associated with two hydroxyethyl starch colloids following acute hypovolaemia in volunteers. *Anaesthesia* 2004; **59**: 738–42.

61 Hankeln K, Senker R, Beez M, Gol'dina OA. A comparative study of the effectiveness of 5% human albumin and 10% hydroxyethyl starch (HAES-steril) for correcting hemodynamics and O_2 transport in surgical interventions. *Anesteziol Reanimatol* 1997; **1**: 23–6.

62 Degremont AC, Ismail M, Arthaud M, *et al.* Mechanisms of postoperative prolonged plasma volume expansion with low molecular weight hydroxethy starch (HES 200/0.62, 6%). *Intensive Care Med* 1995; **21**: 577–83.

63 Boldt J. New light on intravascular volume replacement regimens: what did we learn from the past three years? *Anesth Analg* 2003; **97**: 1595–604.

64 Sirtl C, Laubenthal H, Zumtobel V, Kraft D, Jurecka W. Tissue deposits of hydroxyethyl starch (HES): dose-dependent and time-related. *Br J Anaesth* 1999; **82**: 510–5.

65 Ginz HF, Gottschall V, Schwarzkopf G, Walter K. Excessive tissue storage of colloids in the reticuloendothelial system. *Anaesthesist* 1998; **47**: 330–4.

66 Trop M, Schiffrin EJ, Callahan R, Carter EA. Effect of heta-starch colloidal solutions on reticuloendothelial phagocytic system (RES) function in burned and infected rats. *Burns* 1992; **18**: 463–5.

67 Cittanova ML, Leblanc I, Legendre C, *et al.* Effect of hydroxyethylstarch in brain-dead kidney donors on renal function in kidney-transplant recipients. *Lancet* 1996; **348**: 1620–2.

68 Dehne MG, Muhling J, Sablotzki A, *et al.* Effect of hydroxyethyl starch solution on kidney function in surgical intensive care patients. *Anasthesiol Intensivmed Notfallmed Schmerzther* 1997; **32**: 348–54.

69 Allison KP, Gosling P, Jones S, Pallister I, Porter KM. Randomized trial of hydroxyethyl starch versus gelatine for trauma resuscitation. *J Trauma* 1999; **47**: 1114–21.

70 Boldt J, Heesen M, Padberg W, Martin K, Hempelmann G. The influence of volume therapy and pentoxifylline infusion on circulating adhesion molecules in trauma patients. *Anaesthesia* 1996; **51**: 529–35.

71 Owen HG, Brecher ME. Partial colloid starch replacement for therapeutic plasma exchange. *J Clin Apheresis* 1997; **12**: 87–92.

72 Treib J, Baron JF, Grauer MT, Strauss RG. An international view of hydroxyethyl starches. *Intensive Care Med* 1999; **25**: 258–68.

73 de Jonge E, Levi M, Buller HR, Berends F, Kesecioglu J. Decreased circulating levels of von Willebrand factor after intravenous administration of a rapidly degradable hydroxyethyl starch (HES 200/0.5/6) in healthy human subjects. *Intensive Care Med* 2001; **27**: 1825–9.

74 Jonville-Bera AP, Autret-Leca E, Gruel Y. Acquired type I von Willebrand's disease associated with highly substituted hydroxyethyl starch. *N Engl J Med* 2001; **345**: 622–3.

75 Sanfelippo MJ, Suberviola PD, Geimer NF. Development of a von Willebrand-like syndrome after prolonged use of hydroxyethyl starch. *Am J Clin Pathol* 1987; **88**: 653–5.

76 Michiels JJ, Budde U, van der Planken M, *et al.* Acquired von Willebrand syndromes: clinical features, aetiology, pathophysiology, classification and management. *Best Pract Res Clin Haematol* 2001; **14**: 401–36.

77 Castro VJ, Astiz ME, Rackow EC. Effect of crystalloid and colloid solutions on blood rheology in sepsis. *Shock* 1997; **8**: 104–7.

78 Jamnicki M, Zollinger A, Seifert B, *et al.* Compromised blood coagulation: an *in vitro* comparison of hydroxyethyl starch 130/0.4 and hydroxyethyl starch 200/0.5 using thrombelastography. *Anesth Analg* 1998; **87**: 989–93.

79 Jamnicki M, Bombeli T, Seifert B, *et al*. Low- and medium-molecular-weight hydroxyethyl starches: comparison of their effect on blood coagulation. *Anesthesiology* 2000; **93**: 1231–7.

80 Treib J, Haass A, Pindur G, *et al*. Influence of low molecular weight hydroxyethyl starch (HES 40/0.5-0.55) on hemostasis and hemorheology. *Haemostasis* 1996; **26**: 258–65.

81 Treib J, Haass A. The rheological properties of hydroxyethyl starch. *Dtsch Med Wochenschr* 1997; **122**: 1319–22.

82 Treib J, Haass A, Pindur G. Coagulation disorders caused by hydroxyethyl starch. *Thromb Haemost* 1997; **78**: 974–83.

83 Stoll M, Treib J, Schenk JF, *et al*. No coagulation disorders under high-dose volume therapy with low-molecular-weight hydroxyethyl starch. *Haemostasis* 1997; **27**: 251–8.

84 Entholzner EK, Mielke LL, Calatzis AN, *et al*. Coagulation effects of a recently developed hydroxyethyl starch (HES 130/0.4) compared to hydroxyethyl starches with higher molecular weight. *Acta Anaesthesiol Scand* 2000; **44**: 1116–21.

85 Nearman HS, Herman ML. Toxic effects of colloids in the intensive care unit. *Crit Care Clin* 1991; **7**: 713–23.

86 Gall H, Schultz KD, Boehncke WH, Kaufmann R. Clinical and pathophysiological aspects of hydroxyethyl starch-induced pruritus: evaluation of 96 cases. *Dermatology* 1996; **192**: 222–6.

87 Murphy M, Carmichael AJ, Lawler PG, White M, Cox NH. The incidence of hydroxyethyl starch-associated pruritus. *Br J Dermatol* 2001; **144**: 973–6.

88 Deman A, Peeters P, Sennesael J. Hydroxyethyl starch does not impair immediate renal function in kidney transplant recipients: a retrospective, multicentre analysis. *Nephrol Dial Transplant* 1999; **14**: 1517–20.

89 Neff TA, Doelberg M, Jungheinrich C, *et al*. Repetitive large-dose infusion of the novel hydroxyethyl starch 130/0.4 in patients with severe head injury. *Anesth Analg* 2003; **96**: 1453–9.

90 Alpar EK, Killampalli VV. Effects of hypertonic dextran in hypovolaemic shock: a prospective clinical trial. *Injury* 2004; **35**: 500–6.

91 Moore FA, McKinley BA, Moore EE. The next generation in shock resuscitation. *Lancet* 2004; **363**: 1988–96.

92 Cooper DJ, Myles PS, McDermott FT, *et al*. Prehospital hypertonic saline resuscitation of patients with hypotension and severe traumatic brain injury: a randomized controlled trial. *JAMA* 2004; **291**: 1350–7.

93 Dubick MA, Atkins JL. Small-volume fluid resuscitation for the far-forward combat environment: current concepts. *J Trauma* 2003; **54**(5 Suppl): S43–5.

94 Diebel LN, Tyburski JG, Dulchavsky SA. Effect of hypertonic saline solution and dextran on ventricular blood flow and heart-lung interaction after hemorrhagic shock. *Surgery* 1998; **124**: 642–9.

95 Elgjo GI, Poli de Figueiredo LF, Schenarts PJ, *et al*. Hypertonic saline dextran produces early (8–12 hrs) fluid sparing in burn resuscitation: a 24-hr prospective, double-blind study in sheep. *Crit Care Med* 2000; **28**: 163–71.

96 Tollofsrud S, Tonnessen T, Skraastad O, Noddeland H. Hypertonic saline and dextran in normovolaemic and hypovolaemic healthy volunteers increases interstitial and intravascular fluid volumes. *Acta Anaesthesiol Scand* 1998; **42**: 145–53.

97 Stapley SA, Clasper JC, Horrocks CL, Kenward CE, Watkins PE. The effects of repeated dosing with 7.5% sodium chloride/6% dextran following uncontrolled intra-abdominal hemorrhage. *Shock* 2002; **17**: 146–50.

98 Jarvela K, Koskinen M, Koobi T. Effects of hypertonic saline (7.5%) on extracellular fluid volumes in healthy volunteers. *Anaesthesia* 2003; **58**: 878–81.

99 Svensen CH, Waldrop KS, Edsberg L, Hahn RG. Natriuresis and the extracellular volume expansion by hypertonic saline. *J Surg Res* 2003; **113**: 6–12.

100 Boldt J, Knothe C, Zickmann B, *et al*. Volume loading with hypertonic saline solution: endocrinologic and circulatory responses. *J Cardiothorac Vasc Anesth* 1994; **8**: 317–23.

101 Dubick MA, Davis JM, Myers T, Wade CE, Kramer GC. Dose response effects of hypertonic saline and dextran on cardiovascular responses and plasma volume expansion in sheep. *Shock* 1995; **3**: 137–44.

102 Tollofsrud S, Elgjo GI, Prough DS, *et al*. The dynamics of vascular volume and fluid shifts of lactated Ringer's solution and hypertonic-saline-dextran solutions infused in normovolemic sheep. *Anesth Analg* 2001; **93**: 823–31.

103 Kramer GC. Hypertonic resuscitation: physiologic mechanisms and recommendations for trauma care. *J Trauma* 2003; **54**(5 Suppl): S89–99.

104 Wade CE, Dubick MA, Grady JJ. Optimal dose of hypertonic saline/dextran in hemorrhaged swine. *J Trauma* 2003; **55**: 413–6.

105 Rotstein OD. Novel strategies for immunomodulation after trauma: revisiting hypertonic saline as a resuscitation strategy for hemorrhagic shock. *J Trauma* 2000; **49**: 580–3.

106 Pruitt BA Jr. Does hypertonic burn resuscitation make a difference? *Crit Care Med* 2000; **28**: 277–8.

107 Thomas SJ, Kramer GC, Herndon DN. Burns: military options and tactical solutions. *J Trauma* 2003; **54**(5 Suppl): S207–18.

108 Kinsky MP, Milner SM, Button B, Dubick MA, Kramer GC. Resuscitation of severe thermal injury with hypertonic saline dextran: effects on peripheral and visceral edema in sheep. *J Trauma* 2000; **49**: 844–53.

109 Simma B, Burger R, Falk M, Sacher P, Fanconi S. A prospective, randomized, and controlled study of fluid management in children with severe head injury: lactated Ringer's solution versus hypertonic saline. *Crit Care Med* 1998; **26**: 1265–70.

110 Simma B, Burger R, Falk M, *et al.* The release of antidiuretic hormone is appropriate in response to hypovolemia and/or sodium administration in children with severe head injury: a trial of lactated Ringer's solution versus hypertonic saline. *Anesth Analg* 2001; **92**: 641–5.

111 Berger S, Schurer L, Hartl R, Messmer K, Baethmann A. Reduction of post-traumatic intracranial hypertension by hypertonic/hyperoncotic saline/dextran and hypertonic mannitol. *Neurosurgery* 1995; **37**: 98–107.

112 de Carvalho H, Matos JA, Bouskela E, Svensjo E. Vascular permeability increase and plasma volume loss induced by endotoxin was attenuated by hypertonic saline with or without dextran. *Shock* 1999; **12**: 75–80.

113 Mouren S, Delayance S, Mion G, *et al.* Mechanisms of increased myocardial contractility with hypertonic saline solutions in isolated blood-perfused rabbit hearts. *Anesth Analg* 1995; **81**: 777–82.

114 Kien ND, Moore PG, Pascual JM, Reitan JA, Kramer GC. Effects of hypertonic saline on regional function and blood flow in canine hearts during acute coronary occlusion. *Shock* 1997; **7**: 274–81.

115 Zallen G, Moore EE, Tamura DY, *et al.* Hypertonic saline resuscitation abrogates neutrophil priming by mesenteric lymph. *J Trauma* 2000; **48**: 45–8.

116 Ajito T, Suzuki K, Iwabuchi S. Effect of intravenous infusion of a 7.2% hypertonic saline solution on serum electrolytes and osmotic pressure in healthy beagles. *J Vet Med Sci* 1999; **61**: 637–41.

117 Sirieix D, Hongnat JM, Delayance S, *et al.* Comparison of the acute hemodynamic effects of hypertonic or colloid infusions immediately after mitral valve repair. *Crit Care Med* 1999; **27**: 2159–65.

118 Qureshi AI, Suarez JI. Use of hypertonic saline solutions in treatment of cerebral edema and intracranial hypertension. *Crit Care Med* 2000; **28**: 3301–13.

119 Riddez L, Drobin D, Sjostrand F, Svensen C, Hahn RG. Lower dose of hypertonic saline dextran reduces the risk of lethal rebleeding in uncontrolled hemorrhage. *Shock* 2002; **17**: 377–82.

120 Vassar MJ, Perry CA, Holcroft JW. Prehospital resuscitation of hypotensive trauma patients with 7.5% NaCl versus 7.5% NaCl with added dextran: a controlled trial. *J Trauma* 1993; **34**: 622–32.

121 Gan TJ, Bennett Guerrero E, *et al.* Hextend, a physiologically balanced plasma expander for large volume use in major surgery: a randomized phase III clinical trial. Hextend Study Group. *Anesth Analg* 1999; **88**: 992–8.

122 Behne M, Thomas H, Bremerich DH, *et al.* The pharmacokinetics of acetyl starch as a plasma volume expander in patients undergoing elective surgery. *Anesth Analg* 1998; **86**: 856–60.

123 Thorell A, Nygren J, Ljungqvist O. Insulin resistance: a marker of surgical stress. *Curr Opin Clin Nutr Metab Care* 1999; **2**: 69–78.

CHAPTER 16

The microcirculation

Bryce Randalls

Introduction

Study of the microcirculation in humans is extremely difficult. Much work on the function and control of the microcirculation has been performed on animals, either using preparations or using genetic knockout models (usually mice). In this chapter, a description trying to relate physiological function to the increased knowledge of microvascular mechanisms is discussed. This chapter attempts to apply the principles of these studies in a generic fashion so that an understanding of what may be happening in humans in health and disease can be gained. This is a field that is rapidly moving forward and in which the artificial separation of physiology, biochemistry and molecular biology no longer applies.

Anatomy of the microcirculation

The microcirculation is that area confined within the various organs where metabolic exchange occurs. The microcirculation represents the smallest vessels in the body. It is the site of many complex control mechanisms that have come to light over the last decade. The efficiency of metabolic exchange requires that the microcirculation is in 'diffusion distance' of the cells in each organ; thus, the vast number of cells require a vast number of capillaries to service them. Tissues with the greatest metabolic rates have the greatest capillary densities. In the systemic circulation, a microvasculature unit consists of a network of blood vessels (diameter less than 250 µm) lying between the arteries and veins. Arterioles form a diverging network of vessels ranging from 100–150 µm in diameter to terminal arterioles that approximate 10 µm in diameter; arterioles actively regulate their diameter in response to many stimuli.

Terminal arterioles supply the capillary bed, a network of diverging and converging vascular segments ranging 3–10 µm in diameter and composed of a single layer of endothelial cells. Blood draining from the capillary bed is collected by postcapillary venules which converge into large venules.

The microcirculation is responsible for regulating blood flow in individual organs and for nutrient exchange between blood and tissue. The larger arterioles are completely enveloped in vascular smooth muscle (VSM) and are responsible for regulation of distribution of the cardiac output. The terminal arterioles have discontinuous VSM; these are often termed precapillary sphincters and regulate flow to a capillary bed and are a point of control for capillary bed recruitment. They also possess sensors to monitor shear stress at the blood vessel–wall interface, and monitor circumferential stress in the vessel wall. The arteriolar network consists of cylindrical segments with decreasing diameter and length and increasing number of parallel paths. When an arteriole is dilated, its lumen is circular. During constriction the lumen changes to an irregular star-shaped cross-section (endothelial cells bulge inwards). A twofold change in dilatation can result in a 16-fold change in flow resistance. The capillaries (and postcapillary venules) are the sites of fluid exchange. They consist of a single cellular layer of endothelial cells and their basement membrane. The venules are thin but with greater cross-sectional area and often run adjacent to arterioles. Thus, the flow will be slower and the parallel arrangement may provide for countercurrent exchange (e.g. in the intestine and skin). The different microvascular beds throughout the body differ in the functions they serve and may depend on different control mechanisms.

Capillaries

Capillaries are endothelial cell tubes 6 µm in diameter interconnected by gap junctions. They are surrounded by a basement membrane made up of a collagen support matrix. This matrix interacts with the interstitium or extracellular matrix (ECM). The luminal and junctional surfaces of endothelium are endowed with a glycocalyx surface layer: a network of fibrous, membrane-embedded biomolecules that contains proteoglycans, glycoproteins and glycoaminoglycans. Attached to these are sugar chains with sialic residues stretching into the capillary lumen or the intercellular clefts. This confers the glycocalyx with a net negative electrostatic charge and selectivity of transendothelial pathways to particular molecules. The glycocalyx has an important role in modulating haemodynamic resistance and haematocrit in the capillary and acts as a molecular sieve in its interaction with the flow of plasma and erythrocytes. The glycocalyx is a dynamic structure that can change its charge and its thickness (e.g. in response to mechanical damage of the endothelial surface). The normal function of the endothelial barrier is dependent on plasma proteins. If one removes albumin almost completely from the perfusate (levels <0.1 g/L), large increases in microvascular hydraulic conductance are observed. Other plasma proteins, such as orosomucoid, seem to be needed for the maintenance of a normal capillary permeability. Capillaries in different vascular beds are heterogeneous (i.e. they have varying permeability characteristics as exhibited by the different capillary types in the body).

1 *Continuous capillaries:* form a continuous layer with narrow intercellular clefts between cells. They also contain caveolae.

2 *Fenestrated capillaries:* possess perforated pores containing a fenestrated diaphragm. The fenestrae allow almost free passage of water and low molecular solutes.

3 *Discontinuous capillaries:* consist of wide 'leaky' gaps through which proteins and erythrocytes can freely pass. They have a discontinuity in the underlying basement membrane.

The function of the capillaries is fluid and solute exchange with the interstitium bathing the cells. This is accomplished by a combination of filtration, absorption and diffusion. Only 20–25% capillaries will be open at a time, the rest being collapsed. However, because the potential total capillary surface area is approximately 700 m^2 there is considerable redundancy. When a tissue increases its activity, collapsed capillaries will open up (recruitment) and allow blood passage. Capillaries provide minimal diffusion distance from blood to tissue (less than 25 µm) and maximal opportunity for exchange.

Vascular endothelium physiology

Endothelial cells are a metabolically active monolayer exposed to biochemical and biomechanical stimuli. They exhibit an anticoagulant, anti-inflammatory and antiproliferative phenotype. They are considered a true endocrine–paracrine organ, important not only as a structural semi-permeable membrane between the circulation and surrounding tissue, but also because they maintain vascular homoeostasis; their strategic location allows them to detect changes in haemodynamic forces and blood-borne signals and 'respond' by releasing vasoactive substances, sometimes with opposite function but physiologically balanced. Thus, they have a wide variety of critical roles in control of vascular function.

Endothelial cells contain an actin-myosin cytoskeleton whose role is in cell locomotion, regulation of permeability and, via transmembrane receptors, to detect shear stress of blood flow. The actin–myosin cytoskeleton 'contracts' (more properly, changes shape) via a Ca-calmodulin action on myosin light chain kinase (MLCK). Endothelial cells are linked to each other by different types of adhesive structures or cell–cell junctions of membrane proteins (VE–cadherin, claudin, occluding, platelet–endothelial cell adhesion molecule (PECAM). These junctions are dynamic in that their mechanism of interaction can be rapidly altered by intra- and extracellular signals. These are complex structures formed by transmembrane molecules linked to the network of cytoplasmic/cytoskeletal proteins. There are two major types of junctions: adherens and tight junctions. Permeability to plasma solute is controlled by junction permeation. The organization of these junctions varies throughout the vascular tree. In brain, tight junctions (TJ) are well developed and plentiful, explaining the impermeability to plasma proteins and all but water and electrolytes. In other vascular beds, the postcapillary venules, which allow cell trafficking, TJ are few in number and poorly organized. Paracellular transport via these junctions is entirely passive (contrast with the generally active-type of transmembrane transport), is bidirectional and tends to define the degree of 'leakiness' or permeability of that tissue. In tissues where large volumes of isosmotic fluids are moved (e.g. intestine) the TJ are very leaky. In tissues where large electrosmotic gradients are generated, TJ exist (e.g. collecting ducts of kidney). The TJ do not offer completely free access but act as large pores. These junctional membrane proteins are the basis for pore size, selectivity, charge and conductance properties of the endothelial paracellular path. In some parts of the circulation, proteins called connexins join endothelium to VSM. Electrical signals may be transmitted from cell to cell via this route. Another group of proteins, which act as cell surface receptors, are the integrins. These are heterodimeric glycoproteins which provide for cell–cell adhesion as well as adhesion to the extracellular matrix. There is an increasing body of evidence that, because they bridge the extracellular environment and the cell cytoskeleton, they mediate outside-to-in, and inside-to-out signals. They may have a role in mechanotransduction, tissue injury, permeability and vascular tone.

Endothelium contains membrane-bound vesicles termed caveolae. These are connected to the endothelial cell membrane (invaginations). Transcytosis is one of the functional roles proposed for caveolae. In this process, caveolae transport macromolecules from the luminal side of the blood vessel to the subendothelial space. Transcytosis can be both constitutive (e.g. fluid phase transport) and receptor-mediated (the molecule transported requires the presence of its cognate receptor in caveolae — albumin binds to a membrane protein, albondin, which is present in all capillary beds except brain, and initiates endocytosis of albumin). Caveolae-mediated transcytosis is an important mechanism of transendothelial transport of albumin and of albumin-conjugated nutrients, fatty acids and hormones across the endothelial barrier. Thus, macromolecules move from the blood to interstitial fluid through the cell.

Endothelium also contains large numbers of ion-sensitive channels and pores. Many of these result in calcium entry that, via its action on signal pathways, can alter the actin-myosin cytoskeleton. Endothelial cells have a major role in the regulation of vascular tone, through production of several vasoactive mediators. Nitric oxide, prostacyclin, endothelin (ET) and endothelial-derived hyperpolarizing factor are powerful vasoactive substances released from the endothelium in response to both humoral and mechanical stimuli, and can profoundly affect both the function and structure of the underlying VSM. Both type II (cytokine inducible) and type III (endothelial constitutive) nitric oxide synthase (NOS), which catalyse the conversion of L-arginine to nitric oxide, are found in endothelial cells (Fig. 16.1). Constitutive production of nitric oxide by the endothelium modulates vascular tone. In the endothelium, caveolin-1 regulates nitric oxide signalling by binding to and inhibiting type III NOS; increased cytosolic calcium or activation of a particular kinase leads to NOS activation and its dissociation from caveolin-1.

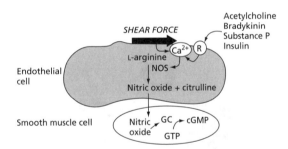

Figure 16.1 Nitric oxide synthase (NOS) type III catalyses the production of nitric oxide from the cationic amino acid L-arginine. The enzyme is activated via changes in intracellular calcium in response to changes in shear forces or via a receptor-mediated process. Released nitric oxide activates soluble guanylate cyclase (GC) in smooth muscle cells, converting guanosine triphosphate (GTP) to cyclic guanosine monophosphate (cGMP). This activates a protein kinase that leads to the inhibition of calcium influx into the smooth muscle cell, and decreased calcium-calmodulin stimulation of myosin light chain kinase. This in turn decreases the phosphorylation of myosin light chains, decreasing smooth muscle tension development and causing vasodilatation. Reproduced with permission from Galley and Webster [1].

Extracellular matrix

The ECM is a structural complex composed mainly of glycoproteins and proteoglycans, which supports and secures cells in the tissues (Fig. 16.2). It can be imagined as a complex aggregation of protein fibres and carbohydrate polymers. The ECM links together to make a solid matrix entangled in a network of collagen fibres. These proteins are all negatively charged. The matrix is able to take up fluid. This combination of proteoglycans and entrapped fluid has the characteristics of a gel and is termed the interstitial fluid. It has an inherent tendency to expand (the electrostatic charges of each fibre causes them to repel each other) when given free access to fluid, a result primarily of the hyaluronan content. This negative charge results in attraction of positive ions (e.g. Na) which sets up via the Gibbs–Donnan effect, an osmotic pressure. This pressure drives the ECM to uptake fluid. This tendency to swell is counteracted by the collagen network interaction with β_1 integrins secreted by fibroblasts, which prevents the matrix proteins uncoiling. The fibroblasts in the ECM affect the gel's swelling characteristics by generating a 'restraining' tension. Any factor causing the integrin to 'decouple'

from the collagen framework allows the interstitial pressure to decrease. The gel itself gives organs and tissues of the body their characteristic shape and protects against impact forces. It also prevents water flowing downwards due to gravity. It has a role in limiting the spread of infection because particles of bacterial size cannot move in the gel. Bacteria such as streptococci, which secrete hyaluronidase, convert the gel into a fluid state, enabling free access. The ECM is subject to constant remodelling (degradation and resynthesis) primarily by matrix metalloproteinases (MMP) which have physiological roles relating to cell behaviour.

The fluid pressure within the gel is negative, such that the cells of the tissue are 'sucked' together and the connective tissue binds firmly around them, retaining a rigid shape (Fig. 16.3). The negative free fluid pressure is generated from the oncotic pressure across the capillary wall and the 'suction' effect of the lymphatics returning fluid to the circulation. Under normal conditions, the interstitial space has a net negative pressure of approximately 3 mmHg. This means that most of our body is held together by a vacuum in the interstitial space. It is neither collagen nor elastin fibres that provide most of the support that keeps tissues firm and of 'normal' consistency but the negative interstitial pressure present in most organs and tissues. If you 'tent' the skin on the back of the hand of a severely dehydrated patient and watch it just sit there standing bolt upright you can begin to grasp the concept of 'net negative interstitial pressure'.

Almost all of the water in the interstitium is present in a gel form because it is bound into the proteogly-

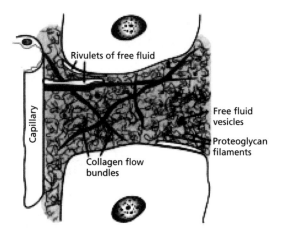

Figure 16.2 The interstitial space between the capillary and the tissue is composed of proteoglycan filaments arranged in a tight non-compliant matrix. Free flow of fluid across the space is limited and occurs through tiny rivulets and vesicles. Reproduced with permission from Guyton and Hall [2].

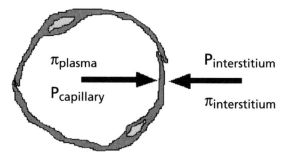

Figure 16.3 Balance between hydrostatic (P) and oncotic (π) pressures within the capillary and interstitium.

can biopolymer brushpile that interweaves between cells. Under normal conditions, virtually no pockets of free or 'unbound' water of more than a few hundredths of a micron in diameter exist. There are small rivulets in the interstitium where fluid can flow freely but this accounts for <1% of the space. Thus, there is a very substantial barrier to free flow of ultrafiltered fluid from the capillaries through the interstitium to the cells. Both the proteoglycan fibres and the collagen filaments that permeate the interstitial spaces not only slow the flow of capillary filtrate, but also act to evenly distribute that flow over the cells. The entangled gel offers resistance to water and solute convective flow and movement is by diffusion.

The interstitium can be divided into two phases: the interstitial fluid and the structural molecules of the extracellular matrix. The latter can be imagined as a three-dimensional network or mesh. The presence of all these macromolecules results in 'crowding'. The constituents of the ECM (e.g. glycosaminoglycans) are negatively charged and further 'exclude' proteins such as albumin. The fluid space available for diffusing species is then less than the total interstitial volume. This steric exclusion effect tends to retard movement of proteins through the interstitium but has minimal effects on water, ion and small solutes.

Lymphatics

Lymphatics in the tissues are likened to blind-ending sacs of endothelial cells tethered loosely together. They are highly permeable, possessing large intercellular pores, which freely accept proteins and fluid. Their function is to clear the interstitium of excess fluid, proteins, lipids and foreign material. Tissue filtrate enters the afferent lymphatic capillaries and because of the presence of valves, smooth muscle and the body's muscle pump, unidirectional flow occurs to the lymph node and onwards via efferent lymphatic vessels to the thoracic duct and return to the circulation. The lymphatic system is, in effect, a sump pump for the tissues, always attempting to propel excess free fluid away from the tissue spaces. Because their walls are attached to the surrounding tissue they tend not to collapse. The lymphatics are

the only mechanism for movement and return of proteins from the interstitial fluid to the circulation. The rate of lymph flow appears to be controlled by the interstitial fluid pressure — the higher the pressure, the higher the lymph flow. Interstitial pressure is influenced by the capillary filtration rate. Normal lymphatic capillaries are tightly adherent to the proteoglycan and collagen brushpile. When this brushpile expands as fluid accumulates, pressure is exerted on the smallest (terminal) ends of the lymphatics and the pores are opened. The frequency of contractions seems to be determined mainly by the amount of fluid in the lymph vessel. When a segment of vessel immediately below a valve becomes distended, it contracts, and the fluid is pushed forward beyond the valve. The excess filling on the upstream side of this value causes the next segment of the lymphatic vessel to contract, thus propelling the fluid forward to another segment. Each segment of lymphatic vessel operates as a separate individual pump and is responsive to the amount of lymph that fills its chamber. Thus, the lymphatic pump activity is defined as active propulsion mechanisms of lymph mediated by rhythmical spontaneous contractions of lymphatic smooth muscles. The larger lymphatics can generate (through peristalsis and native one-way valves) negative pressures of 30 mmHg, and actively pump excess interstitial water in this way.

Mechanism of capillary exchange

Fluid, electrolytes, gases, small and large molecular weight substances traverse the capillary endothelium via different mechanisms. Crossing from the inside to outside of the capillary endothelium can occur by several methods. Non-polar compounds and water can freely diffuse through the cell (transcellular). Movement through intercellular clefts allows water, electrolytes and small molecules access to the interstitial fluid (paracellular). Intracellular vesicles (caveolae) that allow protein and macromolecules to cross through the cell but topologically remain outside it.

Active transport
This is seldom an exchange mechanism between blood and interstitium.

Diffusive flux

Diffusion is the principal mechanism for exchange of oxygen, nutrients and metabolic waste (small solutes). It is the net effect of random movement of small ions and molecules brought about by their thermodynamic energy. Two or more substances can move in opposite directions without affecting each other (e.g. O_2 and CO_2). It is very rapid over small distances for small molecules; for example, the rate at which water molecules diffuse through the capillary membrane is approximately 80 times as great as the rate at which plasma itself flows linearly along the capillary (i.e. water in the plasma is exchanged 80 times as it travels the length of the capillary). It is an extremely poor transfer mechanism over distances >25 μm. The relationship between concentration and rate of flux is described by Fick's Law:

$$Js = PA (Cp - Ct)$$

Solute flux = permeability × surface area × plasma to tissue concentration difference.

Lipid-soluble solutes (e.g. oxygen or anaesthetic gases) can diffuse across the entire capillary surface. The permeability depends on their oil–water partition coefficient.

Small lipid-insoluble solutes, such as sodium ions and glucose, cannot cross the plasma membrane by diffusion, and move across the capillary wall primarily through small pores, probably existing as junctions between endothelial cells. The driving force may be a concentration or electrical gradient (or both). Endothelial cells have 'looser' junctions (contrast epithelial cells) which allow for significant transcellular flow when subjected to a pressure difference. The fibre matrix structure of the glycocalyx poses a barrier to proteins such as albumin. The size and shape of these pores relative to the size of the solute determine the permeability of the wall to that solute. The pores are modelled to be approximately 15–20 nm in diameter in continuous capillaries, they are 1000 nm long and described as being a tortuous cylinder. They occupy less than 0.5% of the capillary surface area.

The permeability of a membrane to a particular solute (P) depends upon the size of the pores in the membrane (radius r), relative to size of the molecule (radius a), the length of the pores (dx, related, but not equal to the thickness of the membrane), the restricted diffusion coefficient of the solute (D′) and the area of the pores relative to the total surface area of the cell membrane (Ap/AT).

$$P = (D' Ap) \Phi (dxAT)$$

where $\Phi = (r - a)^2 / 2r$: the equilibrium partition coefficient. This is a measure of the size of the molecule relative to that of the pore. A high value for Φ means that the molecule is much smaller than the pore and the area available for diffusion within the pore is almost equal to the area of the pore. If Φ is low then the molecule is similar in size to the pore, and therefore the effective size of the pore is smaller than its actual size. *The permeability of a membrane to a solute therefore decreases with increasing solute size.* If the permeability is high, and flow is slow, as the blood passes from the arterial to the venous end of a capillary, the concentration difference decreases, so reducing solute flux. In this case, solute flux is flow limited. A decrease in flow through an individual capillary will therefore limit solute delivery.

Large lipid-insoluble molecules larger than small proteins (10 000 kDa) have a much lower permeability than smaller molecular weight solutes. Albumin, for example, has a diameter of 7 nm, and is therefore almost the same size as the small pores. However, larger molecules >10 nm diameter do cross the capillary wall and have a low, but measurable, permeability. Endocytosis via caveolae appears to be the primary method of their transport. If the permeability is low, there is no great change in Cp–Ct as the blood passes through an individual capillary. Solute flux is limited by the diffusive capacity of the molecule through the membrane and is described as diffusion limited.

Convective flux

Convective flux or bulk flow occurs through pores and intercellular clefts (especially in glomerular capillaries) and follows Poiseuille's equation. The rate of flow of water depends on the balance of pressures inside and outside the capillaries, and their permeability to water. There is a hydrostatic pressure inside the capillaries (Pc; generated by the action of the heart) which must be counteracted by another pressure holding fluid in the blood vessels. This is the oncotic pressure exerted by the plasma proteins (to which the capillaries are not highly permeable). Remembering that there is also an interstitial colloid oncotic pressure and an interstitial tissue pressure (Pi) we can describe filtration rate (Jv) in terms given in the Starling equation (see below).

Oncotic reflection coefficient σ is the probability that a particular molecule will bounce off the sides of a pore rather than go through it: $\sigma = (1 - \Phi)^2$. If the molecule is close to the same size as the pore (e.g. albumin) then it will have a high reflection coefficient (0.95–0.98). If the molecule is larger than the pore then it will have a reflection coefficient of 1.0. If the molecule was very much smaller than the pore (e.g. Na$^+$) then it will have a reflection coefficient close to zero (0.05–0.1).

Solvent drag (also referred to as convective flux) is when water moves through pores it will drag solutes with it. It will in effect increase the velocity of the solute in one direction. For small solutes this will have a negligible effect on solute flux because the additional flux is so small compared with the diffusive flux. For large molecules, however, solvent drag may be a very significant contribution to solute flux. Solvent drag can be calculated as:

Js (conv) = Jv (1 − σ) Cp.

If we include both diffusive and convective fluxes, we can estimate total solute flux.

Js = PA (Cp − Ct) + Jv (1 − σ) Cp

It can be seen from this that for molecules to which P is very low, solute flux is heavily dependent on filtration rate.

The interstitial protein concentration sets the interstitial colloid oncotic pressure, and therefore influences filtration rate. However, interstitial protein concentration is itself set by capillary pressure. Interstitial protein concentration (in mg/mL) depends on the mass of protein crossing the capillary wall (mg/min, solute flux) divided by the volume of fluid crossing the capillary wall (mL/min, filtration rate). If filtration rate increases, the volume of fluid will go up and so protein concentration will go down (solute flux will also go up, but not by as much as a result of reflection of protein molecules at the wall). Con-

versely, if filtration rate decreases then interstitial protein concentration will go up. *If filtration rate falls to zero, then the interstitial protein concentration will rise to equal the plasma protein concentration.*

Throughout most capillary beds there is a continuous overproduction of interstitial fluid (i.e. a net filtration rate into the tissue). This is because the capillary pressure is usually higher than the oncotic pressure difference through most, or all, of the capillary bed. The fraction of plasma filtered per transit is actually very small. The extra fluid that is formed during filtration is removed by the lymphatic system. This drainage ensures that interstitial volume remains stable. However, as net filtration rate increases, lymph flow increases in concert. Eventually, maximal lymph flow is reached. The lymphatics cannot pump any more fluid, the tissue swells and tissue pressure increases. This is oedema.

Transcapillary solute exchange

Hydrostatic and osmotic forces dictate movement of fluid between different compartments of the body across semi-permeable membranes (Fig. 16.3). These forces are described by the Starling equation:

Flow per unit area (J) = L [(Pc − Pt) − σ (πc − πt)]

where L is hydraulic conductivity (degree of permeability of the capillary); Pc is capillary hydrostatic (blood) pressure; Pt is tissue (interstitial fluid) hydrostatic pressure; σ is plasma protein reflection coefficient (varies between different tissues, muscle 0.5, brain 1.0); πc is capillary colloid osmotic pressure; and πt is tissue colloid osmotic pressure.

In health, the net intracapillary pressures are greater than the interstitial pressures, resulting in a pressure gradient that produces a slow continuous flow of fluid from capillary lumen to interstitium, predominantly the perimicrovascular space. This tissue or interstitial fluid drains via the lymphatic system back into the systemic circulation. Capillary hydrostatic pressure falls from approximately 30 mmHg at the arterial end to 15 mmHg at the venous end. The major contribution to the osmotic gradient is the difference in protein and colloid concentration on each side of the endothelium. Protein transfer occurs as described above. Some may occur via gap junctions between cells in health, and this certainly becomes more important in states of capillary leak. Over time, this leads to a net movement of colloid into the interstitium. The second part of the Starling equation is therefore modified by the protein reflection coefficient, σ. This has a value between 0 and 1, and represents the degree to which the membrane prevents the transfer of colloid molecules. Zero indicates free passage of molecules, and 1 represents total impermeability to that colloid. Organ beds have different σ-values. In most capillaries it has a value of 0.95 in relation to plasma proteins, while the pulmonary capillaries have a value of 0.7. The implication is that pulmonary capillaries are inherently more 'leaky' than those in the systemic circulation. The higher interstitial protein protects the lung against oedema formation. The Starling equation has unmeasurable quantities which are interdependent on each other. It should be used with caution in explaining fluid exchange in pathological states. Basically, there is a net driving force for fluid to permeate through the microvascular network (net filtration pressure, NFP) based on the sum of hydrostatic pressures, sum of oncotic pressures and the conductivity of the capillary wall. Capillary pressures average 20–30 mmHg (but vary depending on location, e.g. kidney 60 mmHg, lung 10 mmHg). However, NFP is often found to equal only 1 mmHg.

Contrary to most physiology textbooks, the sum of the hydrostatic and oncotic forces across the capillary membrane results in continual filtration of fluid out of the capillary into the interstitium. It has been found that there is a greater formation of afferent lymph consistent with no reabsorption in the postcapillary venules. The capillaries of all tissues (except brain) are to some degree 'leaky', allowing proteins to move from the circulation to the interstitium. This results in the oncotic forces favouring fluid reabsorption being much less than expected. Similarly, the protein reflection coefficient, σ, reduces the expected oncotic pressure gradient. Further, tissue pressure being negative favours fluid transit into the tissues. The net fluid filtration pressure along a skeletal muscle capillary is approximately 1 mmHg. This results in a net fluid filtration of 12 L/day or a rate of body interstitial fluid turnover in 30 hours.

It has recently been suggested that interstitial oncotic pressure is more important for fluid exchange in most microvascular beds. It is thought that fluid and proteins cross capillary walls by separate routes and the extravascular protein concentration that matters is that in the endothelial intercellular space between the glycocalyx and the tight junction (i.e. there is an oncotic asymmetry). The gradient that determines fluid movement is not between blood and tissue but between the immediate environments of the paracellular cleft. The glycocalyx represents the primary barrier to albumin and other protein movement. At the entrance to the interendothelial cleft, the contribution to flow from the oncotic pressure drop is balanced by the hydrostatic pressure drop. Hence, net flow will be close to zero. Only when capillary pressure exceeds this oncotic pressure across the cleft will there be significant flow into the surrounding interstitial space. This mechanism can act to rapidly attenuate increases in tissue fluid volume caused by sudden increases in capillary hydrostatic pressure. It also can explain that any factor causing a breakdown or separation in the junctions between endothelial cells (increasing cleft size) would dissipate the oncotic gradient and increase transcapillary fluid flux.

The excluded volume of proteins (see above) has important consequences in the dynamics of transcapillary exchange. Albumin (which is responsible for 80% of the oncotic pressure of plasma) is excluded from a large part of the interstitium. This results in the effective concentration of albumin in the interstitium being higher than if it was assumed that all the interstitial fluid was available. As a consequence a more rapid approach to steady-state flow occurs after a change in transcapillary fluid flux (a form of autoregulation). It also implies less transfer of protein to plasma for a given increase in capillary filtration. This principle of interstitial steric exclusion thus acts to influence plasma volume.

There are situations where sustained absorption from interstitial fluid into capillaries does occur. In these situations (kidney, gastrointestinal tract, lymph nodes) the interstitium has a second fluid supply that is able to 'wash away' proteins whose oncotic pressure would increase and oppose absorption.

Control of blood flow in capillaries

Cells respond to their fluid-dynamic environment (e.g. endothelial cells align in the direction of flow). Many of the biological functions of cells are controlled by fluid-dynamic forces. These forces consist of the viscous drag that is generated at the luminal surface of endothelial cells by the streaming blood (wall shear stress) acting parallel to the vessel wall and the cyclic strain of the vascular wall that results from pulsatile changes in blood pressure. The entire endothelial cytoskeleton is under a given tension, even in the absence of an external stimulus. Shear stress or stretch at the endothelial cell surface redistributes these forces across the entire cell so that a stimulus at the cell surface is translated into a chemical signal at the end of a filament or fibre, be it within caveolae, in the vicinity of the cell–cell adhesion points or within the integrin-rich focal adhesion contacts that anchor the cell to the basal membrane.

The cellular constituents of blood influence the rheological properties of whole blood especially in the microcirculation where the diameter of the blood vessel becomes comparable to that of the cell. The microvascular network of an organ is fractal, exhibiting self-similarity and with distance downstream, the vessel diameter and length follow a power-law relationship. This results in a pressure gradient that is most pronounced in the arterioles where the ratio of wall thickness to lumen diameter is greatest. This (anatomical) arrangement enables blood flow regulation primarily by diameter change. At this level of the arteriolar network, where the pressure gradient is steepest, is the region where the greatest active changes in diameter occur.

Blood is a concentrated suspension, consisting of erythrocytes (biconcave discs of 7 µm diameter), leucocytes (a typical neutrophil is circular with a 8-µm diameter) and platelets (discoids of 2 µm diameter). The suspending fluid, or plasma, contains ions and macromolecules up to 1000 kDa. Flow behaviour in the microcirculation is complex because of the branching geometry of the microvascular network, the glycocalyx coating endothelium and the expression of cell receptors that can interact with cells in the blood therefore retarding their flow. In the setting of inflammation, the leucocytes vacate the central or axial stream to the periphery where they come into close mechanical contact to and interact with the endothelial cells. This may induce a strain-dependent increase in matrix permeability which may be important when the leucocyte compresses the layer of glycocalyx.

Erythrocytes tend to form aggregates that can reversibly disaggregate under influence of shear forces. Reduction of viscosity with increased shear rate is termed shear thinning. Erythrocyte aggregation and their ability to deform is a major determinant of blood shear-thinning. This partly accounts for the viscosity minima of blood at capillary diameters of 7 µm, and the observation of red blood cells traversing capillaries in 'single file'.

The glycocalyx or endothelial surface layer (ESL) is increasingly being seen as an important determinant of flow and function control in the capillary. The ESL thickness (0.5–1 µm) depends on local shearing forces and their nature (laminar, turbulent or pulsatile). The composition of the glycocalyx results from a balance of the rate of biosynthesis of glycosoaminoglycans by the endothelial cell, and their removal, which may be mediated by intracellular and/or membrane-bound proteases released or activated by G-protein signalling. This physiological regulation may be lost in inflammation where leucocytes cause not only 'shedding' of the ESL but also by plugging the capillary can induce significant flow changes in the microvasculature.

Activation of leucocytes results in a dramatic increase in microvascular resistance. The expression of adhesion molecules by endothelium causes leucocytes to roll, adhere, then migrate through paracellular pathways. This may cause local obstruction or reduction of capillary flow.

Capillaries are the sites of oxygen supply to the tissues and act as a large surface area–volume system. This delivery of oxygen depends on capillary density, erythrocyte capillary transit time and geometrical distribution of the capillary network. Only 5% of blood volume is in capillaries at any one time. Yet this is its most important role. In the 'average' capillary, flow velocity is 70 mm/s and erythrocyte transit time is 1–2 s, giving adequate time for diffusion to occur. Transfer is multiphase (haemoglobin to plasma, through capillary wall, through interstitium to cell). However, with tissue oedema and cell swelling, oxygen delivery may become diffusion-limited. Diffusive flux from capillary to tissue is given by:

$$QO_2/dt \propto ppO_2 \, (R2 - R1)$$

where R1 is the capillary radius; R2 is the distance to cell; and ppO_2 is the oxygen partial pressure.

Diffusive oxgyen transport between two sites depends on the difference of tissue and blood oxgyen tensions. Oxgyen diffusion, however, is not the process once envisaged, occurring for example only in a capillary bed. Oxygen diffusion also occurs from capillaries to neighbouring capillaries. And, in addition to their role in convective oxgyen transport, arterioles also function as a diffusive source of oxgyen that serves to replenish that lost from the red blood cells as they move along the capillaries. Therefore, while the capillary bed is the primary site of oxgyen exchange within tissues, oxgyen exchange with surrounding tissues occurs in the arteriolar tree, thus leading to a precapillary fall in haemoglobin oxgyen saturation. Reoxygenation of erythrocytes flowing through capillaries by diffusion from nearby arterioles helps provide homogeneous tissue oxygenation despite heterogeneous capillary blood flows.

It is estimated that only 20–25% of available capillaries are perfused in ambient conditions. In stress situations, however, capillaries can be recruited to maintain metabolic homoeostasis. Microcirculatory blood flow is regulated actively by changes in vascular resistance and perfusion pressures, originating from parent arterioles, and alterations of vascular tone within the capillary network. Blood flow within the microcirculation may also exhibit passive control; for example, when influenced by rheologic influences and network geometry (the latter may vary considerably between tissues). Microcirculatory blood flow is typically non-uniform; both temporal heterogeneity (changes over time) and spatial heterogeneity (differences between vessels) of capillary flow are common. Capillary flow heterogeneity is lessened by metabolic stress and increasing erythrocyte supply to the tissue.

Blood flow in the microcirculation is regulated by physiological oxygen gradients which are coupled to vasoconstriction or vasodilatation. This function is usually ascribed to nitric oxide (NO) bioactivity (see

below). Thionitrites, (oxidative formation of NO and sulphydryl groups) including both low molecular weight nitrosothiol (SNO) derivatives of cysteine and glutathione, and also S-nitrosylated proteins such as S-nitrosoalbumin, are among the most potent vasodilatory compounds known. Previously, haemoglobin was seen as a scavenger of NO, inactivating it and forming an Hb-Fe(II)-NO nitrate complex. This only occurs when haemoglobin is free and not compartmentalized within the red blood cell. However, haemoglobin is among the blood proteins that sustain S-nitrosylation, and S-nitrosylated haemoglobin (SNO-Hb) formation is competitive with and/or circumvents the Fe(II)-NO nitrate-forming reaction and concomitant loss of NO bioactivity.

S-nitrosylation of human haemoglobin is linked *in vivo* to oxgyen saturation and occurs at β-Cys-93 of haemoglobin. The reactivity of cysteine toward NO is dependent on the quaternary structure of the haemoglobin tetramer. SNO-Hb forms preferentially in the oxygenated (or R) structure of haemoglobin, whereas conditions favouring deoxygenated or T structure, such as low P_{O_2}, favour release of NO groups. The circulating levels of SNO-Hb are thus partly dependent on the O_2 saturation-governing equilibrium between T and R structures, and not on the P_{O_2}. Crystal structures and molecular models of SNO-Hb provide a rational stereochemical basis for allosterically regulated dispensing of NO bioactivity. Thus, whereas cys-thiol has no access to solvent in R state (and therefore could not dilate blood vessels), it protrudes into solvent in the deoxygenated (or T) structure. Thus, erythrocytes provide a novel NO vasodilator activity in which haemoglobin acts as an oxygen sensor and oxygen-responsive NO signal transducer. S-nitroso haemoglobin has an important role regulating both peripheral and pulmonary vascular tone. Red cell derived relaxing activity may be responsible for autoregulation of blood flow and oxgyen delivery. It appears that SNO can contribute to regulation of vascular resistance under basal conditions and its dysregulation in disorders characterized by tissue oxgyen deficits such as endotoxic shock. This mechanism can also explain the vasoconstriction that occurs during hyperbaric oxgyen treatment.

Central mechanisms of control

Fluid flux through the tissues is controlled by an autoregulatory mechanism (Starling equation) that acts to maintain a steady state. There must also be additional controls to meet, in a coordinated fashion, the functional requirements of that organ. It is known that, as flow through the capillary increases, there is a flow-dependent increase in permeability. Nutrient exchange in the microcirculation is controlled by changes in capillary density. As this increases, the cross-sectional area available for diffusion is also increased and the 'effective' radius increases, resulting in a marked decrease in flow velocity and increased transit time for erythrocytes in the capillaries. Efficient tissue exchange will thus depend on the matching of open capillaries to the metabolic needs of the tissue.

Certain regulatory adjustments of the smooth muscle tone in arterial and venous microvessels are essential for the internal fluid balance in the body by their specific control of net capillary fluid transfer. There are two main objects of the biological control mechanisms that govern this homoeostatic process: some serve to induce net transcapillary fluid shifts with the primary aim of controlling plasma volume (e.g. in hypo- and hypervolaemia); others serve to prevent untoward fluid transfer, as during hydrostatic capillary load or alteration of arterial or venous pressure. The control mechanisms can be at the level of capillary pressure, at the level of interstitium and at the level of the endothelial cell.

On a 'macro' level, blood pressure in the capillaries (Pc is the mean capillary hydrostatic pressure) is determined by upstream arterial pressure (Pa), venous pressure (Pv), and the ratio of postcapillary to precapillary resistance (r_v/r_a) according to the relationship:

$$Pc = \frac{(r_v/r_a)\,Pa + Pv}{1 + (r_v/r_a)}$$

Thus, elevations of arterial pressure, venous pressure or (r_v/r_a) will produce elevations of Pc (a given rise in Pv increases Pc approximately five times the same rise in Pa). Thus, any mechanism which influences either the pre- or postcapillary resistance or

venous pressure may have a profound effect on the capillary pressure and hence transcapillary fluid flux. Under normal physiologic conditions, $(r_v/r_a) \sim 5$ (i.e. in the upright position). In the motionless limb, the ratio (r_v/r_a) increases to about 20 and can lead to oedema formation in the motionless limb. Certain vasomotor reactions, mainly neurogenic ones, contribute to the active regulation of plasma volume by inducing redistributions of fluid between the intra- and extravascular compartments (i.e. net absorption of extravascular fluid into the blood stream during a period of reduced plasma volume and ultrafiltration into the tissues during overfilling of the circulatory system). Capillary pressure, Pc, is the only Starling variable under neurogenic control. Only skeletal muscle and skin, which contain a total interstitial fluid 'reserve' of some 6 L and an intracellular fluid volume of about 16 L, participate in such centrally controlled plasma volume adjustments. They have a large total extravascular fluid volume, their tissue functions are not impaired by even extensive fluid withdrawal, and they are not enclosed by rigid structures which otherwise could limit fluid transfer by pronounced alteration of tissue pressure. This mechanism does not occur in internal organs. Adrenergic nerve fibre excitation constricts the resistance and capacitance vessels, resulting in continuous net transcapillary absorption of extravascular fluid into the blood stream. This is because of a reduction in hydrostatic capillary pressure, and in turn because of a decrease in (r_v/r_a). The rate of such fluid absorption is related to the frequency of nerve excitation. During acute severe haemorrhage this reflex absorption of interstitial fluid from the muscles into the blood stream can occur at the rate of nearly 0.5 L during the first hour of haemorrhagic hypotension. This important plasma volume control, mediated by nervous and also humoral adrenergic mechanisms, seems to be reinforced by a neurogenic β-adrenergic dilator mechanism. The α-adrenergic constrictor mechanism controls capillary pressure via a decrease in r_v/r_a. The reflex β-adrenergic mechanism simultaneously controls the size of the functional capillary surface area by a preferential dilator effect on the smallest precapillary vessels, which in skeletal muscle function as 'sphincters'. The resulting increase in functional capillary surface area in face of a reflexly decreased capillary pressure can facilitate the fluid absorption process markedly. This control of capillary fluid transfer occurs only in skeletal muscle and only at blood pressure levels below the autoregulatory threshold.

Local mechanisms of control

The myogenic response is the autoreflex contraction of VSM when it is stretched. This stabilizes blood flow and capillary filtration in situations of changing blood pressure. When pressure rises in the VSM surrounding an arteriole, a stretch-sensitive cation channel opens which activates an L-type calcium channel and simultaneously activates protein kinase C to increase the cell actinomyosin sensitivity to calcium. The tone in the cell is maintained by a calcium-activated K channel that acts to hyperpolarize the cell and thus minimize the depolarization driving contraction. This mechanism is of importance in blood flow autoregulation. The intracellular concentration of ATP is a determinant to activate and deactivate potassium-ATP (K-ATP) channels. These are located in the plasma membrane of cells including vascular and non-VSM cells and participate in the regulation of the membrane potential. Thus, ATP produced by respiratory activity and metabolic demand in the cells may contribute to feedback mechanisms that control cell functions through an activation of KATP channels and hence membrane electrical activity. Although metabolites are very effective in small terminal arterioles, an accumulation of metabolites alone cannot reduce vascular resistance sufficiently to coordinate the behaviour of upstream and downstream vessel and additional mechanisms are necessary to achieve an adequate conductance down to the tissue supplied by certain capillaries. Such a mechanism is the conducted dilatation, which most probably is based on an electrotonic propagation of local changes in membrane potential via connexion membrane proteins. Conduction of such signals from capillaries to upstream resistance vessels and between downstream arterioles and upstream vessels has been described to have considerable mechanical length constants.

A second mechanism with potential coordinating properties is the 'flow-dependent dilatation' which is caused by a shear stress-induced tonic production of NO by endothelial cells in most tissues. Any dilatation of upstream arterioles will increase flow to some extent and, by the concomitant increase of shear stress, an NO-mediated dilatation of downstream vessels will be subsequently induced. Tonic production of NO by endothelial cells due to shear stress, acts on the VSM to alter flow. This mechanism appears to be important in dilating the supply arteries upstream to an organ, when the arterioles within the organ dilate in response to a rise in other vasodilator signals within the organ itself. Use of L-NMMA (L-N-monomethylarginine), an NO synthase inhibitor, results in an increase in blood pressure with a marked reduction in blood flow. An increase of wall shear stress is an adequate stimulus for the augmentation of endothelial NO release, with increasing flow. The following dilatation tends to bring back the wall shear stress to initial values. The basic mechanism of translation of a mechanical force into biochemical events is still not clear. Shear stress increases intracellular free calcium. This leads to an increase of NO synthesis because type I NOS is a calcium/calmodulin-dependent enzyme. Endothelial NO thus has an important role in coupling resistance and flow in the arterial tree to ensure that demand ensures supply. The shear-induced augmentation of NO release also represents an important mechanism to oppose pressure-induced myogenic constrictions which would otherwise tend to reduce tissue perfusion in a self-augmenting, negative feedback loop. In endothelial cells, mechanotransduction may not occur via a single pathway; rather it reflects the integrated response of multiple signalling networks that are spatially organized throughout the cell. The final effect is a coordinated dilatation along the vascular tree that results in an adaptation of the overall vascular conductance to the new flow load. Because this is a positive feedback mechanism, it is possible that 'preferential flow channels' may be established while other vessels running in parallel may be relatively underperfused ('steal phenomenon'). Therefore additional coordinating mechanisms, especially between different branches of a vessel, are necessary. The above mentioned 'conducted dilatation' may represent such a mechanism.

Tissue metabolism and activity is intrinsically linked to tissue flow. Acidosis, hypoxia, adenosine, K, PO_4 and hyperosmolality can all cause arteriolar dilatation. The importance of each will vary in different tissues and the mechanism while not fully elucidated will probably be similar to above.

Erythrocytes provide a novel NO vasodilator activity in which haemoglobin acts as an oxygen sensor and oxygen-responsive NO signal transducer, influencing vascular tone. There appears to be a pivotal role for SNO haemoglobin in mediating this response and in red cell derived relaxing activity in autoregulation of blood flow and oxgyen delivery (see above).

The increase in vascular permeability is a key early event in an acute inflammatory process. A number of mediators are known to be involved including histamine, 5-hydroxytryptamine (5-HT) and bradykinin, prostaglandins and nitric oxide, followed by entire families of inflammatory cytokines and growth factors. These can be divided into early (preformed) and late (process-induced) mediators. Early mediators, such as histamine and 5-HT, are released quickly in response to an injury because they are preformed and stored in cells. Early mediators also trigger amplification of the signal by synergizing with different, late-phase mediators. Other mediators, including the pro-inflammatory cytokines interleukin-1 and tumour necrosis factor α induce enzymes such as inducible type II NOS (iNOS) and cyclo-oxygenase 2 (COX-2). Nitric oxide and prostanoids produced by these enzymes are involved in increasing vascular flow and permeability.

In a single vascular bed, flow is determined by a combination of the above neural, humoral and local factors. In differing beds, the influence of each will have a varying degree of importance and may well change over time. It appears that control hierarchy is from the bottom up such that local control is the most dominant. Various control mechanisms may override others, especially during times of stress. Thus, heterogeneous responses are to be expected. For example, most vascular beds exhibit autoregulation to maintain a constant Pc. The pulmonary vascular bed does not.

Changes in transcapillary flux

Starling's view of the passive nature of microvascular exchange has been firmly established. Blood–tissue fluid balance is governed by forces generated within the capillary, interstitial and lymphatic compartments. The ECM and myogenic lymph pump automatically control transcapillary fluid movement. The physicochemical properties of the ECM determine the pressure and compliance of the interstitial spaces. In addition, the dependence of interstitial protein exclusion on matrix hydration amplifies the extent of oncotic buffering induced by interstitial volume alterations. Distension of lymph vessels elicits increases in contraction frequency, stroke volume and lymph flow. Thus, the rate of lymphatic removal of interstitial water and protein is geared to the state of hydration of the interstitial matrix. These interstitial and lymphatic compensatory reactions are important safety components in prevention of oedema formation. It has become appreciated that although microvascular exchange is passive, the interstitial pressure and permeability coefficients that determine how much solute and fluid is exchanged are actively regulated under both physiological and pathological conditions.

Change in interstitial fluid pressure

The interstitium has been regarded as having minimal effect on transcapillary fluid flux and regarded as less important than changes in the endothelial barrier permeability. However, interstitial fluid pressure changes are undoubtedly interrelated with those of the endothelium. The interstitial fluid volume is fairly constant at ~20% of body weight. It is maintained at this level by the interstitial fluid's linear compliance at normal tissue pressure. Thus, as fluid accumulates in the interstitium there is only a small increase in interstitial fluid pressure which will act against further fluid influx. Linked with the increased flow in the lymphatics, a buffering mechanism thus exists to minimize oedema formation in the tissues. At a state of overhydration, the fibrillar proteins in the extracellular matrix are extended resulting in the gel becoming a solution. From studies of burn injury and anaphylaxis it is known that there is a rapid increase in net capillary filtration with visible oedema within 5 minutes. This occurs when capillary permeability has only increased by a factor of 2. Tissue pressure decreases to approximately −10 mmHg. This negative pressure is brought about by contraction of the ECM collagen induced by changes in β_1 integrin. The matrix can be thought of as 'contracting' down because of increased tension induced through the β_1 integrin. This acts to 'suck' fluid into the interstitium. Thus, interstitial fluid pressure can make a significant contribution to transcapillary flux and offers a method for dynamic modulation of that flux.

Increased capillary permeability resulting from mediators and calcium signalling

The transendothelial movement of fluid and solutes is a dynamic process regulated by a complex interaction between signalling molecules and structural elements comprising cell cytoskeleton, cell–cell adherence and cell–matrix attachment. The efficient operation of the endothelial barrier requires coordination and integration between different signalling reactions that are triggered by various mediators. Cells appear to respond to fluid shear stress via a complex process involving several potential transduction elements such that at the site of force application any of the following signal pathways may be activated:

1 Stress-activated ion channels for Ca
2 G-protein-linked receptors/guanylate cyclase (GC)
3 Integrin proteins
4 Tyrosine kinase receptors
5 Phospholipase C cGMP-dependent protein kinase (PKG).

The force transduction signal can be transmitted to the cell cytoskeleton leading to alterations in the cell action and function. Disruption of the cytoskeleton inhibits shear stress-mediated signalling and changes gene expression. Signalling events such as phosphorylation and changes in ion concentrations within the cell can lead to protein conformational changes. On one hand, the contractile force generated by the cross-bridge interaction between actin and myosin can cause cytoskeleton reorganization and cell contraction, establishing a morphological basis for intercellular gap formation. On the other hand, the binding between junctional proteins (e.g. VE-cadherin) and cytoskeletal elements via the catenin linking molecules produces an adhesive force

that pulls the adjacent endothelial cells together in close apposition, preventing intercellular leakage. The rise in calcium activates key signalling pathways, which mediate cytoskeletal reorganization, through myosin light chain (MLC) dependent contraction; this leads to cell retraction and disassembly of VE-cadherin and other transmembrane proteins at the adherens junctions. Elevation of calcium also acts on actin-myosin in the cells cytoskeleton to alter the interaction of junctional membrane proteins between adjacent endothelial cells. MLCK activation–mediated MLC phosphorylation can directly result in cell contraction and gap formation. VE-cadherin and β-catenin phosphorylation may induce a dissociation of the junctional proteins and their connection to the cytoskeleton, this process contributing to the barrier dysfunction of microvascular endothelium.

Shear stress increase results in an NO-dependent increase in permeability (Fig. 16.1). This offers a second-to-second ability to increase solute transfer. Here it is thought that proteins in the glycocalyx act to transduce a mechanical stimulus of increased flow into a biochemical signal to increase paracellular flow. Integrins may have a role here as antibodies against β_3 integrin attenuate flow-induced vasodilatation. Cyclic GMP also has a role in altering cell permeability as evidenced by the effects of guanylate cyclase inhibitors, which have similar effects to those of NOS inhibition. Inflammatory mediators, such as thrombin, that bind to heptahelical G-protein-coupled receptors (GPCR) and trigger increased endothelial permeability do so by increasing the intracellular calcium concentration. Similarly, agonists such as atrial naturetic factor (ANP), histamine and ATP act via cell surface receptors that open calcium channels, resulting in ion entry down its electrochemical gradient. The degree of calcium entry can be modified by hyperpolarization of the endothelial membrane. This increase in calcium induced by a variety of agonists is achieved not only by calcium entry via channels, but also by release of calcium from intracellular stores (in the endoplasmic reticulum) under the influence of the generation of inositol 1,4,5-trisphosphate (IP_3). IP_3-sensitive calcium store depletion activates plasma membrane cation channels (store-operated cation channels) to cause calcium influx into endothelial cells. Store-operated calcium influx signals induce an increase in cell permeability, NO production and can provoke changes in gene expression in endothelial cells. Action of these signals on the intracellular motors of actinomyosin stress fibre formation leads to cell retraction and increased vascular leakage. Rather than there being a specific mechanoreceptor expressed on endothelial cells, the entire cytoskeleton itself (which is under tension) may act as a mechanoreceptor and generate chemical signals to alter shape and permeability. Thus, the Ca-NOS-GC-PKG cascade and the PLC-PKC pathway contribute to the signal transduction in enhanced microvascular permeability. While activated PKC may alter the endothelial barrier function partially through the modulation of NOS activity, PKG activation may act as a common signal in the mediation of the hyperpermeability response. Biophysically the reflection coefficient σ becomes zero.

Inflammation

Tissue injury, in its many forms, triggers off a protective mechanism to isolate and repair the damaged tissue. This inflammatory response occurs at the level of the microcirculation. A primary component of the inflammatory response is this increase in microvascular permeability. The initial phase is thought to be mediated primarily by a change in interstitial fluid pressure (as described above). When the inflammatory mediators are histamine, serotonin, etc. then the increase in permeability is confined to the postcapillary venules via a mechanism involving increased gap formation. Only in the latter phases do gaps and fenestrae between endothelial cells open up.

As inflammation progresses, the hydraulic pressure gradient increases via arteriolar vasodilatation and its action on r_v/r_a to increase Pc. The transcapillary oncotic gradient decreases (protein leaks into the interstitial space) and capillary reflection coefficient decreases because of opening of intercellular gaps. Thus, there is an increase in fluid flux across the capillary into the interstitium. Ischaemic endothelial cells express selectins on their membrane which causes leucocytes to adhere to them. This leads to their activation and they migrate between the venu-

lar endothelial cells. This increase in permeability is brought about by release of oxidants and heparin-binding protein by the neutrophil that interacts with the endothelial actinomyosin cytoskeleton, probably via an action on transmembrane proteins. This causes cell contraction to 'open' up the tight and adherent junctions. The mechanism for this is not fully understood but also involves calcium influx, activation of NO synthase and production of cGMP. The end result is, again, an increase in the endothelial permeability (Fig. 16.4). However, this only occurs in the microcirculation. It does not occur in the macrocirculation; the response is designed to remain localized. However, if it becomes unregulated and systemic in nature, this results in a systemic inflammatory response and produces widespread derangements in organ and body physiology.

(a)

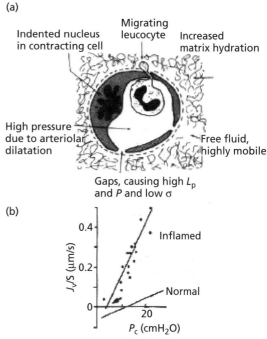

(b)

Figure 16.4 Structural and functional changes in the microcirculation during acute inflammation. The sevenfold increase in slope shows that hydraulic conductance (capillary permeability) increases with inflammation. The decrease in the intercept shows the effective osmotic gradient across the capillary wall ($\sigma\Delta\pi$) is reduced by inflammation.

It can be seen that increases in vascular permeability, while initially caused by a single agent, over time become a result of several agents acting simultaneously and/or in concert. The changes described relate to acute inflammation. Those of chronic inflammation are less well understood.

Microcirculation in different organs

Lung

The primary function of lung is gas exchange. The microcirculation runs in association with the alveoli (blood–gas barrier) to facilitate exchange. The capillary and alveolar cells are thin, to minimize the diffusion barrier. The capillaries form a dense network providing a large surface area. The pulmonary circuit is a low pressure system with very low flow resistance. The lungs have a strong requirement to remain dry yet the capillaries have an inherent 'leakiness', with the protein (albumin) reflection coefficient equaling 0.7. This ensures that the interstitial protein content is high (75% of plasma) and hence a higher interstitial oncotic pressure acts to decrease fluid transfer across the capillary wall. This, in association with an increasingly negative interstitial pressure as fluid moves from the lung periphery to the lung hilum, ensures there is a net outward fluid rate that is efficiently removed (which will equal the pulmonary lymph flow rate of 20 mL/min).

Formation of pulmonary oedema results from increased transcapillary fluid filtration secondary to altered hydrostatic or oncotic pressure gradients or because of increased permeability. However, because 80% of transendothelial protein flux is attributable to convection under physiological conditions, then P_c will determine both passive fluid filtration and protein transport. At the onset of pulmonary oedema, lung interstitial pressure increases rapidly because of its low interstitial compliance. This low compliance, caused by the ECM structure, acts as a protective mechanism to minimize the volume increase of fluid. Fluid absorbed by the ECM glycosaminoglycan and hyaluronan in the extra-alveolar interstitial space prevents fluid flooding alveoli. This system eventually fails because of matrix remodelling by MMP and mechanical stress. Tissue compliance increases over 4–6 hours, promoting oedema progression. Mechanical forces can alter endothelial barrier properties. In the lung, the pulmonary capillaries are exposed to a longitudinal tension in the alveolar wall associated with lung inflation. This tension, if exaggerated (with positive pressure ventilation), may result in endothelial cytoskeleton changes resulting in increased permeability and oedema formation as occurs in ventilator-induced lung injury.

Brain

The blood–brain barrier (BBB) is formed by brain capillary endothelial cells. These cells have at least three properties that distinguish them from their peripheral counterparts:

1 Super-tight junctions (TJ) of extremely low permeability and very low hydraulic conductivity; the paracellular cleft is almost completely sealed. This prevents paracellular macromolecular diffusion driven by their concentration gradient.
2 Low rates of fluid-phase endocytosis.
3 Specific transport and carrier molecules (i.e. the capillary endothelium is not freely permeable to low molecular weight solutes such as glucose, urea or mannitol; these can freely cross the capillary endothelium in the periphery).

Uptake of essential molecules into the central nervous system (CNS) is mediated through specific transport and carrier complexes.

The capillaries of most vascular beds in the body are permeable to low molecular weight solutes and have a low permeability to proteins. In the brain, the capillary is relatively impermeable to most of the low molecular weight solutes and impermeable to proteins. It exhibits a gate function to solute transfer. This infers that the driving filtration force across the capillary membrane is the difference in hydrostatic pressure between blood and brain tissue (ICP; intracranial pressure) and the difference in osmotic pressure of blood and the osmotic pressure in brain. Unlike other capillary beds, where the osmotic pressure difference (because of essentially free permeation of low molecular weight solutes) is generated by the difference in protein concentration (5–10 mmHg), in brain the osmotic gradient is generated by all the plasma constituents. At an osmolality of 290 mOsm/kg the osmotic pressure is 5500 mmHg.

In combination, these features restrict the non-specific flux of ions, proteins and other substances into the CNS environment. These restrictions protect neurones from harmful fluctuations occurring in the blood and thus maintain homoeostasis, yet allow uptake of essential molecules. However, small changes in plasma osmolality (e.g. hypernatraemia resulting from dehydration) can have a marked effect on the fluid volume of the intracranial compartment.

Different mechanisms are involved in TJ-dependent permeability regulation including:

1 Alterations of the architecture of the actin cytoskeleton

2 Post-translational modifications of junctional proteins, by PKC

3 Proteolytic degradation of junctional constituents.

Breakdown of the BBB is associated with a variety of CNS disorders (e.g. traumatic brain injury, infection). Recent work has shown the barrier breakdown to be related to protein disassembly of the endothelial TJ brought about by inflammatory mediators or MMPs.

Microcirculatory pathophysiology

Inflammation

The inflammatory response is a vital process that has a key role in health and disease. The word 'inflammation' can be considered as an umbrella term. Many diseases have an inflammatory component and it is a common theme in several, apparently distinct pathologies. The inflammatory process is initiated by a complex series of events, of which pivotal early steps are vascular changes that start immediately and develop during the first few hours. Vascular changes are regulated by factors that control exudation, which occurs mainly from the postcapillary venules. This phase occurs either concomitantly or is followed by association between neutrophils and the endothelium of postcapillary venules, which contributes to a more prolonged phase of increased vascular permeability. During inflammation, the cytoskeleton of the endothelial cells permits retraction and opening of the tight intercellular junction thus increasing the permeability of vessel walls to plasma proteins and other substances. The protein-rich exudate escapes into the surrounding interstitial space causing localized swelling in the tissues. The increase in fluid in the tissue spaces is further compounded by an increase in hydrostatic pressure at the arteriolar end of the capillary bed because of vasodilatation. The major functions of the various types of exudates are to dilute toxins produced by bacteria, to provide a fluid medium for the movement of immunoglobulins and leucocytes, and to drain bacterial toxins to the lymphatics and thence to lymph nodes, where B and T cells are situated, and an immune response can be initiated.

Inflammation is a condition that exhibits the dynamic and heterogeneous nature of microcirculatory flow and its sensitivity to sepsis. Cells and mediators evoked by sepsis can cause havoc in the microcirculation with vascular dysregulation, loss of barrier function (capillary leak syndrome), endothelial cell dysfunction, as well as a host of blood-associated disturbances such as increased clotting, red blood cell rigidity and leucocyte activation. The upshot of this catastrophe is a complete collapse of microcirculatory functional control which, together with inflammatory mediators, ultimately leads to cell death. Using sublingual orthogonal polarization spectroscopy, microcirculatory blood flow can be examined in humans. During sepsis it has been shown that microcirculatory perfusion is reduced by approximately half, despite overall correction of systemic haemodynamic variables and parameters of oxygen delivery. The severity of this microcirculatory depression is correlated to the patient's outcome as well as to blood lactate levels and severity of illness scores, but not to any of the other usual clinical variables monitored. Depressed microcirculatory flow occurs more severely in the smallest vessels, leaving the larger vessels more or less unaffected. This provides direct support for the idea that shunting of the microcirculation is a prominent feature of sepsis. Microvascular occlusion resulting from leucocytes 'plugging and blocking' the capillary may be the cause. These results also provide an explanation as to why systemic haemodynamic variables are a poor reflection of haemodynamic properties in the microcirculation. In animal models of sepsis, endothelial cell responsiveness to acetylcholine is preserved, which, upon vasodilatation, corrected and restored microcirculatory flow back to normal values and patterns. In a similar study in septic patients, systemic administration of nitroglycerine restored and corrected microcirculatory flow that had previously been depressed. Such a mechanism may account for the improved oxygen extraction seen in septic patients when given the potent vasodilator prostacyclin. It may be that to improve oxgyen extraction in sepsis, what is required is a means of improving microcirculatory flow.

One of the great problems in treating sepsis is the necessary fluid resuscitation (because of the increase in microvascular permeability) that leads to oedema formation.

Oedema

There are two forms of oedema: that secondary to increased permeability in the microcirculation (usually secondary to an inflammatory stimulus), and that resulting in pathological states leading to sodium and water retention resulting from a decreased effective circulating volume or to hypoproteinaemia. Only the former is discussed here.

The primary sites of oedema formation are the skeletal muscle and subcutaneous tissue. Oedema also forms in potential spaces such as peritoneum and pleura. Oedema of the extracellular space occurs when there is derangement of the transcapillary fluid flux such that fluid removal by the lymphatics is overwhelmed by fluid inflow. This results in expansion of the interstitial fluid space. While the collagen gel may contract as described above there is a limit to which this occurs. As fluid leaks into the interstitial fluid space there will be a 'bath-tub' effect beyond which the compliance of the space will increase with formation of large volumes of free fluid. Oedema directly and profoundly interferes with distribution of vital substrates and removal of wastes, cytokines and other undesirables present in capillary leak secondary to endothelial injury. When interstitial oedema occurs there is a mismatch between the number of proteoglycan and collagen filaments and water flux. This results in the creation of large, low resistance channels of fluid with vastly increased rates of flow. The flow rate goes up in the typical oedematous patient's interstitial space by 250 000 times baseline. As proteins migrate through the en-

larged interendothelial gaps, large quantities of fluid are taken along (1 g albumin binds 18 g isotonic fluid). This leads to salt and water retention as interstitial oedema.

This is deleterious for a number of reasons. Under normal physiological conditions, the 'thin-filming' and reduced rate of flow of capillary filtrate allows adequate time for diffusion of nutrients and waste products into and out of cells to occur. It also provides for very uniform delivery of comparatively high molecular weight nutrients such as amino acids and vitamins which cross cell membranes especially slowly. Conversely, it allows for 'wash-out' of large proteins such as cytokines and other regulatory molecules when their jobs are done. In the typical case of serious capillary leak, the interstitial fluid volume can easily double from a normal value of 12–24 L with a pressure increase in the interstitium of as little as +3 mmHg. The curve of increased interstitial fluid volume versus interstitial pressure is roughly exponential, so that a positive interstitial pressure of 6 mmHg could be expected to increase interstitial fluid volume to as much as 50 L. Even in moderate oedema, the net result of this is 'channelling' of fluid through paths of least resistance contributes to inadequate substrate delivery, ionic disturbances and accumulation of cytotoxins in the static pools of fluid that end up surrounding a significant fraction of a patient's cells. The rivulets become rivers, bypassing most cells. Bacteria can move with ease into tissue spaces. The severity of the problem will not be appreciated when only haemodynamic parameters and global measurements of physiological function such as lactate concentration, oxygen consumption are measured as indicators of the disease process. Oedema is therefore not benign. The increase in diffusion distances for solute transfer further disturbs cellular homoeostasis in an already compromised patient. This may lead to a vicious positive feedback cycle that characterizes immune-inflammatory mediated diseases.

Albumin is important for the vascular–interstitial fluid balance in both health and disease. Studies of albumin kinetics during injury have shown lymph flow rate and albumin concentration in lymph decreases. In sepsis, there are indications that both the opening and closing of the lymphatic capillaries and the peristaltic capability of the larger lymphatics are inhibited or abolished. Thus, oedema may impair the ability to organize lymphatic recruitment and it is not inconceivable that interstitial oedema may lead to cellular oedema. Oedema has its own positive feedback system. As more oedema forms and increases the interstitial fluid pressure, there comes a time when this pressure will act to compress the lymphatics and decrease lymph flow. In sick patients confined to bed and immobile, the lack of skeletal muscle compression will further lead to decreased lymph flow and hence favour further oedema formation.

This means that colloid and fluid transport are greatly inhibited. Finally, significant peripheral oedema in the setting of systemic injury such as sepsis is almost always accompanied by pulmonary oedema, because the safety factor against oedema in the lungs is much lower than it is in almost any other tissue. If the patient is bloated with fluid peripherally then it is certain there is pulmonary oedema as well. In a 70-kg adult the pulmonary interstitial fluid volume cannot increase by more than half without alveolar flooding starting to occur. This volume is on average <100 mL. Pulmonary oedema will invariably worsen gas exchange and hence oxgyen delivery to the microcirculation.

Conclusions

The microcirculation was, until recently, seen as a site of passive exchange governed primarily by the haemodynamics of the macrocirculation. Quite to the contrary, it is a site of complex control mechanisms. Net fluid transfer is driven by bulk flow. Metabolic exchange is by diffusion which occurs along the full length of the capillary, depending on concentration gradients, but can be modulated by many factors. The microcirculation will in the future be the site of therapeutic intervention to alter the course of pathological states. These interventions will only arise if the physiology and molecular biology of microcirculatory function and control are elucidated.

References

1 Galley HF, Webster NR. Physiology of the endothelium. *Br J Anaesth* 2004; **93**: 105–13.
2 Guyton AC, Hall JE. The microcirculation and the lymphatic system: capillary fluid exchange, interstitial fluid, and lymph flow. In: *Textbook of Medical Physiology*, 10th edn. Guyton AC, Hall JE, eds. Philadelphia: WB Saunders, 2000: 162–74.

Further reading

Bosman FT, Stamenkovic I. Functional structure and composition of the extracellular matrix. *J Pathol* 2003; **200**: 423–8.
Kamm RD. Cellular fluid mechanics. *Ann Rev Fluid Mech* 2002; **34**: 211–32.
Levick JR. Revision of the Starling principle: new views of tissue fluid balance. *J Physiol* 2004; **557**: 704.
Martinez-Lemus LA, Wu X, Wilson E, *et al*. Integrins as unique receptors for vascular control. *J Vasc Res* 2003; **40**: 211–33.
Michel CC. Fluid exchange and the microcirculation. *J Physiol* 2004; **557**: 701–2.
Michel CC, Curry FE. Microvascular permeability. *Physiol Rev* 1999; **79**: 703–61.
Popel AS, Johnson PC. Microcirculation and hemorheology. *Ann Rev Fluid Mech* 2005; **37**: 43–69.
Wing H, Rubin K, Reed RK. New and active role of the interstitium in control of interstitial fluid pressure: potential therapeutic consequences. *Acta Anaesthesiol Scand* 2003; **47**: 111–21.

CHAPTER 17

Respiratory physiology at the molecular level

Andrew Lumb

Introduction

Non-respiratory functions of the lung and lung function tests are described in Chapters 18 and 28, respectively; this chapter aims to provide a review of some of the remaining topics in respiratory physiology. Our understanding of lung mechanics and gas exchange has remained mostly unchanged for many years, and traditional physiological concepts are described only briefly here. Developments in molecular medicine have recently begun to be applied to respiratory physiology research, and have led either to further elucidation of the mechanisms underlying some aspects of respiratory physiology or have caused us to challenge long-standing dogma about the way the respiratory system functions [1]. The topics covered in this chapter have been selected to illustrate how greater understanding of molecular interactions has impacted on our understanding of respiration.

Control of respiration

Breathing is controlled by groups of neurones in the medulla loosely referred to as the respiratory centre. The output from the respiratory centre is via two pools of neurones corresponding to inspiratory and expiratory muscle activity, and these neurones constitute the primary motor neurones for the respiratory muscles. Inspiratory muscles include the airway dilator muscles, external intercostals, scalene muscles and diaphragm, while the internal intercostals and abdominal muscles are responsible for expiration, and are only active when hyperventilating,

for example during exercise or when breathing out against a resistance.

Central pattern generator

Within the respiratory centre there is a specialized group of neurones, collectively known as the central pattern generator (CPG) [2], that are responsible for initiating the respiratory rhythm. The CPG begins to initiate breathing activity, erratically at first, in early pregnancy, but once established continues to do so for many decades. The origins of rhythmicity are different from the cardiac pacemaker, there being no individual cell responsible for initiating a breath. Instead, there are groups of interconnected neurones, each responsible for a different part of the respiratory cycle, corresponding approximately to inspiration, passive expiration and active expiration. Within each group, intrinsic membrane properties and excitatory and inhibitory effects on nearby neurones allow a series of 'waves' of neuronal activity to progress through the groups of neurones responsible for each phase of the respiratory cycle. For example, spontaneous activity in early inspiratory neurones causes excitatory activity on inspiratory augmenting neurones, which recruit further inspiratory neurones causing a crescendo of inspiratory neurone activity, including those of the inspiratory motor neurone pool. Finally, the secretion of excitatory neurotransmitters reaches a high enough level to activate late-inspiratory neurones which in turn cause inhibition of the inspiratory augmenting neurones and activate expiratory decrementing neurones to reduce inspiratory muscle activity in a slow controlled manner to allow passive expiration. This complex system is necessary to allow the infinite variations that are required of the CPG, as described below. Within the CPG, glutamate acts as the main excitatory neurotransmitter with both γ-aminobutyric acid (GABA) and glycine having inhibitory activity.

Respiratory centre connections

Many different factors influence the rate, depth and pattern of breathing, all of which must ultimately do so by acting on the neurones of the CPG. A wide variety of neuromodulators are involved [3], as summarized in Figure 17.1. The exact role of these neuromodulators in normal human respiration remains unclear, but they are of undoubted relevance in both normal and abnormal breathing. For example, exogenous opioids are known to have a powerful effect in depressing breathing in humans, indicating the presence of opioid receptors in the respiratory centre, but administration of the opioid antagonist naloxone has no effect on breathing in resting normal subjects. Other neuromodulators include acetylcholine, which acts via both muscarinic and nicotinic receptors to mediate the effect of central chemoreceptors on respiration (see below). Glutamate acts as a neuromodulator via both N-methyl-D-aspartate (NMDA) and non-NMDA receptors to mediate the pontine influence on the CPG and is also involved in the modulation of the respiratory pattern by pulmonary stretch receptors and peripheral chemoreceptors. This diverse collection of neuromodulators probably all ultimately act via a common intracellular signalling pathway within CPG neurones, involving protein kinases A and C that in turn influence the activity of GABA, glycine and glutamate linked potassium and chloride channels [4]. The presence in the CPG of receptors for these neuromodulators also explains why some drugs, particularly opioids acting on μ-receptors, have such potent effects on breathing.

There are three physiological systems that influence breathing: the central nervous system, peripheral nervous system and chemical control of breathing.

Central nervous system

The pons is anatomically close to the respiratory centre and has numerous neuronal connections with it, but the functional role of the pons has never been clearly elucidated. Pontine neurones firing in synchrony with different phases of respiration are known to exist, and are referred to as the pontine respiratory group (PRG). The PRG is no longer considered to be essential for the generation of the respiratory rhythm, but does nevertheless influence the medullary respiratory neurones via a multisynaptic pathway contributing to fine control of the respiratory rhythm as, for example, in setting the lung

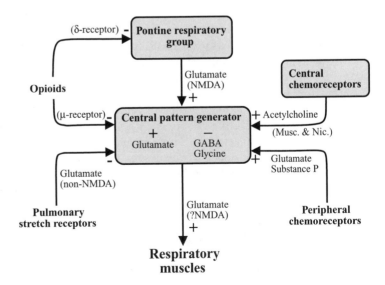

Figure 17.1 Central and peripheral connections to the respiratory centre, and the neurotransmitters and neuromodulators involved. Shaded boxes indicate functional neuronal groups and bold type represents influences on the central pattern generator. Substances involved in neurotransmission are shown with the most likely receptor subtype, in parentheses, if known. + indicates excitatory effect increasing respiratory activity; − indicates inhibitory activity decreasing respiration. Many of the connections shown may not be active during normal resting conditions.

volume at which inspiration is terminated. There are many central neuronal pathways to the PRG, including connections to the hypothalamus, the cortex and the nucleus tractus solitarius. It is now thought that the pons acts as a coordinator for the wide range of other central nervous system influences on the respiratory centre; for example, coughing, laughing, hiccups, sneezing and other expulsive efforts all require major alterations to respiratory centre function.

The cerebral cortex also influences breathing, probably acting via the pons. Considering what a vital function breathing is, it is surprising that we can, under conscious control, hold our breath for some minutes. Another more complex example of cortical control over breathing is for speech [5]. During prolonged conversation, respiratory rate and tidal volume must be maintained approximately normal to prevent biochemical disturbance. In addition, for speech to be easily understood, pauses to allow inspiration must occur at appropriate boundaries in the text; for example, between sentences. To achieve this, the brain performs complex assessments of the forthcoming speech to select appropriate size breaths to prevent cumbersome interruptions. This is easier to achieve during reading aloud when 88% of breaths are taken at appropriate boundaries in the text, compared with only 63% during spontaneous speech.

Peripheral nervous input

A variety of receptors are present in the mucosa of the airway from the nasal cavity to the small bronchi [6]. These receptors provide information to the respiratory centre that influences breathing pattern, and are of three types:

1 *Irritant receptors:* respond to inhalation of potentially toxic chemicals such as the constituents of cigarette smoke or inhaled anaesthetics. Stimulation of irritant receptors in the upper airway results in cough, laryngeal closure and bronchoconstriction, while irritation of the lower airways may also cause hypertension, tachycardia and secretion of mucus.

2 *Cold receptors:* found superficially on the vocal folds. Activation generally results in depression of ventilation. The importance of this reflex in adult humans is uncertain, but these receptors may pro-

duce bronchoconstriction in susceptible individuals.

3 *Mechanoreceptors:* found mostly above the larynx, particularly in the oropharynx, and respond to changes in transmural pressure. Stimulation occurs in response to negative airway pressures and results in increased pharyngeal dilator muscle activity, particularly during airway obstruction.

The lung parenchyma also contains numerous receptors that provide sensory input to the respiratory centre [6]. These receptors are relatively silent during normal breathing but are stimulated under various pathological conditions. Irritant receptors are found in the lung, with similar stimulants and effects to those already described for the airway above. They also respond to mediators and cytokines released following tissue damage, which results in accumulation of interstitial fluid. For the control of breathing, the most important pulmonary receptors are the stretch receptors, which are sensitive to inflation and deflation of the lung. Slowly adapting stretch receptors (SARs) are found in the small airways rather than in the alveoli. Lung inflation stimulates the SARs receptors, which are named 'slowly adapting' because of their ability to maintain their firing rate when lung inflation is maintained, thus acting as a form of lung volume sensor. Conversely, rapidly adapting stretch receptors (RARs) are located in the superficial mucosal layer, and are stimulated by changes in tidal volume, respiratory frequency or changes in lung compliance.

The reflexes associated with these pulmonary stretch receptors have attracted much attention since the associated inflation and deflation reflexes were described by Hering and Breuer in 1868. The inflation reflex describes the inhibition of inspiration in response to an increased pulmonary pressure (as in sustained inflation of the lung), but the significance of the Hering–Breuer reflex in humans is controversial [7]. There appears to be an important species difference between laboratory animals, in which the reflex is easy to demonstrate, and humans, in whom the reflex is very weak. For example, patients have essentially normal ventilatory patterns after bilateral lung transplant, when both lungs must be totally denervated. Although the Hering–Breuer inflation reflex therefore appears to have minimal functional significance in humans, its existence has been demonstrated in adults, and it is widely accepted as being present in neonates and infants.

Chemical control of breathing

Carbon dioxide (CO_2) partial pressure in the blood has a major influence on breathing, controlling the normal arterial P_{CO_2} within narrow limits despite wide physiological variations in CO_2 production. The relationship between minute volume of ventilation and arterial P_{CO_2} is linear, with an average slope of 15 L/min/kPa, although there are wide interindividual variations in the response, with some subjects showing almost no response at all. Carbon dioxide influences breathing at the central chemoreceptors, which are located in the anterior medulla, just 0.2 mm below its surface. An elevation of arterial P_{CO_2} causes an approximately equal rise of cerebrospinal fluid (CSF), cerebral tissue and jugular venous P_{CO_2}. In the short term, and without change in CSF bicarbonate, a rise in CSF P_{CO_2} causes a fall in CSF pH. The blood–brain barrier (operative between blood and CSF) is permeable to CO_2 but not hydrogen ions, so CO_2 crosses the barrier and hydrates to carbonic acid, which then ionizes to give a pH inversely proportional to the log of the P_{CO_2}. A hydrogen ion sensor is thus made to respond to P_{CO_2}. The mechanism by which a change in pH causes stimulation of chemoreceptor neurones is not firmly established, but it could clearly influence the action of an enzyme. Acetylcholine (ACh) is the neuromodulator involved in the interaction between the central chemoreceptors and the CPG (Fig. 17.1) and its metabolism by cholinesterase is inhibited at decreased pH.

Although required less frequently, the ventilatory response to arterial hypoxaemia is also vital, representing a potentially life-saving reflex. The acute phase of this response occurs within a few seconds of the onset of a reduced arterial P_{O_2}, and this response is non-linear, with ventilation being approximately doubled at an arterial P_{O_2} of 8 kPa, and quadrupled at 5 kPa. The response originates in the peripheral chemoreceptors that are located in the carotid bodies. Reduced arterial P_{O_2} (not reduced blood oxygen content) or hypoperfusion of the carotid bodies causes the glomus cells to release a variety of neurotransmitters that increase the firing rate in the carotid sinus nerves, which in turn release glutamate or substance P to stimulate the CPG. The molecular basis of this highly efficient oxygen sensor has been the subject of much research, and several possible mechanisms are now suggested [8]. In glomus cells, arterial hypoxaemia causes a reduction in the intracellular level of adenosine triphosphate (ATP) at levels of P_{O_2} that have little effect elsewhere in the body. In addition, in response to hypoxia there is a graded increase in intracellular calcium concentration following its release from mitochondria. Calcium release is brought about by changes to mitochondrial membrane potassium channels, some of which are themselves directly sensitive to low P_{O_2}. However, many other mechanisms have also been shown to alter potassium channel function, including activation by haem-based mitochondrial cytochromes, NADPH+-oxidase enzyme systems, and the levels of reactive oxygen species found within the mitochondria, all of which are greatly influenced by changes in local P_{O_2}.

If arterial hypoxia is sustained for more than a few minutes, the ventilatory response subsides to a value just above normoxic levels, an observation referred to as hypoxic ventilatory decline (Fig. 17.2). The sensitivity of the carotid bodies is unchanged, so the decline in ventilation must be mediated by a reduction in the response of the CPG to the sensory input from the carotid, and increased release of GABA is implicated [9]. With even more prolonged hypoxia (several hours), and isocapnic conditions, ventilation again begins to increase (Fig. 17.2). However, if arterial P_{CO_2} is not controlled (poikilocapnia), the reduced P_{CO_2} caused by the continued small degree of hyperventilation exactly balances the effect of hypoxia and minute ventilation remains constant and slightly above normoxic levels. This response is believed to represent reduced sensitivity of the carotid bodies to hypoxia.

Lung compliance

If the chest cavity is opened or air allowed into the pleura, the lung contained within will contract until eventually all the contained air is expelled. In contrast, when the thoracic cage is opened it tends to expand to a volume approximately 1 L greater than functional residual capacity. Thus, in a relaxed

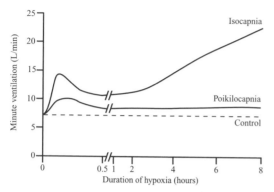

Figure 17.2 Time course of the ventilatory response to sustained hypoxia ($SaO_2 \approx 80\%$). When arterial P_{CO_2} is maintained at normal levels (isocapnia) the response is triphasic with an initial acute hyperventilation, quickly followed by hypoxic ventilatory decline, and a final increase in ventilation over several hours. When arterial P_{CO_2} is not controlled (poikilocapnia) the magnitude of the response is damped because the hypoxia-induced hyperventilation reduces P_{CO_2} and therefore respiratory drive.

subject with an open airway and no air flowing (e.g. at the end of expiration or inspiration), the inward elastic recoil of the lungs is exactly balanced by the outward recoil of the thoracic cage.

Lung compliance is defined as the change in lung volume per unit change in transmural pressure gradient (i.e. between the alveolus and pleural space) and normal lungs have a compliance of 1.5 L/kPa (150 mL/cmH$_2$O). The tendency of the lungs to contract has two origins: the elastic nature of the lung tissue itself and the surface forces at the alveolar gas–liquid interface. In both cases, the rate at which a change in lung volume occurs influences the elastic behaviour of the lungs.

Time dependency of pulmonary elastic behaviour

If lung tissue is rapidly inflated and then held at the new volume, the inflation pressure quickly falls from its initial value to a lower level that is attained after just a few seconds. This also occurs in the intact subject, and is readily observed during an inspiratory pause in a patient receiving artificial ventilation. It is broadly true to say that the volume change divided by the initial change in pressure corresponds to the

dynamic compliance (measured during normal breathing), while the volume change divided by the ultimate change in pressure (measured after it has become steady) corresponds to the static compliance. Static compliance will thus be greater than the dynamic compliance by an amount determined by the degree of time dependence in the elastic behaviour of a particular lung.

There are many possible explanations of the time dependence of pulmonary elastic behaviour, the relative importance of which may vary in different circumstances.

• Surfactant activity (see below) is probably the most important cause of the observed time dependent behaviour of the intact lung. The complex changes described below in the molecular configuration of surfactant that occur with changes in lung volume must take some time to become established.

• Stress relaxation is an inherent property of all elastic bodies. For example, if a spring is pulled out to a fixed increase in its length, the resultant tension is maximal at first and then declines exponentially to a constant value. Thoracic tissues display stress relaxation and these 'viscoelastic' properties contribute significantly to the difference between static and dynamic compliance [10]. The crinkled structure of collagen in the lung is likely to favour stress relaxation and excised strips of human lung show stress relaxation when stretched.

• Redistribution of gas occurs between areas of lung with differing compliance or resistance when inflation pressure is held constant. This observation is traditionally described in terms of 'fast' and 'slow' alveoli (the term 'alveoli' here referring to functional units rather than the anatomical entity). The 'fast' alveolus has a low airway resistance and/or low compliance (or both) while the 'slow' alveolus has a high airway resistance and/or a high compliance. These properties mean that the fast alveoli are preferentially filled during a short inflation. A slow or sustained inflation permits increased distribution of gas to slow alveoli and so tends to distribute gas in accord with the compliance of the different functional units. Extreme differences between fast and slow alveoli only occur in diseased lungs and gas redistribution is therefore unlikely to be a major factor in healthy subjects.

Surface forces in the lung

For many years it was thought that the recoil of the lung was due entirely to stretching of the yellow elastin fibres present in the lung tissue until, in 1929, von Neergaard showed that a lung completely filled with and immersed in water had an elastance that was much less than the normal value obtained when the lung was filled with air. He correctly concluded that much of the 'elastic recoil' was caused by surface tension acting throughout the vast air–water interface lining the alveoli.

Surface tension at an air–water interface produces forces that tend to reduce the area of the interface. Thus, the gas pressure within a bubble is always higher than the surrounding gas pressure because the surface of the bubble is in a state of tension. The pressure inside a bubble is higher than the surrounding pressure by an amount depending on the surface tension of the liquid and the radius of curvature of the bubble according to the Laplace equation:

$$P = \frac{2T}{R}$$

where P is the pressure within the bubble, T is the surface tension of the liquid and R is the radius of the bubble. Using this analogy, smaller alveoli would have a higher pressure within them and thus gas would tend to flow from smaller alveoli into larger alveoli and lungs would be unstable which, of course, is not the case. Similarly, the retractive forces of the alveolar lining fluid would increase at low lung volumes, and tend to further empty the lung, and decrease at high lung volumes, tending to fill the lung, which is exactly the reverse of what is observed. These paradoxes were clear to von Neergaard who concluded that the surface tension of the alveolar lining fluid must be considerably less than would be expected from the properties of simple liquids and that its value must be variable. These properties of alveolar lining fluid are now known to result from the presence of surfactant.

Alveolar surfactant

The secretion of surfactant by type II alveolar cells [11,12], and its chemical nature, have been described elsewhere in this book (Chapter 18). To maintain the stability of alveoli, surfactant must alter the surface tension in the alveoli as their size varies with inspiration and expiration. A simple explanation of how this occurs is that during expiration, as the surface area of the alveolus diminishes, the surfactant molecules are packed more densely and so reduce surface tension to a greater degree. In reality, the situation is considerably more complex, and at present poorly elucidated [13]. Surfactant phospholipid is known to exist *in vivo* in both monolayer and multilayer forms [12], and it is possible that in some areas of the alveoli the phospholipid alternates between these two forms as alveolar size changes during the respiratory cycle. This aspect of surfactant function is entirely dependent on the presence of SP-B, a small hydrophobic protein, which can be incorporated into a phospholipid monolayer, and SP-C, a larger protein with a hydrophobic central portion allowing it to span a lipid bilayer. When alveolar size reduces and the surface film is compressed, SP-B molecules may be squeezed out of the lipid layer so changing its surface properties, while SP-C may serve to stabilize bilayers of lipid to act as a reservoir from which the surface film may reform when alveolar size increases.

Alternative models to explain lung recoil

Treating surfactant-lined alveoli as bubbles that obey Laplace's law has aided the understanding of lung recoil in health and disease for many decades, but this simplistic approach is now being challenged [14]. Arguments against the so-called bubble model include the following:

- The air contained within alveoli is connected to the exterior by the air passages — a bubble cannot exist with a section of its side missing
- Differing surface tensions in adjacent alveoli theoretically cannot occur if the liquid lining the alveoli is connected by a continuous liquid layer, within which fluid can flow
- When surfactant layers are compressed at 37°C, multilayered 'rafts' of dry surfactant form, although inclusion of surfactant proteins reduces this physico-chemical change
- Alveoli are not shaped like perfect spheres with a single entrance point — they are variable polyhedrons with convex bulges in their walls where pulmonary capillaries bulge into them.

Two very different alternative models have been proposed.

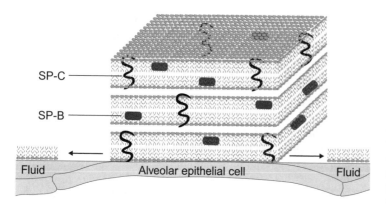

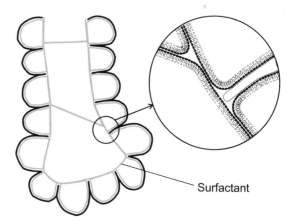

Figure 17.3 Morphological model of surfactant function. Multilayered 'rafts' of surfactant are adsorbed directly onto the alveolar epithelium, interspersed with fluid pools. Smaller globular SP-B lies within a single lipid layer while the larger SP-C molecules span lipid bilayers, both proteins controlling the formation and dispersion of the surfactant rafts to modify the surface forces between the liquid and less wettable areas.

Morphological model

For many years it has been suggested that the surfactant lining alveoli results in a 'discontinuous' liquid lining [15]. Based on knowledge of the physical chemistry of surfactants, this model shows that surfactant phospholipids are adsorbed directly onto the epithelial cell surface so causing patches of the surface to become less wettable, these patches being interspersed with fluid pools. Surface forces generated by the interaction between these 'rafts' of surfactant and the areas of liquid are theoretically large enough to maintain alveolar stability. The rafts of surfactant, several layers of phospholipid deep (Fig. 17.3), may form and disperse with each breath, their function almost certainly being dependent on SP-B and SP-C as described above.

Foam model

A more radically different model for the maintenance of alveolar stability has been proposed by Scarpelli [16]. By maintaining tissue in a more natural state than previous studies, including keeping lung volume close to normal, he has described a 'new anatomy' for alveoli. Scarpelli's findings suggest that *in vivo* alveoli have bubble films across their entrances, with similar lipid bilayer films also existing across alveolar ducts and respiratory bronchioles (Fig. 17.4). In this model, each group of alveoli may be considered as a series of interconnected, but closed, bubbles so forming a stable 'foam'. The bubble films are estimated to be less than 7 nm thick so will offer little resistance to gas diffusion, the normal

Figure 17.4 Schematic representation of the 'foam' model of alveolar structure [16]. Surfactant lines the alveoli, and forms films that span both the alveolar openings and the alveolar ducts. Inset: detail of the surfactant layer showing connection between phospholipid monolayer and bilayer (not to scale).

mechanism by which gas movement occurs in a single pulmonary acinus.

More research is clearly needed to confirm or refute each of these models, but the well-established bubble model of alveolar recoil is no longer as universally accepted as previously.

Respiratory system resistance

When breathing takes place, the impedance to gas flowing into and out of the lung must be overcome. This non-elastic resistance has three components:

1 Frictional resistance to gas flowing through the airways

2 Viscoelastic tissue resistance from deformation of lung and thoracic tissues

3 Inertia associated with the initiation of movement of gas and tissues.

These last two are of little significance during normal breathing in a healthy subject, but may become important in disease states; for example, abnormalities of the chest wall tissues may cause very high viscoelastic resistance to gas flow, or inertia of respiratory gases may become significant during high frequency ventilation.

Frictional resistance to gas flow in the airways is therefore the major cause of resistance during breathing. The resistance offered to gas flow through a tube depends on whether the flow is laminar, turbulent or a mixture of both. Flow in the nose, pharynx, larynx and large airways is turbulent, and so determined by the density of the inhaled gas and the fifth power of the radius of the airway. As gas reaches more distal airways, its velocity decreases and flow becomes predominantly laminar, and is now determined by the viscosity of the gas and the fourth power of the radius of the airway. In both these types of flow, airway radius is by far the most important factor affecting resistance, and control of airway size is therefore the major physiological determinant of airway resistance.

Control of airway diameter
Passive changes in airway size

The trachea and main bronchi have U-shaped cartilage in their walls and are therefore almost impossible to narrow without applying substantial external pressures. Irregular-shaped sections of cartilage are present in the walls of airways from the main bronchi until the 11th generation from the trachea (small bronchi), again offering resistance to compression. Beyond this, in the respiratory bronchioles and alveolar ducts, the airways have no supporting tissue in their walls and are held open only by the surrounding elastic tissue of the lung parenchyma.

As a result, lung volume is a major determinant of airway resistance, this being a hyperbolic relationship with airways resistance being maximal at

residual volume and minimal at total lung capacity. At low lung volumes, airway size is reduced to such an extent that in some regions of lung airway closure occurs, leading to gas trapping in the alveoli beyond the closed airway, and significant impairment of gas exchange. The lung volume at which this occurs is the closing capacity, and is usually mid-way between residual volume and functional residual capacity, but with increasing age the closing capacity increases and airway closure begins to occur in some regions of lung even in healthy subjects.

Reduced airway size and airway collapse may also occur with high air flows during expiration. A forced expiration will generate a positive intrathoracic pressure, and as air moves along the airways down its pressure gradient there will come a point at which the intrathoracic and airway pressure are equal, and the normal forces keeping the small airways open are lost. This phenomenon is much more likely to occur at low lung volumes when airway size is already reduced, and so can easily be demonstrated when a forced expiration to residual volume is performed.

Active control of airway size

There are four systems for controlling muscle tone in small bronchi and bronchioles:

1 Neural pathways [17] influence bronchomotor tone by three different nervous pathways:

- Parasympathetic nerves have a powerful bronchoconstrictor effect and when activated can completely obliterate the lumen of small airways. Both afferent and efferent fibres travel to the lung in the vagus nerve. Afferents arise from receptors in the bronchial epithelium and respond either to noxious stimuli in the airway or to cytokines released by cellular mechanisms such as mast cell degranulation. Efferent nerves release ACh, which acts at M_3 muscarinic receptors to cause contraction of bronchial smooth muscle while also stimulating M_2 prejunctional muscarinic receptors to exert negative feedback on ACh release. A complex series of second messengers is involved in bringing about smooth muscle contraction in response to ACh (see below). Stimulation of any part of the reflex arc results in bronchoconstriction. Some degree of resting tone is normally present and may therefore permit some bron-chodilatation when vagal tone is reduced in a similar fashion to vagal control of heart rate.

• Sympathetic nerves exist in the lung but are not yet proven to be of major importance in humans. It appears unlikely that there is any direct sympathetic innervation of the airway smooth muscle, although there may be an inhibitory effect on cholinergic neurotransmission in some species.

• Non-adrenergic non-cholinergic (NANC) nerves [18] provide a third system for autonomic control of the airway smooth muscle, and this system is the only potential bronchodilator nervous pathway in humans, although its exact role remains uncertain. The efferent fibres run in the vagus nerve and pass to airway smooth muscle where they cause prolonged relaxation of bronchi. The neurotransmitter is vasoactive intestinal peptide (VIP), which produces airway smooth muscle relaxation by promoting the production of nitric oxide (NO) [19]. Resting airway tone involves bronchodilation by NO, but whether this is from local cellular production of NO or NANC and VIP-mediated release of NO is not clear [13]. There is also a bronchoconstrictor part of the NANC system [19], with important effects in airways disease, but the contribution of this system to normal airway tone is unknown.

2 Humoral control also occurs in normal lung [20]. Despite the minimal significance of sympathetic innervation, bronchial smooth muscle has plentiful β_2-adrenergic receptors, which are highly sensitive to circulating adrenaline, and act via complex second messenger systems (see below). Basal levels of adrenaline probably do not contribute to bronchial muscle tone, but this mechanism is brought into play during exercise or during the sympathetic 'stress response'.

3 Direct physical and chemical stimulation of the respiratory epithelium activates the parasympathetic reflex described above causing bronchoconstriction. Activation of the bronchoconstrictor path of the NANC system may also play a part. Physical factors known to produce bronchoconstriction include mechanical stimulation of the upper air passages by laryngoscopy and the presence of foreign bodies in the trachea or bronchi. Inhalation of particulate matter, an aerosol of water or just cold air may cause bronchoconstriction, the latter being used as a simple provocation test. Many chemical stimuli result in bronchoconstriction including liquids with low pH such as gastric acid, and gases such as sulphur dioxide, ammonia, ozone and nitrogen dioxide.

4 Local cellular mechanisms involve inflammatory cells in the lung such as mast cells, eosinophils, neutrophils, macrophages and lymphocytes. These inflammatory cells are stimulated by a variety of pathogens, but some may also be activated by the direct physical factors described in the previous paragraph. Once activated, cytokine production causes amplification of the response, and a variety of mediators are released that can cause bronchoconstriction (Table 17.1) [21]. These mediators are produced in normal individuals, but patients with airway disease are usually 'hyper-responsive' and so develop symptoms of bronchospasm more easily.

Molecular mechanisms controlling airway smooth muscle

The prevalence of asthma has now reached dramatic proportions in many areas of the world and the disease now affects 15–30% of children in developed countries [22]. With so many patients affected, the search for new and more efficacious bronchodilator drugs has led to huge efforts to elucidate the molecular mechanisms of airway smooth muscle contraction. Three main receptors exist in the airway, and all have been targeted for therapeutic effects.

Acetylcholine receptor

Stimulation of M_3 ACh receptors activates a G-protein, characterized as Gq. This in turn activates phospholipase C to stimulate the production of inositol triphosphate (IP_3), which then binds to sarcoplasmic reticulum receptors causing release of calcium from intracellular stores. The elevation of intracellular calcium activates myosin light chain kinase, which phosphorylates part of the myosin chain to activate myosin ATPase and initiate cross-bridging between actin and myosin [21]. IP_3 is converted into the inactive inositol diphosphate by IP_3 kinase. Tachykinin, histamine and leukotriene receptors responsible for bronchoconstriction from other mediators (Table 17.1) act by a very similar mechanism, being

Table 17.1 Mediators involved in alteration of bronchial smooth muscle tone during airway inflammation.

Source	Bronchoconstriction		Bronchodilatation	
	Mediator	Receptor	Mediator	Receptor
Mast cells & other pro-inflammatory cells	Histamine	H_1	Prostaglandin E_2	EP
	Prostaglandin D_2	TP	Prostacyclin (PGI_2)	EP
	Prostaglandin $F_{2\alpha}$	TP		
	Leukotrienes $C_4 D_4 E_4$	$CysLT_1$		
	PAF	PAF		
	Bradykinin	B_2		
C-fibres (e-NANC)	Substance P	NK_2		
	Neurokinin A	NK_2		
	CGRP	CGRP		
Endothelial and epithelial cells	Endothelin	ET_B		

CGRP, calcitonin gene-related peptide; e-NANC, excitatory non-adrenergic non-cholinergic; PAF, platelet activating factor.

linked to G-protein–phospholipase C complexes, which lead to IP_3 formation.

Anticholinergic drugs used in the airway are classified into short-acting (e.g. ipratropium) or long-acting (e.g. tiotropium) types. These drugs have similar binding affinities for both prejunctional inhibitory M_2 and postjunctional M_3 receptors, giving rise to opposing effects on the degree of stimulation of airway smooth muscle. Differences in relative numbers of M_2 and M_3 receptors between individuals and in different disease states [17] will therefore explain the variability in response seen with inhaled anticholinergic drugs. Tiotropium, a recently introduced anticholinergic, has a long duration of therapeutic effect because of faster dissociation of the drug from M_2 compared with M_3 receptors, leaving only the M_3 receptors antagonized.

β_2-Adrenoreceptor

The molecular basis of the functional characteristics of the β_2-adrenoceptor are now clearly elucidated [23]. It contains 413 amino acids and has seven transmembrane helices (Fig. 17.5). The agonist binding site is within this hydrophobic core of the protein, which sits within the lipid bilayer of the cell membrane. Receptors exist in either activated or inactivated form, the former state occurring

when the third intracellular loop is bound to guanosine triphosphate (GTP) and the α subunit of the Gs-protein. β_2-Receptor agonists probably do not induce a significant conformational change in the protein structure but simply stabilize the activated form, allowing this to predominate.

Activation of the G-protein by the β_2-receptor in turn activates adenylate cyclase to convert ATP to cyclic adenosine monophosphate (cAMP) [23]. cAMP causes relaxation of the muscle cell by inhibition of calcium release from intracellular stores and probably also activates protein kinase A to phosphorylate some of the regulatory proteins involved in the actin–myosin interaction.

Two β_2-receptor genes are present in humans, with a total of 13 polymorphisms described, giving rise to a large number of possible phenotypes. Studies of these phenotypes are at an early stage, but some genetic differences have been shown to be associated with worse nocturnal falls in peak flow and varying degrees of receptor desensitization by β_2-agonists [23].

Currently available inhaled β_2-adrenoceptor agonists are highly specific for the β_2-receptors, with cardiac (β_1) effects only occurring at very high doses. Recent developments have involved the introduction of long-acting β_2-agonists (e.g. salmeterol).

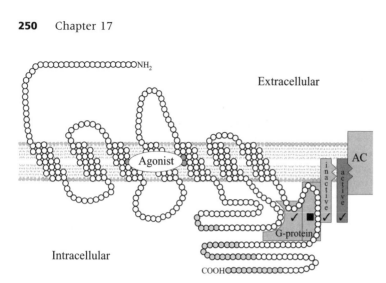

Figure 17.5 Molecular mechanisms of β_2-adrenoceptor action. The receptor exists in activated and inactivated states according to whether or not the α subunit of the G-protein is bound to adenyl cyclase (AC). The agonist binds to the third and fifth transmembrane domains within the lipid bilayer, and by doing so stabilizes the receptor G-protein complex in the activated state. The intracellular C-terminal region of the protein (shaded) is the area of the receptor that is susceptible to phosphorylation by intracellular kinases, causing inactivation and down-regulation of the receptor.

These drugs are more lipophilic than the shorter acting drugs and so form a depot in the lipid bilayer from which they can repeatedly interact with the binding site of the receptor, producing a much longer duration of action than hydrophilic drugs. The therapeutic effect of β_2-agonists is more complex than simple relaxation of airway smooth muscle as they are also known to inhibit the secretion of inflammatory cytokines and most of the bronchoconstrictor mediators shown in Table 17.1.

After its production following β_2-receptor stimulation, cAMP is rapidly hydrolysed by the intracellular enzyme phosphodiesterase (PDE), inhibition of which will therefore prolong the smooth muscle relaxant effect of β_2-receptor stimulation. Seven subgroups of PDE have now been identified, with subgroups PDE3 and PDE4 occurring in airway smooth muscle, but the PDE inhibitors currently used in asthma, such as theophylline, are non-specific for the different subgroups [21]. This lack of specificity of currently used PDE inhibitors also accounts for their wide ranging side-effects, which continue to limit their therapeutic use.

There are now believed to be many molecular interactions between the IP$_3$ and cAMP signalling pathways. Activation of phospholipase C by protein Gq also liberates intracellular diacylglycerol which activates another membrane-bound enzyme, protein kinase C. This enzyme is able to phosphorylate a variety of proteins including G-proteins and the β_2-receptor itself (Fig. 17.5) causing uncoupling of the receptor from the G-protein and down-regulation of the transduction pathway [21,23].

Receptors for arachidonic acid derivatives

Inflammatory mediators released in the airway stimulate phospholipase A$_2$ to produce arachidonic acid from the lipids of the nuclear membrane [24]. Arachidonic acid may then enter either the cyclo-oxygenase pathway, producing a variety of prostaglandins, or the lipo-oxygenase pathway, producing leukotrienes. These mediators are mostly bronchoconstrictors, although some prostaglandins can cause bronchodilatation (Table 17.1).

Even in non-asthmatic individuals, leukotrienes are potent bronchoconstrictors, so the therapeutic potential of leukotriene antagonists has been extensively investigated. In the lung, leukotrienes all act via a single receptor (CysLT$_1$) on airway smooth muscle cells to cause contraction via the G-protein–IP$_3$ system described above. Leukotrienes have a wide range of activities apart from bronchoconstriction, in particular amplification of the inflammatory response by chemotaxis of eosinophils.

The opposing effects of prostaglandins on bronchial smooth muscle mean that drugs that block bronchoconstrictor effects induced by this pathway must be very receptor-specific, and appropriate agents have not been developed. Inhibition of prostaglandin production by non-specific inhibitors of cyclo-oxygenase (COX) has harmful effects in some asthmatic patients, with aspirin, and the closely related non-steroidal anti-inflammatory drugs, sometimes causing bronchospasm in asthma patients, referred to as aspirin-induced asthma (AIA) [25]. Based on patient history alone, only 2.7% of asthma patients report wheezing in response to aspirin, but when provocation with oral aspirin is carried out, 21% of patients develop a reduction in forced expiratory volumes [26]. Inhibiting the COX pathway in the airway will reduce synthesis of the bronchodilator prostaglandin PGE_2, so potentially causing bronchospasm. Reduced synthesis of PGE_2 cannot alone account for AIA; patients with AIA also have increased production of leukotriene E_4 (LTE_4), a potent bronchoconstrictor. This effect on the lipo-oxygenase pathway is not mediated by aspirin itself, and possibly results from loss of inhibition of lipo-oxygenase by PGE_2. Genetic polymorphisms for the enzymes involved in leukotriene production may explain why some patients are aspirin sensitive [27]. Multiple isoforms of COX exist: COX-1 seems to be responsible for most cases of AIA, so the recently introduced COX-2 inhibitors should be safe for use in AIA patients [25].

Oxygen and carbon dioxide carriage in the red blood cell

At a very basic level, the carriage of oxygen by haemoglobin in the red blood cell (RBC) and the carriage of CO_2 as bicarbonate ion in the blood may be considered as two separate physiological processes. Christian Bohr, in 1904, was the first to demonstrate a connection between the two processes when he demonstrated that the CO_2 concentration of blood affected the reaction between haemoglobin and oxygen. Better understanding of protein function at the molecular level has demonstrated that CO_2 and oxygen transport processes are linked much more closely than the simple Bohr effect.

Carriage of carbon dioxide

Blood contains approximately 50 mL/dL of CO_2, with three systems contributing to its transport. The first of these involves CO_2 being physically dissolved in the blood. The solubility of CO_2 in blood is affected by temperature, but at 37°C there is approximately 2.5 mL/dL carried in this form.

Carbamino carriage of carbon dioxide

This describes CO_2 combining with uncharged amino groups found in proteins. The only amino groups in a protein that are free to bind CO_2 are the one terminal amino group in each protein chain and the side chain amino groups of lysine and arginine. Because both hydrogen ions and CO_2 compete to react with uncharged amino groups, the ability to combine with CO_2 is markedly pH dependent. Only very small quantities of CO_2 are carried in carbamino compounds with plasma protein. Almost all is carried by haemoglobin, and deoxyhaemoglobin is approximately 3.5 times as effective as oxyhaemoglobin, this being a major component of the Haldane effect. The Haldane effect is the difference in the quantity of CO_2 carried, at constant P_{CO_2}, in oxygenated and deoxygenated blood. Although the amount of CO_2 carried in the blood by carbamino carriage is small, the *difference* between the amount carried in venous and arterial blood is approximately one-third of the total arterial–venous difference. This therefore accounts for the major part of the Haldane effect, the remainder being due to the increased buffering capacity of reduced haemoglobin, which is described below.

Transport of carbon dioxide as bicarbonate

Hydration of CO_2 to form carbonic acid and its subsequent dissociation to bicarbonate ions are crucial reactions for transporting CO_2. The first of these reactions is slow, requiring some minutes for equilibrium to be reached, which is far too slow for the time available for gas exchange in pulmonary and systemic capillaries if the reaction were not catalysed in both directions by the enzyme carbonic anhydrase (CA). The enzyme exists as seven isozymes of which two are involved in blood CO_2 transport. Red blood cells contain large amounts of CA II, one of the fastest enzymes known, while CA IV is a membrane-bound isozyme present in pulmonary capillaries. Carbonic anhydrase is a zinc-containing enzyme of low molecular weight, and there is now extensive knowledge of the molecular mechanisms of CA [28]. First, the zinc atom hydrolyses water to a reactive Zn–OH⁻ species, while a nearby histidine residue acts as a 'proton shuttle', removing the H⁺ from the metal-ion centre and transferring it to any buffer molecules near the enzyme. Carbon dioxide then combines with the Zn–OH⁻ species and the HCO_3^- formed rapidly dissociates from the zinc atom. The maximal rate of catalysis is determined by the buffering power in the vicinity of the enzyme, as the speed of the enzyme reactions are so fast that its kinetics are determined mostly by the ability of the surrounding buffers to provide/remove H⁺ ions to or from the enzyme. Carbonic anhydrase is inhibited by a large number of compounds of which acetazolamide is the most well known. Acetazolamide is nonspecific for the different CA isozymes and has been used extensively in the study of carbonic anhydrase, and has revealed the surprising fact that it is not essential to life. The quantity and efficiency of RBC CA is such that more than 98% of activity must be blocked before there is any discernable change in CO_2 transport, although when total inhibition is achieved, $P\text{co}_2$ gradients between tissues and alveolar gas are increased, pulmonary ventilation is increased and alveolar $P\text{co}_2$ is decreased.

There is no CA activity in plasma, so the production of bicarbonate occurs within the RBC. For the CA to function effectively, the H⁺ ions produced must be quickly removed from the active site of the enzyme by buffering. Proteins are generally inefficient buffers, with most of the possible reactions occurring only at pH values far removed from the physiologi-cal range. Histidine residues, with their imidazole side chains, have buffering power at normal blood pH, and haemoglobin contains numerous histidine groups in all four of its constituent chains. The change in conformational state of haemoglobin that occurs when binding or releasing oxygen (see below) significantly changes the buffering capacity of the histidine such that better buffering occurs in deoxygenated blood, allowing greater CO_2 carriage.

Hamburger shift and the band 3 protein

Apart from rapid buffering of H⁺ ions, efficient CA function also requires the bicarbonate to be removed from the vicinity of the CA. In the RBC this is achieved by actively exporting bicarbonate ions out of the cell into the plasma, in exchange for chloride ions to maintain electrical neutrality across the RBC membrane. This ionic exchange was first suggested by Hamburger in 1918, and believed to be a passive process. It is now known to be facilitated by a com-

plex membrane-bound protein that has been extensively studied and named band 3 after its position on a gel electrophoresis plate [29,30]. Band 3 exchanges bicarbonate and chloride ions by a 'ping-pong' mechanism in which one ion first moves out of the RBC before the other ion moves inwards, in contrast to most other ion pumps, which simultaneously exchange the two ions (Fig. 17.6). Band 3 is also closely associated with carbonic anhydrase, and the protein complex formed is believed to act as a metabolon, a term describing the channelling of a substrate directly between proteins that catalyse sequential reactions in a metabolic pathway [29]. In this case the substrate is bicarbonate, which, after its formation by CA, is transferred directly to band 3, which rapidly exports it from the cell.

Carriage of oxygen

As for CO_2, oxygen is carried in blood in simple solution. At 37°C, there is 0.0225 mL/dL/kPa oxygen dissolved, which equates to 0.25 mL/dL at normal arterial $P\text{o}_2$, or less than 1% of total oxygen carriage. The remainder is carried in combination with haemoglobin.

Molecular basis of haemoglobin function

In the most common type of adult human haemoglobin (HbA) there are four protein chains, two α-chains and two β-chains, each of which binds to a haem group via one of the numerous histidine residues found in haemoglobin [31,32].

The four chains of the haemoglobin molecule lie in a ball like a crumpled necklace. However, the form is not as random as this analogy suggests, and the actual shape (the quaternary structure) is of critical importance and governs the reaction with oxygen. The shape is maintained by loose electrostatic bonds between specific amino acids on different chains and also between some amino acids on the same chain. One consequence of these bonds is that the haem groups lie in crevices formed by electrostatic bonds between the haem groups and histidine residues, other than those to which they are attached by normal valency linkages. For example, in the α-chain the haem group is attached to the iron atom, which is bound to the histidine residue in position 87. However, the haem group is also attached by an

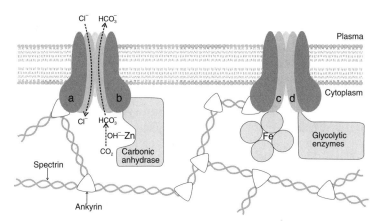

Figure 17.6 Proteins associated with band 3 in the red blood cell membrane. Band 3 has 12 trans-membrane domains forming the bicarbonate–chloride exchange ion channel, and four globular cytoplasmic domains (a–d), each of which is associated with different groups of intracellular proteins. a, Ankyrin and spectrin, to maintain and possibly alter red cell shape; b, carbonic anhydrase, with which band 3 acts as a metabolon to directly transfer bicarbonate ions into and out of the red cell; c, haemoglobin, with which band 3 may act as a metabolon to export nitric oxide; d, glycolytic enzymes — the functional significance of this association is unknown.

electrostatic bond to the histidine residue in position 58 and also by non-polar bonds to many other amino acids. This forms a loop in the protein chain and places the haem group in a crevice, the shape of which controls the ease of access for oxygen molecules.

In deoxyhaemoglobin, the electrostatic bonds within and between the protein chains are stronger, holding the haemoglobin molecule in a tense (T) conformation, in which the molecule has a relatively low affinity for oxygen. In oxyhaemoglobin, the electrostatic bonds are weaker, and the haemoglobin adopts its relaxed (R) state, in which the crevices containing the haem groups can open and bind oxygen, and the molecule's affinity for oxygen becomes 500 times greater than in the T state. Binding of oxygen to just one of the four protein chains induces a conformational change in the whole haemoglobin molecule, which increases the affinity of the other protein chains for oxygen. This 'cooperativity' between oxygen binding sites is fundamental to the physiological role of haemoglobin, and affects the kinetics of the reaction between haemoglobin and oxygen, giving rise to the well-known S-shaped dissociation curve. The conformational state (R or T) of the haemoglobin molecule is also altered by other factors that influence the strength of the electrosta-tic bonds; such factors include CO_2, pH and temperature.

The Bohr effect describes the alteration in haemoglobin oxygen affinity that arises from changes in hydrogen ion or CO_2 concentrations, and is generally considered in terms of its influence upon the dissociation curve. Changes in pH affect the numerous electrostatic bonds that maintain the quaternary structure of haemoglobin, and so stabilizes the molecule in the T conformation, reducing its affinity for oxygen. Similarly, CO_2 binds to the N-terminal amino acid residues of the α-chain to form carbaminohaemoglobin (see above), and this small alteration in the function of the protein chains stabilizes the T conformation and facilitates release of the oxygen molecule from haemoglobin.

Conversely, the Haldane effect describes the smaller amount of CO_2 that can be carried in oxygenated blood compared with deoxygenated blood. Crystallographic studies have shown that in deoxyhaemoglobin the histidine in position 146 of the β-chain is loosely bonded to the aspartine residue at position 94, and that when haemoglobin binds oxygen and changes to the R conformation the histidine 146 moves 1 nm further away from the aspartine, which is sufficient distance to change its pK value [33]. Once again, this small change in one area of the β-chain has widespread effects on electrostatic bonds throughout the molecule, changing the quaternary structure of the entire molecule and altering its ability to buffer hydrogen ions and form carbamino compounds with CO_2.

Haemoglobin and nitric oxide

It has been known for some time that NO binds to haemoglobin very rapidly, and this observation is fundamental to its therapeutic use when inhaled NO exerts its effects in the pulmonary vasculature but is inactivated by binding to haemoglobin before it reaches the systemic circulation [34,35]. There are two quite separate chemical reactions between NO and the haemoglobin molecule [36]:

1 NO binds to the haem moiety of each haemoglobin chain, but the resulting reaction differs with the state of oxygenation. For deoxyhaemoglobin, in the T conformation, a fairly stable Hb–NO complex is rapidly formed, which has little vasodilator activity, while for oxyhaemoglobin, in the R conformation, the oxygen is displaced by NO and in doing so the iron atom is oxidized to methaemoglobin and a nitrate ion produced:

$$Hb\,[Fe^{2+}] + NO \rightarrow Hb\,[Fe^{2+}]\,NO$$

or

$$Hb\,[Fe^{2+}]\,O_2 + NO \rightarrow Hb\,[Fe^{3+}] + NO_3^-$$

These reactions are so rapid that there is doubt that endogenous NO itself can exert any effects within blood (e.g. on platelets) before being bound by haemoglobin, and must therefore act via an intermediate substance.

2 Nitric oxide is also known to form stable compounds with sulphydryl groups termed S-nitrosothiols, this reaction occurring with sulphur-containing amino acid residues within proteins. Nitrosothiols retain biological activity as vasodilators and can survive for longer than free NO within the blood vessels. NO forms a nitrosothiol group with the cysteine residue at position 93 on the haemoglobin β-chains, producing S-nitrosohaemoglobin (SNO-Hb). As a result of conformational changes in haemoglobin the reaction is faster with R-state oxyhaemoglobin and under alkaline conditions [36].

Thus, *in vivo* NO in arterial blood is predominantly in the form of SNO-Hb, while in venous blood haem bound HbNO predominates. It has been proposed that as haemoglobin passes through the pulmonary capillary, changes in oxygenation, P_{CO_2} and pH drive the change from the deoxygenated T conformation to the oxygenated R conformation, and this change in quaternary structure of haemoglobin causes the intramolecular transfer of NO from the haem to cysteine bound positions. In the peripheral capillaries, the opposite sequence of events occurs, which encourages release of NO from the RSNO group, where it may again bind to the haem group, or be released from the RBC to act as a local vasodilator, effectively improving flow to vessels with the greatest demand for oxygen [37]. Export of NO activity from the RBC is believed to occur via a complex mechanism. Deoxygenated T conformation haemoglobin binds to one of the cytoplasmic domains of the RBC transmembrane band 3 protein (Fig. 17.6), which may again act as a metabolon and directly transfer the NO, via a series of nitrosothiol reactions, to the outside of the cell membrane where it can exert its vasodilator activity. The biological implications of this series of events are yet to be determined. The suggestion that haemoglobin is acting as a nitric oxide carrier to regulate capillary blood flow and oxygen release from the RBC represents a fundamental advance in our understanding of the delivery of oxygen to tissues [34,35].

The RBC membrane and oxygen carriage

For oxygen to transfer from the alveolus to the haemoglobin within the RBC it must diffuse across multiple barriers:

• *Alveolar lining fluid:* including the complex arrangements of fluid pools and varying thickness layers of surfactant described above.

• *Tissue barrier:* which includes the alveolar epithelial cell, its basement membrane, the interstitial space and the pulmonary capillary endothelium. In the region where alveolar capillaries are in close proximity to the alveoli, these structures are all very thin, presenting an overall thickness of approximately 0.5 μm.

• *Plasma layer:* human pulmonary capillaries have a mean thickness of 7 μm, so to reach the middle of the capillary oxygen must diffuse 3.5 μm, or seven times further than the tissue barrier. Alveolar lining fluid and the tissue barrier therefore offer little resistance to diffusion in comparison with the long and slow diffusion path through plasma.

• *Diffusion into and within the RBC* [38]: confining haemoglobin within the RBC reduces oxygen uptake by haemoglobin by 40% in comparison with free haemoglobin solution. There are three possible explanations for this observation. First, the rapid uptake of O_2 by RBCs causes depletion of gas in the plasma layer immediately surrounding the RBC. Referred to as the 'unstirred layer', this phenomenon is most likely to occur at low packed cell volume when adjacent RBCs in the pulmonary capillary have more plasma between them [39]. Secondly, oxygen must diffuse across the RBC membrane, although this is not normally believed to be a significant diffusion barrier. Thirdly, once in the cell, oxygen must diffuse through a varying amount of intracellular fluid before combining with haemoglobin, a process that is aided by mass movement of the haemoglobin molecules caused by the deformation of the RBC as it passes through the capillary bed, in effect 'mixing' the oxygen with the haemoglobin.

Red blood cells change shape as they pass through capillaries (both pulmonary and systemic) and this has an important role in the uptake and release of oxygen [38]. The dependence of diffusing capacity on RBC shape changes may result from reducing the unstirred layer by 'mixing' the plasma around the RBC, from changes in the cell membrane surface area to RBC volume ratio or from assisting the mass movement of haemoglobin within the cell. This has led to further studies in which the deformability of RBCs is reduced (using chlorpromazine) or increased (using sodium salicylate), which have demonstrated that diffusing capacity is increased with greater RBC deformability [39]. Of more clinical significance are recent studies of the effect of plasma cholesterol on RBC function [40]. Elevated cholesterol concentration in the plasma causes increased cholesterol in the RBC membrane, a change that is known to make the membrane thicker and less deformable, both of which lead to reduced efficiency of diffusion across the membrane. Oxygen uptake by RBCs in the lung, and its release in the tissues, are both believed to be significantly impaired by hypercholesterolaemia,

particularly in tissues with high oxygen extraction ratios such as the heart.

Furthermore, studies of the band 3 RBC membrane, described above in relation to CO_2 carriage and the transfer of nitric oxide activity, suggest yet another role for this protein in facilitating oxygen carriage by altering RBC cytoskeleton function (Fig. 17.6). The cytoplasmic domain of band 3 acts as an anchoring site for many of the proteins involved in the maintenance of cell shape and membrane stability such as ankyrin and spectrin. A genetically engineered deficiency of band 3 in animals results in small, fragile, spherical RBCs [41]. This association between band 3 and the RBC cytoskeleton raises the intriguing possibility that changes in CO_2 or oxygen tension occurring in pulmonary or systemic capillaries could alter red cell shape or deformability. This would allow more of the red cell membrane to make contact with the capillary wall and so facilitate rapid gas exchange without the need for diffusion across the plasma layer.

References

1 Lumb AB. *Nunn's Applied Respiratory Physiology*, 6th edn. London: Elsevier Butterworth Heinemann, 2005.

2 Bianchi AL, Denavit-Saubie M, Champagnat J. Central control of breathing in mammals: neuronal circuitry, membrane properties, and neurotransmitters. *Physiol Rev* 1995; **75**: 1–31.

3 Ramirez JM, Telgkamp P, Elsen FP, Quellmalz UJA, Richter DW. Respiratory rhythm generation in mammals: synaptic and membrane properties. *Respir Physiol* 1997; **110**: 71–85.

4 Richter DW, Lalley PM, Pierrefiche O, *et al.* Intracellular signal pathways controlling respiratory neurons. *Respir Physiol* 1997; **110**: 113–23.

5 Winkworth AL, Davis PJ, Adams RD, Ellis E. Breathing patterns during spontaneous speech. *J Speech Hear Res* 1995; **38**; 124–44.

6 Widdicombe J. Airway receptors. *Respir Physiol* 2001; **125**: 3–15.

7 Gaudy JH. The Hering–Breuer reflex in man? *Br J Anaesth* 1991; **66**: 627–8.

8 Prabhakar NR. Oxygen sensing by the carotid body chemoreceptors. *J Appl Physiol* 2000; **88**: 2287–95.

9 Soto-Arape I, Burton MD, Kazemi H. Central amino acid neurotransmitters and the hypoxic ventilatory response. *Am J Respir Crit Care Med* 1995; **151**: 1113–20.

10 Milic-Emili J, Robatto FM, Bates JHT. Respiratory mechanics in anaesthesia. *Br J Anaesth* 1990; **65**: 4–12.

11 Hamm H, Kroegel C, Hohlfeld J. Surfactant: a review of its functions and relevance in adult respiratory disorders. *Respir Med* 1996; **90**: 251–70.

12 Whitsett JA, Weaver TE. Hydrophobic surfactant proteins in lung function and disease. *N Engl J Med* 2002; **347**: 2141–8.

13 Weaver TE, Conkright JJ. Functions of surfactant proteins B and C. *Annu Rev Physiol* 2001; **63**: 555–78.

14 Dorrington KL, Young JD. Development of the concept of a liquid pulmonary alveolar lining layer. *Br J Anaesth* 2001; **86**: 614–7.

15 Hills BA. An alternative view of the role(s) of surfactant and the alveolar model. *J Appl Physiol* 1999; **87**: 1567–83.

16 Scarpelli EM. The alveolar surface network: a new anatomy and its physiological significance. *Anat Rec* 1998; **251**: 491–527.

17 Canning BJ, Fischer A. Neural regulation of airway smooth muscle tone. *Respir Physiol* 2001; **125**: 113–27.

18 Widdicombe JG. Autonomic regulation: i-NANC/e-NANC. *Am J Respir Crit Care Med* 1998; **158**: S171–5.

19 Drazen JM, Gaston B, Shore SA. Chemical regulation of pulmonary airway tone. *Annu Rev Physiol* 1995; **57**: 151–70.

20 Thomson NC, Dagg KD, Ramsay SG. Humoral control of airway tone. *Thorax* 1996; **51**: 461–4.

21 Barnes PJ. Pharmacology of airway smooth muscle. *Am J Respir Crit Care Med* 1998; **158**: S123–32.

22 Holgate ST. The epidemic of asthma and allergy. *J R Soc Med* 2004; **97**: 103–10.

23 Johnson M. The β-adrenoceptor. *Am J Respir Crit Care Med* 1998; **158**: S146–53.

24 Drazen JM, Isreal E, O'Byrne PM. Treatment of asthma with drugs modifying the leukotriene pathway. *N Engl J Med* 1999; **340**: 197–206.

25 Szczeklik A, Stevenson DD. Aspirin-induced asthma: advances in pathogenesis, diagnosis, and management. *J Allergy Clin Immunol* 2003; **111**: 913–21.

26 Jenkins C, Costello J, Hodge L. Systematic review of prevalence of aspirin induced asthma and its implications for clinical practice. *Br Med J* 2004; **328**: 434–7.

27 Szczeklik A, Sanak M. Genetic mechanisms in aspirin-induced asthma. *Am J Respir Crit Care Med* 2000; **161**: S142–6.

28 Chegwidden WR, Carter ND, Edwards YH, eds. *The Carbonic Anhydrase: New Horizons*. Basel: Birkhäuser Verlag, 2000.

29 Tanner MJA. Band 3 anion exchanger and its involvement in erythrocyte and kidney disorders. *Curr Opin Hematol* 2002; **9**: 133–9.

30 Zhang D, Kiyatkin A, Bolin JT, Low PS. Crystallographic structure and functional interpretation of the cytoplasmic domain of erythrocyte membrane band 3. *Blood* 2000; **96**: 2925–33.

31 Hsia CCW. Respiratory function of hemoglobin. *N Engl J Med* 1998; **338**: 239–47.

32 Russo R, Benazzi L, Perrella M. The Bohr effect of hemoglobin intermediates and the role of salt bridges in the tertiary/quaternary transitions. *J Biol Chem* 2001; **276**: 13628–34.

33 Ho C, Perussi JR. Proton nuclear magnetic resonance studies of haemoglobin. *Methods Enzymol* 1994; **232**: 97–139.

34 Hobbs AJ, Gladwin MT, Patel RP, Williams DLH, Butler AR. Haemoglobin: NO transporter, NO inactivator or none the above. *Trends Pharmacol Sci* 2002; **23**: 406–11.

35 Gross SS. Targeted delivery of nitric oxide. *Nature* 2001; **409**: 577–8.

36 Jia L, Bonaventura C, Bonaventura J, Stamler JS. S-nitrosohaemoglobin: a dynamic activity of blood involved in vascular control. *Nature* 1996; **380**: 221–6.

37 Shen W, Hintze TH, Wolin MS. Nitric oxide: an important signaling mechanism between vascular endothelium and parenchymal cells in the regulation of oxygen consumption. *Circulation* 1995; **92**: 3505–12.

38 Sarelius I. Invited editorial on 'Effect of RBC shape and deformability on pulmonary O_2 diffusing capacity and resistance to flow in rabbit lungs'. *J Appl Physiol* 1995; **78**: 763–4.

39 Betticher DC, Reinhart WH, Geiser J. Effect of RBC shape and deformability on pulmonary O_2 diffusing capacity and resistance to flow in rabbit lungs. *J Appl Physiol* 1995; **78**: 778–83.

40 Buchwald H, O'Dea TJ, Menchaca HJ, Michalek VN, Rohde TD. Effect of plasma cholesterol on red blood cell oxygen transport. *Clin Exp Pharmacol Physiol* 2000; **27**: 951–5.

41 Jay DG. Role of band 3 in homeostasis and cell shape. *Cell* 1996; **86**: 853–4.

CHAPTER 18

Non-respiratory functions of the lung

Andrew Lumb and Susan Walwyn

Introduction

For over 1400 years, the writings of Galen described the lungs as having two principal functions: to act as a protective sponge to cushion the heart and to cool the heart, which was believed to be the source of the body's innate heat [1]. In the 17th century, a group of physiologists from Oxford, who founded the Royal Society of London, used a series of scientific experiments to demonstrate that the lung was responsible for transferring gases to and from the blood as it passed through the lung tissue. A relatively short time later, advances in the new science of chemistry led to the discovery of oxygen, carbon dioxide and nitrogen, and improved understanding of the primary role of the lungs as organs of gas exchange.

Over the years, other functions of the lungs have emerged. As a filter of inhaled substances it has a large surface area of respiratory epithelium, which is well designed to remove or inactivate the enormous range of pathogens, particles and gases that enter the lung during normal breathing. The airway lining also humidifies the gas entering the lungs to reduce damage to the delicate, thin alveolar cells that facilitate gas exchange. The pulmonary circulation receives almost the whole of the cardiac output and is thus well suited to act as a safety net, filtering any venous emboli to prevent them gaining access to the arterial circulation. Finally, the endothelial lining of the pulmonary circulation is metabolically active, having a variety of metabolic and endocrine roles, and, as a consequence, affecting the pharmacokinetics of some drugs.

Respiratory epithelium

To facilitate efficient gas exchange, the barrier between alveolar gas and the pulmonary capillary blood has a large surface area and is extremely thin, and so offers a huge potential for the ingress of harmful substances into the body's tightly regulated internal milieu. Before inspired air reaches the alveoli it must be humidified, and airborne particles, pathogens and irritant chemicals removed. These tasks are undertaken by the respiratory epithelium. Before considering in detail how these functions are carried out, it is helpful to consider the cellular components found lining the airways.

Cell types
Ciliated columnar cells

These ciliated cells are the most abundant cell type in the respiratory epithelium [2]. In the nose, pharynx and larger airways the epithelial cells are pseudo-stratified, gradually changing to a single layer of columnar cells in bronchi, cuboidal cells in bronchioles, and finally thinning further to merge with the type I alveolar epithelial cells. They are differentiated from either basal or secretory cells (see below) and are characterized by the presence of approximately 300 cilia per cell. The movement of cilial action is towards the trachea. Cilial beat frequency is 12–14 beats per second and can be affected by pollutants, smoke, anaesthetic agents and infection. The cilia are thought to beat by a relative shift in the skeletal tubules as they slide over one another. The recovery stroke involves a slow whip-like return to the normal position. Cilia have been extensively studied as they freeze for up to a month without any hindrance in functional recovery. The presence of numerous mitochondria within these cells is a feature of their high metabolic rate, with large amounts of energy being required for the activity of cilia and for the active control of airway surface liquid volume and composition (see below).

Goblet cells

These are differentiated columnar epithelial cells containing membrane-bound acidic mucin granules [3]. In the trachea, goblet cells are present at a density of about $6000/mm^2$ and are responsible, along with submucosal secretory cells, for producing the mucous layer of the airway surface liquid. Mucin, the principal glycoprotein in mucus, is released by rapid (<150ms) exocytosis from the mucus-secreting cells in response to a range of stimuli. These include direct chemical irritation (e.g. by tobacco smoke), inflammatory cytokines and neuronal stimulation, predominantly by cholinergic nerves. Stimulation of these cholinergic neurones may occur via parasympathetic nerves (carried in the vagus nerve) or from a reflex arc following stimulation of nearby airway irritant receptors [4]. Both goblet cell numbers and secretions increase in many airway diseases such as asthma, bronchitis and cystic fibrosis.

Submucosal secretory cells

These can be subdivided into serous cells and mucous cells. The serous cells are found in the gland acinus, while mucous cells are found closer to the collecting duct. The whole submucosal gland structure can be found in the larger bronchi and in the trachea; in the latter there are approximately 10 submucosal openings per millimetre [2]. The serous cells have the highest levels of membrane-bound cystic fibrosis transmembrane conductance regulator (CFTR) in the lung (see below).

Basal cells

These cells lie underneath the columnar cells, giving rise to the pseudo-stratified appearance, and are absent in the bronchioles and beyond. They are believed to be the stem cell responsible for producing new epithelial and goblet cells.

Clara cells

Clara cells are non-ciliated columnar cells that are found mostly in the epithelium of terminal bronchioles. They are the most metabolically active epithelial cell and have been compared to Paneth cells in the gut. Clara cells are responsible for the secretion of surfactant proteins, antiprotease enzymes and a variety of other airway surface liquid proteins whose functions are mostly unknown [5] although some are involved in the metabolism of chemical toxins. Some Clara cells are able to act as local stem cells at times of injury.

Neuroepithelial cells

These cells are found throughout the bronchial tree, but occur in larger numbers in the intrapulmonary and terminal bronchioles. They may be found individually or in clusters as neuroepithelial bodies, and are of uncertain function in the adult lung [6,7]. Present in fetal lung tissue in a greater number, they may be responsible for controlling lung development. Similar cells elsewhere in the body secrete a variety of amines and peptides with diverse effects such as calcitonin, gastrin releasing peptide, calcitonin gene-related peptide and serotonin.

Mast cells

The lungs contain numerous mast cells, which are located underneath the epithelial cells of the airways as well as in the alveolar septa. Some also lie free in the lumen of the airways and may be recovered by bronchial lavage. They are important in mediating bronchoconstriction in patients with airway disease.

Macrophages

Macrophages are phagocytic cells found throughout the lung, although they are more abundant in the alveoli than the airways. Macrophages form the major component of host defence within the alveoli. They are derived either from monocyte stem cells that differentiate in the lung or from circulating phagocytes that pass freely from the circulation, through the interstitial space and thence through the gaps between alveolar epithelial cells to lie on their surface within the alveolus (Fig. 18.1) [8]. They can re-enter the body, but are remarkable for their ability to live and

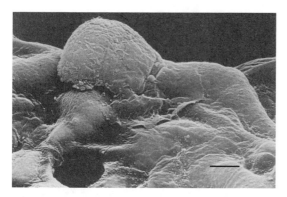

Figure 18.1 Scanning electron micrograph of an alveolar macrophage advancing to the right over type I alveolar epithelial cells. The scale bar is 5 μm. (From Weibel [8] with permission of the author and the publishers; © Harvard University Press.)

function outside the body. Macrophages are active in combating infection and scavenging foreign bodies such as small dust particles. Phagocytosis can be sub-divided into chemotaxis, adherence, ingestion and digestion. Chemotaxis is enabled by the presence of microbial cell wall products, complement or sur-factant protein A. Recognition of foreign particulate matter, microorganisms and debris is followed by adherence and ingestion. Presence of antibodies, complement and other opsonins will enhance the recognition process. Following adherence, ingestion occurs in two ways: either by active adenosine tri-phosphate (ATP)-dependent phagocytosis or passive endocytosis. In the latter, the particle is transported in a phagosome and combined with a lysosome to undergo oxidative or non-oxidative killing. Lung macrophages are much more effective than their blood counterparts. This process is effective in eradi-cating Gram-positive organisms such as *Staphylococcus aureus* but ineffective against Gram-negative bacteria.

Neutrophils and eosinophils may also participate in phagocytosis but only during lung inflammation.

Type I alveolar epithelial cells

These cells line the alveoli and exist as a thin sheet approximately 0.1 μm in thickness, except where expanded to contain nuclei. Each cell covers several capillaries and is joined to neighbouring cells by tight

junctions with a gap of only approximately 1 nm. There is now evidence that alveolar epithelial cells are involved in active clearance of fluid from the al-veoli in normal human lungs [9,10]. On the alveolar side of these cells, the cell membrane contains epi-thelial sodium channels (ENaC) and CFTR channels, which actively pump sodium and chloride ions, re-spectively, into the cell [10]. On the interstitial bor-der of the cells, chloride moves passively out of the cell and the Na^+/K^+-ATPase channel actively re-moves sodium from the cell. Water from the alveolus follows these ion transfers down an osmotic gradi-ent into the interstitium. Aquaporins are found in human alveolar epithelial cells, suggesting that water movement may be facilitated by these water channel proteins, but their role in normal adult lung remains unclear [10]. A small amount of active clearance of fluid from the alveoli occurs under normal circum-stances, but these systems become vital when pul-monary oedema develops.

Type II alveolar epithelial cells

These cuboidal cells are found in clusters at points of alveolar convergence and are the stem cells from which type I cells arise. Their most important func-tion is the production of surfactant, which is stored in osmiophilic lamellar bodies that are characteristic of type II cells (Fig. 18.2) [11]. Some 90% of surfactant consists of lipids, mostly comprising dipalmitoyl phosphatidyl choline, the main constituent respon-sible for the effect on surface tension. The fatty acids are hydrophobic and generally straight, lying paral-lel to each other and projecting into the gas phase. The other end of the molecule is hydrophilic and lies within the alveolar lining fluid. The molecule is thus confined to the surface where, being detergents, they lower surface tension in proportion to the concen-tration at the interface.

Approximately 2% of surfactant by weight con-sists of surfactant proteins (SP), of which there are four types A–D [12]. SP-B and SP-C are small pro-teins that are vital to the stabilization of the surfactant monolayer (see below); a congenital lack of SP-B results in severe and progressive respiratory failure [12]. SP-A, and to a lesser extent SP-D, are involved in the control of surfactant release. Stored surfactant is released into the alveolus from the lamellar bodies

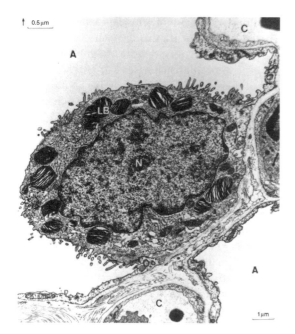

Figure 18.2 Electron micrograph of a type II alveolar epithelial cell. Note the large number of osmiophilic lamellar bodies containing surfactant components awaiting release. A, alveolus; C, capillary; LB, lamellar bodies; N, nucleus. (From Weibel [11] with permission of Professor E.R. Weibel and the Editors of *Physiological Reviews*.)

by exocytosis in response to high volume lung inflation, increased ventilation rate or endocrine stimulation. After release, surfactant initially forms areas of a lattice structure termed tubular myelin, which is then reorganized into mono- or multilayered surface films. This conversion into the functionally active form of surfactant is believed to be critically dependent on SP-B and SP-C (see below) [12]. The alveolar half-life of surfactant is 15–30 hours, with most of its components being recycled by type II alveolar cells. SP-A is intimately involved in controlling the surfactant present in the alveolus with type II alveolar cells having SP-A surface receptors, stimulation of which exerts a negative feedback on surfactant secretion and increases reuptake of surfactant components into the cell.

Type II cells are involved in pulmonary defence mechanisms in that they may secrete cytokines and contribute to pulmonary inflammation. SP-A and, to a lesser extent, SP-D, have specific antimicrobial activity. In addition to enhancing macrophage recognition of pathogens, the molecules themselves are directly antimicrobial. Type II alveolar epithelial cells also have metabolic functions, which are described in more detail below.

Airway surface liquid

Within the airway surface liquid there are two distinct layers [13,14]: a periciliary or 'sol' layer which is of low viscosity containing water and solutes and in which the cilia are embedded, and a mucous or 'gel' layer above.

Mucociliary function

Mucus is produced by the goblet and submucosal secretory cells described above. It has an important role in pathogen entrapment and removal, and also contains a variety of antimicrobial proteins, which are described in more detail below. Mucus is composed mostly of glycoproteins called mucins, which determine the viscoelastic properties of the mucus. They have a core composed of glycoprotein subunits joined by disulphide bonds and their length may extend up to 6 µm. The core is 80% glycosylated with side chains attached via O-glycosidic bonds. Almost all terminate in sialic acid and possess microorganism binding sites. Large airways are completely lined by a mucous layer, while in smaller, more distal, airways the mucus is found in 'islands', and a mucous layer is absent in small bronchioles and beyond. The mucous layer is propelled cephalad by the ciliated epithelial cells at a rate of 4 mm/min before being removed by expectoration on reaching the larynx. The cilia beat mostly within the low-viscosity periciliary layer of airway lining fluid, with the cilia tips intermittently gripping the underside of the mucous layer, so propelling the mucous layer along the airway wall (Fig. 18.3) [15].

For this propulsion system to work effectively, it is crucial that the depth of the periciliary layer be closely controlled [14,16], particularly when it is realized that there is an increasing amount of mucus converging on larger airways as the mucus passes up towards the trachea. The depth of both layers of the airway surface liquid is controlled by changes in the volume of secretions and the speed of their reabsorption. If the periciliary layer reduces in depth, the gel layer will compensate for this by donating liquid to the periciliary layer to maintain the correct depth of fluid, an effect probably mediated by simple osmotic gradients between the two (Fig. 18.4). The mucous layer may donate fluid to the periciliary layer until its volume is diminished by 70%. The reverse happens as the mucus converges on the larger airways, with the mucous layer absorbing excess periciliary water (Fig. 18.4). The volume of periciliary fluid is therefore effectively determined by its salt concentration, which is in turn controlled by active ion transport on the surface of the epithelial cells. The ion channels responsible for active control are amiloride sensitive Na^+ and Cl^- channels, the latter better known as the CFTR protein. CFTR is likely to be partially active at rest but is stimulated when Na^+ channels are inhibited. The factors responsible for this are unknown.

In patients with cystic fibrosis, an inherited defect of CFTR leads to dysfunction in the regulation of airway surface liquid production. This, in turn, causes abnormal physical characteristics of the airway lining fluid layers, ciliary malfunction and severely impaired defence against inhaled pathogens. Production of normally functioning airway surface liquid is a poorly understood, but clinically important, aspect of lung function, which is likely to be intensively researched in future.

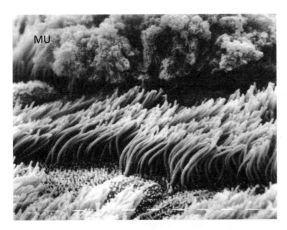

Figure 18.3 Scanning electron micrograph of ciliated epithelial cells beating in the fluid layer beneath the mucus (MU). (From Jeffery [15] with permission of Dr P.K. Jeffery, Imperial College School of Science, Technology and Medicine, London and the publishers of *Respiratory Medicine*.)

Functions of the respiratory epithelium

Humidification

Respiratory epithelium and the airway lining fluid act as heat and moisture exchangers [17]. During inspiration, relatively cool, dry air causes evaporation of surface water and cooling of the airway wall, then on expiration moisture condenses on the surface of the airway wall and warming occurs. Thus, only

Figure 18.4 Schematic drawing of the mucous layer of airway surface liquid acting as a fluid reservoir. With variations in the amount of water present in the airway surface liquid the mucous layer absorbs fluid from, or donates fluid to, the periciliary layer to maintain it at the correct depth for normal ciliary function. Changes in electrolyte concentrations in the periciliary layer will then stimulate fluid absorption or secretion by the epithelial cells. (After Boucher [16].)

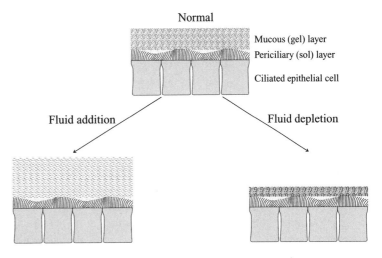

about half of the heat and moisture needed to condition (fully warm and saturate) each breath is lost to the atmosphere. With quiet nasal breathing, air is conditioned before reaching the trachea, but as ventilation increases smaller airways are recruited until at minute volumes of over 50 L/min airways of 1 mm diameter are involved in humidification.

Removal of inhaled particles

Where in the respiratory tract inhaled particles are deposited depends on both their size and the breathing pattern during inhalation. Three mechanisms cause deposition: inertial impaction, sedimentation and diffusion.

Inertial impaction

This occurs with large particles (>3 µm). Inertial impaction occurs when the airway has a sharp corner (e.g. the pharynx or nose) or when gas flow becomes turbulent (e.g. at bifurcations): the turbulent flow at bifurcation points in the airway causes a 100-fold increase in particle deposition. Thus, particles with a size >8 µm rarely reach further than the pharynx before impaction on to the nasal mucosa. Smaller particles (3–8 µm) penetrate further into the respiratory tract. Inertial impaction is greatly influenced by the velocity of the particles, so a slower rate of inspiration by the subject will increase the penetration into the lungs by particles of this size.

Sedimentation

This occurs with particles of 1–3 µm, and is seen in the smaller airways or alveoli where slow gas velocity allows the particles to fall out of suspension and be deposited on lung tissue. Breath holding after inhalation of an aerosol encourages sedimentation.

Diffusion

For small particles (<0.5–1 µm) Brownian motion occurs, leading to deposition on any surrounding structures. Aiding these processes is the inherently high humidity within the respiratory tract. Absorption of water by the particle during its journey along the airways will increase particle weight, and so encourage both inertial impaction and sedimentation to occur. Naturally, this affects hygroscopic particles to a greater degree.

The fate of inhaled particles

Large particles (>10 µm) such as atmospheric dust or the particulate products of diesel combustion are trapped by the airway lining fluid and removed from the lung by the mucociliary transport mechanism already described [18]. Small particles (1–3 µm) pass into the alveoli and may either diffuse back out of the alveolus to be exhaled, or be deposited on the alveolar walls where they will be ingested by alveolar macrophages. Different dust types have variable persistence in the lung, some being rapidly cleared and others persisting within the pulmonary macrophage for many years. Differing particle types activate the macrophage to a varying extent, but may stimulate cytokine release causing lung inflammation that then proceeds to lung tissue repair, the deposition of collagen and pulmonary fibrosis. For example, occupational exposure to asbestos fibres (asbestosis) or silica (silicosis) for many years leads to pulmonary fibrosis. Organic dusts may also cause lung inflammation by an immune mechanism, the allergen normally being derived from a fungus to which the patient has had occupational exposure (e.g. farmer's lung).

Delivery of inhaled drugs

Recent advances in our understanding of particle deposition in the respiratory tract have been driven by potential pharmaceutical benefits [19,20] (e.g. delivery of insulin). The aim may be to deliver drugs that are intended to act on the airway directly to the airway, such as bronchodilators, antibiotics or antiviral agents. Alternatively, the lung may be used as a route of administration for drugs intended to act systemically, examples of this application include insulin, heparin, ergotamine and calcitonin. Pulmonary administration of a drug that is intended to work systemically offers many advantages over other routes, such as very rapid delivery into the circulation and avoidance of first-pass metabolism in the liver.

For delivery of a drug to the alveoli, particles around 3 µm are the optimal size, as larger particles tend to deposit in the airways, and smaller particles tend to be inhaled and exhaled without being deposited in lung tissue at all. Targeted delivery of drugs to specific regions of the respiratory tract should be possible, for example, by modifying the particle size, the timing of its addition to the breath or the breathing pattern during inhalation [20]. In practice, most delivery devices in clinical use produce aerosols containing a wide range of particle sizes, the most commonly used metered-dose inhaler used to treat asthma generating particles of 1–35 μm. Use of a spacer device before inhalation allows the largest particles to fall out of the aerosol before inhalation, and so reduces their impaction in the pharynx, where they are responsible for many of the side-effects of inhaled drugs.

Defence against inhaled pathogens

As an interface with the outside environment the lung is exposed to a great many organisms carried by up to 20 000 L air breathed per day. Pulmonary defence mechanisms have evolved to protect the respiratory tract from invasion by microorganisms. They can be subdivided into direct removal of the pathogen, chemical inactivation of the invading organism and, if these fail, immune defences.

Direct removal of pathogens

With normal nasal breathing, a majority of inhaled pathogens impact on the nasal mucosa, which is swept backwards by the ciliated nasal epithelium and swallowed. At higher inspiratory flow rates, for example when dyspnoeic, pathogens will penetrate deeper into the airways and be trapped by the airway surface liquid, transferred to the larynx and expectorated or swallowed.

Chemical inactivation of pathogens

Airway surface liquid is more than a simple transport mechanism for impacted microorganisms [21,22]. Some smaller particles will penetrate far into the bronchial tree and take some time to be transported out of the respiratory tract. To prevent these organisms from causing damage during this time, the airway surface liquid contains multiple systems for directly killing pathogens.

Surfactant

In addition to its crucial role in reducing lung compliance, surfactant also acts as part of the innate defences in the lung [23]. Surfactant proteins A–D are members of the collectin family, a large group of proteins defined by their common dual structure and their ability to opsonize pathogens and regulate production of inflammatory mediators. SP-A is the most important surfactant protein in pulmonary defence. Not only does it enhance bacterial clearance but it also stimulates macrophage migration, production of reactive oxygen species and the synthesis of immunoglobulin and cytokines. Recent research has found that both SP-A and SP-D are directly bactericidal [24]. The mechanism involves a calcium-dependent reaction between the lipid A domain of the lipopolysaccharide in the cell wall and the C-terminal domain of SP-A. There is increased bacterial cell wall permeability, release of intracellular microbial proteins and bacterial agglutination as a result. SP-A has specific antimicrobial activity against *Streptococcus pneumonia*, *Staphylococcus aureus*, *Haemophilus*, *Escherichia coli*, *Klebsiella*, *Mycobacterium*, *Cryptococcus*, *Herpes simplex* and *Aspergillus*.

Lactoferrin

This is an iron-binding protein found in neutrophil granules and epithelial secretions. It inhibits bacterial growth by sequestering the iron necessary for bacterial metabolism.

Lysozyme

This is an enzyme, secreted by neutrophils, that is capable of destroying microbial cell walls by acting on the acetylglucosamine and acetylmuramic acid components of the peptidoglycan. In addition to enzymatic lysis of cell walls it is also effective in non-enzymatic lysis. It is active against Gram-positive bacteria but less so against Gram-negative species, although the presence of cofactors such as lactoferrin enhances the activity of lysozyme against the latter.

Defensins

These are small molecular weight (3–5 kDa) peptides that have a wide antimicrobial range. They are able to aggregate, and on doing so create defects in the bacterial cell wall, and also stimulate respiratory epithelial cells to release chemokines to recruit inflammatory cells. α-Defensins are present in the α-granules of neutrophils. These human neutrophil peptides 1, 2, 3 and 4 constitute approximately 5% of neutrophil intracellular protein. They are active against *Staphylococcus, E. coli, Pseudomonas aeruginosa* and some viruses such as *Herpes simplex*. β-Defensins are derived from epithelial lining and at least four human β-defensins (HBD) have been identified. HBD-1 is found in lung secretions in normal individuals while HBD-2 is found in secretions of cystic fibrosis patients as well as those with inflammatory lung disease. These small peptides contribute to inflammation and repair. Inactivation of HBDs by abnormal electrolyte concentrations in the airway lining fluid may contribute to chronic airway infection in cystic fibrosis.

Cathelicidins

These are part of a large family of antimicrobial peptides. They have a highly conserved N-terminal structure, but a varied C-terminal end containing 10–40 amino acids. Cleavage of the C-terminal end from the inactive molecule activates the cathelicidin to act against a broad spectrum of pathogens. The only known human cathelicidin is named LL37 and is found in human neutrophil granules and in airway epithelium.

Protease–antiprotease system

Protease enzymes such as neutrophil elastase and metalloproteinases are normally released in the lung following activation of neutrophils or macrophages in response to tobacco smoke or pathogens [25]. These enzymes are powerful antimicrobial molecules in the airway surface liquid. However, if left unchecked, these enzymes will damage lung tissue. For example, protease enzymes with activity against elastin are likely to be responsible for generating emphysema. Elastin deposition in the lung occurs early in life, and is minimal beyond late adolescence. Later, any pulmonary elastin lost through smoking or inflammation is likely to be replaced with collagen, so reducing lung elasticity and probably explaining the general decline in lung recoil throughout life [26].

There are at least two mechanisms that protect the lung from damage by its own protease enzymes. First, the proteases are mostly confined to the mucous layer of the airway surface liquid, so avoiding close contact with underlying epithelial cells while being in close proximity to inhaled microorganisms.

Secondly, they are inactivated by conjugation with antiprotease enzymes present in the lung [27]. Antiprotease enzymes active in the lung include α_1-antitrypsin, α_2-macroglobulin and α_1-chymotrypsin. α_1-Antitrypsin is manufactured in the liver and transported to the lung. It constitutes a major proportion of antiprotease activity in the alveoli and is the most active inhibitor of neutrophil elastase. A deficiency of α_1-antitrypsin allows protease activity to remain unchecked, and is a significant risk factor for early development of emphysema [27]. The combination of smoking (known to reduce antitrypsin levels and increase protease production) and α_1-antitrypsin deficiency leads to the development of more severe airways disease. Disturbances of less well understood protease–antiprotease systems, such as the matrix metalloproteases group of enzymes, are now also believed to be involved in the generation of emphysema, as these proteases are normally involved in remodelling of the extracellular lung matrix [25].

Lung protease activity is increased during lung inflammation, and under these conditions α_2-macroglobulin enters the alveolus through the leaky alveolar capillary membrane. It is effective against both neutrophil elastase and metalloproteases.

Immune systems

Direct removal of pathogens and their inactivation in the airway surface liquid are efficient defence systems. If pathogens successfully breach these defences, immunological systems then come into play.

Humoral immunity

Immunoglobulins are found in the airway lining fluid. IgA is the major type present in the nasopharyngeal area and large bronchi. Its role seems to be to prevent the binding of bacteria to the nasal mucosa, and specific IgA has the ability to act as an opsonin and induce complement. Deeper in the respiratory tract IgG is present in larger relative volumes, becoming the most prevalent immunoglobulin in the alveoli.

Cellular immunity

Respiratory epithelial cells and macrophages present in normal airways have considerable activity as immunological active cells. In response to a variety of stimuli, bronchial epithelial cells may secrete numerous molecules to initiate an inflammatory response:

- *Adhesion molecules* (e.g. intracellular adhesion molecule-1; ICAM-1) to induce margination of inflammatory cells in nearby pulmonary capillaries
- *Chemokines* (e.g. interleukin-8; IL-8) to recruit inflammatory cells into the lung tissue
- *Cytokines* (e.g. IL-1, IL-6 and tumour necrosis factor; TNF) to amplify the inflammatory response by further stimulation of inflammatory cells
- *Growth factors* (e.g. transforming growth factor β, epithelial growth factor; TGF-β, EGF) to stimulate the cells responsible for tissue repair such as fibroblasts
- *Extracellular matrix proteins* (e.g. collagen, hyalouronan) to begin the tissue repair process.

Once initiated, this response causes large numbers of phagocytic cells to enter the lung tissue. The presence of immunoglobulins, complement and other opsonins enhances the phagocytic cells' recognition process. In severe infections, the reactive oxygen species used in the killing of microorganisms by phagocytic cells may spill out of the lysosome and into the lung tissue, exacerbating the tissue injury.

In patients with asthma, the inflammatory cells responsible for airway inflammation are eosinophils and mast cells, while in those with chronic obstructive pulmonary disease and other forms of lung inflammation, neutrophils predominate.

Inactivation of inhaled xenobiotics

Droplet size will influence the distance that inhaled chemicals penetrate into the lungs. Once deposited on the airway lining, water solubility will influence the speed at which the chemical dissolves in the airway surface liquid to gain access to the underlying epithelial cells. Lipophilic substances and gases cross cell membranes easily — these include organic solvents, anaesthetic gases, bronchodilators and many constituents of tobacco smoke. Once incorporated into the lung tissue, water solubility affects the rate at which chemicals are cleared from the lung, with water-soluble substances taking longer than lipid-soluble ones to be absorbed into the blood for disposal elsewhere.

Metabolism of inhaled chemicals occurs in all cell types of the respiratory mucosa, but in animals is particularly well developed in Clara cells, endothelial cells and type II alveolar cells. As in the liver, metabolism of toxic chemicals involves two stages.

1 *Phase I metabolism,* in which the toxic molecule is converted into a different compound, usually by oxidative reactions. The lung has a full complement of phase I enzymes (cytochrome P450, NADPH cytochrome P450 reductase, flavin-dependent mono-oxygenase, epoxide hydrolase and dihydrodiol dehydrogenase) of which cytochrome P450 mono-oxygenase is by far the most important. The lung is one of the major extrahepatic sites of mixed function oxidation by the cytochrome P450 systems, but, gram-for-gram, remains considerably less active than the liver.

2 *Phase II metabolism* involves conjugation of the resulting compounds to 'carrier' molecules, which render them less biologically active, more water-soluble and therefore easier to excrete. Enzymes participating in conjugative pathways in the human lung include glutathione S-transferase, glutathione peroxidase, UDP-glucuronosyltransferase, N-acetyltransferase, N-methyltransferase and sulphotransferase. Most pulmonary phase II metabolism reactions involve conjugation with glucuronide or glutathione [28]. Despite this range of phase II enzymes, the ability of human lung to perform phase II reactions is limited, having only 1% of the activity of liver in phase II reactions. The ability to metabolize in this manner is easily induced but negatively influenced by tobacco smoke inhalation.

Metabolic changes to inhaled chemicals may not be beneficial, especially with many synthetic organic compounds and several chemicals in cigarette smoke. Bioactivation by phase I metabolism converts some quite innocuous compounds into potent carcinogens, while slightly different metabolic conversions may do the reverse [28,29]. The balance between activating and inactivating pathways varies between species. What few data are available on human lungs indicates that we are fortunate in having a very favourable ratio, the inactivation of potential carcinogens being 100-fold greater than in rodents. Presumably, without this evolutionary advantage, the history of cigarette smoking would have been considerably different.

Detrimental pulmonary metabolic activity also occurs in the cases of paraquat and bleomycin where the metabolic process produces toxic metabolites.

Some Clara cells do not possess the P450 enzyme complex. It is postulated that this has a beneficial effect in that these cells are unaffected by toxic metabolites produced during normal metabolism of xenobiotics, and so form a pool of surviving Clara cells to act as stem cells following damage to the airway epithelium.

Filtration

Sitting astride the whole output of the right ventricle, the lung is ideally situated to filter out particulate matter from the systemic venous return. Without such a filter, there would be a constant risk of emboli entering the arterial system.

Pulmonary capillaries have a diameter of approximately 7 µm, but this does not appear to be the effective pore size of the pulmonary circulation when considered as a filter. Animal studies have demonstrated the passage through perfused lungs of glass beads up to 500 µm diameter and small quantities of gas and fat emboli may gain access to the systemic circulation in patients without intracardiac shunting. Emboli may bypass the alveoli via some of the precapillary anastomoses that are known to exist in the pulmonary circulation. More extensive invasion of the systemic arteries may occur in the presence of an overt right-to-left intracardiac shunt, which is now known to be quite common. Postmortem studies show that over 25% of the population have a 'probe-patent' foramen ovale, usually in the form of a slit-like defect that acts as a valve, and which is therefore normally kept closed by the left atrial pressure being slightly greater than the right [30]. In 10% of normal subjects, a simple valsalva manoeuvre or cough results in easily demonstrable blood flow between the right and left atria [31]. Paradoxical embolism may therefore result from a relative increase in right atrial pressure caused by physiological events or pulmonary embolus.

So far as the survival of the lung is concerned, the pulmonary microcirculation is well adapted for maintaining alveolar perfusion in the face of quite large degrees of embolization. Large numbers of pulmonary capillaries tend to arise at right angles from metarterioles and there are abundant anastomoses throughout the microcirculation. This tends to preserve circulation distal to the impaction of a small

embolus. Similarly, the ability of the pulmonary circulation to passively dilate or recruit pulmonary capillaries, responses designed to minimize pulmonary arterial pressure during physiological increases in cardiac output, also serves to minimize dangerous pulmonary hypertension following pulmonary embolus. However, a significant degree of embolization inevitably blocks the circulation to parts of the lung, disturbing the balance between ventilation and perfusion, and ultimately disturbing gas exchange.

Thromboembolism

Pulmonary microembolism with small clumps of fibrin and/or platelets will not have a direct effect on gas exchange until it is very extensive. Plugging of pulmonary capillaries by microemboli, however, initiates neutrophil activation in the area, leading to an increase in endothelial permeability and alveolar oedema. Thrombi are cleared more rapidly from the lungs than from other organs. The lung possesses well-developed proteolytic systems not confined to the removal of fibrin. Pulmonary endothelium is known to be rich in plasmin activator, which converts plasminogen into plasmin, which in turn converts fibrin into fibrin degradation products. However, the lung is also rich in thromboplastin, which converts prothrombin to thrombin. To complicate the position further, the lung is a particularly rich source of heparin, and bovine lung is used in its commercial preparation. The lung can thus produce high concentrations of substances necessary to promote or delay blood clotting and also for fibrinolysis.

Three mechanisms give rise to the physiological changes seen in pulmonary embolism [32]:
• Physical occlusion of the pulmonary vascular system (Fig. 18.5)
• Platelet activation within the thrombus leads to release of 5-hydroxytryptamine (5-HT) and thromboxane A_2, causing a further increase in pulmonary vascular resistance
• Right ventricular failure occurs when the heart is unable to overcome the raised pulmonary vascular resistance.

The primary respiratory lesion is an increase in alveolar dead space with an increased arterial–end-tidal P_{CO_2} gradient. Carbon dioxide elimination is therefore reduced and if ventilation remains un-

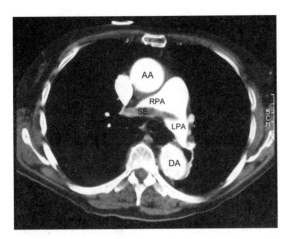

Figure 18.5 Spiral computed tomographic scan of pulmonary thomboembolus. Intravenous contrast injected immediately before scanning makes the blood vessels appear white. Emboli then appear as darker areas within the blood vessel lumen. A saddle embolus (SE) can be seen, situated mainly in the right pulmonary artery (RPA). AA, ascending aorta; DA, descending aorta; LPA, left pulmonary artery.

changed, arterial P_{CO_2} slowly climbs, until elimination is restored in spite of the large dead space. However, in awake patients hypercapnia is unusual because hyperventilation is almost always present and arterial P_{CO_2} is usually below the normal range [33]. The cause of respiratory stimulation is unclear, but may involve stimulation of J receptors by mediators released in the pulmonary circulation, or stimulation by hypoxia if present.

Arterial P_{O_2} is also decreased. This results from derangement of normal ventilation–perfusion relationships, the effects of which are exacerbated by low cardiac output causing reduced pulmonary perfusion and low mixed venous oxygen content [33].

Bronchospasm is a well-recognized complication of pulmonary embolism and has been attributed to the 5-HT released from platelets and also to local hypocapnia in the part of the lung without effective pulmonary circulation.

Endocrine lung

An endocrine organ must, by definition, release substances into the circulation that bring about a useful physiological response in a distant tissue. In spite of its wide-ranging metabolic activities already described, the endocrine functions of the lung remain ill-defined.

Inflammatory mediators such as histamine, endothelin, serotonin, platelet activating factor (PAF), adenosine and eicosanoids may all be released from the lung following immunological activation by inhaled allergens. These mediators are undoubtedly responsible for cardiovascular and other physiological changes in the rest of the body, such as a rash, peripheral vasodilatation and a reduction in blood pressure. However, it is doubtful if this can really be regarded as a desirable physiological effect.

Hypoxic endocrine responses may occur in the lung [34]. Animal studies have demonstrated the presence of clusters of peptide and amine secreting cells in lung tissue. These cells degranulate in the presence of acute hypoxia, but the substances secreted and their effects are not known. The cells belong to the 'diffuse endocrine system' and are present in humans, but their role is extremely unclear.

Nitric oxide has an important role in the regulation of airway smooth muscle and pulmonary vascular resistance, and is well known for its effects on platelet function and the systemic vasculature. There is no evidence that pulmonary endothelium secretes nitric oxide into the blood in order to exert an effect elsewhere, mainly because of the rapid uptake of nitric oxide by haemoglobin. However, this does not rule out an indirect effect of pulmonary nitric oxide production in influencing peripheral blood flow, which may be controlled by the balance between different forms of nitric oxide haemoglobin complexes.

Metabolism of endogenous compounds

The endothelial cells are specially adapted to the dual functions of gas exchange and metabolic activity. There is almost $70\,m^2$ of endothelial surface present in the blood vessels of the lung and therefore it is the most metabolically active component of the respiratory tract. The activity depends on blood flow, perfusion and transit time. Perfused area is under active control and recruitment of pulmonary vessels may increase the surface area to 90 m². Individual endothelial cells are structurally similar to type I alveolar epithelial cells. Multiple vesicles are present within the cytoplasm. Some of these are seen abutting the endothelial lumen, termed caveolae. The cells themselves have multiple invaginations and projections. Tight junctions are found between the endothelial cells, these junctions forming part of the physical barrier between blood and the exterior. On the surface of the endothelium are found enzymes responsible for the conversion of angiotensin I to angiotensin II, and the inactivation of bradykinin and adenosine compounds. Within the cytoplasm are enzyme systems necessary for production of arachidonic acid products, degradation of certain prostaglandins, breakdown of 5-HT and other amines.

A summary of the metabolic activities of the pulmonary endothelium is shown in Table 18.1.

Amine metabolism

Noradrenaline is actively transported into the endothelial cell by highly specific transport proteins found on the capillary surface of pulmonary endothelium. Uptake is saturable, energy and temperature dependent and inhibited by a variety of drugs. Around one-third of circulating noradrenaline is removed in one circulation. Once within the cell, noradrenaline is degraded via the monoamine oxidase and catechol-*O*-methyl transferase enzymes.

5-HT is found in the human brain, platelets and chromaffin cells of the gut. In the lungs the sources include mast cells and neuroendocrine cells. The clearance of blood 5-HT is almost complete with as much as 98% being removed from the circulation following a single pass through the pulmonary circulation. Uptake is again thought to be active, involving carrier-mediated transport into the cell.

Table 18.1 Summary of metabolic changes to hormones and drugs on passing through the pulmonary circulation [35,36].

Group	Effect of passing through pulmonary circulation		
	Activated	No change	Inactivated
Amines		Dopamine Adrenaline Histamine	5-Hydroxytryptamine Noradrenaline
Peptides	Angiotensin I	Angiotensin II Oxytocin Vasopressin Atrial natriuretic peptide	Bradykinin Endothelins
Arachidonic acid derivatives	Arachidonic acid	PGI$_2$ (prostacyclin) PGA$_2$	PGD$_2$ PGE$_2$ PGF$_{2\alpha}$ Leukotrienes
Purine derivatives			Adenosine ATP, ADP, AMP
Steroids	Cortisone		Progesterone Beclometasone
Basic drugs		Morphine Isoprenaline	Fentanyl Lidocaine Propranolol

ADP, adenosine diphosphate; AMP, adenosine monophosphate; ATP, adenosine triphosphate.

Metabolism is similar to that for noradrenaline, involving metabolism by monoamine oxidase. Although similar, the metabolism of these two amines is not mutually exclusive and does not use exactly the same pathways. Other amines such as histamine, dopamine and adrenaline are not removed from the pulmonary circulation because of a lack of specific transmembrane carrier proteins.

Angiotensin converting enzyme

The lung is a major site for conversion of angiotensin I to angiotensin II by angiotensin converting enzyme (ACE). Some 80% of angiotensin I passing through the lungs is converted to angiotensin II in a single pass. Angiotensin II acts directly on smooth muscle cells to cause vasoconstriction and also binds to receptors on the zona glomerulosa cells in the adrenal gland to promote the synthesis and release of aldosterone, which accelerates renal sodium reabsorption.

Bradykinin is a vasoactive nonapeptide that is also inactivated by ACE. Bradykinin dilates normal pulmonary vessels, but may be a vasoconstrictor in the presence of pulmonary injury. It has a half-life of 17 s in blood but less than 4 s in the lung. ACE is found free in the plasma, but is also bound to the surface of endothelium. This appears to be a general property of endothelium but ACE is present in abundance on the vascular surface of pulmonary endothelial cells, also lining the inside of the caveolae and extending onto the projections into the lumen. Angiotensin converting enzyme is a zinc containing carboxypeptidase with two active sites, each located within a deep groove in the side of the protein [37]. Binding sites in the groove attach the substrate firmly to the protein and the zinc moiety then cleaves either a phenylalanine-histidine bond (angiotensin I) or a phenylalanine-arginine bond (bradykinin).

Drugs that inhibit ACE (see below) do so by binding to the protein deep within the groove above the active site, simply preventing the substrate gaining access to the active site [37]. It follows that inhibition of ACE will increase levels of bradykinin in the blood. This may explain some of the adverse effects seen with ACE inhibitors such as increased incidence of angioneurotic oedema and cough.

Endothelins

Endothelins are a group of 21 amino acid peptides with diverse biological activities including prolonged pulmonary vasoconstriction in response to hypoxia. They have a plasma half-life of just a few minutes, being cleared by the kidney, liver and lungs. The pulmonary enzymes responsible are not clearly defined, but there are believed to be several different types in humans [38].

Platelet activating factor

The most important sources of PAF are leucocytes and platelets, but pulmonary endothelium is also known to release PAF in response to stimulation by phospholipase A_2. PAF has multiple pro-inflammatory functions and is believed to act as an important mediator in chronic obstructive pulmonary disease. Effects include increased airway reactivity, pulmonary hypertension and increased inflammatory cell accumulation.

Adenosine nucleotides

Purine derivatives are metabolized on the endothelial surface by 5-nucleotidase and ATPase. Adenosine has potent effects on the circulation but is rapidly inactivated by uptake into the pulmonary endothelial cells. This uptake is an active and saturable process that is inhibited by dipyridamole. Adenosine may be subsequently released in response to acute hypoxia or become incorporated into adenosine monophosphate (AMP), adenosine diphosphate (ADP) or ATP.

Arachidonic acid derivatives

The lung is a major site of synthesis, metabolism, uptake and release of arachidonic acid metabolites. The group as a whole are 20-carbon carboxylic acids, generically known as eicosanoids. The initial stages of eicosanoid synthesis involve the conversion, by phospholipase A_2, of membrane phospholipids into arachidonic acid. Metabolism of arachidonic acid involves its oxygenation by two main pathways for which the enzymes are cyclo-oxygenase (COX) and lipoxygenase.

Cyclo-oxygenase pathway

Oxygenation and cyclization of arachidonic acid by COX produces the prostaglandin PGG_2 (the subscript 2 indicates two double bonds in the carbon chain). A non-specific peroxidase then converts PGG_2 to PGH_2, which is the parent compound for synthesis of the many important derivatives shown in Figure 18.6. The rate limiting step in the production of eicosanoids is the availability of arachidonic acid. It is known that steroids reduce the availability of this substrate, the effect of which can be bypassed with the introduction of exogenous arachidonic acid.

Eicosanoids are not stored preformed, but are synthesized as required by many cell types in the lung, including endothelium, airway smooth muscle, mast cells, epithelial cells and vascular muscle. Production of arachidonic acid by activation of phospholipase initiates the pathway, and results from a variety of stimuli such as inflammatory cytokines, complement activation, hormones, allergens or mechanical stimuli. The enzyme for the next step of the pathway,

COX, exists in multiple isoforms, including COX-1, which is a constitutive enzyme present at low concentrations, and COX-2, which is induced by inflammatory cytokines. In the normal lung, the physiological role of these COX isoforms is uncertain, but in some patients with asthma, inhibition of COX-1 by aspirin induces bronchospasm, while inhibition of COX-2 does not.

$PGF_{2\alpha}$, PGD_2, PGG_2, PGH_2 and thromboxane are bronchial and tracheal constrictors, $PGF_{2\alpha}$ and PGD_2 being much more potent in asthmatic patients compared with normal subjects. PGE_1 and PGE_2 are bronchodilators, particularly when administered by aerosol. Prostacyclin (PGI_2) has different effects in different species. In humans, it has no effect on airway calibre in doses that have profound cardiovascular effects. Prostacyclin and PGE_1 are pulmonary vasodilators, while PGH_2 and $PGF_{2\alpha}$ are pulmonary vasoconstrictors.

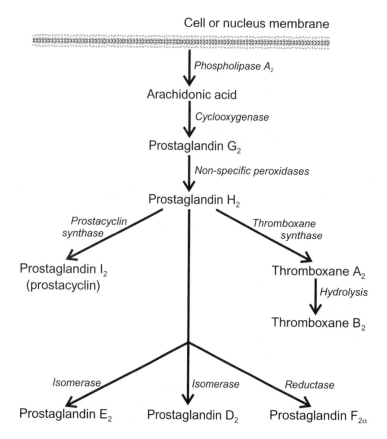

Figure 18.6 The prostaglandin pathway.

Various specific enzymes in the lung are responsible for extensive metabolism of PGE_2, PGE_1 and $PGF_{2\alpha}$, but PGA_2 and PGI_2 pass through the lung unchanged. As for catecholamine metabolism, specificity for pulmonary prostaglandin metabolism is in the uptake pathways rather than with the intracellular enzymes.

Leukotrienes are also eicosanoids derived from arachidonic acid but by the lipoxygenase pathway (Fig. 18.7) [39]. The leukotrienes LTC_4 and LTD_4 are mainly responsible for the bronchoconstrictor effects of what was formerly known as slow-reacting substance of anaphylaxis or SRS-A. SRS-A also contains LTB_4, which is a less powerful bronchoconstrictor but increases vascular permeability. These compounds, which are synthesized by the mast cell, have an important role in asthma and drugs that inhibit leukotriene synthesis are now used in the treatment of asthma.

Aspirin-induced asthma

The involvement of arachidonic acid derivatives in the normal control of bronchial smooth muscle predicts that drugs blocking these pathways may influence the airways of asthma patients [40]. This is indeed the case with aspirin and the closely related non-steroidal anti-inflammatory drugs, sometimes causing bronchospasm in asthma patients. Based on patient history alone, only 2.7% of asthma patients report wheezing in response to aspirin, but when provocation with oral aspirin is carried out 21% of patients develop a reduction in forced expiratory volume in 1 s (FEV_1) [41]. Many asthmatic patients who are sensitive to aspirin have a characteristic clinical presentation. Typically, aspirin-induced asthma (AIA) develops in patients at around 30 years of age, is associated with rhinitis and nasal polyps, and occurs in more female than male patients [40].

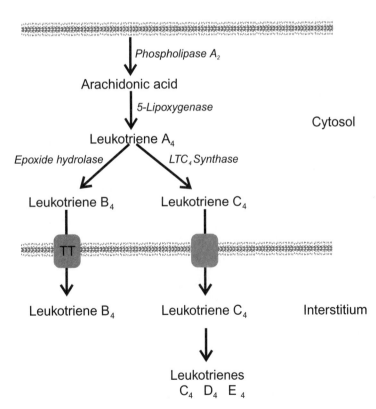

Figure 18.7 The leukotriene pathway in the lung. Inflammatory mediators stimulate phospholipase A_2 to produce arachidonic acid from the phospholipid of the nuclear membrane. Leukotrienes B_4 and C_4 leave the cell via a specific transmembrane transporter (TT) protein. Non-specific peptidases in the interstitium convert leukotriene C_4 into D_4 and E_4, all of which stimulate the $CysLT_1$ receptor to cause intense broncho-constriction. (After Drazen *et al.* [39].)

The mechanism of aspirin sensitivity is beginning to be elucidated. Inhibitors of the COX pathway in the airway will reduce synthesis of the bronchodilator prostaglandin PGE_2. Reduced synthesis of PGE_2 cannot alone account for AIA; patients with AIA also have increased production of LTE_4, a potent bronchoconstrictor. This effect on the lipoxygenase pathway is not mediated by aspirin itself, and possibly results from loss of inhibition of lipoxygenase by PGE_2. Multiple isoforms of COX exist and COX-1 seems to be responsible for most cases of AIA. A recently introduced group of drugs, known as coxibs, are highly specific inhibitors of COX-2 and seem to be safe for use in AIA patients [40]. The analgesic effects of paracetamol (acetaminophen) may be mediated by inhibition of COX-3 [42], and a small subset of patients with AIA develop bronchospasm in response to paracetamol [41]. This sensitivity to paracetamol usually involves only a mild reaction in response to high doses of the drug, and occurs in less than 2% of asthmatic patients.

Drug metabolism

The lung is ideally positioned to metabolize both inhaled and intravenous drugs. Its large epithelial and endothelial surface areas maximize contact between the drug and the cells. Examples of drugs that are metabolized in the lung are shown in Table 18.1.

Inhaled drugs
These will be subjected to the same metabolic activity in the airway and alveolar cells as other toxic chemicals described above. Mixed function oxidase and cytochrome P450 systems are active in the lung and so are presumed to metabolize drugs in the same way as in hepatocytes. Inhalational anaesthetics, in particular older agents that undergo significant metabolism elsewhere in the body such as methoxyflurane and halothane, undergo biotransformation in the airways by similar pathways to those in the liver, producing fluoride ions.

Intravenous drugs
Many drugs are removed from the circulation on passing through the lungs [36]. However, in the majority of cases this occurs by retention of the drug in lung tissue rather than actual metabolism. This low activity of metabolic enzymes found in the lung occurs for two reasons. First, access to the metabolic enzymes in endothelial cells is closely controlled by specific uptake mechanisms that are vital to allow the highly selective metabolism of endogenous compounds already described. Secondly, it is possible that the oxidative systems responsible for drug metabolism elsewhere in the body are located mostly in the airways thus preventing bloodborne drugs gaining access to them. Drugs that are basic (pKa >8) and lipophilic tend to be taken up in the pulmonary circulation while acidic drugs preferentially bind to plasma proteins [43]. Examples of drugs with significant pulmonary uptake that are of importance to anaesthetists include opiates such as fentanyl, pethidine and methadone, and amide local anaesthetics such as bupivacaine and lidocaine. Drug binding in the pulmonary circulation may act as a first-pass filter for any drug administered intravenously [44]. This drug reservoir within the lung may then be released slowly, or even give rise to rapid changes in plasma drug levels when the binding sites either become saturated or when one drug is displaced by a different drug with greater affinity for the binding site.

Pulmonary toxicity of drugs
Accumulation of some drugs and other toxic substances in the lung may cause dangerous local toxicity [29]. Paraquat is an outstanding example; it is slowly taken up into alveolar epithelial cells where it promotes the production of reactive oxygen species with resulting lung damage. Some drugs cause pulmonary toxicity by a similar mechanism, including nitrofurantoin and bleomycin, toxicity from the latter being strongly associated with exposure to high oxygen concentrations. Amiodarone, a highly effective and commonly used antiarrhythmic agent, is also associated with pulmonary toxicity, which occurs in 6% of patients given the drug. When toxicity occurs it may be severe and is fatal in up to 10% of cases. The cause is unknown, but formation of reactive oxygen species, immunological activation and direct cellular toxicity are all believed to contribute [45].

References

1 Lumb AB. The history of respiratory physiology. In: Lumb AB. *Nunn's Applied Respiratory Physiology*, 6th edn. Oxford: Butterworth-Heinemann, 2005.

2 Knight DA, Holgate ST. The airway epithelium: structural and functional properties in health and disease. *Respirology* 2003; **8**: 432–6.

3 Rogers DF. Airway goblet cells: responsive and adaptable frontline defenders. *Eur Respir J* 1994; **7**: 1690–706.

4 Rogers DF. Motor control of airway goblet cells and glands. *Respir Physiol* 2000; **125**: 129–44.

5 Singh G, Katyal SL. Clara cell proteins. *Ann N Y Acad Sci* 2000; **923**: 43–58.

6 Cutz E. Introduction to pulmonary neuroendocrine cell system, structure–function correlations. *Microsc Res Tech* 1997; **37**: 1–3.

7 Gosney J. Pulmonary neuroendocrine cell system in pediatric and adult lung disease. *Microsc Res Tech* 1997; **37**: 107–13.

8 Weibel ER. *The Pathway for Oxygen.* Cambridge, MA: Harvard University Press, 1984.

9 Matthay MA, Clerici C, Saumon G. Active fluid clearance from the distal air spaces of the lung. *J Appl Physiol* 2002; **93**: 1533–41.

10 Matthay MA, Folkesson HG, Clerici C. Lung epithelial fluid transport and the resolution of pulmonary edema. *Physiol Rev* 2002; **82**: 569–600.

11 Weibel ER. Morphological basis of alveolar–capillary gas exchange. *Physiol Rev* 1973; **53**: 419.

12 Weaver TE, Conkright JJ. Functions of surfactant proteins B and C. *Annu Rev Physiol* 2001; **63**: 555–78.

13 Widdicombe JH, Bastacky SJ, Wu DX-Y, Lee CY. Regulation of depth and composition of airway surface liquid. *Eur Respir J* 1997; **10**: 2892–7.

14 Widdicombe JH. Regulation of the depth and composition of airway surface liquid. *J Anat* 2002; **201**: 313–8.

15 Jeffery PK. Microscopic structure of normal lung. In: Brewis RAL, Corrin B, Geddes DM, Gibson GJ, eds. *Respiratory Medicine.* London: WB Saunders, 1995: 54–72.

16 Boucher RC. Regulation of airway surface liquid volume by human airway epithelia. *Pflugers Arch* 2003; **445**: 495–8.

17 McFadden ER Jr. Heat and water exchange in the human airways. *Am Rev Respir Dis* 1992; **146**: S8–10.

18 Mossman BT, Churg A. Mechanisms in the pathogenesis of asbestosis and silicosis. *Am J Respir Crit Care Med* 1998; **157**: 1666–80.

19 Groneberg DA, Witt C, Wagner U, Chung KF, Fischer A. Fundamentals of pulmonary drug delivery. *Respir Med* 2003; **97**: 382–7.

20 Bennett WD, Brown JS, Zeman KL, *et al.* Targeting delivery of aerosols to different lung regions. *J Aerosol Med* 2002; **15**: 179–88.

21 Ganz T. Antimicrobial polypeptides in host defense of the respiratory tract. *J Clin Invest* 2003; **109**: 693–7.

22 Ganz T. Antimicrobial polypeptides. *J Leukoc Biol* 2004; **75**: 34–8.

23 Wright JR. Pulmonary surfactant: a front line of lung host defense. *J Clin Invest* 2003; **111**: 1453–5.

24 Wu H, Kuzmenko A, Wan S, *et al.* Surfactant proteins A and D inhibit the growth of Gram-negative bacteria by increasing membrane permeability. *J Clin Invest* 2003; **111**: 1589–602.

25 Hogg JC, Senior RM. Chronic obstructive pulmonary disease 2: Pathology and biochemistry of emphysema. *Thorax* 2002; **57**: 830–4.

26 Pierce RA, Mariani TJ, Senior RM. Elastin in lung development and disease. *Ciba Found Symp* 1995; **192**: 199–214.

27 Carrell RW, Lomas DA. Alpha$_1$-antitrypsin deficiency: a model for conformational diseases. *N Engl J Med* 2002; **346**: 45–53.

28 Bond JA. Metabolism and elimination of inhaled drugs and airborne chemicals from the lungs. *Pharmacol Toxicol* 1993; **72** (Suppl 3): 36–47.

29 Foth H. Role of the lung in accumulation and metabolism of xenobiotic compounds: implications for chemically induced toxicity. *Crit Rev Toxicol* 1995; **25**: 165–205.

30 Kerut EK, Norfleet WT, Plotnick GD, Giles TD. Patent foramen ovale: a review of associated conditions and the impact of physiological size. *J Am Coll Cardiol* 2001; **38**: 613–23.

31 Fisher DC, Fisher EA, Budd JH, Rosen SE, Goldman ME. The incidence of patent foramen ovale in 1000 consecutive patients. *Chest* 1995; **107**: 1504–9.

32 Goldhaber SZ, Elliott CG. Acute pulmonary embolism: Part I. Epidemiology, pathophysiology, and diagnosis. *Circulation* 2003; **108**: 2726–9.

33 Santolicandro A, Prediletto R, Fornai E, *et al.* Mechanisms of hypoxemia and hypocapnia in pulmonary embolism. *Am J Respir Crit Care Med* 1995; **152**: 336–47.

34 Gosney JR. The endocrine lung and its response to hypoxia. *Thorax* 1994; **49**: S25–6.

35 Iervasi G, Clerico A, Pilo A, *et al.* Atrial natriuretic peptide is not degraded by the lungs in humans. *J Clin Endocrinol Metab* 1998; **83**: 2898–906.

36 Bahkle YS. Pharmacokinetic and metabolic properties of the lung. *Br J Anaesth* 1990; **65**: 79–93.

37 Brew K. Structure of human ACE gives new insights into inhibitor binding and design. *Trends Pharmacol Sci* 2003; **24**: 391–4.

38 Michael JR, Markewitz BA. Endothelins and the lung. *Am J Respir Crit Care Med* 1996; **154**: 555–81.

39 Drazen JM, Isreal E, O'Byrne PM. Treatment of asthma with drugs modifying the leukotriene pathway. *N Engl J Med* 1999; **340**: 197–206.

40 Szczeklik A, Stevenson DD. Aspirin-induced asthma: advances in pathogenesis, diagnosis, and management. *J Allergy Clin Immunol* 2003; **111**: 913–21.

41 Jenkins C, Costello J, Hodge L. Systematic review of prevalence of aspirin induced asthma and its implications for clinical practice. *Br Med J* 2004; **328**: 434–7.

42 Schwab JM, Schluesener HJ, Laufer S. COX-3: just another COX or the solitary elusive target of paracetamol? *Lancet* 2003; **361**: 981–2.

43 Boer F. Drug handling by the lungs. *Br J Anaesth* 2003; **91**: 50–60.

44 Upton RN, Doolette DJ. Kinetic aspects of drug deposition in the lungs. *Clin Exp Pharmacol Physiol* 1999; **26**: 381–91.

45 Reasor MJ, Kacew S. An evaluation of possible mechanisms underlying amiodarone-induced pulmonary toxicity. *Proc Soc Exp Biol Med* 1996; **212**: 297–305.

CHAPTER 19

The brain as a site of inflammation after acute injury

Jonathan Rhodes and Peter Andrews

Introduction

Injury to the brain is common, associated with high mortality and survivors frequently have significant residual disability. Traumatic brain injury is the leading cause of death in individuals under the age of 45 years in Europe and the USA. Worldwide, stroke is the second most common cause of death after coronary heart disease.

Although the aetiology of traumatic destruction of cerebral tissue and focal or global ischaemia are quite different, their pathologies are linked by a common process. It is clear that the extent of injury in each case is not limited to that caused by the primary insult, be it traumatic or ischaemia induced neuronal death. Instead, there will always be secondary damage, the magnitude of the injury increasing with time. This is illustrated in traumatic brain injury by the large numbers of patients who are able to talk, implying preserved higher function, and then die as a result of their brain injury (Fig. 19.1) [1].

Cerebral tissue hypoxia is central to the progression of brain injury and can arise as a result of multiple interacting processes. This results in harmful derangements of neurochemistry and the induction of reactive cascades of chemical mediators each capable of adversely prejudicing neuronal survival [2,3]. These insults include excitatory amino acid release, derangement of calcium homoeostasis, free radical production and activation of the inflammatory process (Fig. 19.2). It is likely that this chemical injury is responsible for the inexorable deterioration seen in many patients despite compliance with guidelines for the maintenance of cerebral perfusion [4,5].

This chapter examines the role of inflammation as a secondary injury process, with particular reference to traumatic brain injury. Because there are tremendous similarities in the pathophysiology of traumatic brain injury and primary ischaemic cerebral injury (stroke), many important lessons can be gained from the stroke literature, which is also discussed.

Inflammation

Inflammation is defined as a local reaction at the microvessel interfaces that results in fluid and cell translocation from the intravascular medium into the tissue in order to 'wall off' and sequester injurious agents and protect and repair the tissue [6]. The central nervous system (CNS) was traditionally considered an immune privileged site lacking a lymphoid system and antigen presenting dendritic cells [7]. However, it has become apparent that injury to the brain, including trauma and ischaemia, is followed by glial cell activation, the expression of cytokines and leucocyte migration into areas of damage. However, many features of this response are atypical when compared with stereotyped inflammation in the periphery. In the CNS, mast cells, required for the rapid release of preformed mediators, are absent. Leucocytes appear reluctant to cross the blood–brain barrier and the resident macrophages, the microglia, are quiescent [8]. These differences appear to develop in the postnatal period [9]. To date, the induction and function of the inflammatory process remains poorly understood. The remainder of this review describes this inflammatory reaction in more detail, concentrating on the major pro-inflammatory mediators. The significance of inflammation as a

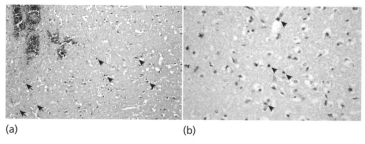

(a)   (b)

Figure 19.1 Primary injury to the central nervous system damages neurones and induces profound changes in the neurochemical environment. The expression of inflammatory mediators and infiltration of inflammatory cells constitute part of this derangement and potentially lead to further neuronal injury. (a) Coronal section through a cerebral contusion at 4 hours after surgery. Numerous shrunken necrotic neurones are apparent (arrow heads) and may be contrasted with neurones with normal morphology (arrows). Traumatic haemorrhage is present in the upper left corner of the section. ×100. (b) By 24 hours after injury polymorphonuclear leucocytes (arrow heads) can be seen infiltrating the contused tissue. ×200.

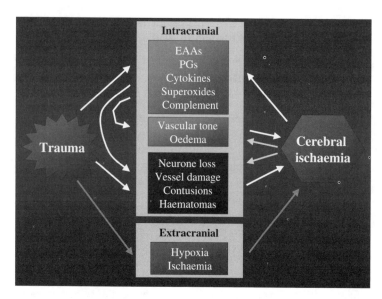

Figure 19.2 Acute brain injury leads to neuronal loss both directly and indirectly. Both trauma and ischaemia can lead to early neuronal death. Oedema, space occupying lesions, changes in cerebral vascular tone and the effects of extracranial injuries result in further cerebral ischaemia which either directly or via the activation of diverse chemical systems such as inflammation causes secondary neuronal injury. EAA, excitatory amino acids; PG, prostaglandins.

chemical injury process and the potential for therapies designed to modulate it is considered.

Inflammatory cytokine expression

The mediators central to the inflammatory process are the cytokines. The cytokine family is a diverse group of polypeptides, the precise function of which often depends upon the organ or species studied. Within the CNS, some of the inflammatory cytokines are expressed at constitutively low levels. However, following injury, expression can increase signifi-cantly. While there is evidence to suggest that some cytokines have positive effects on neuronal homoeo-stasis, unchecked release of pro-inflammatory mediators can prejudice cell survival following brain injury [10].

Clinical expression

In patients with acute ischaemic stroke, interleukin-1β (IL-1β) is transiently elevated in the cerebrospinal fluid (CSF) after the onset of symptoms [11] while tumour necrosis factor α (TNF-α) is increased in serum after stroke, peaking at 7 days [12]. IL-6 level is elevated in both the serum/plasma and CSF of patients, both peaking within 48 hours of onset [11,13,14]. Serum/plasma and CSF IL-6 levels correlate poorly with outcome [13,15].

Increases in CSF and serum TNF [16,17], IL-1 [18] and IL-6 [19,20] have been reported following both elective neurosurgical procedures and traumatic brain injury. Levels are either raised on admission, or peak within 24 hours of injury. In 1997, our group published a report describing a transcranial gradient of serum IL-6, in patients with traumatic brain injury or subarachnoid haemorrhage, supporting an intracerebral source of production of this cytokine [21].

Animal models

Early expression of tissue pro-inflammatory cytokine levels above background has been found in both ischaemic and traumatic experimental brain injuries. TNF-α mRNA and protein is detectable in ischaemic tissue within an hour of either permanent or transient ischaemia and peak within 24 hours of injury [22,23]. Similarly, in both permanent and transient focal ischaemia, IL-1β mRNA is induced in the ischaemic cortex and deeper structures including hippocampus and thalamus as early as 15 minutes after the onset of ischaemia and has been shown to peak within 3–6 hours [24,25]. Permanent ischaemia also induced IL-1β protein expression in the ischaemic cortex of rats from 4 hours, peaking at 3 days [26]. Permanent and transient ischaemia leads to significant induction of IL-6 mRNA in the ischaemic cortex from 3 hours, peaking at 12–24 hours [27,28], and permanent injuries induced IL-6 protein expression in the ischaemic cortex from 12 hours and peaking at 24 hours [26].

Non-penetrating traumatic injury to the cortex induces TNF-α mRNA expression in the ipsilateral tissue as early as 1 hour following injury and returns to baseline by 24 hours [29]. In the same injury, ipsilateral cortical TNF-α protein peaked at 3–8 hours [30]. In similar studies TNF levels increased significantly in the injured cortex at 1 and 4 hours after severe trauma [31,32].

Experimental trauma also induces IL-1β mRNA expression [33] and IL-1β protein in the injured hemisphere, peaking at 8 hours after injury [30] and increased IL-1β mRNA has also been detected following penetrating injury to the striatum. In this injury the mRNA expression was widespread and bilateral, peaking at 4 hours after injury. At the injury site, IL-1β protein was also recovered by microdialysis [34,35].

IL-6 mRNA and protein is increased in the injured hemisphere following blunt trauma, peaking at 8 hours after injury [30,32,36]. Penetrating injury to the striatum also induced IL-6 mRNA, peaking at 6 hours, and IL-6 protein expression has also been confirmed by immunohistochemistry and microdialysis [34,35].

Cellular expression of inflammatory cytokines

Local synthesis by resident glial and neuronal cells of the CNS has been described in a growing number of both *in vitro* and *in vivo* studies. Constitutive expression appears to occur predominantly in neurones.

In vitro

Cell culture experiments have demonstrated that activated microglial cells express IL-1 [37]. Following fluid percussion trauma to cultured human astrocytes, increased IL-6 protein production has been found [38]. Cytokine interactions have also been studied: IL-1β has been shown to stimulate production of other cytokines, including TNF and IL-6 in astrocytes [39,40], whereas TNF has been shown to cause the release of cytokines including IL-6, from human astrocytes [40].

In vivo

TNF-α has been localized at low levels to cells with features resembling neurones, in normal cerebral cortex [23]. Following permanent focal ischaemic injury, TNF-α immunopositive cells were identifiable within and around the ischaemic area. Neurones, astrocytes, glia and infiltrating peripheral mononuclear cells expressing TNF-α have been identified [22,41,42].

Following severe lateral traumatic brain injury, immunohistochemistry localized the early increase in TNF-α to neurones of injured cerebral cortex [31]. TNF-α positive astrocytes have been localized to focal lesions and this expression occurred relatively late after injury and was maximal at 6 days [43].

The constitutive expression of IL-1β mRNA and IL-1β activity in the normal adult rat brain is neuronal, although in the striatum and septum much lower levels of IL-1β mRNA have been observed and are possibly of glial origin [44].

IL-1β mRNA positive cells resembling glia or macrophages have been identified after permanent focal ischaemia in the rat [45]. Similarly after transient focal ischaemia, the cells expressing IL-1β mRNA were interpreted as being glia and vascular endothelial cells [46]. Holmin *et al.* [43] studied expression of cytokine mRNA in a contusional injury using a weight drop model. Contrary to the findings of the majority of the studies, no cytokine mRNA was seen within the first 2 days of injury. However, expression of IL-1β by mononuclear cells and astrocytes was described in and around the lesion by days 4–6 post-trauma. The dominant source of IL-1β was thought to be resident microglia and invading monocytes.

The constitutive expression of IL-6 mRNA also appears to be neuronal [47,48]. After transient ischaemia, IL-6-positive cells resembling microglia and neurones have been observed from 24 hours in the ischaemic penumbra [49]. In diffuse traumatic brain injury, increased IL-6 expression occurs in neurones, although a few IL-6 mRNA positive cells were also localized to the meninges and were assumed to be macrophages [50]. Following focal traumatic injury, mononuclear cells expressing IL-6 mRNA have also been described [43].

Significance of cytokine expression

Cytokines have diverse local effects including the control of cell growth and differentiation, orchestration of inflammatory responses and migration of leucocytes, control of cytotoxic and phagocytic cells, wound healing and tissue remodelling. They are also important mediators of the whole body metabolic response to trauma and infection. Such systemic activities include induction of fever, adrenocorticotrophic hormone (ACTH) release, muscle catabolism, neutrophilia and production of acute phase reactants such as C-reactive protein and decreased synthesis of albumin.

Interleukin-1

IL-1 appears to act as an endogenous mediator of host responses to injury such as fever, anorexia, sickness behaviour, slow wave sleep and alterations in neuroendocrine, cardiovascular and immune systems. These actions are mediated mainly through the hypothalamus and can be blocked by local injection of interleukin-1 receptor antagonist (IL-1ra) or antibodies to IL-1β [51]. IL-1 has been shown to induce a wide variety of responses, many of which could exacerbate neural damage. These include blood–brain barrier dysfunction, adhesion molecule expression, recruitment of immune cells, damage to the cerebral vasculature and the release of substances such as eicosanoids, β amyloid precursor protein, corticotrophin releasing factor, nitric oxide, free radicals and activated complement components, growth factor and neurotrophin induction, as well as modulation of calcium currents, have also been reported and might be beneficial [51].

Exposure of a monolayer of rat cerebral endothelial cells to IL-1β induces a decline in the trans-endothelial resistance suggesting increased permeability. This can be completely abolished by cyclo-oxygenase inhibition or the introduction of IL-1ra [52]. Intracisternal recombinant IL-1 induces peripheral mononuclear cell accumulation in the CSF and significantly increased blood–brain barrier permeability within 3 hours [53]. Increased IL-1β observed after trauma might be responsible for oedema formation occurring after head injury.

Cultured astrocytes release eicosanoids, predominantly prostaglandin E and thromboxane B_2, in response to IL-1β [54]. IL-1β also induces the production of nitric oxide by astrocytes in culture [55], which has been implicated in the generation of free radicals after acute brain injury.

On its own, the application to neuronal cultures of IL-1β does not result in overt cell death until high concentrations are reached. The effect of IL-1β on cell viability can depend on the environment cells are exposed to. *In vitro*, cells subjected to hypoxia, TNF-α or with withdrawal of nerve growth factor (NGF) undergo apoptosis and this can be reduced by blocking the IL-1 system [56,57]. Similarly, *in vivo*, if combined with another injurious event such as ischaemia or excitotoxicity, intracerebroventricular or parenchymal injection exacerbates neuronal damage [58,59]. It has been suggested that the net effect of IL-1 depends on either the presence of threatened neurones or other factors with which it interacts [51].

Intracerebroventricular (ICV) injection of IL-1β either prior to or following permanent ischaemia, enhances the infarct volume and is associated with a significant increase in temperature [59,60]. Following 60 minutes of transient ischaemia, IL-1β significantly increased oedema over that caused by ischaemia alone and this was also associated with significant increases in infarction size and numbers of parenchymal and endothelial cells. Administration of anti-IL-1β antibody or zinc protoporphyrin, an IL-1 blocker, by injection reduced infarction size, neutrophil number and brain water content. Radiation induced leucopenia further and augmented the reduction in oedema associated with anti-IL-1β antibody administration [61].

Further evidence for a pathological role of IL-1β comes from experiments using IL-1ra, an endogenous inhibitor of IL-1β. ICV IL-1ra administration can result in a >50% reduction in infarction volume after both permanent and transient ischaemic injuries. Furthermore, the delay in the administration of IL-1ra to 3 hours after the onset of transient ischaemia sustained a significant reduction in lesion volume by 46%, an effect that may be clinically useful [58,60,62]. Intravenous administration of IL-1ra during permanent middle cerebral artery occlusion has also been shown to be protective with significant reductions in weight loss, neuronal necrosis, lesion size and leucocyte recruitment in the ischaemic hemisphere in rats. Neurological function in the treated animals also improved significantly with time [63].

Similarly, the administration of IL-1ra ICV immediately following fluid percussion injury and continuing for 48 hours reduced cortical damage by 40%. When the first administration was delayed until 4 hours after injury, the reduction in damage remained significant at 28% [64].

Tumour necrosis factor-α

The role of TNF-α in brain injury as a whole is controversial. Harmful effects of TNF include induction of inflammatory mediators, breakdown of the blood–brain barrier and exacerbation of ischaemic insults. However, protective effects against excitatory amino acids (EAA) and oxidative stress have been observed.

In vitro studies of TNF-α function have generated conflicting results, some studies suggesting harmful effects of this cytokine and others beneficial effects. Some of the observed differences may occur because of differences in the maturity of cells used in culture, the concentration of TNF-α administered or the timing of the TNF-α administration.

In cultured fetal neurones, addition of TNF-α potentiates glutamate toxicity and is associated with reduced glutamate metabolism and uptake [65]. TNF-α also induces necrotic changes in oligodendrocytes and degeneration of myelin [66–68]. Damage to oligodendrocytes in culture can be prevented by inhibitors of nitric oxide and TNF-α. Anti-TNF-α inhibits nitric oxide production, implying a toxic mechanism for TNF-α via nitric oxide [68]. TNF-α may cause direct damage to the endothelium, because high concentrations have been found to alter cell morphology in cerebral endothelial cells. TNF-α also induces nitric oxide and endothelin expression in endothelial cell cultures. This would suggest a possible role for it in the altered cerebrovascular responsiveness after acute brain injury [69]. Endothelial cells and astrocytes cultured with TNF-α also express intercellular adhesion molecule 1 (ICAM-1) [70]. Conversely, pretreatment of rat embryonic neurones with TNF-α is protective against glucose deprivation and excitatory amino acids, stabilizing the elevation of intracellular calcium [71]. TNF-α pretreatment also protects neurones from oxidative stress [72,73] through induction of manganese superoxide dismutase and inhibits mitochondrial peroxynitrite formation and lipid peroxidation [73]. TNF-α also induces proliferation of astrocytes in culture and has been implicated in gliosis associated with brain injury [74].

A possible explanation for the inconsistency in the *in vitro* results presented could be because of the limitations of studying the effects of single agonists on a single cell type, cultured in isolation. The inflammatory response clearly involves multiple mediators acting simultaneously. In human fetal brain cell cultures composed of neurones and glia, individually neither IL-1β nor TNF-α were toxic. However, in combination they caused marked neuronal injury and substantial amounts of nitric oxide were produced. Blockade of nitric oxide production was accompanied by a marked reduction in neuronal injury, suggesting that the production of nitric oxide by astrocytes [55] has a role in cytokine-induced neurotoxicity. The addition of N-methyl-D-aspartate (NMDA) receptor antagonists to the cell cultures also blocked toxicity, implicating these receptors in the response. Treatment of brain cell cultures with IL-1β plus TNF-α was found to inhibit glutamate uptake and astrocyte glutamine synthase activity, two major pathways involved in NMDA receptor-related neurotoxicity [75]. Taken together, these findings provide some indication of how multiple mediators might interact in disease. The combined administration of cytokines augmented NMDA-mediated toxicity, and this was associated with nitric oxide generation and lipid peroxide damage to cell membranes [76,77].

In vitro exposure of cerebral endothelial cell monolayers to TNF results in increased permeability which, like IL-1β, is abolished by cyclo-oxygenase inhibition [52]. Intracisternal TNF-α resulted in CSF inflammation [78].

The role of TNF-α in stroke has been widely investigated. Pretreatment of rats with intracisternal TNF-α, 24 hours before either permanent or transient ischaemia, significantly increased infarct size assessed at 24 hours [79]. However, pretreatment of mice intracisternally with a much larger dose of TNF-α, 48 hours prior to permanent middle cerebral artery occlusion was found to reduce infarct volume at 24 hours [80]. Blocking endogenous TNF-α with repeated doses of either monoclonal antibody or soluble TNF-receptor I, prior to injury, reduced focal ischaemic injury 24 hours after permanent middle cerebral artery occlusion [79]. Intracortical administration of anti-TNF-α antibodies and topical TNF binding protein (TBP) after onset of ischaemia also significantly reduced lesion size [81,82]. Similarly, antagonizing the TNF-α system reduces lesion volume after transient ischaemia [83].

However, there is evidence that TNF-α can also be supportive. Pretreatment with intracisternal TNF-α 48 hours prior to permanent middle cerebral

artery occlusion reduced infarct volume [80]. In animals deficient in TNF receptors, damage to neurones caused by focal ischaemia and seizures was increased. Oxidative stress was increased and levels of antioxidant enzymes reduced, suggesting that TNF protects neurones by stimulating antioxidant pathways [84]. Chronic deficiency in TNF-α function might lead to the loss of neuroprotective mechanisms but acute overexpression could be equally detrimental.

In trauma models, the acute expression of TNF-α also appears harmful. Both prevention of TNF production by pentoxifylline (PTX) and the administration of TBP have been used to reduce the activity of TNF-α, resulting in significantly less peak oedema formation at 24 hours and improved recovery of motor function over the first 4 days. TBP also attenuated disruption of the blood–brain barrier and protected hippocampal cells [85]. ICV administration of a selective TNF antagonist improved performance in a series of standardized motor tasks at 7 and 14 days after injury [31].

In animals chronically deficient in TNF, the benefits of a lack of TNF at the time of the injury are also seen. However, TNF may also have an important role in recovery from injury. In genetically modified TNF deficient animals, mortality was significantly decreased at 1 week compared with wild-types in an experimental trauma model. In the 24 hours after injury, no significant differences in the degree of blood–brain barrier dysfunction, infiltration of neutrophils or cell death were found between the deficient and wild-type animals. Neurological outcome assessed over 7 days was not significantly different between the two groups, although the TNF knockouts trended towards better recovery at 7 days [86]. In another study, mice genetically deficient in both TNF-α and lymphotoxin-α (LT-α or TNF-β) were subjected to controlled trauma. These animals also had significantly less severe neurological deficits when compared with brain injured wild-types at 48 hours post-injury. However, at 7 days post-injury there was no difference in motor scores between the knockouts and the wild-types and by 2–3 weeks the wild-type motor score had recovered to baseline while the TNF deficient mice had persistent deficit. Histological examination showed that initially there was no difference in the cortical injury cavity volume at 1 week post-injury between TNF deficient and wild-type animals. However, the injury volume increased more in the TNF deficient mice, becoming significantly greater by 4 weeks post-injury [87]. Acute TNF expression would therefore appear harmful, but in the longer term the ability to express TNF-α is associated with less histological damage and better recovery.

Interleukin-6

The precise role of IL-6 in the response of the brain to injury remains unclear. Interleukin-6 has been shown to have a neurotrophic action, supporting the survival of catecholaminergic and cholinergic neurones in culture [88–90]. *In vivo* infusion of excitotoxic amounts of NMDA into the rat striatum resulted in a reduction in the number of cholinergic and GABAergic neurones at 2 days post-injection. Co-infusion of IL-6 reduced the loss of cholinergic but not GABAergic neurones [91]. The CSF of patients after traumatic brain injury has been shown to contain IL-6 and to induce NGF production in astrocytes. The induction of NGF was inhibited by the addition of anti-IL-6 antibodies, implying a protective role for IL-6. However, chronic overexpression of IL-6 in mice leads to the development of severe neurological disease with neurodegeneration, astrocytosis and angiogenesis [92]. As with IL-1β and TNF-α, IL-6 increases endothelial monolayer permeability *in vitro* [52,53,93].

Cytokines and leucocyte recruitment

Injury to the brain is associated with infiltration of leucocytes and activation of microglia. However, this differs with respect to the kinetics and nature of the cellular infiltrate compared with that seen out with the CNS, the brain parenchyma appearing resistant to leucocyte recruitment. For example, the neuronal degeneration induced by intracerebral injection of kainic acid or the introduction of pro-inflammatory stimuli such as lipopolysaccharide (LPS), IL-1β or TNF-α, fails to induce an acute inflammatory response in the parenchyma. In the first 24–48 hours, polymorphonuclear cells accumulate in blood vessels and local activation of microglia occurs. In contrast to the parenchyma, numerous leucocytes were localized to the meninges, choroid plexus and ventricles [94].

In peripheral tissue such as skin, IL-1β induces TNF-α and vice versa and there is a similar accumulation of neutrophils and monocytes within hours [95–97]. In the CNS, more specific responses to injury have been reported which tend to be delayed and related to the area studied. Microinjection of IL-β into the striatum induces *de novo* IL-1β but not TNF-α and TNF-α did not induce TNF-α or IL-1β production [97]. IL-1β tended to be associated with recruitment of mononuclear cells, whereas TNF-α injection led to the recruitment of monocytes although this developed slowly over 24 hours [98].

Both ischaemic injuries and traumatic lesions to the brain are associated with characteristic patterns of leucocyte infiltration and glial activation. Focal ischaemia to the brain may be either permanent, or transient with reperfusion. This distinction is associated with variation in the temporal pattern of leucocyte recruitment in to the affected tissue. Polymorphonuclear cells, mainly neutrophils, are the predominant leucocytes to infiltrate the parenchyma initially after ischaemia. These are then followed by monocytes and lymphocytes [99,100]. In human stroke and ischaemia models, maximal neutrophil infiltration occurs within 72 hours of ischaemia onset [101], whereas monocyte infiltration peaks at 7 days [102]. In addition to infiltrating monocytes, resident cerebral microglia, derived from the same origins as monocytes and macrophages, become reactive.

Traumatic injury to the brain occurs either as direct 'focal' tissue destruction or the result of acceleration–deceleration injury, stretching neurones and leading to temporary dysfunction or permanent disconnection, a process known as 'diffuse axonal injury' [103]. Leucocyte recruitment and cytokine expression appears to be more significant in focal rather than diffuse injuries [104,105]. Focal injuries are characterized by marked invasion of neutrophils and mononuclear phagocytes. In diffuse injury, leucocyte invasion of the parenchyma is much less significant, the dominant reactive cells being resident microglia.

Following cerebral contusion, neutrophil accumulation peaks within the first 2 days. Monocytes, macrophages and reactive microglia also accumulate in and around the lesion within the first 2 days of injury. Thereafter, marked increases in these cells occurs until days 4–6 and then declines by day 8. T lymphocytes and natural killer (NK) cells are also reported in lower numbers but in a similar temporal profile. Reactive astrocytes are seen from day 2 onwards [106,107].

The effect of leucocyte accumulation
Blood flow

Accumulation of circulating leucocytes after injury is generally considered harmful, impairing perfusion and releasing toxic mediators. Neutrophils and monocytes have been observed plugging capillaries and venules after both transient and permanent ischaemic insults [108]. Deficient microvascular perfusion, 'no-reflow', was reported to occur in >60% of capillaries within 1 hour of reperfusion following middle cerebral artery occlusion [108]. Induction of neutropenia with mechlorethamine or antineutrophil antibody or a reduction in leucocyte adherence to the endothelium preserves cerebral blood flow and function after ischaemia [109]. Following 45 minutes of ischaemia in neutropenic mice, infarct volume was reduced by 67%. Neurological deficit was significantly reduced, while cerebral blood flow was significantly increased [109].

Polymorphonuclear leucocytes

Polymorphonuclear leucocytes contain numerous potentially toxic agents such as myeloperoxidase and elastase and are potent generators of free radicals. *In vitro* co-culture of neutrophils with hippocampal neurones is associated with increased cell death [110]. Intracerebral accumulation of neutrophils is associated with the breakdown of the blood–brain barrier — an effect prevented by the induction of neutropenia [111]. Following transient ischaemia, depletion of circulating neutrophils with an antineutrophil antibody (RP3) inhibited the increase in extracellular radical concentration after reperfusion, reduced infarct size and the extent of oedema [112].

Monocytic cell lines

Microglia are the resident macrophages of the brain, phagocytosing damaged cells and scavenging debris [113]. Monocytes and resident microglial cells have been implicated in free radical generation and excitatory amino acid-like toxin production. Microglia are a source of superoxide [114] and nitric oxide [115]. In addition, drugs such as chloroquine and colchicine have been found to inhibit mononuclear cell secretion and phagocytic function and administration of these compounds following transient middle cerebral artery occlusion has been shown to reduce the number of reactive mononuclear phagocytes in infarcted tissue — an effect that was associated with a reduction in the neurone killing activity. The increase in reactive mononuclear cells and neurotoxic activity was not seen until 2 days after the insult [113].

Adhesion molecules

The recruitment of leucocytes from the blood into inflamed parenchyma requires interaction between the leucocytes and the vascular endothelium. Three major protein families have been identified that have a role in these leucocyte–endothelial interactions: the selectins, β_2-integrins, and the intracellular adhesion molecules (ICAMs) [3].

The selectin family includes E-selectin, P-selectin and L-selectin. These mediate adhesion by binding to carbohydrate residues on glycoproteins and glycolipids [3]. P-selectin and E-selectin are unregulated on activated endothelium, while L-selectin is constitutively expressed on leucocytes. The β_2-integrins are heterodimeric proteins consisting of a common β-chain, CD18 and differing α-chains, CD11a, b or c. Members of this family include lymphocyte function-associated antigen (LFA; CD11a/CD18), Mac-1 (CD11b/CD18) and p150.95 (CD11c/CD18). The integrins expressed by leucocytes bind to endothelial surface proteins of the immunoglobulin superfamily (ICAM-1, ICAM-2, ICAM-3, VCAM-1).

Under the action of pro-inflammatory mediators, endothelial cells up-regulate factors associated with leucocyte transmigration [104]. For instance, both TNF-α and γ-interferon (IFN-γ) can increase ICAM-1 expression in microglia culture [116]. Similarly,

TNF-α, IL-1β and IFN-γ increase ICAM-1 expression in cultured human brain microvessel endothelial cells [117]. TNF-α also induces expression of vascular cell adhesion molecule 1 (VCAM-1) and E-selectin in CNS endothelial cells *in vitro* [118].

During recruitment to sites of inflammation, leucocytes initially tether 'loosely' to the endothelium, rolling along it with the haemodynamic shear forces, an interaction mediated by the selectin family. Leucocyte activation then leads to integrin–ICAM interaction and firm adherence to the endothelium prior to migration across the vessel wall (Fig. 19.3) [119]. ICAM-1 and E-selectin mRNA are induced in the ischaemic cortex within hours of experimental injury

[120], while ICAM-1 and P-selectin have been localized to blood vessels of ischaemic cerebral tissue [109,121]. ICAM-1 positive vessels have also been identified in human cerebral cortical infarcts along with LFA positive cells [122].

The significance of adhesion molecules in the pathology of the inflammatory process is indicated by the reduction in leucocyte recruitment and parenchymal damage following administration of anti-adhesion molecules in ischaemic and traumatic injuries. Following 2 hours of ischaemia, administration of anti-CD11b antibody, repeated at 22 hours, significantly reduced infarct volume by 43%. Tissue neutrophil numbers assessed at microscopy were

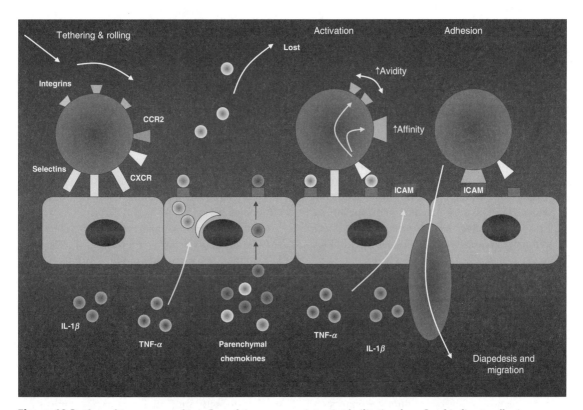

Figure 19.3 Chemokines expressed in inflamed tissue lead to the recruitment of circulating leucocytes. Circulating white cells roll across the endothelium, tethered loosely by selectins. Chemokines on the endothelial surface interact with receptors on the leucocytes resulting in conformational changes in integrins facilitating there firm binding to adhesion molecules. The leucocytes now held on the endothelial surface can then migrate into the damaged tissue. CCR, CC, chemokine receptor; CXC, CXCR, chemokine receptor; ICAM, intercellular adhesion molecule 1; IL, interleukin; TNF-α, tumour necrosis factor α.

also significantly reduced, as were neurological function scores [123]. When the initial dose of anti-CD11b antibody was delayed for 1 hour, the lesion volume was still significantly reduced by 28% [124]. Further work by the same group examined the effect of anti-integrins given as a single, but larger, dose of anti-CD11b antibody administered only on reperfusion. This resulted in an approximately 53% reduction in infarct volume [125]. The effect of anti-ICAM antibodies has also been investigated and showed a beneficial effect on infarct size, neutrophil accumulation and oedema [126]. However, although effective, increasing the duration of the ischaemic insult prior to reperfusion and delaying the time of administration appears to reduce the effectiveness of anti-adhesion molecule therapy.

In trauma, the administration of ICAM-1 antibody was associated with the finding of improved motor function and reduced neutrophil accumulation when administered to rats after trauma (from 1 hour post-injury) [127]. However, it is noteworthy that in this study, some protection was also seen when a non-specific antibody was given. In ICAM-1 gene deficient animals the situation is even less clear. Although ICAM-1 could be detected in the choroid plexus and cerebral endothelium of wild-type mice at 24 hours post-injury, there was no difference in neutrophil accumulation, lesion volume or outcome between ICAM-1 knockouts and wild-type animals [128]. This may reflect the difficulties in using knockout animals to represent wild-type acute pathology.

Chemokines

In addition to the expression of adhesion molecules, another group of peptides, the chemokines, have been found to be required for the recruitment and parenchymal infiltration of leucocytes. Chemokines are a subgroup of the cytokine family known to be chemotactic for leucocytes. This family consists of over 50 ligands acting on multiple receptors. All members contain a conserved sequence of 2–4 cysteine units. The position of the first two cysteines of this grouping has been used to further divide the chemokines into subgroups, the CXC, CC, C and CX3C or α, β, γ and δ chemokines. The largest and most comprehensively described subgroups are the

CXC and CC families. The CXC are further subclassified based on the presence of a glutamic acid-leucine-arginine tripeptide motif (ELR). The α-CXC-ELR positive chemokines, IL-8, growth regulated oncogene (GRO) and macrophage inflammatory protein (MIP-2) are predominantly neutrophil chemoattractants. The α-CXC-ELR negative chemokines such as interferon inducible protein-10 (IP-10) attract lymphocytes and monocytes. The β-CC chemokines, monocyte chemoattractant protein (MCP-1), regulated on activation normal T cells expressed and secreted (RANTES) and macrophage inflammatory protein-1α and β (MIP-1α, MIP-1β) principally attract monocytes, lymphocytes, eosinophils and basophils [129].

Chemokine expression

Significant elevation of IL-8 has been measured in the CSF of children early after traumatic brain injury. Levels were equivalent to those seen in bacterial meningitis and there was a strong association with CSF IL-8 concentrations and mortality [130]. In adults with severe traumatic brain injury, significantly elevated IL-8 concentrations were measurable in CSF from the first 24 hours and up to 21 days after injury. CSF from patients was found to induce NGF expression in cultured mouse astrocytes, an effect reduced by pre-incubation of CSF with anti-IL-8 antibodies [131].

Chemokine expression has been described in *in vitro* experiments using a wide variety of cells pertinent to the CNS. Astrocytes produce MIP-2 and IL-8 when incubated with pro-inflammatory cytokines such as TNF-α or IL-β [40,41,132,133]. Brain microvascular endothelial cells also release MIP-2 in culture with TNF-α, although compared with the astrocytes, the other major component of the blood–brain barrier, this is substantially less.

Human microglia also express IL-8 and this can be significantly reduced in *in vitro* experiments by pre-incubation with anti-inflammatory cytokines such as IL-4, IL-10 and tissue growth factor β1 (TGF-β1) [133]. Microglia, but not astrocytes, subjected to 8 hours of hypoxia and 24 hours of reoxygenation, express MIP-2. With a more severe hypoxic injury of 12 hours, microglial death was observed and no increase in MIP-2 detected. In contrast, although an increase in MIP-2 was not observed in astrocyte cultures, these cells maintained their viability even with 12 hours of hypoxia. Although MIP-2 expression was not observed until 12 hours of hypoxia, it increased further with longer durations of insult. Immunohistochemistry localized the MIP-2 production to the microglia [134].

Microglia express MIP-1α and MIP-1β but not MCP-1 in response to inflammatory mediators [135]. CNS endothelial cells display up-regulation of MCP-1 on culture with TNF-α and IL-1β, which can be inhibited by co-treatment with dexamethasone. Aortic endothelial cells were found to have a greater baseline expression of MCP-1 than CNS endothelial cells. This is possibly in keeping with the relative resistance of the CNS to inflammation [136].

In rabbits subjected to transient focal ischaemia, tissue IL-8 levels were increased after 6 hours of reperfusion and IL-8 was localized to vessels and infiltrating neutrophils [137]. MCP-1 mRNA induction has been described following both permanent and transient middle cerebral artery occlusion [138–140]. MCP-1 and MIP-1α mRNA are induced in ischaemic rat cortex within hours of injury [138,140]. Double-labelling hybridization identified astrocytes and microglia/macrophages as the source of MCP-1. MIP-1α was localized to microglia/macrophages only [140].

Following a penetrating traumatic injury, astrocytes express MCP-1 mRNA and protein. Messenger RNA is present within 5 hours and protein levels are elevated 10–24 hours after injury [141]. Removal of a segment of cerebral cortex induces, in the remaining tissue, MCP-1 mRNA and expression peaks at 12–24 hours. This is associated with localized microglial activation and macrophage accumulation at the site of the lesion, which increases in the days after injury [142].

Following closed head injury in mice, increased MIP-2 protein was increased and peaked at 4 hours and was significantly less in TNF/LT-α knockout animals. Regulation by TNF/LT-α was therefore implied [143].

In an attempt to identify how CNS damage induces chemokine expression, treatment of brain slice cultures has been compared with astrocyte cultures. When corticostriatal slice cultures were subjected to an excitotoxic injury with NMDA, MCP-1 was induced in astrocytes, with MCP-1 release into the culture medium. In contrast, NMDA treatment of astrocyte cultures did not induce production of MCP-1. This suggests that damage to neurones leads to signal transmission to astrocytes inducing MCP-1 production [140].

In common with cytokines, the chemokine family displays a diverse range of functions within the CNS. Many of these are incompletely characterized. Chemokine receptors have been identified on neurones, glia and endothelial cells of normal brains. In addition to chemotactic effects on leucocyte populations, important roles in the migration of multipotent progenitor cells and cell proliferation during CNS development have been described. Chemokine modulation of synaptic activity, neurotrophic effects, induction of the febrile response and anorexia have also been reported [129].

Intrahippocampal microinjection of chemokines has been studied in mice. Both MIP-2 and IL-8 induce predominant neutrophil recruitment by 24 hours and some monocytic cells were also present by 48 hours. Endothelial activation indicated by ICAM-1 expression was also noted. MIP-2 evoked a widespread response compared to IL-8. This would be consistent with species differences in the dominant α-chemokine. The recruitment of neutrophils was associated with increased blood–brain barrier permeability. Mice rendered leucopenic by prior irradiation did not display leucocyte recruitment or blood–brain barrier breakdown. MCP-1 was the most potent monocyte chemoattractant of the β chemokines tested in this study. Monocyte recruitment was associated with limited blood–brain barrier breakdown and with ICAM-1 expression. RANTES and IP-10 were associated with minimal monocytic infiltration [145].

This study supports the role of chemokines in the recruitment of leucocytes to the CNS after injury and is consistent with studies in animals overexpressing chemokines [146]. In addition it also demonstrates some additional features of the uniqueness of the cerebral inflammatory response compared to peripheral inflammation. Most noteworthy is that, consistent with observations that acute inflammatory stimuli provoke a diminished response in the

CNS, the effect of the α-chemokines on neutrophil recruitment is delayed [94,96,146]. Whereas IL-8 causes maximal recruitment of neutrophils into the skin of rabbits after 30 minutes [147], in this study neutrophil recruitment was not evident 6 hours after administration, the earliest time point studied. Similarly, despite the introduction of MCP-1, monocyte chemotaxis was also delayed compared to peripheral models of inflammation. Furthermore, although RANTES and IP-10 are chemotactic for lymphocytes after dermal injection only occasional cells were seen in the brain [111].

Antagonism of chemokine function

Some limited evidence for the potential benefit of the inhibition of chemokine function exists at present. In rabbits subjected to transient focal ischaemia, the administration of an anti-IL-8 antibody reduced oedema and infarct size compared with controls [137]. Viral macrophage inflammatory protein-2 (vMIP-2) is a chemokine-like peptide with a broad spectrum of antagonistic activity against chemokine receptors [148]. ICV administration of vMIP-2 1 hour prior to ischaemia results in a dose-dependent reduction in infarct volume at 2 days post-ischaemia. The number of activated microglia/macrophages were significantly decreased in the vMIP-II treated group [140].

Anti-inflammatory strategies

Following injury to the brain, multiple derangements in neurochemistry occur. It is now clear that, via complex interrelated processes, much of this derangement is potentially harmful to the surviving neurones. Logically, neurological recovery could only benefit from attenuation of this chemical secondary injury. This approach is supported by laboratory studies antagonizing pro-inflammatory mediators and leucocyte recruitment. However, these benefits have not yet been translated into clinical practice. In the final part of this review we examine some of the anti-inflammatory strategies that are topical or likely to be so in the near future.

Steroids

Steroid molecules have been used in the treatment of traumatic brain injury for over 30 years. This use has been largely empirical and has concerns, such as the increased risk of pneumonia and gastrointestinal haemorrhage in critically ill patients. Until recently, neither moderate benefits nor moderate harmful effects of steroid administration to patients with traumatic brain injury could be excluded [149,150].

Although the precise biochemistry of inflammation has not yet been fully defined, laboratory work with antagonists of pro-inflammatory cytokines supports the concept of modulating the inflammatory response in order to improve outcome after brain injury. Glucocorticoids inhibit many aspects of the inflammatory response including the expression of pro-inflammatory cytokines by monocytic cell lines [151]. Therefore, it is entirely reasonable to suppose that the antagonism of inflammation via corticosteroid administration might improve outcome in acute brain injury. Laboratory data supporting the use of steroid molecules in both ischaemic and traumatic injuries are available. However, the available clinical data do not support the routine use of steroids.

Following middle cerebral artery occlusion, both protective and deleterious effects of steroid action have been reported. Methylprednisolone given intravenously starting 30 minutes after commencement of 4 hours of ischaemia, and continuing for 23 hours, produced evidence of neuroprotection. Experimental and control animals showed similar early mortality rates, but in the surviving methylprednisolone treated animals mean infarct size was more than six times smaller than in the control group. The methylprednisolone treated animals also had a less marked reduction in cerebral blood flow during ischaemia [152]. In contrast to this finding, metyrapone, an 11-β-hydroxylase inhibitor of glucocorticoid production, significantly reduces infarct volume and cell loss when given intravenously 30 minutes prior to middle cerebral artery occlusion, transient global forebrain ischaemia or kainic acid induced excitotoxic insult. A harmful effect of intact glucocorticoid production on neuronal viability was implied [153]. Differences in the timing of the glucocorticoid administration and the steroid concentrations achieved might account for the differing results obtained. Dexamethasone administered to neurones in culture prior to oxygen-glucose deprivation exaggerated injury, whereas continuous application prior to, during and after insult protected neurones [154].

In a mouse model of closed head injury, the administration of a large (30 mg/kg) intravenous dose of methylprednisolone within 5 minutes of the injury significantly improved motor function when assessed at 1 hour. A 15-mg/kg dose was less effective and larger doses ineffective. A 60 mg/kg dose of prednisolone was also beneficial, while hydrocortisone was of no benefit [155]. High-dose methylprednisolone (30 mg/kg initially) given to severely head injured patients within 6 hours of injury has been associated with a significant reduction in mortality from 52% in the low dose and placebo group to 39% in the high dose group. In patients less than 40 years of age this reduction was greater: 43% in the low dose and placebo groups compared with 6% in those receiving the high dose. No significant difference in outcome was seen in the low dose methylprednisolone group compared with placebo [156]. A lower dose of methylprednisolone also failed to produce a significant difference in outcome at 6 months after injury [157]. Triamcinolone has also been shown to improve outcome after severe traumatic brain injury. However, this improvement in outcome was significant in a subgroup of patients who had a focal lesion and were Glasgow coma score (GCS) <8 on admission [158].

Unfortunately, clinical benefit of steroid treatment in traumatic brain injury has not been a consistent finding. Dexamethasone administered to head injured patients failed to statistically improve mortality at 1 month or outcome at 6 months and no beneficial effect on intracranial pressure (ICP) was seen in the steroid treated groups [159–162].

Compared with controlled animal models, clinical trials involve varying severities and complexities of head injury and so have much greater intersubject variability. Many of the trials conducted so far have therefore lacked the power to detect a meaningful effect of steroid administration. Indeed, until recently the aggregate total of patients in previous studies was only approximately 2300 [163]. In an attempt to address some of these issues, the corticosteroid randomization after significant head injury (CRASH) trial was undertaken. After recruiting 10 008 patients, interim analysis suggested the trial be stopped and early outcome data published. Patients with a head injury and a GCS of 14 or less were randomized to receive either a methylprednisolone infusion for 48 hours or placebo. The mortality within 14 days was significantly higher in the steroid treated group than placebo, 21.1% versus 17.9%, respectively (relative risk 1.18; 95% confidence interval 1.09–1.27; $P = 0.0001$) [164].

One explanation for a failure to demonstrate a beneficial effect of steroid treatment in clinical traumatic brain injury could be that the immune response to brain trauma is not uniform. Focal injuries are characterized by marked leucocyte recruitment [43,104,106,145,165,166]. In diffuse injuries, the dominant response is microglial activation [105]. The anti-inflammatory effect of steroid molecules might therefore be greater in some patients than others and more difficult to detect in a mixed group of brain injuries.

Hypothermia

Mild hypothermia (body temperatures of 32–34°C) is associated with modulation of the inflammatory process. Clinical examples of neuroprotection exist, although the effect has not yet been shown to be a universal one. Hypothermia reduces tissue damage in both permanent and transient models of ischaemic stroke. However, benefit is lost the longer the delay between ischaemia onset and cooling [167]. In animals subjected to lateral fluid percussion injury, early cooling of the brain — within minutes — to 30°C for 3 hours reduced neuronal necrosis, contusion volume and suppressed the increase in hydroxyl radicals and glutamate [168,169]. Similarly, following controlled cortical impact, reducing the brain temperature within 10 minutes, to 32°C for 4 hours, reduced neutrophil accumulation at that time [170]. For survivors of out-of-hospital cardiac arrest, 12–24 hours of hypothermia at 32–34°C significantly improved survival with good neurological function compared with normothermia [171,172]. In patients with traumatic brain injury, moderate hypothermia was associated with a reduction in CSF glutamate and IL-1β [173], and both systemic and jugular venous IL-6 [174].

A small randomized controlled phase II trial of hypothermia (32–33°C) versus normothermia for 48 hours in 46 patients with severe traumatic brain injury concluded that hypothermia was safe. However, no statistically significant improvement in outcome was seen, possibly because of the small sample size [175]. In a subsequent trial, 87 patients were again randomized to receive moderate hypothermia or normothermia. The patients were prospectively stratified by GCS: 3–4 and 5–7 at randomization. Cooling was achieved for an average of 10 hours post-injury and maintained for a further 24 hours. Outcome was assessed by Glasgow outcome scale (GOS) at 3, 6 and 12 months after injury. GCS 3–4 patients at initial presentation did not benefit from hypothermia, whereas GCS 5–7 patients had significantly better GOS scores at 3 and 6 months and a tendency to better recovery at 12 months [172]. In the largest multicentre clinical trial to date of moderate hypothermia, 392 patients with severe traumatic brain injury were randomized to receive either hypothermia or normothermia for 48 hours. No significant benefit of treatment on outcome was found. Hypothermic patients had a greater incidence of bleeding, sepsis and pneumonia [176]. However, it should be noted that the time to reach target temperature in the hypothermia group was approximately 8 hours after injury. Because inflammatory events occur early after injury, the delay in reaching the target temperatures in these two studies might have significantly undermined the effectiveness of the hypothermia. The latter trial might have been further weakened by significant intercentre differences in the incidence of low mean arterial blood pressure and cerebral perfusion pressure, use of vasopressors and incidence of dehydration [177]. The National Acute Brain Injury Study: Hypothermia II (NABISH II) is currently recruiting patients to repeat these studies concentrating on early cooling [178].

Interleukin-1 receptor antagonist

Intracerebroventricular or peripheral IL-1ra inhibits ischaemic [58,60,63,80] and traumatic damage [64]. It can be administered as late as 4 hours after the onset of insult with significant reduction in lesion volume [62,64]. IL-1ra is licensed for the treatment of rheumatoid arthritis [179] and is currently undergoing phase II trials in stroke [180]. However, it is a large molecule (17 kDa) and while it can cross the blood–brain barrier in rodents, concern has been expressed about the adequacy of this in brain injury [181].

Conclusions

The interplay of pathological mediators initiated by trauma to the brain is by no means adequately described. However, it is already apparent that this process is diverse and extremely complex. It is therefore unlikely that one single class of agent will be sufficient to modulate the pathology enough to improve outcome. Instead, time-specific administration of diverse agents, analogous to chemotherapy, might be required. In the meantime, newer classes of agents and therapies aimed at targeting multiple aspects of the inflammatory response are being evaluated both in experimental models and in clinical trials.

References

1 Reilly PL, Graham DI, Adams JH, Jennett B. Patients with head injury who talk and die. *Lancet* 1975; 375–7.

2 McIntosh TK, Smith DH, Meaney DF, *et al.* Neuropathological sequelae of traumatic brain injury: relationship to neurochemical and biomechanical mechanisms. *Lab Invest* 1996; 315–42.

3 Sharkey J, Kelly JS, Butcher SP. Inflammatory responses to cerebral ischaemia. In: Ter Horst GJ, Korf J, eds. *Clinical Pharmacology of Cerebral Ischaemia*. Totowa, NJ: Humana Press, 1997; 235–62.

4 Bullock R, Chesnut RM, Clifton G, *et al.* Guidelines for the management of severe head injury. Brain Trauma Foundation. *Eur J Emerg Med* 1996; 109–27.

5 Maas AI, Dearden M, Teasdale GM, *et al.* EBIC-guidelines for management of severe head injury in adults. European Brain Injury Consortium. *Acta Neurochir (Wien)* 1997; 286–94.

6 Gallin JL, Goldstein IM, Snyderman R. *Inflammation: Basic Principles and Clinical Correlates*. New York: Raven Press, 1988.

7 Perry VH, Gordon S. Macrophages and microglia in the nervous system. *Trends Neurosci* 1988; 273–7.

8 Perry VH, Bell MD, Brown HC, Matyszak MK. Inflammation in the nervous system. *Curr Opin Neurobiol* 1995; 636–41.

9 Lawson LJ, Perry VH. The unique characteristics of inflammatory responses in mouse brain are acquired

during postnatal development. *Eur J Neurosci* 1995; 1584–95.

10 Rothwell NJ, Relton JK. Involvement of cytokines in acute neurodegeneration in the CNS. *Neurosci Biobehav Rev* 1993; 217–27.

11 Tarkowski E, Rosengren L, Blomstrand C, *et al.* Early intrathecal production of interleukin-6 predicts the size of brain lesion in stroke. *Stroke* 1995; 1393–8.

12 Intiso D, Zarrelli MM, Lagioia G, *et al.* Tumor necrosis factor alpha serum levels and inflammatory response in acute ischemic stroke patients. *J Neurol Sci* 2004; 390–6.

13 Fassbender K, Rossol S, Kammer T, *et al.* Pro-inflammatory cytokines in serum of patients with acute cerebral ischemia: kinetics of secretion and relation to the extent of brain damage and outcome of disease. *J Neurol Sci* 1994; 135–9.

14 Beamer NB, Coull BM, Clark WM, Hazel JS, Silberger JR. Interleukin-6 and interleukin-1 receptor antagonist in acute stroke. *Ann Neurol* 1995; 800–5.

15 Smith CJ, Emsley HC, Gavin CM, *et al.* Peak plasma interleukin-6 and other peripheral markers of inflammation in the first week of ischaemic stroke correlate with brain infarct volume, stroke severity and long-term outcome. *BMC Neurol* 2004; 2.

16 Goodman JC, Robertson CS, Grossman RG, Narayan RK. Elevation of tumor necrosis factor in head injury. *J Neuroimmunol* 1990; 213–7.

17 Ross SA, Halliday MI, Campbell GC, Byrnes DP, Rowlands BJ. The presence of tumour necrosis factor in CSF and plasma after severe head injury. *Br J Neurosurg* 1994; 419–25.

18 McClain CJ, Cohen D, Ott L, Dinarello CA, Young B. Ventricular fluid interleukin-1 activity in patients with head injury. *J Lab Clin Med* 1987; 48–54.

19 McClain C, Cohen D, Phillips R, Ott L, Young B. Increased plasma and ventricular fluid interleukin-6 levels in patients with head injury. *J Lab Clin Med* 1991; 225–31.

20 Hans VH, Kossmann T, Joller H, Otto V, Morganti-Kossmann MC. Interleukin-6 and its soluble receptor in serum and cerebrospinal fluid after cerebral trauma. *Neuroreport* 1999; 409–12.

21 McKeating EG, Andrews PJ, Signorini DF, Mascia L. Transcranial cytokine gradients in patients requiring intensive care after acute brain injury. *Br J Anaesth* 1997; 520–3.

22 Liu T, Clark RK, McDonnell PC, *et al.* Tumor necrosis factor-alpha expression in ischemic neurones. *Stroke* 1994; 1481–8.

23 Ohtaki H, Yin L, Nakamachi T, *et al.* Expression of tumor necrosis factor alpha in nerve fibers and oligodendrocytes after transient focal ischemia in mice. *Neurosci Lett* 2004; 162–6.

24 Minami M, Kuraishi Y, Yabuuchi K, Yamazaki A, Satoh M. Induction of interleukin-1 beta mRNA in rat brain after transient forebrain ischemia. *J Neurochem* 1992; 390–2.

25 Hill JK, Gunion-Rinker L, Kulhanek D, *et al.* Temporal modulation of cytokine expression following focal cerebral ischemia in mice. *Brain Res* 1999; 45–54.

26 Legos JJ, Whitmore RG, Erhardt JA, *et al.* Quantitative changes in interleukin proteins following focal stroke in the rat. *Neurosci Lett* 2000; 189–92.

27 Wang X, Yue TL, Young PR, Barone FC, Feuerstein GZ. Expression of interleukin-6, c-fos, and zif268 mRNAs in rat ischemic cortex. *J Cereb Blood Flow Metab* 1995; 166–71.

28 Ali C, Nicole O, Docagne F, *et al.* Ischemia-induced interleukin-6 as a potential endogenous neuroprotective cytokine against NMDA receptor-mediated excitotoxicity in the brain. *J Cereb Blood Flow Metab* 2000; 956–66.

29 Fan L, Young PR, Barone FC, *et al.* Experimental brain injury induces differential expression of tumor necrosis factor-alpha mRNA in the CNS. *Brain Res Mol Brain Res* 1996; 287–91.

30 Taupin V, Toulmond S, Serrano A, Benavides J, Zavala F. Increase in IL-6, IL-1 and TNF levels in rat brain following traumatic lesion. Influence of pre- and post-traumatic treatment with Ro5 4864, a peripheral-type (p site) benzodiazepine ligand. *J Neuroimmunol* 1993; 177–85.

31 Knoblach SM, Fan L, Faden AI. Early neuronal expression of tumor necrosis factor-alpha after experimental brain injury contributes to neurological impairment. *J Neuroimmunol* 1999; 115–25.

32 Shohami E, Novikov M, Bass R, Yamin A, Gallily R. Closed head injury triggers early production of TNF alpha and IL-6 by brain tissue. *J Cereb Blood Flow Metab* 1994; 615–9.

33 Fan L, Young PR, Barone FC, *et al.* Experimental brain injury induces expression of interleukin-1 beta mRNA in the rat brain. *Brain Res Mol Brain Res* 1995; 125–30.

34 Yan HQ, Banos MA, Herregodts P, Hooghe R, Hooghe-Peters EL. Expression of interleukin (IL)-1 beta, IL-6 and their respective receptors in the normal rat brain and after injury. *Eur J Immunol* 1992; 2963–71.

35 Woodroofe MN, Sarna GS, Wadhwa M, *et al.* Detection of interleukin-1 and interleukin-6 in adult rat brain, following mechanical injury, by *in vivo* microdialysis: evidence of a role for microglia in cytokine production. *J Neuroimmunol* 1991; 227–36.

36 Rhodes JK, Andrews PJ, Holmes MC, Seckl JR. Expression of interleukin-6 messenger RNA in a rat model of diffuse axonal injury. *Neurosci Lett* 2002; 1–4.

37 Giulian D, Baker TJ, Shih LC, Lachman LB. Interleukin 1 of the central nervous system is produced by ameboid microglia. *J Exp Med* 1986; 594–604.

38 Hariri RJ, Chang VA, Barie PS, *et al.* Traumatic injury induces interleukin-6 production by human astrocytes. *Brain Res* 1994; 139–42.

39 Chung IY, Benveniste EN. Tumor necrosis factor-alpha production by astrocytes: induction by lipopolysaccharide, IFN-γ, and IL-1β. *J Immunol* 1990; 2999–3007.

40 Aloisi F, Care A, Borsellino G, *et al.* Production of hemolymphopoietic cytokines (IL-6, IL-8, colony-stimulating factors) by normal human astrocytes in response to IL-1β and tumor necrosis factor-α. *J Immunol* 1992; 2358–66.

41 Botchkina GI, Meistrell ME III, Botchkina IL, Tracey KJ. Expression of TNF and TNF receptors (p55 and p75) in the rat brain after focal cerebral ischemia. *Mol Med* 1997; 765–81.

42 Buttini M, Appel K, Sauter A, Gebicke-Haerter PJ, Boddeke HW. Expression of tumor necrosis factor alpha after focal cerebral ischaemia in the rat. *Neurosci* 1996; 1–16.

43 Holmin S, Schalling M, Hojeberg B, *et al.* Delayed cytokine expression in rat brain following experimental contusion. *J Neurosurg* 1997; 493–504.

44 Bandtlow CE, Meyer M, Lindholm D, *et al.* Regional and cellular codistribution of interleukin 1β and nerve growth factor mRNA in the adult rat brain: possible relationship to the regulation of nerve growth factor synthesis. *J Cell Biol* 1990; 1701–11.

45 Buttini M, Sauter A, Boddeke HW. Induction of interleukin-1β mRNA after focal cerebral ischaemia in the rat. *Brain Res Mol Brain Res* 1994; 126–34.

46 Yabuuchi K, Minami M, Katsumata S, Yamazaki A, Satoh M. An *in situ* hybridization study on interleukin-1β mRNA induced by transient forebrain ischemia in the rat brain. *Brain Res Mol Brain Res* 1994; 135–42.

47 Schobitz B, de KE, Sutanto W, Holsboer F. Cellular localization of interleukin 6 mRNA and interleukin 6 receptor mRNA in rat brain. *Eur J Neurosci* 1993; 1426–35.

48 Gadient RA, Otten U. Identification of interleukin-6 (IL-6)-expressing neurones in the cerebellum and hippocampus of normal adult rats. *Neurosci Lett* 1994; 243–6.

49 Block F, Peters M, Nolden-Koch M. Expression of IL-6 in the ischemic penumbra. *Neuroreport* 2000; 963–7.

50 Hans V, Kossmann T, Lenzlinger PM, *et al.* Experimental axonal injury triggers interleukin-6 MRNA, protein synthesis and release into cerebrospinal fluid. *J Cereb Blood Flow Metab* 1999; **19**: 184–94.

51 Rothwell NJ. Annual review prize lecture cytokines: killers in the brain? *J Physiol* 1999; 3–17.

52 de Vries HE, Blom-Roosemalen MC, van Oosten M, *et al.* The influence of cytokines on the integrity of the blood–brain barrier *in vitro*. *J Neuroimmunol* 1996; 37–43.

53 Quagliarello VJ, Wispelwey B, Long WJ Jr, Scheld WM. Recombinant human interleukin-1 induces meningitis and blood–brain barrier injury in the rat: characterization and comparison with tumor necrosis factor. *J Clin Invest* 1991; 1360–6.

54 Hartung HP, Schafer B, Heininger K, Toyka KV. Recombinant interleukin-1β stimulates eicosanoid production in rat primary culture astrocytes. *Brain Res* 1989; 113–9.

55 Lee SC, Dickson DW, Liu W, Brosnan CF. Induction of nitric oxide synthase activity in human astrocytes by interleukin-1β and interferon-γ. *J Neuroimmunol* 1993; 19–24.

56 Friedlander RM, Gagliardini V, Rotello RJ, Yuan J. Functional role of interleukin 1β (IL-1β) in IL-1β-converting enzyme-mediated apoptosis. *J Exp Med* 1996; 717–24.

57 Troy CM, Stefanis L, Prochiantz A, Greene LA, Shelanski ML. The contrasting roles of ICE family proteases and interleukin-1β in apoptosis induced by trophic factor withdrawal and by copper/zinc superoxide dismutase down-regulation. *Proc Natl Acad Sci U S A* 1996; 5635–40.

58 Loddick SA, Rothwell NJ. Neuroprotective effects of human recombinant interleukin-1 receptor antagonist in focal cerebral ischaemia in the rat. *J Cereb Blood Flow Metab* 1996; 932–40.

59 Lawrence CB, Allan SM, Rothwell NJ. Interleukin-1β and the interleukin-1 receptor antagonist act in the striatum to modify excitotoxic brain damage in the rat. *Eur J Neurosci* 1998; 1188–95.

60 Relton JK, Rothwell NJ. Interleukin-1 receptor antagonist inhibits ischaemic and excitotoxic neuronal damage in the rat. *Brain Res Bull* 1992; 243–6.

61 Yamasaki Y, Matsuura N, Shozuhara H, *et al.* Interleukin-1 as a pathogenetic mediator of ischemic brain damage in rats. *Stroke* 1995; 676–80.

62 Mulcahy NJ, Ross J, Rothwell NJ, Loddick SA. Delayed administration of interleukin-1 receptor antagonist

protects against transient cerebral ischaemia in the rat. *Br J Pharmacol* 2003; 471–6.

63 Garcia JH, Liu KF, Relton JK. Interleukin-1 receptor antagonist decreases the number of necrotic neurones in rats with middle cerebral artery occlusion. *Am J Pathol* 1995; 1477–86.

64 Toulmond S, Rothwell NJ. Interleukin-1 receptor antagonist inhibits neuronal damage caused by fluid percussion injury in the rat. *Brain Res* 1995; 261–6.

65 Chao CC, Hu S. Tumor necrosis factor-α potentiates glutamate neurotoxicity in human fetal brain cell cultures. *Dev Neurosci* 1994; 172–9.

66 Selmaj K, Raine CS. Tumor necrosis factor mediates myelin damage in organotypic cultures of nervous tissue. *Ann N Y Acad Sci* 1988; 568–70.

67 Selmaj KW, Raine CS. Tumor necrosis factor mediates myelin and oligodendrocyte damage *in vitro*. *Ann Neurol* 1988; 339–46.

68 Merrill JE, Ignarro LJ, Sherman MP, Melinek J, Lane TE. Microglial cell cytotoxicity of oligodendrocytes is mediated through nitric oxide. *J Immunol* 1993; 2132–41.

69 Estrada C, Gomez C, Martin C. Effects of TNF-α on the production of vasoactive substances by cerebral endothelial and smooth muscle cells in culture. *J Cereb Blood Flow Metab* 1995; 920–8.

70 Otto VI, Heinzel-Pleines UE, Gloor SM, *et al.* sICAM-1 and TNF-α induce MIP-2 with distinct kinetics in astrocytes and brain microvascular endothelial cells. *J Neurosci Res* 2000; 733–42.

71 Cheng B, Christakos S, Mattson MP. Tumor necrosis factors protect neurones against metabolic-excitotoxic insults and promote maintenance of calcium homeostasis. *Neurone* 1994; 139–53.

72 Barger SW, Horster D, Furukawa K, *et al.* Tumor necrosis factors α and β protect neurones against amyloid β-peptide toxicity: evidence for involvement of a κB-binding factor and attenuation of peroxide and Ca²⁺ accumulation. *Proc Natl Acad Sci U S A* 1995; 9328–32.

73 Mattson MP, Goodman Y, Luo H, Fu W, Furukawa K. Activation of NF-κB protects hippocampal neurones against oxidative stress-induced apoptosis: evidence for induction of manganese superoxide dismutase and suppression of peroxynitrite production and protein tyrosine nitration. *J Neurosci Res* 1997; 681–97.

74 Selmaj KW, Farooq M, Norton WT, Raine CS, Brosnan CF. Proliferation of astrocytes *in vitro* in response to cytokines: a primary role for tumor necrosis factor. *J Immunol* 1990; 129–35.

75 Chao CC, Hu S, Ehrlich L, Peterson PK. Interleukin-1 and tumor necrosis factor-α synergistically mediate neurotoxicity: involvement of nitric oxide and of *N*-methyl-ᴅ-aspartate receptors. *Brain Behav Immunol* 1995; 355–65.

76 Love S. Oxidative stress in brain ischemia. *Brain Pathol* 1999; 119–31.

77 Gilgun-Sherki Y, Rosenbaum Z, Melamed E, Offen D. Antioxidant therapy in acute central nervous system injury: current state. *Pharmacol Rev* 2002; 271–84.

78 Kim KS, Wass CA, Cross AS, Opal SM. Modulation of blood–brain barrier permeability by tumor necrosis factor and antibody to tumor necrosis factor in the rat. *Lymphokine Cytokine Res* 1992; 293–8.

79 Barone FC, Arvin B, White RF, *et al.* Tumor necrosis factor-α: a mediator of focal ischemic brain injury. *Stroke* 1997; 1233–44.

80 Nawashiro H, Tasaki K, Ruetzler CA, Hallenbeck JM. TNF-α pretreatment induces protective effects against focal cerebral ischemia in mice. *J Cereb Blood Flow Metab* 1997; 483–90.

81 Meistrell ME, III, Botchkina GI, Wang H, *et al.* Tumor necrosis factor is a brain damaging cytokine in cerebral ischemia. *Shock* 1997; 341–8.

82 Nawashiro H, Martin D, Hallenbeck JM. Inhibition of tumor necrosis factor and amelioration of brain infarction in mice. *J Cereb Blood Flow Metab* 1997; 229–32.

83 Yang GY, Gong C, Qin Z, *et al.* Inhibition of TNF-α attenuates infarct volume and ICAM-1 expression in ischemic mouse brain. *Neuroreport* 1998; 2131–4.

84 Bruce AJ, Boling W, Kindy MS, *et al.* Altered neuronal and microglial responses to excitotoxic and ischemic brain injury in mice lacking TNF receptors. *Nat Med* 1996; 788–94.

85 Shohami E, Bass R, Wallach D, Yamin A, Gallily R. Inhibition of tumor necrosis factor α (TNF-α) activity in rat brain is associated with cerebroprotection after closed head injury. *J Cereb Blood Flow Metab* 1996; 378–84.

86 Stahel PF, Shohami E, Younis FM, *et al.* Experimental closed head injury: analysis of neurological outcome, blood–brain barrier dysfunction, intracranial neutrophil infiltration, and neuronal cell death in mice deficient in genes for pro-inflammatory cytokines. *J Cereb Blood Flow Metab* 2000; 369–80.

87 Scherbel U, Raghupathi R, Nakamura M, *et al.* Differential acute and chronic responses of tumor necrosis factor-deficient mice to experimental brain injury. *Proc Natl Acad Sci U S A* 1999; 8721–6.

88 Hama T, Miyamoto M, Tsukui H, Nishio C, Hatanaka H. Interleukin-6 as a neurotrophic factor for promoting the survival of cultured basal forebrain cholinergic neurones from postnatal rats. *Neurosci Lett* 1989; 340–4.

89 Hama T, Kushima Y, Miyamoto M, *et al.* Interleukin-6 improves the survival of mesencephalic catecholaminergic and septal cholinergic neurones from postnatal, two-week-old rats in cultures. *Neurosci* 1991; 445–52.

90 Kushima Y, Hama T, Hatanaka H. Interleukin-6 as a neurotrophic factor for promoting the survival of cultured catecholaminergic neurones in a chemically defined medium from fetal and postnatal rat midbrains. *Neurosci Res* 1992; 267–80.

91 Toulmond S, Vige X, Fage D, Benavides J. Local infusion of interleukin-6 attenuates the neurotoxic effects of NMDA on rat striatal cholinergic neurones. *Neurosci Lett* 1992; 49–52.

92 Campbell IL, Abraham CR, Masliah E, *et al.* Neurologic disease induced in transgenic mice by cerebral over-expression of interleukin 6. *Proc Natl Acad Sci U S A* 1993; 10061–5.

93 Maruo N, Morita I, Shirao M, Murota S. IL-6 increases endothelial permeability *in vitro*. *Endocrinol* 1992; 710–4.

94 Andersson PB, Perry VH, Gordon S. Intracerebral injection of proinflammatory cytokines or leucocyte chemotaxins induces minimal myelomonocytic cell recruitment to the parenchyma of the central nervous system. *J Exp Med* 1992; 255–9.

95 Luger TA, Schwarz T. Evidence for an epidermal cytokine network. *J Invest Dermatol* 1990; (Suppl): 104S.

96 Andersson PB, Perry VH, Gordon S. The acute inflammatory response to lipopolysaccharide in CNS parenchyma differs from that in other body tissues. *Neurosci* 1992; 169–86.

97 Blond D, Campbell SJ, Butchart AG, Perry VH, Anthony DC. Differential induction of interleukin-1beta and tumour necrosis factor-alpha may account for specific patterns of leucocyte recruitment in the brain. *Brain Res* 2002; 89–99.

98 Schnell L, Fearn S, Schwab ME, Perry VH, Anthony DC. Cytokine-induced acute inflammation in the brain and spinal cord. *J Neuropathol Exp Neurol* 1999; 245–54.

99 Garcia JH, Kamijyo Y. Cerebral infarction: evolution of histopathological changes after occlusion of a middle cerebral artery in primates. *J Neuropathol Exp Neurol* 1974; 408–21.

100 Jander S, Kraemer M, Schroeter M, Witte OW, Stoll G. Lymphocytic infiltration and expression of intercellular adhesion molecule-1 in photochemically induced ischemia of the rat cortex. *J Cereb Blood Flow Metab* 1995; 42–51.

101 Kochanek PM, Hallenbeck JM. Polymorphonuclear leucocytes and monocytes/macrophages in the pathogenesis of cerebral ischemia and stroke. *Stroke* 1992; 1367–79.

102 Garcia JH, Liu KF, Yoshida Y, *et al.* Influx of leucocytes and platelets in an evolving brain infarct (Wistar rat). *Am J Pathol* 1994; 188–99.

103 Povlishock JT, Christman CW. The pathobiology of traumatically induced axonal injury in animals and humans: a review of current thoughts. *J Neurotrauma* 1995; 555–64.

104 Soares HD, Hicks RR, Smith D, McIntosh TK. Inflammatory leukocytic recruitment and diffuse neuronal degeneration are separate pathological processes resulting from traumatic brain injury. *J Neurosci* 1995; 8223–33.

105 Csuka E, Hans VH, Ammann E, *et al.* Cell activation and inflammatory response following traumatic axonal injury in the rat. *Neuroreport* 2000; 2587–90.

106 Biagas KV, Uhl MW, Schiding JK, Nemoto EM, Kochanek PM. Assessment of posttraumatic polymorphonuclear leucocyte accumulation in rat brain using tissue myeloperoxidase assay and vinblastine treatment. *J Neurotrauma* 1992; 363–71.

107 Holmin S, Soderlund J, Biberfeld P, Mathiesen T. Intracerebral inflammation after human brain contusion. *Neurosurg* 1998; 291–8.

108 del Zoppo GJ, Schmid-Schonbein GW, Mori E, Copeland BR, Chang CM. Polymorphonuclear leucocytes occlude capillaries following middle cerebral artery occlusion and reperfusion in baboons. *Stroke* 1991; 1276–83.

109 Connolly ES Jr, Winfree CJ, Springer TA, *et al.* Cerebral protection in homozygous null ICAM-1 mice after middle cerebral artery occlusion: role of neutrophil adhesion in the pathogenesis of stroke. *J Clin Invest* 1996; 209–16.

110 Dinkel K, Dhabhar FS, Sapolsky RM. Neurotoxic effects of polymorphonuclear granulocytes on hippocampal primary cultures. *Proc Natl Acad Sci U S A* 2004; 331–6.

111 Bell MD, Taub DD, Perry VH. Overriding the brain's intrinsic resistance to leucocyte recruitment with intraparenchymal injections of recombinant chemokines. *Neurosci* 1996; 283–92.

112 Matsuo Y, Kihara T, Ikeda M, *et al.* Role of neutrophils in radical production during ischemia and reperfusion

of the rat brain: effect of neutrophil depletion on extracellular ascorbyl radical formation. *J Cereb Blood Flow Metab* 1995; 941–7.

113 Giulian D, Vaca K. Inflammatory glia mediate delayed neuronal damage after ischemia in the central nervous system. *Stroke* 1993; (Suppl 90).

114 Colton CA, Gilbert DL. Production of superoxide anions by a CNS macrophage, the microglia. *FEBS Lett* 1987; 284–8.

115 Chao CC, Hu S, Molitor TW, Shaskan EG, Peterson PK. Activated microglia mediate neuronal cell injury via a nitric oxide mechanism. *J Immunol* 1992; 2736–41.

116 Zielasek J, Archelos JJ, Toyka KV, Hartung HP. Expression of intercellular adhesion molecule-1 on rat microglial cells. *Neurosci Lett* 1993; 136–9.

117 Wong D, Dorovini-Zis K. Upregulation of intercellular adhesion molecule-1 (ICAM-1) expression in primary cultures of human brain microvessel endothelial cells by cytokines and lipopolysaccharide. *J Neuroimmunol* 1992; 11–21.

118 Dore-Duffy P, Washington RA, Balabanov R. Cytokine-mediated activation of cultured CNS microvessels: a system for examining antigenic modulation of CNS endothelial cells, and evidence for long-term expression of the adhesion protein E-selectin. *J Cereb Blood Flow Metab* 1994; 837–44.

119 Johnston B, Butcher EC. Chemokines in rapid leucocyte adhesion triggering and migration. *Semin Immunol* 2002; 83–92.

120 Wang X, Yue TL, Barone FC, Feuerstein GZ. Demonstration of increased endothelial-leucocyte adhesion molecule-1 mRNA expression in rat ischemic cortex. *Stroke* 1995; 1665–8.

121 Okada Y, Copeland BR, Mori E, *et al.* P-selectin and intercellular adhesion molecule-1 expression after focal brain ischemia and reperfusion. *Stroke* 1994; 202–11.

122 Sobel RA, Mitchell ME, Fondren G. Intercellular adhesion molecule-1 (ICAM-1) in cellular immune reactions in the human central nervous system. *Am J Pathol* 1990; 1309–16.

123 Chen H, Chopp M, Zhang RL, *et al.* Anti-CD11b monoclonal antibody reduces ischemic cell damage after transient focal cerebral ischemia in rat. *Ann Neurol* 1994; 458–63.

124 Chopp M, Zhang RL, Chen H, Li Y, Jiang N, Rusche JR. Postischemic administration of an anti-Mac-1 antibody reduces ischemic cell damage after transient middle cerebral artery occlusion in rats. *Stroke* 1994; 869–75.

125 Zhang ZG, Chopp M, Tang WX, Jiang N, Zhang RL. Postischemic treatment (2–4 h) with anti-CD11b and anti-CD18 monoclonal antibodies are neuroprotective after transient (2 h) focal cerebral ischemia in the rat. *Brain Res* 1995; 79–85.

126 Matsuo Y, Onodera H, Shiga Y, *et al.* Role of cell adhesion molecules in brain injury after transient middle cerebral artery occlusion in the rat. *Brain Res* 1994; 344–52.

127 Knoblach SM, Faden AI. Administration of either anti-intercellular adhesion molecule-1 or a nonspecific control antibody improves recovery after traumatic brain injury in the rat. *J Neurotrauma* 2002; 1039–50.

128 Whalen MJ, Carlos TM, Dixon CE, *et al.* Effect of traumatic brain injury in mice deficient in intercellular adhesion molecule-1: assessment of histopathologic and functional outcome. *J Neurotrauma* 1999; 299–309.

129 Bajetto A, Bonavia R, Barbero S, Florio T, Schettini G. Chemokines and their receptors in the central nervous system. *Front Neuroendocrinol* 2001; 147–84.

130 Whalen MJ, Carlos TM, Kochanek PM, *et al.* Interleukin-8 is increased in cerebrospinal fluid of children with severe head injury. *Crit Care Med* 2000; 929–34.

131 Kossmann T, Stahel PF, Lenzlinger PM, *et al.* Interleukin-8 released into the cerebrospinal fluid after brain injury is associated with blood–brain barrier dysfunction and nerve growth factor production. *J Cereb Blood Flow Metab* 1997; 280–9.

132 Oh JW, Schwiebert LM, Benveniste EN. Cytokine regulation of CC and CXC chemokine expression by human astrocytes. *J Neurovirol* 1999; 82–94.

133 Ehrlich LC, Hu S, Sheng WS, *et al.* Cytokine regulation of human microglial cell IL-8 production. *J Immunol* 1998; 1944–8.

134 Wang JY, Shum AY, Chao CC, Kuo JS, Wang JY. Production of macrophage inflammatory protein-2 following hypoxia/reoxygenation in glial cells. *Glia* 2000; 155–64.

135 Peterson PK, Hu S, Salak-Johnson J, Molitor TW, Chao CC. Differential production of and migratory response to beta chemokines by human microglia and astrocytes. *J Infect Dis* 1997; 478–81.

136 Harkness KA, Sussman JD, Davies-Jones GA, Greenwood J, Woodroofe MN. Cytokine regulation of MCP-1 expression in brain and retinal microvascular endothelial cells. *J Neuroimmunol* 2003; 1–9.

137 Matsumoto T, Ikeda K, Mukaida N, *et al.* Prevention of cerebral edema and infarct in cerebral reperfusion injury by an antibody to interleukin-8. *Lab Invest* 1997; 119–25.

138 Wang X, Yue TL, Barone FC, Feuerstein GZ. Monocyte chemoattractant protein-1 messenger RNA expression in rat ischemic cortex. *Stroke* 1995; 661–5.

139 Kim JS, Gautam SC, Chopp M, *et al.* Expression of monocyte chemoattractant protein-1 and macrophage inflammatory protein-1 after focal cerebral ischemia in the rat. *J Neuroimmunol* 1995; 127–34.

140 Minami M, Satoh M. Chemokines and their receptors in the brain: pathophysiological roles in ischemic brain injury. *Life Sci* 2003; 321–7.

141 Glabinski AR, Balasingam V, Tani M, *et al.* Chemokine monocyte chemoattractant protein-1 is expressed by astrocytes after mechanical injury to the brain. *J Immunol* 1996; 4363–8.

142 Hausmann EH, Berman NE, Wang YY, *et al.* Selective chemokine mRNA expression following brain injury. *Brain Res* 1998; 49–59.

143 Otto VI, Stahel PF, Rancan M, *et al.* Regulation of chemokines and chemokine receptors after experimental closed head injury. *Neuroreport* 2001; 2059–64.

144 Fuentes ME, Durham SK, Swerdel MR, *et al.* Controlled recruitment of monocytes and macrophages to specific organs through transgenic expression of monocyte chemoattractant protein-1. *J Immunol* 1995; 5769–76.

145 Clark RS, Schiding JK, Kaczorowski SL, Marion DW, Kochanek PM. Neutrophil accumulation after traumatic brain injury in rats: comparison of weight drop and controlled cortical impact models. *J Neurotrauma* 1994; 499–506.

146 Andersson PB, Perry VH, Gordon S. The CNS acute inflammatory response to excitotoxic neuronal cell death. *Immunol Lett* 1991; 177–81.

147 Colditz I, Zwahlen R, Dewald B, Baggiolini M. *In vivo* inflammatory activity of neutrophil-activating factor, a novel chemotactic peptide derived from human monocytes. *Am J Pathol* 1989; 755–60.

148 Kledal TN, Rosenkilde MM, Coulin F, *et al.* A broad-spectrum chemokine antagonist encoded by Kaposi's sarcoma-associated herpesvirus. *Science* 1997; 1656–9.

149 Alderson P, Roberts I. Corticosteroids in acute traumatic brain injury: systematic review of randomised controlled trials. *Br Med J* 1997; 1855–9.

150 Alderson P, Roberts I. Corticosteroids for acute traumatic brain injury (Cochrane Review). Oxford: Update Software [2]. 2001.

151 Almawi WY, Beyhum HN, Rahme AA, Rieder MJ. Regulation of cytokine and cytokine receptor expression by glucocorticoids. *J Leukoc Biol* 1996; 563–72.

152 de Court, Kleinholz M, Wagner KR, Xi G, Myers RE. Efficacious experimental stroke treatment with high-dose methylprednisolone. *Stroke* 1994; 487–92.

153 Smith-Swintosky VL, Pettigrew LC, Sapolsky RM, *et al.* Metyrapone, an inhibitor of glucocorticoid production, reduces brain injury induced by focal and global ischemia and seizures. *J Cereb Blood Flow Metab* 1996; 585–98.

154 Flavin MP. Influence of dexamethasone on neurotoxicity caused by oxygen and glucose deprivation in vitro. *Exp Neurol* 1996; 34–8.

155 Hall ED. High-dose glucocorticoid treatment improves neurological recovery in head-injured mice. *J Neurosurg* 1985; 882–7.

156 Giannotta SL, Weiss MH, Apuzzo ML, Martin E. High dose glucocorticoids in the management of severe head injury. *Neurosurg* 1984; 497–501.

157 Saul TG, Ducker TB, Salcman M, Carro E. Steroids in severe head injury: a prospective randomized clinical trial. *J Neurosurg* 1981; 596–600.

158 Grumme T, Baethmann A, Kolodziejczyk D, *et al.* Treatment of patients with severe head injury by triamcinolone: a prospective, controlled multicenter clinical trial of 396 cases. *Res Exp Med (Berl)* 1995; 217–29.

159 Cooper PR, Moody S, Clark WK, *et al.* Dexamethasone and severe head injury: a prospective double-blind study. *J Neurosurg* 1979; 307–16.

160 Braakman R, Schouten HJ, Blaauw-van Dishoeck M, Minderhoud JM. Megadose steroids in severe head injury: results of a prospective double-blind clinical trial. *J Neurosurg* 1983; 326–30.

161 Dearden NM, Gibson JS, McDowall DG, Gibson RM, Cameron MM. Effect of high-dose dexamethasone on outcome from severe head injury. *J Neurosurg* 1986; 81–8.

162 Gaab MR, Trost HA, Alcantara A, *et al.* 'Ultrahigh' dexamethasone in acute brain injury. Results from a prospective randomized double-blind multicenter trial (GUDHIS). German Ultrahigh Dexamethasone Head Injury Study Group. *Zentralbl Neurochir* 1994; 135–43.

163 Alderson P, Roberts I. Corticosteroids for acute traumatic brain injury. *Cochrane Database Syst Rev* 2000; CD000196.

164 Roberts I, Yates D, Sandercock P, *et al.* Effect of intravenous corticosteroids on death within 14 days in 10008 adults with clinically significant head injury (MRC CRASH trial): randomised placebo-controlled trial. *Lancet* 2004; 1321–8.

165 Toulmond S, Duval D, Serrano A, Scatton B, Benavides J. Biochemical and histological alterations induced by fluid percussion brain injury in the rat. *Brain Res* 1993; 24–31.

166 Hausmann R, Kaiser A, Lang C, Bohnert M, Betz P. A quantitative immunohistochemical study on the time-dependent course of acute inflammatory cellular response to human brain injury. *Int J Legal Med* 1999; 227–32.

167 Krieger DW, Yenari MA. Therapeutic hypothermia for acute ischemic stroke: what do laboratory studies teach us? *Stroke* 2004; 1482–9.

168 Dietrich WD, Alonso O, Busto R, Globus MY, Ginsberg MD. Post-traumatic brain hypothermia reduces histopathological damage following concussive brain injury in the rat. *Acta Neuropathol (Berl)* 1994; 250–8.

169 Globus MY, Alonso O, Dietrich WD, Busto R, Ginsberg MD. Glutamate release and free radical production following brain injury: effects of posttraumatic hypothermia. *J Neurochem* 1995; 1704–11.

170 Whalen MJ, Carlos TM, Clark RS, *et al*. The effect of brain temperature on acute inflammation after traumatic brain injury in rats. *J Neurotrauma* 1997; 561–72.

171 Bernard SA, Gray TW, Buist MD, *et al*. Treatment of comatose survivors of out-of-hospital cardiac arrest with induced hypothermia. *N Engl J Med* 2002; 557–63.

172 Hypothermia after Cardiac Arrest Study Group. Mild therapeutic hypothermia to improve the neurologic outcome after cardiac arrest. *N Engl J Med* 2002; **346**: 549–56.

173 Marion DW, Penrod LE, Kelsey SF, *et al*. Treatment of traumatic brain injury with moderate hypothermia. *N Engl J Med* 1997; **336**: 540–6.

174 Aibiki M, Maekawa S, Ogura S, *et al*. Effect of moderate hypothermia on systemic and internal jugular plasma IL-6 levels after traumatic brain injury in humans. *J Neurotrauma* 1999; 225–32.

175 Clifton GL, Allen S, Barrodale P, *et al*. A phase II study of moderate hypothermia in severe brain injury. *J Neurotrauma* 1993; 263–71.

176 Clifton GL, Miller ER, Choi SC, *et al*. Lack of effect of induction of hypothermia after acute brain injury. *N Engl J Med* 2001; 556–63.

177 Clifton GL, Choi SC, Miller ER, *et al*. Intercenter variance in clinical trials of head trauma: experience of the National Acute Brain Injury Study: Hypothermia. *J Neurosurg* 2001; 751–5.

178 Relton JK, Martin D, Thompson RC, Russell DA. Peripheral administration of interleukin-1 receptor antagonist inhibits brain damage after focal cerebral ischemia in the rat. *Exp Neurol* 1996; 206–13.

179 Bresnihan B. The safety and efficacy of interleukin-1 receptor antagonist in the treatment of rheumatoid arthritis. *Semin Arthritis Rheum* 2001; Suppl-20.

180 Allan SM, Rothwell NJ. Inflammation in central nervous system injury. *Phil Trans R Soc Lond B Biol Sci* 2003; 1669–77.

181 Gutierrez EG, Banks WA, Kastin AJ. Blood-borne interleukin-1 receptor antagonist crosses the blood–brain barrier. *J Neuroimmunol* 1994; 153–60.

CHAPTER 20

Heart failure

Sze-Yuan Ooi, Christopher Pepper and Stephen Ball

Introduction

Heart failure is a common and deadly disorder. It affects approximately 900 000 people in the UK today and costs the National Health Service an estimated £905 million per annum [1,2]. Community-based echocardiographic studies have revealed that only 50% of people with impaired left ventricular systolic function are symptomatic [3,4], such that what is seen in clinical practice is the tip of the iceberg and there are large numbers of people at risk of developing heart failure and who would potentially benefit from treatment.

Overt clinical heart failure carries a poor prognosis; from the time of first admission to hospital with heart failure the reported median survival time is 16 months and the 5-year survival rate is 25%. This prognosis is strongly age-related and is similar to that of colorectal carcinoma and worse than that of breast cancer [5].

Despite advances in the treatment of ischaemic heart disease and hypertension (the leading causes of heart failure in Western populations) and in the treatment of heart failure, the incidence of heart failure is rising and the risk of death remains static [1,6]. This is partly accounted for by the ageing population, as the elderly are at greater risk of both heart failure and death from non-cardiovascular causes. However, this trend is also symptomatic of the failure to identify and treat those at risk of developing heart failure, and the suboptimal treatment of those with established heart failure [7,8]. Heart failure is common and carries high risk, but it is treatable and, in some instances, preventable.

This chapter covers developments in the classification, pathogenesis and evidence-based treatment of chronic heart failure.

Defining heart failure

Heart failure syndrome

Heart failure is a syndrome, not a disease. The diagnosis is clinical and is based on a constellation of symptoms and signs that result from the impaired ability of the heart to fulfil its role as a pump. While transthoracic echocardiography is an important tool in the assessment of patients with breathlessness, the demonstration of structural heart disease is neither diagnostic of, nor synonymous with, heart failure. The most common cause of heart failure is left ventricular dysfunction; however, severe heart failure may be present despite normal left ventricular contractile function (e.g. mitral stenosis).

The causes of heart failure are many and varied (Table 20.1). However, in Western populations, ischaemic heart disease is the predominant underlying aetiology. In a Scottish community-based echocardiographic study, McDonagh *et al.* [4] demonstrated that 83% of people with left ventricular impairment had ischaemic heart disease. The recent EuroHeart survey reported coronary disease as the underlying aetiology in two-thirds of people admitted to hospital with heart failure [9]. In both of these studies, hypertension was identified as a frequent comorbidity. Hypertension can cause heart failure either directly by imposing a chronic haemodynamic burden, or indirectly through the promotion of atherosclerotic disease. Valvular heart disease and idiopathic dilated cardiomyopathy are important causes of heart failure; other aetiologies are uncommon in Western populations.

Reclassification of heart failure

Previous methods of classifying heart failure have been based on functional status (e.g. New York Heart

Table 20.1 Causes of heart failure.

Ischaemic heart disease

Hypertension

Valvular disease

Cardiomyopathy*
- Dilated cardiomyopathy
  e.g. familial or idiopathic
- Hypertrophic obstructive cardiomyopathy

Viral myocarditis

Infiltrative diseases
- Haemochromatosis
- Amyloidosis

Connective tissue diseases

Drug-induced, e.g. anthracyclines, clozapine

Alcohol

Tachycardia-induced cardiomyopathy

Nutritional/endocrine diseases, e.g. beri beri, thyrotoxicosis

---

* The term 'cardiomyopathy' is often used to cover 'damage of the heart', whatever the underlying cause (e.g. ischaemic cardiomyopathy, hypertensive cardiomyopathy, cardiomyopathy secondary to infiltrative disease).

Association [NYHA] classification). However, recognition of the fluctuating nature of symptoms, their dependence on treatment and poor correlation with underlying structural disease, prompted the development of a new classification scheme [10]. Patients are divided into four strata:
- *Stage A:* Patients at high risk of developing heart failure, but with no evidence of structural or functional heart disease, or symptoms or signs of heart failure
- *Stage B:* Patients with asymptomatic structural heart disease that is strongly associated with the development of heart failure
- *Stage C:* Patients with prior or current symptoms of heart failure and underlying structural heart disease
- *Stage D:* Patients with advanced structural heart disease and marked symptoms at rest despite optimal medical therapy.

This new approach emphasizes the importance of identifying those at high-risk of developing heart failure and those with asymptomatic structural heart disease. There is robust evidence that blood pressure lowering in patients with hypertension [11], and angiotensin-converting enzyme (ACE) inhibition in patients with either coronary disease or at high vascular risk, reduce the risk of developing heart failure [12,13]. In addition, there is growing evidence that ACE inhibition and β-blockade reduce adverse outcomes in patients with asymptomatic left ventricular systolic impairment [14,15]. Although people categorized as either Stage A or B do not, by definition, have heart failure, their inclusion in this classification scheme is an important step in the prevention of heart failure.

Pathophysiology of heart failure

Pathological processes leading to heart failure vary widely depending on the underlying aetiology. This section focuses on the pathogenesis of *systolic* heart failure secondary to myocardial injury because this is the most studied and understood. While diastolic dysfunction is as prevalent as systolic dysfunction, it is uncommon in the absence of some systolic impairment, and there is a spectrum of dysfunction between patients (Fig. 20.1). Diastolic heart failure is discussed separately.

The pathogenesis of systolic heart failure is a complex process, triggered by a cardiac insult and culminating in a dilated, incoordinate and ineffective ventricle. This process has been termed 'adverse remodelling'. Current hypotheses implicate the long-term deleterious effects of acute adaptive responses to cardiac injury as the driving force behind this deterioration.

Acute response to cardiac injury

Through evolution, the body has developed mechanisms to maintain circulatory integrity, protecting against catastrophic blood loss and also providing day-to-day, hour-to-hour, beat-to-beat blood pressure homoeostasis.

The Frank–Starling mechanism explains the heart's ability to cope with varying volumetric loads. When presented with an increase in blood volume,

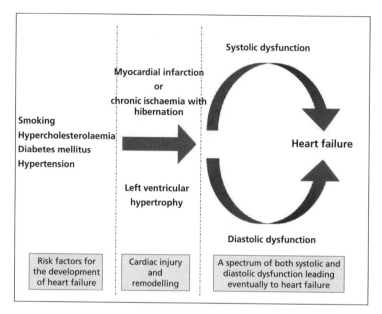

Figure 20.1 The progression to heart failure.

the heart responds by pumping harder. An increase in preload results in myocardial stretch and a subsequent increase in myocardial contractility. Following acute cardiac injury, ventricular dilatation enables retention of a greater blood volume, thereby increasing contractility and leading to an increase in stroke volume.

A fall in blood pressure is sensed by arterial baroceptors in the carotid body and the aortic arch, resulting in vasopressin release from the neurohypophysis and an increase in central sympathetic neural outflow. Vasopressin, also known as antidiuretic hormone, acts principally to increase water resorption in the renal collecting ducts. Sympathetic activation increases both heart rate and contractility, and in the short-term this increases cardiac output, but also augments peripheral vasoconstriction, diverting blood flow to critical organs and bolstering blood pressure.

Sympathetic stimulation also contributes to renin release from the cells of the renal juxtaglomerular apparatus, although the principal stimulant for this is renal hypoperfusion. Renin is the key regulator of the renin–angiotensin system. It catalyses the proteolysis of the propeptide angiotensinogen to form angiotensin I. Angiotensin I is subsequently converted to the biologically active angiotensin II by ACE. An-

giotensin II is a powerful vasoconstrictor and promotes renal sodium retention through both direct renal actions and the stimulation of aldosterone secretion from the adrenal cortex. Thus, the cumulative actions of angiotensin II result in a rise in blood pressure.

In the context of cardiac injury, together these various mechanisms maintain perfusion to vital organs by optimizing cardiac output, increasing intravascular volume and increasing peripheral vascular resistance.

When adaptive mechanisms become maladaptive

It is now recognized that while these mechanisms are important acutely, in the long-term, mechanical remodelling and neurohormonal activation become maladaptive (Fig. 20.2). In the setting of heart failure there is no blood loss as a cause of reduced cardiac output and the result is volume overload driven by angiotensin II, aldosterone and vasopressin. Coupled with sympathetic mediated venoconstriction, this leads to a rise in preload and adrenergic and angiotensin II-driven arterial vasoconstriction causes a rise in afterload. Although, in the short term, this has the cumulative effect of maintaining blood pressure, in the long term it imposes an increasing haemody-

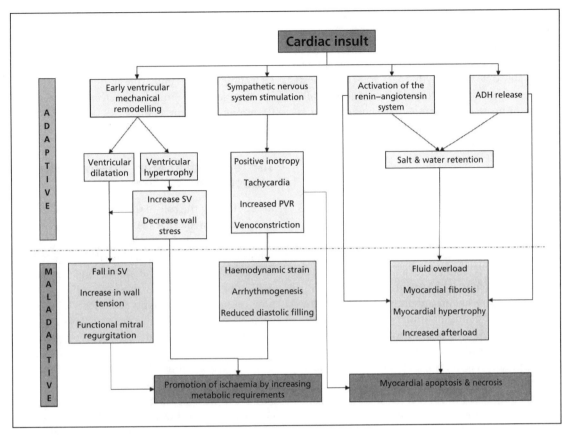

Figure 20.2 The pathogenesis of systolic heart failure. ADH, antidiuretic hormone; PVR, peripheral vascular resistance; SV, stroke volume.

namic burden on the heart [16]. Continuing volume overload leads to progressive ventricular dilatation. This is mediated by serial myocyte hypertrophy (myocyte lengthening), myocyte slippage and interstitial expansion, while at the same time there is parallel myocyte hypertrophy (myocyte thickening — see below) [17,18]. At first this may improve stroke volume according to the Frank–Starling mechanism, but the degree of inotropic gain decreases with each increment until eventually stroke volume declines. This relationship is represented in the Frank–Starling curve. Ventricular dilatation has two other important sequelae: (i) the development of functional mitral regurgitation; and (ii) in accordance with Laplace's law, a rise in wall tension. Increasing wall tension impairs the energy efficiency of the heart, increasing metabolic requirements and thus

promoting ischaemia [17]. This is further exacerbated by the tachycardia associated with sympathetic overdrive.

In response to either rising wall tension or to primary pressure overload (e.g. aortic stenosis or hypertension) the myocardium becomes hypertrophied and thickened, although it may not appear so because of cavity enlargement. This is mediated through parallel myocyte hypertrophy [17]. As Laplace's law indicates, increased wall thickness confers the acute benefit of reduction in wall tension, but ultimately this process also leads to a rise in myocardial metabolic requirements.

Myocardial stretch is an important catalyst for the remodelling process, but it is now recognized that activation of the renin–angiotensin system also has an integral role. Angiotensin II promotes myocyte hypertrophy and apoptosis, and both angiotensin II and aldosterone mediate local fibroblastic proliferation and subsequent myocardial fibrosis [19–21]. Myocardial fibrosis impairs contractility and is a potential substrate for arrhythmogenesis [17]. These effects suggest that angiotensin II is produced locally within the heart, and experimental data showed that the production of angiotensin II is increased in cardiac injury and that it is predominantly formed locally via both ACE-dependent and ACE-independent pathways [22,23]. There is growing evidence supporting the role of other factors such as oxidative stress, tumour necrosis factor-α and endothelin in the development of heart failure but the clinical and therapeutic importance of these are as yet unclear [19,24,25].

Ongoing cardiac ischaemia

Ischaemic injury has an important role in the progression of heart failure; coronary artery disease is a persistent potential source of further cardiac insult. Myocardial infarction may precipitate an acute decompensation in patients with chronic heart failure. In addition, chronic cardiac ischaemia without infarction may result in myocardial hibernation and reversible impairment of systolic function. The CHRISTMAS trial [26] demonstrated that the degree of improvement of left ventricular ejection fraction with carvedilol therapy was dependent on the quantity of hibernating myocardium. This finding not only reiterates the importance of cardiac ischaemia in the pathogenesis of systolic heart failure, but also supports the role of anti-ischaemic therapy in the treatment of patients with heart failure and underlying coronary disease.

Ultimately, cardiac injury and subsequent myocardial remodelling lead to a self-perpetuating downward spiral in ventricular function and, together with the continued inappropriate retention of salt and water in the setting of an already expanded intravascular volume, are largely responsible for the symptoms of heart failure.

The role of diuretics

Diuretics are the mainstay of treatment of overt clinical heart failure. Their appropriate and logical use has been frequently reviewed, yet in practice this knowledge is not always applied optimally. Many patients with severe heart failure tread a narrow path between breathlessness and oedema and overdiuresis leading to renal impairment. Inevitably, diuretic use stimulates the renin–angiotensin system, and aldosterone antagonists and Na^+/K^+ pump inhibitors play a pivotal part in this (see below).

Targeting the renin–angiotensin–aldosterone system

Recognition of the role of the renin–angiotensin–aldosterone system (RAAS) in the pathogenesis of heart failure has led to the development of pharmacological agents designed to block the deleterious effects of angiotensin II and aldosterone. The role of ACE inhibitors is well established, and their use is now routine for all patients with heart failure. The evidence is summarized in a meta-analysis that compiled data from five long-term trials investigating the effect of ACE inhibitors in 12 763 patients with documented heart failure [27]. ACE inhibition was associated with a reduction in all-cause mortality, readmission for heart failure and myocardial infarction. These benefits were seen in all patients regardless of their baseline ejection fraction, although greatest benefit was conferred to those in the lowest stratum. The protection against myocardial infarction conferred by ACE inhibitors, whatever the mechanism, is an interesting observation because the prevention of further infarction is important to avoiding further damage and worsening heart failure.

Aldosterone-receptor blockade has been shown to confer additional benefit in patients already receiving an ACE inhibitor [28]. The RALE study of 1663 patients with NYHA class III or IV heart failure, randomized patients to receive either spironolactone or placebo. Spironolactone reduced all-cause mortality, cardiovascular mortality and the frequency of hospitalization for cardiac causes. A subanalysis of 261 patients demonstrated that spironolactone therapy was associated with a reduction in serum levels of markers of collagen synthesis [29], suggesting that spironolactone may confer benefit through antifibrotic mechanisms, which may be independent of its haemodynamic effects. Given that 95% of patients were on optimal doses of ACE inhibitors prior to randomization, the results of this trial highlighted the inadequacy of ACE inhibitors in the long-term suppression of aldosterone production.

A similar rationale has led to a flurry of recent trials evaluating the efficacy of angiotensin II type-1 (AT_1) receptor antagonists. It has been observed that despite chronic optimal dosing, ACE inhibitors do not completely suppress the production of angiotensin II. The mechanism of this 'angiotensin escape' is not fully understood, although ACE-independent pathways, the loss of feedback suppression of angiotensin II on renin release and the up-regulation of ACE transcription are thought to be instrumental [22]. It has been hypothesized that complete blockade of the RAAS with AT_1 receptor blockers may confer additional benefit when used either instead of, or in addition to, ACE inhibitors.

This hypothesis has been tested in two clinical settings: chronic heart failure and heart failure following acute myocardial infarction. There have been four large trials evaluating various AT_1-receptor antagonists in patients with chronic heart failure and documented left ventricular systolic dysfunction: ELITE II, Val-HEFT, CHARM-alternative and CHARM-added [30–33]. In ELITE II, 3152 patients were to receive either losartan or captopril. It was designed as a superiority study and failed to establish superiority for both its primary endpoint (all-cause mortality) and secondary endpoints (combined endpoint of sudden cardiac death or resuscitated cardiac arrest). In the Val-HEFT trial, 5010 patients were to receive either valsartan or placebo. Approximately 92% of patients were already established on ACE inhibitor therapy. A 13% reduction in the primary combined endpoint was reported, although this was largely attributable to a 24% reduction in hospitalization for heart failure. No mortality advantage was demonstrated. The CHARM-alternative and CHARM-added trials assessed candesartan versus placebo in patients intolerant of ACE inhibitors and patients receiving concomitant ACE inhibitors, respectively. Candesartan significantly reduced the risk of the primary endpoint (cardiovascular death or admission for heart failure) in both the CHARM-alternative and the CHARM-added populations.

All-cause mortality was not significantly reduced in either study.

Further trials have also been undertaken: the VALIANT and OPTIMAAL trials recruited patients with heart failure post acute myocardial infarction [34,35]. In the VALIANT study, 14 808 patients were randomized to receive valsartan, captopril or both. Both primary (total mortality) and secondary (combined endpoint of death from cardiovascular causes, recurrent myocardial infarction or hospitalization for heart failure) endpoints were similar in all three groups. In a prospectively defined subgroup analysis, valsartan was demonstrated to be non-inferior to captopril. Rates of hospital admission were lower in the group receiving valsartan and captopril compared with those receiving captopril alone. In OPTIMAAL, 5477 patients were randomized to losartan or captopril. No significant differences in all-cause mortality, sudden or resuscitated cardiac death or re-infarction rates were demonstrated. Prospectively defined criteria for non-inferiority were not met.

Interpretation of these trails is difficult, given their heterogeneity. However, the CHARM-alternative and VALIANT studies have established AT_1 receptor antagonists as safe and effective alternatives in patients intolerant of ACE inhibition. The losartan trials (ELITE II, OPTIMAAL) failed to establish non-inferiority, although there is evidence suggesting that this may be attributable to inadequate dosing of the AT_1 antagonist [36]. While the results of the CHARM-added study are encouraging, concerns remain over the use of combination ACE inhibitor/AT_1 receptor blocker therapy. *Post hoc* analysis of the Val-HEFT population revealed an adverse effect on mortality in patients receiving an ACE inhibitor plus valsartan and a β-blocker. This observation was not verified in subgroup analyses of the CHARM-added and VALIANT studies. A recent meta-analysis confirmed that the addition of an AT_1 receptor antagonist to ACE inhibitor therapy confers a morbidity, but not a mortality benefit [37]. In VALIANT, Val-HEFT and CHARM-added, this was achieved at the expense of an increased risk of drug-related adverse events. Certainly, the literature reinforces the use of ACE inhibitors as first-line therapy in patients with heart failure and supports the use of AT_1 receptor blockade in those unable to tolerate this therapy.

There is, as yet, no clear consensus with respect to the use of combination therapy.

β-Blockade in heart failure

The use of the β-adrenergic antagonists metoprolol, bisoprolol and carvedilol are now firmly established in the treatment of heart failure. Their benefit is summarized in a recent meta-analysis that involved 14 857 patients from 16 randomized controlled trials [38]. β-Blockade was associated with a reduction in all-cause mortality, sudden cardiac death and the frequency of hospitalization for heart failure. Further analysis of data from the CIBIS I, CIBIS II, MERIT-HF and COPERNICUS trials demonstrated that this benefit did not differ between NYHA class III and IV patients, nor between patients with an ejection fraction less than 25% or above 25%.

There have been many mechanisms proposed to explain the beneficial effects of β-blockers. β-Blockers have antiarrhythmic properties, which may explain the reduction in risk of sudden cardiac death. They are also thought to prevent adverse ventricular remodelling by blocking β_1-receptor mediated myocyte hypertrophy, apoptosis and necrosis. In addition, β-blockers may also reduce cardiac metabolic requirements by reducing heart rate and improving diastolic coronary blood flow [39].

Considerable debate has arisen over the importance of specific pharmacological attributes of the various β-blockers. The β-Blocker Evaluation of Survival Trial (BEST) was notable in its failure to demonstrate a mortality benefit in patients randomized to receive bucindolol [40]. Despite an overlap in the confidence interval around the primary endpoint in other positive trials, and a significant reduction in the secondary endpoints of cardiovascular death and hospitalizations for heart failure, there has been much speculation regarding the adverse characteristics of bucindolol. The intrinsic sympathomimetic activity of bucindolol and central sympatholytic effects have been cited as potentially undesirable qualities [40–42]. In the COMET trial, the only head-to-head β-blocker trial in heart failure, carvedilol was associated with a reduction in all-cause mortality in comparison with metoprolol [43]. Metoprolol and bisoprolol are β_1-selective antagonists, while carvedilol is a non-selective β-blocker. In addition, carvedilol acts as a radical scavenger, displays α_1-receptor antagonism and improves insulin sensitivity [39,43]. However, despite the results of COMET, the importance of these properties remains controversial; in particular there has been much debate over the adequacy of metoprolol dosing and therefore the equivalence of β_1-blockade between study groups in the COMET study [44].

Pharmacotherapy: use with caution

While the results of the ACE inhibitor, spironolactone and β-blocker trials have revolutionized the treatment of heart failure patients, it is important to recognize their limitations. Trial populations do not reflect everyday clinical practice because of stringent inclusion and exclusion criteria and possible recruitment bias. In addition, the trial environment is an artificial one, and often the degree of patient monitoring in practice falls short of that stipulated in a strict study protocol. As such, extrapolation of trial data in the treatment of the general heart failure population can be fraught with difficulty. This was recently illustrated by Juurlink et al. [45] who demonstrated a rise in hyperkalaemia-related hospital admissions and deaths following the publication of the RALE study, attributed in part to the use of higher doses of spironolactone than in the RALE study. However, it was also thought to be related to the treatment of patients with lower glomerular filtration rates and to the wider coadministration of β-blockers and higher doses of ACE inhibitors [46]. It is important to state that the association of the publication of RALE and the rise in hyperkalaemia-related events was assumed, not proven. Nevertheless, this observation serves as an important reminder of the limitations of pharmacotherapy.

ACE inhibitors, AT_1 receptor blockers and spironolactone should be used with caution in the elderly, in patients with diabetes mellitus and in those with known renal impairment. Renal function and potassium levels should be monitored closely, especially if several of these agents are used in combination. β-Blockers should only be introduced in stable patients who are already rendered euvolaemic with diuretic therapy and established on either an ACE inhibitor or AT_1 receptor antagonist. Careful implementation of therapeutic approaches leading from trial data should ensure that the promised benefits of these drugs are realized, without an accompanying rise in related adverse reactions.

New drugs or the use of established agents in new ways have not been the only innovations to reduce mortality in the modern treatment of heart failure. Device therapy has emerged as an important adjunct to pharmacotherapy.

Cardiac resynchronization therapy

The concept of cardiac resynchronization therapy evolved from the observation that up to one-third of heart failure patients have a prolonged QRS dura-

tion, and that this is associated with incoordinate cardiac contraction. Prolongation of the QRS complex usually manifests as left bundle branch block. In left bundle branch block, ventricular depolarization does not occur uniformly, but instead commences in the anterior septum and spreads finally to the inferolateral heart. This results in abnormal ventricular septal motion, delayed left ventricular lateral wall contraction, functional mitral regurgitation, a delay in aortic valve closure and a delay in mitral valve opening, with a consequent fall in ejection fraction [47]. Biventricular pacing technology was developed then in the hope of negating the haemodynamic effects of both inter- and intraventricular mechanical dyssynchrony (Fig. 20.3).

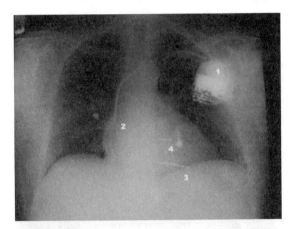

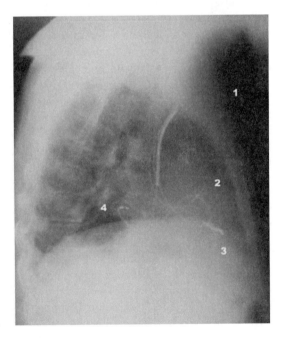

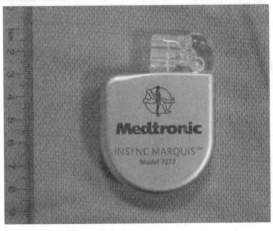

Figure 20.3 Combined biventricular pacemaker and cardioconverter-defibrillator device (BiV-ICD). 1, Pulse generator; 2, atrial lead; 3, right ventricular lead; 4, left ventricular lead (coursing through the coronary sinus and into a posterior cardiac vein).

The efficacy of biventricular pacing in improving symptoms and exercise capacity has been demonstrated in several randomized controlled trials, although the earliest trials are small, single-blind and cross-over by design. These studies have all recruited patients with documented ejection fractions less than 35%, NYHA class III or IV symptoms and QRS prolongation on 12-lead electrocardiography (ECG). However, the lower cut-off point for QRS duration varies between the studies, ranging from 120 to 150 ms. These studies consistently reported an improvement in qualitative and quantitative measures of morbidity [47]. In the recently published COMPANION trial, Bristow *et al.* [48] reported that cardiac resynchronization therapy was associated with a significant reduction in the primary combined endpoint of all-cause mortality or hospitalization. A significant reduction in the secondary combined endpoint of death from or hospitalization for cardiovascular causes or heart failure was also demonstrated. However, while there was a trend towards a reduction in all-cause mortality, this did not achieve statistical significance ($P = 0.059$). A meta-analysis of data from the CONTAK-CD, InSync ICD, MIRACLE and MUSTIC trials and prepublication preliminary data from COMPANION reported that all-cause mortality may be reduced by biventricular pacing [49]. This has now been confirmed following publication of the CARE-HF study in 2005 [50].

CARE-HF randomized 813 patients with NYHA class III–IV heart failure resulting from left ventricular dysfunction and evidence of dyssynchrony between medical therapy and cardiac resynchronization without implantable cardioverter defibrillator (ICD) therapy. All-cause mortality was reduced from 30% to 20% by cardiac resynchronization therapy after a mean of 29.4 months (hazard ratio 0.64; $P < 0.002$) and improved quality of life and indices of left ventricular dysfunction [50].

Although there is a growing argument for the implantation of biventricular pacing devices in patients with heart failure and dyssynchronous cardiac contraction, it must be emphasized that the evidence is restricted to this specific subset of patients. The vast majority of patients enrolled in these trials were in sinus rhythm and had left bundle branch block. However, patients with right bundle branch block may have an element of left intraventricular dyssynchrony that is not detectable on surface 12-lead ECG [51]. Subsets of patients with right bundle branch block in the MIRACLE and CONTAK-CD studies appeared to derive benefit from biventricular pacing [47], but this has not been formally assessed in a randomized controlled trial. Similarly, while there are preliminary data supporting the efficacy of this therapy in patients with atrial fibrillation, this is yet to be verified [52,53]. Moreover, it is now recognized that QRS prolongation does not necessarily reflect the degree of ventricular asynchrony, and indeed is a relatively insensitive marker [54,55]. Tissue Doppler imaging is emerging as a valuable tool in the assessment of ventricular synchrony and the expectation is that this technology will prove more accurate than QRS duration in identifying those who will benefit most from resynchronization therapy.

Implantable cardioverter defibrillators

Approximately 50% of individuals with left ventricular dysfunction die from ventricular arrhythmia [56,57]. This observation, along with the disappointing results of antiarrhythmic drug trials, has led to the development and utilization of ICDs. A number of landmark trials have established that ICD implantation reduces mortality in individuals who are at a high risk of arrhythmic death [58]. Initial studies concentrated on survivors of aborted sudden death or malignant ventricular tachycardia [59–62]. However, this approach addresses a minority of the population at risk of sudden cardiac death (SCD) and ICD therapy is now being extended to individuals yet to experience major arrhythmia.

The widespread utilization of these devices is principally limited by their technical complexity and financial cost. Consequently, a considerable amount of work has gone into the identification of high risk individuals likely to benefit most. The risk of SCD is proportional to the severity of left ventricular systolic impairment, irrespective of whether this is caused by an ischaemic or non-ischaemic aetiology. Unsurprisingly then, most ICD studies have shown that benefit from the ICD is proportional to the degree of left ventricular systolic dysfunction. Indeed, subanalysis of the AVID study revealed negligible mortality benefit in patients with preserved left ventricular function [59]. The MADIT and MUSST studies, although significantly different in design, used a combination of risk markers including the presence of coronary artery disease, marked reduction in left ventricular ejection fraction, the presence of spontaneous non-sustained ventricular tachycardia (VT) and the presence of inducible sustained VT during electrophysiological testing [63,64]. Employing these inclusion criteria identified a group with a 2-year mortality rate as high as 32%. These studies demonstrated that the number of devices needed to be implanted to save one life (i.e. number needed to treat) is as low as 4 over a 2-year period [65]. This is markedly fewer than any other proven intervention in heart failure patients.

The MADIT II study attempted to simplify the selection process and widen the applicability of the ICD technology by including patients with coronary disease and a left ventricular ejection fraction of ≤30% [66]. Importantly, documentation of a spontaneous or inducible ventricular arrhythmia was not required. Predictably, the MADIT II population was at lower risk of SCD compared with the MADIT patients. However, their absolute risk was still high with a 20% mortality rate after 20 months' follow-up. A statistically and clinically significant benefit was demonstrated in those who received an ICD although, as would be expected, the number needed to treat was higher (17 over 2 years) [65].

The role of ICD implantation is less certain in patients with non-ischaemic cardiomyopathies [67–69]. This has been attributed to the lower mortality rates in the control arms of these studies and their consequent underpowering. However, two recent studies suggest that there may yet be a rationale for ICD use in such patients. The SCD-HeFT study randomized 2521 individuals with symptomatic heart failure of any aetiology to standard medical care, antiarrhythmic prophylaxis with oral amiodarone or ICD therapy [70]. The ICD significantly reduced overall mortality and this benefit was seen in patients with both ischaemic and non-ischaemic cardiomyopathies. Importantly, amiodarone conferred no mortality benefit beyond standard medical therapy.

In addition to assessing the impact of cardiac resynchronization pacing, the COMPANION study included an arm randomized to receive biventricular pacing combined with an ICD. A total of 1520 patients with NYHA class III/IV heart failure, an ejection fraction ≤35% and a QRS duration ≥120 ms were randomized to receive either conventional medical therapy, a biventricular pacemaker or a biventricular pacemaker-defibrillator. The results from the biventricular group have been mentioned earlier. Implantation of a biventricular pacemaker-defibrillator device further reduced the risk of the primary combined endpoint of all-cause mortality or hospitalization, as well as the secondary endpoint of all-cause mortality [48]. Forty-one per cent of the patients randomized to medical therapy and 45% of those receiving a pacing-defibrillator device had non-ischaemic cardiomyopathy. Subgroup analysis revealed that survival benefit was conferred to this subpopulation, although it is difficult to determine what portion of benefit is due to the defibrillator rather than the biventricular pacing component. This finding is consistent with the results of SCD-HeFT [70].

Evolving guidelines for ICD implantation

In 2001, the European Society of Cardiology published guidelines on the indications for ICD therapy (Table 20.2) [71]. This publication preceded the release of the MADIT II data, and inducible ventricular arrhythmia was cited as a prerequisite for the prophylactic implantation of an ICD. In contrast, the joint American guidelines (published after MADIT II) listed post-infarction patients with an ejection fraction ≤30% as a class IIa indication for ICD therapy [58]. The guidelines define class IIa indications as 'conditions for which there is conflicting evidence and/or a divergence of opinion about the usefulness/efficacy of a procedure or treatment, [and] the weight of evidence and opinion is in favour of usefulness/efficacy'. Certainly, there has been much divergence over this issue. While greater than in MADIT I (number needed to treat 2.0 at 3 years) and MUSTT (number needed to treat 2.5 at 3 years), the number needed to treat to gain 1 life-year in MADIT II is still an impressive 8, if examined over 3 years [65]. However, this benefit comes at a small risk of morbidity

Table 20.2 Indications for implantable cardioverter defibrillator therapy related to clinical presentation. (Study Group on Guidelines on ICDs of the Working Group on Arrhythmias and the Working Group on Cardiac Pacing of the European Society of Cardiology.)

Cardiac arrest
- Electrocardiographically documented VT/VF not due to transient or reversible cause
- VT/VF not electrocardiographically documented, but presumed based on successful external defibrillation and/or inducible VT/VF, and/or other relevant clinical data, and arrhythmia not due to transient, reversible or treatable cause

Electrocardiographically documented VT without cardiac arrest
- Sustained VT with severe haemodynamic compromise
- Sustained VT without haemodynamic compromise and LVEF ≤ 40%
- LVEF ≤ 40%, 4 days or more after myocardial infarction with inducible VF or sustained VT at electrophysiological study

Syncope without documented VT
- Inducible VF or VT at electrophysiological study with severe haemodynamic compromise when drug therapy is ineffective, not tolerated or not preferred

Prophylactic indication
- Non-sustained VT ≥ 4 days after myocardial infarction with a LVEF ≤ 40% and inducible VF or sustained VT at electrophysiological study

related to the implantation procedure, and a risk of psychological trauma resulting from inappropriate defibrillations [72]. In addition, adopting MADIT II indications for ICD implantation would also have enormous cost implications for health services — implications that are probably unsustainable in the UK context. However, it is clear that pharmacological therapy is ineffective in preventing SCD and that secondary preventative ICD implantation is helpful in an albeit small number of patients at risk. Attempts to stratify risk within this large group of patients without increasing the complexity of patient selection are on-going. The challenge is to ensure that ICD therapy is distributed as effectively and equitably as possible.

The importance of atrial fibrillation

The relationship between atrial fibrillation (AF) and heart failure is important. AF that is poorly rate controlled is thought to contribute to the development of cardiomyopathy, and a 'tachycardia-induced' cardiomyopathy can result. More usually, heart failure resulting from either left ventricular systolic impairment or diastolic dysfunction predisposes to the de-

velopment of AF, and left ventricular systolic impairment increases the risk of AF fivefold. Heart failure-related atrial stretch, and catecholamine and angiotensin II-induced atrial fibrosis are thought to be the mechanisms responsible [73].

Simplistically, there are three potential clinically important sequelae of AF: (i) rapid ventricular conduction with fast irregular heart rate; (ii) impaired cardiac function; and (iii) thromboembolism. In young people with structurally normal hearts, the development of AF may be unnoticed or minimally symptomatic. In patients with heart failure and minimal cardiac reserve, the onset of AF can be disastrous.

Heart failure is exacerbated by the development of AF because of the loss of the contribution of atrial contraction and tachycardia-related shortening of diastolic filling time. Treatment strategies have therefore centred on the restoration of sinus rhythm and the maintenance of adequate rate control. The AFFIRM, RACE and PIAF trials compared the efficacy of a rhythm-control strategy with that of rate-control and all three concluded that a rhythm control strategy was not superior [74–76]. However, it must be emphasized that patients with heart failure were a minority in all three trials. In the AFFIRM trial, 4060 patients were recruited, of whom only 23.1% had a history of congestive heart failure. Transthoracic echocardiography was performed routinely at enrolment and 74% of participants had a normal left ventricular ejection fraction. Heart failure symptomatology was not recorded. Amongst the 522 RACE trial participants, approximately 50% had a history of heart failure. However, no patients with NYHA class IV symptoms were enrolled and only 3% of patients had NYHA class III symptoms. Finally, in the small PIAF study, only 17% of the 252 recruited patients had a history of dilated cardiomyopathy and 12% had a history of myocardial infarction. Left ventricular ejection fractions and NYHA classifications were not given. Thus, these studies are not representative of the heart failure population, and their findings should be extrapolated with caution to these patients. In particular, there remains a strong rationale for rhythm control in heart failure patients who are very symptomatic. The ongoing AF-CHF study will hopefully offer guidance in the treatment of this population [77].

A devastating complication of AF is stroke. The risk of thromboembolism in heart failure patients is high, and higher still in the setting of concomitant hypertension, coronary artery disease, thyrotoxicosis or diabetes mellitus. Long-term anticoagulation with warfarin is mandatory unless a contraindication exists [78]. In addition, there is now strong evidence that anticoagulation therapy should be continued even after reversion to sinus rhythm as the risk of stroke remains high [74,75].

The role of revascularization

The recognition of the potential reversibility of ventricular impairment resulting from chronic ischaemia, so-called 'myocardial hibernation', has provided a rationale for the revascularization of patients with heart failure resulting from coronary disease [79]. This concept is supported by observational data [80], although randomized controlled trials testing this hypothesis are lacking. Previous trials, comparing surgical revascularization to medical therapy in coronary patients, have included few patients with significant left ventricular impairment [81]. *Post hoc*

analysis of the Coronary Artery Surgery Study (CASS) reported a significant reduction in mortality in patients with an ejection fraction between 34% and 50% and triple vessel disease [82]. However, this subanalysis included a small number of patients and medical therapy has advanced significantly since then.

Assessment of myocardial viability is the key to the logical management of patients with ventricular systolic impairment and significant coronary disease. Demonstration of large areas of viable but ischaemic myocardium suggests that revascularization may result in a significant improvement in ventricular function. Conversely, the lack of myocardial viability indicates that there is little benefit to be gained by attempting revascularization. Currently, dobutamine stress echocardiography (DSE) and various scintigraphic techniques, including fluorodeoxyglucose-positron emission tomography (^{18}F-PET), are the principal techniques employed in the assessment of myocardial viability. However, cardiac magnetic resonance imaging (MRI) techniques, in particular delayed enhancement MRI and low-dose dobutamine MRI, are now emerging as important alternatives. Early studies suggest that cardiac MRI is as accurate as DSE and PET in detecting myocardial viability, with the advantage of superior spatial resolution. In particular, cardiac MRI is superior in its ability to detect subendocardial myocardial infarction [83]. Improved assessment of myocardial ischaemia and viability raises the prospect of better patient selection for revascularization procedures, and thus better clinical outcomes.

Percutaneous or surgical revascularization should be considered in patients who are limited by angina despite optimal medical therapy, and in whom there is objective evidence of myocardial viability and reversible ischaemia. Revascularization in patients without angina is controversial, and is the subject of the ongoing Surgical Treatments for Ischaemic Heart failure (STICH) and Heart Failure Revascularization (HEART-UK) trials [84,85].

Evolving concepts: diastolic heart failure

The concept of diastolic impairment is not new, but

the definition of diastolic heart failure, its diagnosis and its management are still evolving.

Terminology

It is now well documented that a significant proportion of patients with heart failure have normal left ventricular ejection fractions on echocardiography or using other techniques. The reported prevalence in heart failure populations varies from 40% to 71%, depending predominantly on the mean population age [86]. This subpopulation has been dubbed as having 'heart failure with preserved systolic function' (PSF). Heart failure with PSF is not synonymous with diastolic heart failure. The term 'preserved systolic function' does not imply a cause for heart failure, but merely excludes measurable left ventricular systolic impairment. Conversely, diastolic heart failure is a syndrome characterized by clinical symptoms and signs of heart failure and abnormal diastolic function.

Diastolic heart failure is not synonymous with left ventricular diastolic dysfunction, just as systolic heart failure is not synonymous with left ventricular systolic impairment. Diastolic dysfunction denotes a mechanical abnormality that impairs ventricular filling in diastole and may or may not cause symptoms. Community-based echocardiographic studies report a 3.1% incidence of diastolic dysfunction in the general 'healthy' population [87]. Importantly, diastolic and systolic heart failure are not mutually exclusive and approximately 35% of heart failure patients with impaired left ventricular systolic function have evidence of concomitant diastolic dysfunction on echocardiography [88].

Aetiology and pathogenesis

Impairment of ventricular filling can be caused by intrinsic cardiac pathology or extrinsic cardiac compression. However, excluding cardiac tamponade secondary to a pericardial collection, non-myocardial aetiologies are uncommon. In the vast majority of cases, diastolic dysfunction results from impaired relaxation and increased passive stiffness of the myocardium [89]. The development of this abnormality is associated with cardiac ischaemia, hypertension and increasing age [90].

Several processes have been postulated as important mechanisms in the development of diastolic dysfunction. Intrinsic myocytic abnormalities such as perturbed calcium homoeostasis, relative adenosine triphosphate deficiency and alterations in cytoskeletal morphology may affect both active myocardial relaxation and passive myocardial stiffness. Qualitative and quantitative changes in extracellular fibrillar collagen are thought to be pivotal in the development of diastolic dysfunction. These changes are driven by haemodynamic stresses (e.g. pressure overload in hypertension) and chronic activation of RAAS [91].

The diagnostic dilemma

There is no clear consensus on what constitutes diastolic heart failure. Some claim that demonstration of raised left ventricular end-diastolic pressures, in the absence of systolic impairment, on cardiac catheterization is the gold-standard [92,93]. In 1998, the European Study Group on Diastolic Heart Failure published diagnostic guidelines that were based heavily on echocardiographic parameters [94]. These have been criticized for their poor sensitivity [95,96], and their reliance on a test that is dependent on operator skill and multiple fluctuating haemodynamic variables [97]. Zile and Brutsaert [98] suggest that objective measures of diastolic function are impractical and unnecessary. They have proposed that the diagnosis of diastolic heart failure should be made on the basis of: (i) symptoms and signs of heart failure as per Framingham criteria; and (ii) a left ventricular ejection fraction greater than 50% [98]; in essence then, a diagnosis of exclusion.

Treatment

There is a distinct lack of evidence guiding the treatment of diastolic heart failure. Treatment is therefore largely empiric, and based on theoretical mechanisms of benefit. The fundamental aims are to reduce diastolic pressures, prevent tachycardia and prevent cardiac ischaemia and hypertrophy [91]. Initially, reduction of diastolic pressures with the use of diuretics and nitrates should achieve symptomatic improvement in the majority of patients.

Tachycardia is thought to exacerbate the symptoms of diastolic heart failure through various mechanisms including: (i) the promotion of cardiac ischaemia by increasing myocardial oxygen consumption and reducing coronary perfusion time; (ii) the restriction of ventricular diastolic filling time; and (iii) a direct adverse effect on the rate of myocardial relaxation [91]. Theoretically, therefore, β-blockers, calcium antagonists and digitalis may be beneficial. The DIG study [99] evaluated the efficacy of digoxin in the treatment of heart failure, and in an ancillary trial recruited 988 patients with an ejection fraction >45%. Overall, digoxin reduced the rate of hospitalization but not of death, and the findings in the ancillary trial were deemed consistent with these findings. The SWEDIC study demonstrated a marginal improvement in echocardiographic features of diastolic dysfunction in patients randomized to receive carvedilol compared with placebo [100]. There have been no randomized controlled trials assessing the effect of β-blockers or calcium antagonists on clinical outcomes.

Recognition of the importance of myocardial hypertrophy and fibrosis has provided the rationale for various trials evaluating the efficacy of ACE inhibitors and AT$_1$ receptor blockers in diastolic heart failure. To date, only one such study has been published. In the CHARM-Preserved trial, 3020 patients with NYHA class II–IV heart failure and an ejection fraction >40% were randomized to receive either candesartan or placebo [101]. No effect on mortality was observed and the reduction in admissions for heart failure was of borderline significance (P = 0.047). Results of the PEP-CHF (perindopril), I-PRESERVE (irbesartan) and Hong Kong (ramipril, irbesartan) trials are pending.

It is important to emphasize that both the DIG ancillary study and the CHARM-Preserved study recruited patients with heart failure and preserved systolic function. No attempt was made in either study to assess objective measures of diastolic function.

Prognosis

It is generally accepted in the literature that patients with heart failure and PSF have a worse prognosis than the 'healthy' population [86,92,98], although evidence supporting this notion is scant. The majority of studies assessing mortality have recruited small numbers of patients with a correspondingly small number of endpoints [88,102–109]. In addition, many studies have not been case-controlled [102–104], have not been hospital-based [104,105] or have failed to adjust for important variables [88]. In a substudy derived from the EuroHeart Failure Survey, Lenzen *et al.* [110] reported a high rate of morbidity and mortality in patients with heart failure and preserved left ventricular function. However, this observational study has several significant limitations, not least the lack of an appropriate control group to enable a comparison of outcome data. Preserved left ventricular function was defined rather loosely as 'a LVEF ≥40%, as well as patients with a normal or mildly depressed systolic left ventricular function, as assessed by echocardiography'. The inclusion of hospitals in this survey was voluntary and, in addition, 36% of patients were not included in this subanalysis because of the lack of echocardiographic data. Combined with the observational nature of this study, the potential for selection bias is significant. The prognosis of heart failure with PSF therefore remains uncertain.

Evolving concepts: B-type natriuretic peptide — a biomarker for the future?

Originally isolated by Sudoh *et al.* [111] in 1988, B-type natriuretic peptide (BNP) has emerged as an important biomarker in patients with heart failure. BNP is secreted principally by ventricular myocytes in response to myocardial stretch [112]. Tachycardia and circulating glucocorticoids are other important stimuli [113]. It is released as a propeptide (pro-BNP) via a constitutive mechanism, and is subsequently cleaved to produce active BNP and the inactive N-terminal peptide (NT-proBNP). Animal experiments have demonstrated that BNP increases glomerular filtration rate, reduces sodium resorption in the collecting duct and inhibits the activation of the renin–angiotensin system. It is also thought to have antifibrotic actions [114].

Levels of circulating BNP are elevated in patients with heart failure, and the degree of elevation is proportional to NYHA functional class [114]. In response to this observation, assays measuring both BNP and NT-proBNP have been developed. The usefulness of these assays has been studied in various clinical settings: (i) the diagnosis of heart failure in patients with dyspnoea; (ii) as a prognostic marker in patients with known heart failure; and (iii) in screening the asymptomatic population.

Studies assessing the usefulness of BNP and NT-proBNP in the diagnosis of heart failure have been encouraging [114]. They have examined the role of these markers in both the community and acute hospital settings. Cumulatively, the literature suggests that these markers have a high negative predictive value, but with poor specificity. However, the sensitivity of these markers is impressive, and may be useful in the exclusion of heart failure as cause of dyspnoea. This hypothesis was recently tested in a prospective, randomized, emergency department-based trial [115]. In total, 452 patients presenting with dyspnoea were randomized into two groups. The first group had their BNP levels measured, whereas the second group were treated without this knowledge. Incorporation of the measurement of BNP as part of the diagnostic strategy was shown to reduce emergency waiting times, hospitalization rates, the need for admission to the intensive care unit, length of stay and the consequent cost of treatment. This practical demonstration of the benefits of measuring BNP is interesting, although it is limited by the exclusion of the critically ill and patients with significant renal impairment. Further trials are required in this promising area.

There is also growing evidence for the utility of BNP and NT-proBNP measurement in assessing the prognosis of patients with heart failure. Levels of these markers correlate with both qualitative and quantitative measures of cardiac function. They have been shown to be independent predictors of mortality in patients with asymptomatic left ventricular impairment, patients with chronic heart failure and patients admitted for acute decompensation of their heart failure [114]. In addition, Wang *et al.* [116] recently demonstrated in a large community-based trial involving 3346 'healthy' individuals, that raised BNP levels were predictive of all-cause mortality and associated with the risk of a first major cardiovascular event, heart failure, atrial fibrillation and stroke, after adjustment for traditional risk factors. McDonagh *et al.* [117] suggested that elevated levels of these markers should be regarded as a sign of 'cardiorenal distress' that prompts further investigation. The cost effectiveness of widespread screening with BNP and

strategies in managing people with elevated BNP levels need further evaluation.

BNP therefore appears to be a promising biomarker, and in addition to the uses mentioned BNP may also be a helpful tool in the monitoring of heart failure treatment. Preliminary studies suggest that its diagnostic and prognostic abilities extend to those with heart failure and preserved left ventricular function [118,119].

Strategies for the future

Despite the advances in pharmacological therapy and the promise of improved morbidity and mortality with the judicious use of device technology, the prognosis in severe heart failure remains poor. The viability of cardiac transplantation as a solution is hindered by the shortage of donor organs, and thus the search for novel therapeutic strategies continues.

Left ventricular assist devices (LVAD) represent one such strategy. These devices were originally developed as a bridge to transplantation, and to recovery in patients with reversible causes of heart failure (e.g. viral myocarditis). However, their role has since expanded and long-term 'destination' therapy is now a reality [120]. In the REMATCH study, 129 patients with end-stage heart failure were randomly assigned to receive either an LVAD or optimal medical therapy [121]. All patients had NYHA class IV heart failure and were deemed ineligible for cardiac transplantation. The mean left ventricular ejection fraction in both groups was 17%. Implantation of a LVAD was associated with a 48% reduction in all-cause mortality and an improved quality of life. However, this was at the expense of device-related adverse events, including bleeding, infection and device malfunction. Nevertheless, these results are encouraging and it remains to be seen whether improvements in techniques and technology will reduce the frequency of adverse events, and whether left ventricular assist devices will be applicable to a wider spectrum of heart failure patients.

Myocytic regeneration through stem cell transplantation is another interesting stratagem in development. Bone marrow and embryonic stem cells have been successfully transplanted into both experiment myocardial models and in humans with heart failure [122,123]. In a recent randomized controlled trial involving 60 patients presenting with acute ST-elevation myocardial infarction, the intracoronary transfer of autologous bone-marrow cells was associated with an improvement in left ventricular systolic function compared with the control group [124]. However, this technology is still in its infancy and much uncertainty remains. Little is known about the long-term bioavailability of transplanted cells, and the ability of these progenitor cells to adopt a cardio-myocytic phenotype is controversial [125,126]. In addition, there are concerns over the ability of these cells to differentiate into other harmful cell types that may have important clinical implications, such as neoplastic and pro-arrhythmic cells. Despite these concerns, myocardial regeneration remains an exciting prospect for the future.

Conclusions

Heart failure is responsible for significant morbidity and mortality in the community today. However, therapeutic strategies to combat this disorder are ever increasing. The efficacy of neurohormonal inhibition with ACE inhibitors, AT_1-receptor antagonists, spironolactone and β-blockers is well established. The role of device therapy is evolving rapidly with the promise of improving mortality rates further. Prevention of hypertension and ischaemic damage remains paramount. An immediate challenge is to translate trial evidence into safe practice.

References

1 National Institute for Clinical Excellence. NICE clinical guidelines for the care of people who have heart failure. 2003. Available at: http://www.nice.org.uk/pdf/PressRelease_2003_033_heart_failure_guideline.pdf

2 Stewart S, Jenkins A, Buchan S, *et al.* The current cost of heart failure to the National Health Service in the UK. *Eur J Heart Fail* 2002; **4**: 361–71.

3 Davies MK, Hobbs F, Davis R, *et al.* Prevalence of left-ventricular systolic dysfunction and heart failure in the Echocardiographic Heart of England Screening study: a population based study. *Lancet* 2001; **358**: 439–44.

4 McDonagh TA, Morrison CE, Lawrence A, *et al.* Symptomatic and asymptomatic left-ventricular systolic dysfunction in an urban population. *Lancet* 1997; **350**: 829–33.

5 Stewart S, MacIntyre K, Hole DJ, Capewell S, McMurray JJ. More 'malignant' than cancer? Five year survival following a first admission for heart failure. *Eur J Heart Fail* 2001; **3**: 315–22.

6 Jessup M, Brozena S. Heart failure. *N Engl J Med* 2003; **348**: 2007–18.

7 Primatesta P, Brookes M, Poulter NR. Improved hypertension management and control: results from the health study for England 1998. *Hypertension* 2001; **38**: 827–32.

8 Komajda M, Follatt F, Swedberg K, *et al.* The Euro-Heart Survey programme — a survey on the quality of care among patients with heart failure in Europe: Part 2. Treatment. *Eur Heart J* 2003; **24**: 464–74.

9 Cleland JGF, Swedberg K, Follatt F, *et al.* The Euro-Heart Survey programme — a survey on the quality of care among patients with heart failure in Europe: Part 1. Patient characteristics and diagnosis. *Eur Heart J* 2003; **24**: 442–63.

10 Hunt SA, Baker DW, Chin MH, *et al.* ACC/AHA guidelines for the evaluation and management of chronic heart failure in the adult. 2001. American College of Cardiology website. Available at: http://www.acc.org/clinical/guidelines/failure/hf_index.htm

11 Psaty BM, Lumley T, Furberg CD. Health outcomes associated with various antihypertensive therapies used as first-line agents: a network meta-analysis. *JAMA* 2003; **289**: 2534–44.

12 Heart Outcomes Prevention Evaluation Study Investigators. Effects of an ACE inhibitor, ramipril, on cardiovascular events in high risk patients. *N Engl J Med* 2000; **342**: 145–53.

13 European Trial on Reduction of Cardiac Events with Perindopril in Stable Coronary Artery Disease Investigators. Efficacy of perindopril in reduction of cardiovascular events among patients with stable coronary artery disease: randomized, double-blind, placebo-controlled, multi-centre trial. *Lancet* 2003; **362**: 782–8.

14 SOLVD Investigators. Effect of enalapril on mortality and the development of heart failure in asymptomatic patients with reduced left ventricular ejection fractions. *N Engl J Med* 1992; **327**: 685–91.

15 Vantrimpont P, Rouleau JJ, Wun CC, *et al.* Additive beneficial effects of β-blockers to ACE inhibitors in the

Survival and Ventricular Enlargement (SAVE) study. *J Am Coll Cardiol* 1997; **29**: 229–36.

16 Schrier RW, Abraham WT. Hormones and haemodynamics in heart failure. *N Engl J Med* 1999; **341**: 577–85.

17 Baig MK, Mahon N, McKenna WJ, *et al.* The pathophysiology of advanced heart failure. *Heart Lung* 1999; **28**: 87–101.

18 Jugdutt BI. Ventricular remodelling after infarction and the extracellular collagen matrix. *Circulation* 2003; **108**: 1395–403.

19 Cohn JN, Ferrari R, Sharpe N. Cardiac remodelling: concepts and clinical implications: a consensus paper from an international forum on cardiac remodelling. *J Am Coll Cardiol* 2000; **35**: 569–82.

20 Weber KT. Extracellular matrix remodelling in heart failure. *Circulation* 1997; 96: 4065-82.

21 Weber KT. Aldosterone in congestive heart failure. *N Engl J Med* 2001; **345**: 1689–97.

22 Zaman MA, Oparil S, Calhoun DA. Drugs targeting the renin–angiotensin–aldosterone system. *Nat Rev Drug Discov* 2002; **1**: 621–36.

23 Dzau VJ, Bernstein K, Celermajer D, *et al.* Pathophysiologic and therapeutic importance of tissue ACE: A consensus report. *Cardiovasc Drugs Ther* 2002; **16**: 149–60.

24 Anand I, McMurray J, Cohn JN, *et al.* Long-term effects of darusentan on left-ventricular remodelling and clinical outcomes in the Endothelin$_A$ receptor antagonist trial in heart failure (EARTH): randomised, double-blind, placebo-controlled trial. *Lancet* 2004; **364**: 347–53.

25 Mann DL. Inflammatory mediators and the failing heart. *Circ Res* 2002; **91**: 988–98.

26 Cleland JGF, Pennell DJ, Ray SG, *et al.* Myocardial viability as a determinant of the ejection fraction response to carvedilol in patients with heart failure (CHRISTMAS trial): randomised controlled trial. *Lancet* 2003; **362**: 14–21.

27 Flather MD, Yusuf S, Kaber L, *et al.* Long-term ACE-inhibitor therapy in patients with heart failure or left-ventricular dysfunction: a systemic overview of data from individual patients. *Lancet* 2000; **355**: 1575–81.

28 Pitt B, Zannad F, Renne WJ, *et al.* The effect of spironolactone on morbidity and mortality in patients with severe heart failure. *N Engl J Med* 1999; **341**: 709–17.

29 Zannad F, Alla F, Dousset B, Perez A, Pitt B. Limitation of excessive extracellular matrix turnover may contribute to survival benefit of spironolactone therapy in patients with congestive cardiac failure. *Circulation* 2000; **102**: 2700–6.

30 Pitt B, Poole-Wilson PA, Segal R, *et al.* Effect of losartan compared with captopril on mortality in patients with symptomatic heart failure: randomised trial. The losartan heart failure survival study ELITE II. *Lancet* 2000; **355**: 1582–7.

31 Cohn JN, Tognoni G. A randomised trial of the angiotensin-receptor blocker valsartan in chronic heart failure. *N Engl J Med* 2001; **345**: 1667–75.

32 Granger CB, McMurray JJ, Yusuf S, *et al.* Effects of candesartan in patients with chronic heart failure and reduced left-ventricular systolic function intolerant to ACE inhibitors: the CHARM-alternative trial. *Lancet* 2003; **362**: 772–6.

33 McMurray JJV, Ostergren J, Swedberg K, *et al.* Effects of candesartan in patients with chronic heart failure and reduced left-ventricular systolic function taking ACE inhibitors: the CHARM-added trial. *Lancet* 2003; **362**: 767–71.

34 Pfeffer MA, McMurray JJ, Velazquez EJ, *et al.* Valsartan, captopril or both in myocardial infarction complicated by heart failure, left ventricular dysfunction, or both. *N Engl J Med* 2003; **349**: 1893–906.

35 Dickstein K, Kjekshus J and the OPTIMAAL steering committee. Effects of losartan and captopril on mortality and morbidity in high-risk patients after acute myocardial infarction: the OPTIMAAL randomised trial. *Lancet* 2002; **360**: 752–60.

36 Mann DL, Deswal A. Angiotensin-receptor blockade in acute myocardial infarction: a matter of dose. *N Engl J Med* 2003; **349**: 1963–5.

37 Coletta AP, Cleland JG, Freemantle N, *et al.* Clinical trials update from the European Society of Cardiology: CHARM, BASEL, EUROPA and ESTEEM. *Eur J Heart Fail* 2003; **5**: 697–704.

38 Bouzamondo A, Hulot JS, Sanchez P, Lechat P. β-Blocker benefit according to severity of heart failure. *Eur J Heart Fail* 2003; **5**: 281–9.

39 Lohse M, Engelhardt S, Eschenhagen T. What is the role of β-adrenergic signalling in heart failure? *Circ Res* 2003; **93**: 896–906.

40 The β-Blocker Evaluation of Survival Trial Investigators. A trial of the β-blocker bucindolol in patients with advanced chronic heart failure. *N Engl J Med* 2001; **344**: 1659–67.

41 Bristow M. Antiadrenergic therapy of chronic heart failure. *Circulation* 2003; **107**: 1100–2.

42 Andreka P, Aiyar N, Olson LC, *et al.* Bucindolol displays intrinsic sympathomimetic activity in human myocardium. *Circulation* 2002; **105**: 2429–34.

43 Poole-Wilson PA, Swedburg K, Cleland JG, *et al.* Comparison of carvedilol and metoprolol on clinical outcomes in patients with chronic heart failure in the Carvedilol or Metoprolol European Trial (COMET): randomised controlled trial. *Lancet* 2003; **362**: 7–13.

44 Dargie HJ. β-Blockers in heart failure. *Lancet* 2003; **362**: 2–3.

45 Juurlink DN, Mamdani MM, Lee DS, *et al.* Rates of hyperkalaemia after publication of the Randomised Aldactone Evaluation Study. *N Engl J Med* 2004; **351**: 543–51.

46 McMurray JJV, O'Meara E. Treatment of heart failure with spironolactone: trials and tribulations. *N Engl J Med* 2004; **351**: 526–8.

47 Abraham WT, Hayes DL. Cardiac resynchronization therapy for heart failure. *Circulation* 2003; **108**: 2596–603.

48 Bristow MR, Saxon LA, Boehmer J, *et al.* Cardiac resynchronization therapy with or without an implantable defibrillator in advanced chronic heart failure. *N Engl J Med* 2004; **350**: 2140–50.

49 Salukhe TV, Dimopoulos K, Francis D. Cardiac resynchronization may reduce all-cause mortality: meta-analysis of preliminary COMPANION data with CONTAK-CD, Insync ICD, MIRACLE and MUSTIC. *In J Cardiol* 2004; **93**: 101–3.

50 Cleland JGF, Daubert J-C, Erdmann E, *et al.* The effect of cardiac resynchronization on morbidity and mortality in heart failure. *N Engl J Med* 2005; **352**: 1539–49.

51 Garrigue S, Reuter S, Labeque JN, *et al.* Usefulness of biventricular pacing in patients with congestive heart failure and right bundle branch block. *Am J Cardiol* 2001; **88**: 1436–41.

52 Leclercq C, Walker S, Linde C, *et al.* Comparative effects of permanent biventricular and right-univentricular pacing in heart failure patients with chronic atrial fibrillation. *Eur Heart J* 2002; **23**: 1780–7.

53 Leon AR, Greenberg JM, Kanura N, *et al.* Cardiac resynchronization in patients with congestive cardiac failure and chronic atrial fibrillation. *J Am Coll Cardiol* 2002; **39**: 1258–63.

54 Yu C-M, Lin H, Zhang Q, Sanderson JE. High prevalence of left ventricular systolic and diastolic asynchrony in patients with congestive heart failure and normal QRS duration. *Heart* 2003; **89**: 54–60.

55 Yu C-M, Yang H, Lau CP, *et al.* Regional left ventricular mechanical asynchrony in patients with heart disease and normal QRS duration: implications for biventricular pacing therapy. *PACE* 2003; **26** (Part 1): 562–70.

56 Huikuri HV, Castellanos A, Myerburg RJ. Sudden death due to cardiac arrhythmias. *N Engl J Med* 2001; **345**: 1473–82.

57 Zipes DP, Wellens HJJ. Sudden cardiac death. *Circulation* 1998; **98**: 2334–51.

58 Gregoratos G, Abrams J, Epstein AE, *et al.* ACC/AHA/NASPE 2002 guideline update for implantation of cardiac pacemakers and antiarrhythmia devices: summary article. *Circulation* 2002; **106**: 2145–61.

59 AVID Investigators. A comparison of anti-arrhythmic drug therapy with implantable defibrillators in patients resuscitated from near fatal ventricular arrhythmias. *N Engl J Med* 1997; **337**: 1576–83.

60 Connolly SJ, Gent M, Roberts RS, *et al.* Canadian implantable defibrillator study (CIDS). *Circulation* 2000; **101**: 1297–302.

61 Kuck KH, Cappato R, Siebels J, Ruppel R. Randomised comparison of antiarrhythmic drug therapy with implantable defibrillators in patients resuscitated from cardiac arrest (CASH). *Circulation* 2000; **102**: 748–54.

62 Connolly SJ, Hallstrom AP, Cappato R, *et al.* Meta-analysis of the implantable cardioverter defibrillator secondary prevention trials. *Eur Heart J* 2000; **21**: 2071–8.

63 Moss AJ, Hall WJ, Cannom DS, *et al.* Improved survival with an implantable defibrillator in patients with coronary disease at high risk for ventricular arrhythmias. *N Engl J Med* 1996; **335**: 1933–40.

64 Buxton AE, Lee KL, Fisher JD, *et al.* A randomised study of the prevention of sudden death in patients with coronary artery disease. *N Engl J Med* 1999; **341**: 1882–90.

65 Salukhe TV, Dimopoulos K, Sutton R, *et al.* Life-years gained from defibrillator implantation. *Circulation* 2004; **109**: 1848–53.

66 Moss AJ, Zareba W, Hall WJ, *et al.* Prophylactic implantation of a defibrillator in patients with myocardial infarction and reduced ejection fraction. *N Engl J Med* 2002; **346**: 877–83.

67 Bansch D, Antz M, Boczor S, *et al.* Primary prevention of sudden cardiac death in idiopathic dilated cardiomyopathy. *Circulation* 2002; **105**: 1453–8.

68 Strickberger SA, Hummel JD, Bartlett TG, *et al.* Amiodarone versus implantable cardioverter defibrillator: randomised trial in patients with non-ischaemic dilated cardiomyopathy and non-sustained ventricular tachycardia—AMIOVIRT. *J Am Coll Cardiol* 2003; **41**: 1707–12.

69 Kadish A, Dyer A, Daubert JP, *et al.* Prophylactic defibrillator implantation in patients with non-ischaemic

dilated cardiomyopathy. *N Engl J Med* 2004; **350**: 2151–8.

70 Bardy GH. The Sudden Cardiac Death in Heart Failure Trial. Available at: http://www.sicr.org/scdheft_results_acc_lbcc.pdf

71 Hauer RNW, Aliot E, Block M, *et al.* Indications for implantable cardioverter defibrillator (ICD) therapy. *Eur Heart J* 2001; **22**: 1074–81.

72 DiMarco JP. Implantable cardioverter-defibrillators. *N Engl J Med* 2003; **349**: 1836–47.

73 Cha Y, Redfield MM, Shen WK, Gersch BJ. Atrial fibrillation and ventricular dysfunction. *Circulation* 2004; **109**: 2839–43.

74 AFFIRM investigators. A comparison of rate control and rhythm control in patients with atrial fibrillation. *N Engl J Med* 2002; **347**: 1825–33.

75 Van Gelder IC, Hagens VE, Bosker HA, *et al.* A comparison of rate control and rhythm control in patients with recurrent persistent atrial fibrillation. *N Engl J Med* 2002; **347**: 1834–40.

76 Hohnloser SH, Kuck K, Lilienthal J. Rhythm or rate control in atrial fibrillation: pharmacological intervention in atrial fibrillation (PIAF): a randomised trial. *Lancet* 2000; **356**: 1789–94.

77 Roy D. Rationale for the atrial fibrillation and congestive heart failure trial. *Card Electrophysiol Rev* 2003; **7**: 208–10.

78 Fuster V, Ryden LE, Asinger RW, *et al.* ACC/AHA/ESC guidelines for the management of patients with atrial fibrillation: executive summary. *Circulation* 2001; **104**: 2118–50.

79 Wijns W, Vatner SF, Camici PG. Hibernating myocardium. *N Engl J Med* 1998; **339**: 173–81.

80 Allman KC, Shaw LJ, Hachamovitch R, Udelson JE. Myocardial viability testing and impact of revascularization on prognosis in patients with coronary artery disease and left ventricular dysfunction: a meta-analysis. *J Am Coll Cardiol* 2002; **39**: 1151–8.

81 Cleland JGF, John J, Dhawan J, Clark A. What is the optimal medical management of ischaemic failure? *Br Med Bull* 2001; **59**: 135–58.

82 Passamani E, Davis KB, Gillespie MJ, Killip T. A randomized trial of coronary artery bypass surgery: survival of patients with a low ejection fraction. *N Engl J Med* 1985; **312**: 1665–71.

83 Shan K, Constantine G, Sivananthan M, Flamm SD. Role of cardiac magnetic resonance imaging in the assessment of myocardial viability. *Circulation* 2004; **109**: 1328–34.

84 Cleland JGF, Freemantle N, Ball SG, *et al.* The heart failure revascularization trial (HEART): rationale, design and methodology. *Eur J Heart Fail* 2003; **5**: 295–303.

85 Information about the Surgical Treatments for Ischaemic Heart Failure (STICH) trial available at: www.stichtrial.org

86 Hogg K, Swedberg K, McMurray J. Heart failure with preserved left ventricular systolic function. *J Am Coll Cardiol* 2004; **43**: 317–27.

87 Fischer M, Baessler A, Hense HW, *et al.* Prevalence of left ventricular diastolic dysfunction in the community. *Eur Heart J* 2003; **24**: 320–8.

88 Redfield MM, Jacobsen SJ, Burnett JC, *et al.* Burden of systolic and diastolic ventricular dysfunction in the community. *JAMA* 2003; **289**: 194–202.

89 Zile MR, Baicu CF, Gaasch WH. Diastolic heart failure: abnormalities in active relaxation and passive stiffness of the left ventricle. *N Engl J Med* 2004; **350**: 1953–9.

90 Angeja BG, Grossman W. Evaluation and management of diastolic heart failure. *Circulation* 2003; **107**: 659–63.

91 Zile MR, Brutsaert DL. New concepts in diastolic dysfunction and diastolic heart failure: Part II. *Circulation* 2002; **105**: 1503–8.

92 Banerjee P, Banerjee T, Khand A, Clark AL, Cleland JG. Diastolic heart failure: neglected or misdiagnosed? *J Am Coll Cardiol* 2002; **39**: 138–41.

93 Vasan RS, Levy D. Defining diastolic heart failure: a call for standardized diagnostic criteria. *Circulation* 2000; **101**: 2118–21.

94 European Study Group on Diastolic Heart Failure. How to diagnose diastolic heart failure. *Eur Heart J* 1998; **19**: 990–1003.

95 Cahill JM, Horan M, Quigley P, Maurer B, McDonald K. Doppler-echocardiographic indices of diastolic function in heart failure admissions with preserved left ventricular systolic function. *Eur J Heart Fail* 2002; **4**: 473–8.

96 Dahlstrom U. Can natriuretic peptides be used for the diagnosis of diastolic heart failure? *Eur J Heart Fail* 2004; **6**: 281–7.

97 Grodecki PV, Klein AL. Pitfalls in echo-doppler assessment of diastolic dysfunction. *Echocardiography* 1993; **10**: 213–34.

98 Zile MR, Brutsaert DL. New concepts in diastolic dysfunction and diastolic heart failure: Part I. *Circulation* 2002; **105**: 1387–93.

99 Digitalis Investigation Group. The effect of digoxin on mortality and morbidity in patients with heart failure. *N Engl J Med* 1997; **336**: 525–33.

100 Bergstrom A, Andersson B, Edner M, *et al.* Effect of carvedilol on diastolic function in patients with diasto-

lic heart failure and preserved systolic function. Results of the Swedish Doppler-echocardiographic study. *Eur J Heart Fail* 2004; **6**: 453–61.

101 Yusuf S, Pfeffer MA, Swedberg K, *et al*. Effects of candesartan in patients with chronic heart failure and preserved left-ventricular ejection fraction: the CHARM-Preserved trial. *Lancet* 2003; **362**: 777–81.

102 Setaro JF, Soufer R, Remetz MS, Perlmutter RA, Zaret BL. Long-term outcome in patients with congestive heart failure and intact systolic left ventricular performance. *Am J Cardiol* 1992; **69**: 1212–6.

103 Brogan WC, Hillis LD, Flores ED, Lange RA. The natural history of isolated left ventricular diastolic dysfunction. *Am J Med* 1992; **92**: 627–30.

104 Philbin EF, Rocco TA, Lindenmutt NW, Ulrich K, Jenkins PL. Systolic versus diastolic heart failure in community practice: clinical features, outcomes, and the use of ACE inhibitors. *Am J Med* 2000; **109**: 605–13.

105 Pernenkil R, Vinison JM, Shah AS, *et al*. Course and prognosis in patients ≥70 years of age with congestive heart failure and normal versus abnormal left ventricular ejection fraction. *Am J Cardiol* 1997; **79**: 216–9.

106 Vasan RS, Larson MG, Benjamin EJ, *et al*. Congestive heart failure in subjects with normal versus reduced left ventricular ejection fraction. *J Am Coll Cardiol* 1999; **33**: 1948–55.

107 Kupari M, Lindroos M, Iivanainen AM, Heikkila J, Tilvis R. Congestive heart failure in old age: prevalence, mechanisms and 4-year prognosis in the Helsinki Ageing Study. *J Intern Med* 1997; **241**: 387–94.

108 Gottdiener JS, McClelland RL, Marshall R, *et al*. Outcome of congestive heart failure in elderly persons: influence of left ventricular systolic function. *Ann Intern Med* 2002; **137**: 631–9.

109 Senni M, Tribouilloy CM, Rodeheffer RJ, *et al*. Congestive heart failure in the community: a study of all incident cases in Olmsted County, Minnesota, in 1991. *Circulation* 1998; **98**: 2282–9.

110 Lenzen MJ, Scholte op Reimer WJ, Boersma E, *et al*. Differences between patients with preserved and a depressed left ventricular function: a report from the EuroHeart Failure survey. *Eur Heart J* 2004; **25**: 1214–20.

111 Sudoh T, Kangawa K, Minamino N, Matsuo H. A new natriuretic peptide in porcine brain. *Nature* 1988; **332**: 78–81.

112 Hall C. Essential biochemistry and physiology of (NT-pro)BNP. *Eur J Heart Fail* 2004; **6**: 257–60.

113 Vanderheyden M, Bartunek J, Goethals M. Brain and other natriuretic peptides: molecular aspects. *Eur J Heart Fail* 2004; **6**: 261–8.

114 Cowie MR, Jourdain P, Maisel A, *et al*. Clinical applications of B-type natriuretic peptide (BNP) testing. *Eur Heart J* 2003; **24**: 1710–8.

115 Mueller C, Scholer A, Laule-Kilian K, *et al*. Use of BNP in the evaluation and management of acute dyspnoea. *N Engl J Med* 2004; **350**: 647–4.

116 Wang TJ, Larson MG, Levy D, *et al*. Plasma natriuretic peptide levels and risk of cardiovascular events and death. *N Engl J Med* 2004; **350**: 655–63.

117 McDonagh TA, Holmer S, Raymond I, *et al*. NT-proBNP and the diagnosis of heart failure: a pooled analysis of three European epidemiological studies. *Eur J Heart Fail* 2004; **6**: 269–3.

118 Lubien E, De Maria A, Krishnaswamy P, *et al*. Utility of B-natriuretic peptide in detecting diastolic dysfunction. *Circulation* 2002; **105**: 595–601.

119 Kirk V, Bay M, Parner J, *et al*. NT-proBNP and mortality in hospitalized patients with heart failure and preserved versus reduced systolic function: data from the prospective Copenhagen Hospital Heart Failure Study (CHHF). *Eur J Heart Fail* 2004; **6**: 335–41.

120 Stevenson LW, Rose EA. Left ventricular assist devices: bridges to transplantation, recovery and destination for whom? *Circulation* 2003; **108**: 3059–63.

121 Rose EA, Gelljns AC, Moskowitz AJ, *et al*. Long-term use of a left ventricular assist device for end-stage heart failure. *N Engl J Med* 2001; **345**: 1435–43.

122 Hassink RJ, Brutel de la Riviere A, Mummery CL, Doevendans PA. Transplantation of cells for cardiac repair. *J Am Coll Cardiol* 2003; **41**: 711–7.

123 Perin EC, Dohmann HF, Borojevic R, *et al*. Transendocardial, autologous bone marrow cell transplantation for severe, chronic ischaemic heart failure. *Circulation* 2003; **107**: 2294–302.

124 Wollert KC, Meyer GP, Lotz J, *et al*. Intracoronary autologous bone-marrow cell transfer after myocardial infarction: the BOOST randomised controlled clinical trial. *Lancet* 2004; **364**: 141–8.

125 Murry CE, Soonpaa MH, Reinecke H, *et al*. Haemopoietic stem cells do not transdifferentiate into cardiac myocytes in myocardial infarcts. *Nature* 2004; **428**: 664–8.

126 Balsam LB, Wagers AJ, Christensen JL, *et al*. Haemopoietic stem cells adopt mature haemopoietic fates in ischaemic myocardium. *Nature* 2004; **428**: 668–73.

CHAPTER 21

The hormonal and metabolic response to anaesthesia, surgery and trauma

Grainne Nicholson and George M. Hall

Introduction

The stress response refers to the series of hormonal, inflammatory, metabolic and psychological changes, which occur in response to trauma or surgery. Surgery serves as a useful model of the stress response because the changes that occur can be observed from a well-defined starting point, but similar features occur in trauma, burns, severe infection and strenuous exercise. Furthermore, patients sustaining major trauma have an initial stress response but then are subjected to further physiological challenges during surgery. These changes result in substrate mobilization, muscle protein loss and sodium and water retention. Such changes may have evolved to aid survival in a more primitive environment, when fluid retention together with glucose, lipid and protein mobilization would be beneficial to an injured animal that was unable to drink and eat. In modern surgical practice, where such physiological disturbances may be easily prevented or rapidly corrected, the benefits of the stress response are less obvious [1]. These physiological changes are accompanied by complex psychological and behavioural changes, which result in postoperative malaise and fatigue. The underlying causes are poorly understood but personality and preoperative mental status, change of environment, anxiety and fear, immobilization and alterations in normal diurnal rhythms may all have a role [2].

Recently, it has been suggested that multiorgan failure following infection, major trauma or other critical illness may also be a potentially protective mechanism, because reduced cellular metabolism could increase the chances of survival of cells and thus organs, so multiorgan failure may be considered a functional rather than structural abnormality, which occurs as a result of acute phase changes in hormones and inflammatory mediators [3].

It has been argued that attenuating the metabolic and endocrine changes associated with surgery may reduce postoperative morbidity and expedite recovery. However, there is no strict definition of recovery. Many studies have looked at outcomes following major surgery, but this commonly refers to serious morbidity or mortality. There is no agreement on how recovery is best defined or how it can be measured, although time to eating and drinking, return to activities of daily living (ADL) and return to work have all been used [4].

One of the first formal descriptions of the stress response was by Cuthbertson [5] who, in 1932, documented the metabolic responses of four patients with lower limb injuries. He described the physiological changes that occurred and introduced the terms 'ebb' and 'flow' to illustrate the initial decrease, and subsequent increase, in metabolic activity. The early descriptive studies were soon replicated and extended by further investigators [6] but attempts to link the systemic stress response with hormonal changes were initially hampered by difficulties in accurately measuring so-called 'stress hormones' [7–10].

Measurement of corticosteroids in the 1950s confirmed increased glucocorticoid secretion following injury and, in 1959, Hume [11] and Egdahl [12] demonstrated that afferent neuronal input from the surgical site activated hypothalamic–pituitary hormone secretion and the sympathetic nervous system. In animals with an intact sciatic nerve or spinal cord, operative injury or superficial burns to a limb caused a rapid and sustained increase in adrenal hormones. If the nerve or spinal cord was transected, these changes were prevented.

The development of reliable assay techniques for catecholamines by von Euler and colleagues enabled the physiological effects of increased sympathetic nervous system activity following surgery to be studied [13–15]. Hypothalamic activation of the autonomic nervous system results in increased secretion from the adrenal medulla and presynaptic nerve terminals leading to the well-recognized cardiovascular effects of hypertension and tachycardia, as well as some of the metabolic aspects of the stress response such as hyperglycaemia.

The existence of 'wound hormones' has been postulated since the 1950s. The hypothesis that local substances can influence many of the changes associated with surgery was advanced by the discovery of cytokines and their role in the perioperative stress response. Early studies of cytokines from the 1950s to the 1970s involved the description of numerous protein factors produced by different cells that mediated particular functions *in vitro*. The second phase of cytokine research involved the purification of many individual cytokines and, in the past two decades, molecular cloning and the production of highly specific assays have resulted in the precise identification of the structure and properties of individual cytokines [16].

Initiation of the stress response

Hormones

The hypothalamic–pituitary axis and the sympathetic nervous system are activated by afferent neuronal input from the operative or injured site (both somatic and autonomic) and by the release of cytokines from the damaged area. The pituitary response is characterized by an increase in the secretion of adrenocorticotrophin (ACTH), growth hormone (GH), β endorphin and prolactin from the anterior pituitary. The secretion of luteinizing hormone (LH), follicle-stimulating hormone (FSH) and thyroid-stimulating hormone (TSH) also changes, but these

hormones have been studied in much less detail. Arginine vasopressin (AVP) is released from the posterior pituitary. The increased pituitary hormone secretion has secondary effects on target organs. Corticotrophin (ACTH) from the anterior pituitary stimulates cortisol secretion from the adrenal gland and AVP increases the permeability of the collecting ducts in the kidney. In general, the magnitude of the response is proportional to the severity of the trauma and there is a failure of the normal feedback mechanisms that control hormone secretion. For example, hypercortisolaemia fails to inhibit further production of ACTH and, similarly, hyperglycaemia fails to inhibit GH secretion. Enhanced secretion of catabolic hormones predominates, whereas anabolic hormone secretion, such as insulin and testosterone, is suppressed.

Sympathoadrenal response

Hypothalamic activation of the sympathetic autonomic nervous system results in increased secretion of catecholamines from the adrenal medulla and release of noradrenaline (norepinephrine) from presynaptic nerve terminals. Noradrenaline serves predominantly as a neurotransmitter, but some of that released from nerve terminals spills over into the circulation. This increased sympathetic activity results in the well-recognized cardiovascular effects of tachycardia, hypertension and hyperglycaemia. Recently, strenuous efforts have been made to reduce perioperative cardiac morbidity by obtunding the increase in sympathetic activity with perioperative β-blockade [17–19], or by the use of α_2-adrenergic agonists [20–23].

In addition, the function of certain visceral organs, including the liver, pancreas and kidneys, is modified directly by efferent sympathetic stimulation and by circulating catecholamines [24]. Sympathetic stimulation of the pancreas results in an increase in glucagon secretion and inhibition of insulin secretion. Glucagon release stimulates glycogen breakdown in the liver and muscle leading to increased glucose and lactate concentrations. There is mobilization of free fatty acids from triglyceride stores. Renin is released from the kidneys leading to the conversion of angiotensin I to angiotensin II. The latter stimulates the secretion of aldosterone from the adrenal cortex, which, in turn, increases sodium absorption from the distal convoluted tubule of the kidney.

Cortisol

Corticotrophin (ACTH) from the anterior pituitary is secreted in response to corticotrophin-releasing hormone (CRH), a 41 amino acid peptide synthesized in the hypothalamus and secreted into the hypophyseal–portal system. The onset of surgery is associated with the rapid secretion of ACTH, which is synthesized as part of a large precursor molecule, pro-opiomelanocortin (POMC). In the human anterior pituitary, POMC is cleaved by a serine endoprotease, predominantly into ACTH, β-lipotropin and an N-terminal precursor. AVP has an important role in the control of ACTH secretion during stress, by directly stimulating the release of ACTH and acting synergistically with CRH, as well as regulating pituitary CRH receptor expression.

ACTH acts on the adrenal gland through a specific cell surface receptor, a member of the G-protein-coupled receptor family. Feedback inhibition by cortisol normally prevents any further increases in CRH or ACTH production. Cortisol is a C^{21} corticosteroid with both glucocorticoid and mineralocorticoid activity [25]. Endogenous cortisol production is 25–30 mg/day and circulating concentrations vary in a circadian pattern, with a half-life in the circulation of 60–90 minutes [26].

Plasma cortisol concentrations increase rapidly in response to surgical stimulation and remain elevated for a variable time following surgery. Peak values are achieved 4–6 hours after surgery or injury and return towards baseline after 24 hours [27]; this increase in plasma cortisol may, however, be sustained for up to 48–72 hours following major surgery, such as cardiac surgery. The magnitude and duration of the cortisol response reflect the severity of surgical trauma, as well as the occurrence of postoperative complications, and values >1500 nmol/L are not uncommon [28,29]. Increased cortisol production is secondary to ACTH secretion, but the plasma ACTH concentration is far greater than that required to produce a maximal adrenocortical response. Furthermore, the normal pituitary adrenocortical feedback mechanism is no longer effective, as both hormones remain increased simultaneously. The administration of ACTH during surgery does not cause a further increase in cortisol secretion [27].

The amount of cortisol secreted following major surgery, such as abdominal or thoracic surgery, is 75–100 mg on the first day [30–32]. Minor surgery, such as herniorrhaphy, induces less than 50 mg cortisol secretion during the first 24 hours [33]. However, because of changes in volume of distribution and half-life of cortisol during surgery, these calculations may be an overestimation [34].

Cortisol has complex effects on the intermediate metabolism of carbohydrate, fat and protein [35]. It causes an increase in blood glucose concentration by stimulating protein catabolism and promoting glucose production in the liver and kidney by gluconeogenesis from the mobilized amino acids. Cortisol reduces peripheral glucose utilization by an anti-insulin effect. Glucocorticoids inhibit the recruitment of neutrophils and monocyte–macrophages into the area of inflammation [36,37] and also have well-described anti-inflammatory actions, mediated by a decrease in the production of inflammatory mediators such as leukotrienes and prostaglandins [38]. In addition, there is immunoregulatory feedback between the glucocorticoid hormones and interleukin-6 (IL-6); the production and action of IL-6 are inhibited by ACTH and cortisol [39].

Growth hormone

The secretion of GH, a 191 amino acid protein, is controlled by growth hormone releasing hormone (GRH) and somatostatin released by the hypothalamus. GRH secretion is episodic and surges in growth hormone secretion usually coincide with increases in its secretion. Somatostatin secretion is more tonic. Somatostatin is also found in the endocrine pancreas, where it inhibits secretion of insulin and other pancreatic hormones, and in the gastrointestinal tract where it is an important inhibitory gastrointestinal hormone. Growth hormone, also known as somatotrophin, has a major role in growth regulation. The anabolic effects of growth hormone are mediated through polypeptides synthesized in the liver, muscle and other tissues. These are called somatomedins or insulin-like growth factors (because of their structural similarity to insulin) and act on cartilage, bone and skeletal muscle. Several insulin-like growth factors (IGFs) have been isolated; the main polypeptide is somatomedin C or IGF-1. In addition to its effects on growth, GH has many effects on metabolism. In particular, it stimulates protein synthesis and inhibits protein breakdown. Other metabolic effects of GH include stimulation of lipolysis and an anti-insulin effect. This results in inhibition of glucose uptake and oxidation by cells, thus sparing it for use by tissues that have obligatory requirements for glucose such as brain, renal medulla, retina and red blood cells. GH also stimulates glycogenolysis in the liver; however, the diabetogenic effects of GH are not thought to be significant during surgery and hormones such as cortisol and catecholamines have a more significant role in perioperative hyperglycaemia. Growth hormone has enjoyed a resurgence of interest as its potential for promoting anabolism after injury has been explored. Attempts have been made to use recombinant growth hormone, IGF-1 or both to reduce muscle catabolism and improve wound healing in severely catabolic states and in critically ill patients, but as yet the evidence is inconclusive [40–42]. In some patients the use of GH was associated with increased mortality [42].

β-Endorphin and prolactin

β-Endorphin is an opioid, a 31 amino-acid peptide produced from the cleavage of POMC and increased concentrations during surgery reflect anterior pituitary stimulation. The secretion of prolactin is under tonic inhibitory control via prolactin-release-inhibitory-factor (dopamine) and increased prolactin secretion occurs by release of inhibitory control. Increased circulating prolactin concentrations are found after surgery and exercise. Prolactin has a major role during pregnancy and lactation. The physiological effects of increased secretion of both hormones during surgery are unknown, but they may alter immune function.

Insulin and glucagon

Insulin is a polypeptide hormone secreted by β cells of the pancreas. Its structure consists of a 21 amino acid and a 30 amino acid peptide chain linked by di-

sulphide cross-bridges. It is the key anabolic hormone and is normally released after food intake, when blood glucose and amino acid concentrations increase (Table 21.1). Insulin promotes the uptake of glucose into muscle, liver and adipose tissue and its conversion into glycogen and triglycerides. Hepatic glycogenolysis and hepatic and renal gluconeogenesis are inhibited, but at higher concentrations of insulin than those that mediate the peripheral effects.

The hyperglycaemic response to surgical stress is characterized by the failure of insulin secretion to respond to the glucose stimulus [43]. This is caused partly by α_2-adrenergic inhibition of β-cell secretion and also by insulin resistance, where a normal or even elevated concentration of insulin produces a subnormal biological response. Insulin resistance has been defined as 'the unresponsiveness of anabolic processes to the normal effects of insulin' [44]. The precise mechanisms underlying the development of insulin resistance following surgery or trauma remain unclear, but are not simply elevated concentrations of counter-regulatory hormones such as cortisol and excessive cytokine secretion [45]. Enthusiastic attempts have been made to con-

Table 21.1 Key metabolic effects of insulin.

Carbohydrate metabolism
Increases uptake of glucose into skeletal muscle and adipose tissue

Increases storage of glucose as glycogen in muscle and liver

Reduces rate of breakdown of glycogen in muscle and liver

Reduces conversion of amino acids to glucose in liver and kidney (gluconeogenesis)

Lipid metabolism
Increases lipogenesis in the liver

Reduces lipolysis in adipose tissue

Decreases ketone body production by the liver

Protein metabolism
Increases uptake of amino acids by skeletal muscle and liver

Reduces rate of protein breakdown in skeletal muscle

---

trol perioperative hyperglycaemia, particularly because the clinical benefits of returning blood glucose
concentrations to normal in surgical intensive care
patients has been shown clearly by van den Berghe
et al. [46]. It has been suggested that postoperative or
post-traumatic insulin resistance can be prevented
or attenuated by previous glucose loading via the
oral or intravenous route [47–49].

Glucagon is produced in the α cells of the pancreas.
In contrast to insulin, glucagon release promotes hepatic glycogenolysis and gluconeogenesis; it also has
lipolytic activity. Concentrations increase briefly
in response to surgical procedures, but it is not
thought to contribute significantly to perioperative
hyperglycaemia.

Thyroid-stimulating hormone and thyroid hormones

Thyrotropin or thyroid-stimulating hormone (TSH),
secreted by the anterior pituitary, promotes the
production and secretion of thyroxine (T3) and
triiodothyronine (T4) from the thyroid gland. The
secretion of TSH is controlled by a tripeptide, thyro-
tropin-releasing hormone (TRH) from the hypothalamus, and the blood concentration of free T3 and
T4. Small amounts of metabolically inactive reverse
T3 (rT3) are also produced. T3 is formed in the tissues
by deiodination of T4 and it is 3–5 times more active
than T4. Both hormones are extensively protein
bound, to albumin, thyroxine-binding pre-albumin
and thyroid-binding globulin, and have a long half-
life (T3, 24 h; T4, 7 days). The free thyroid hormones
in the circulation are metabolically active and their
concentrations are in equilibrium with bound hormones [50]. Free T3 and T4 exert negative feedback
on TSH secretion at the anterior pituitary. Thyroid
hormones stimulate oxygen consumption in most of
the metabolically active tissues of the body, with the
exception of brain, spleen and anterior pituitary.
Consequently, metabolic rate and heat production
are also increased. There is rapid cellular uptake of
glucose, increased glycolysis and gluconeogenesis
and enhanced carbohydrate absorbtion from the gut
in order to fuel increased metabolic activity. Thyroxine increases lipid mobilization from adipose tissue
causing an increase in free fatty acids but a decrease
in plasma cholesterol, phospholipids and triglycerides. In physiological concentrations T3 and T4 have
a protein anabolic effect, but in larger doses their
effects are catabolic.

The activity of thyroid hormones is closely associated with that of catecholamines. Adrenaline and
noradrenaline also increase the metabolic rate and
thyroid hormones increase the sensitivity of the
heart to catecholamines by increasing the number
and affinity of cardiac β receptors.

Concentrations of TSH increase during surgery, or
immediately afterwards, but this effect is not prolonged. However, there is usually a pronounced and
prolonged decrease in T3 concentrations (both free
and protein-bound) and an increase in rT3. This is
caused partly by cortisol, which has a suppressive effect on TSH secretion and which induces preferential
formation of metabolically inactive rT3 [3]. Changes
in thyroid hormone metabolism may represent
adaptive responses to limit increases in metabolic
rate in the presence of increased sympathetic
activity.

Gonadotrophins

The gonadotrophins LH and FSH are secreted from
the anterior pituitary. FSH is responsible for development of ovarian follicles in women and maintenance of the spermatic epithelium in males. LH
stimulates growth and development of the Leydig
cells of the testis, which produce testosterone. In
females, LH promotes maturation of the ovarian
follicle and the secretion of oestrogen. It also stimulates formation of the corpus luteum from the
follicles after ovulation. Testosterone is a C19 steroid, synthesized from cholesterol in the Leydig cells
of the testis. Small amounts are also produced from
the adrenal cortex. Testosterone has a negative feedback effect on LH secretion from the anterior pituitary. In addition to its reproductive effects,
testosterone has important effects on protein anabolism and growth. Following surgery, testosterone
concentrations are decreased for several days, although LH concentrations show variable changes
[51]. Oestrogen concentrations have also been
shown to decrease for up to 5 days following surgery
[52]. This may be caused, in part, by changes in cortisol and prolactin [3]. The significance of these changes is uncertain, but the decline in testosterone

secretion is another example of the failure of anabolic hormone secretion.

Arginine vasopressin

The posterior pituitary is an extension of the hypothalamus and secretes two hormones, AVP and oxytocin. Both hormones are synthesized in the cell bodies of the supraoptic nucleus and the paraventricular nucleus of the hypothalamus. They are bound to a specific transport protein, neurophysin, and transported in vesicles along the axons to coalesce into storage vesicles in the nerve terminals of the posterior pituitary. AVP is a nonapeptide with a biological half-life of 16–20 minutes. Three receptors have been identified: V_{1A}, V_{1B} and V_2. All are G-protein-coupled. The V_{1A} and V_{1B} receptors act through phosphotidylinositol hydolysis to increase intracellular Ca^{2+} concentration. V_2 receptors act through Gs to increase cyclic adenosine monophosphate (cAMP) concentrations. The V_{1A} receptors mediate vasoconstriction. Vasopressin is a potent stimulator of vascular smooth muscle *in vitro* but large amounts are required to raise blood pressure *in vivo* because vasopressin also acts at the area postrema to cause a decrease in cardiac output. Haemorrhage is a potent stimulus to vasopressin secretion. V_{1A} receptors also occur in the liver and brain. Vasopressin causes glycogenolysis in the liver and serves as a neurotransmitter in the brain and spinal cord. V_{1B} receptors (also known as V_3 receptors) are found in the anterior pituitary and increase ACTH release. Vasopressin exerts its antidiuretic effect via V_2 receptors by activating protein water channels in the luminal membranes of the principal cells of the collecting ducts. In certain physiological situations, simple diffusion of water is augmented by movement through water channels called aquaporins. Five of these have now been identified and the vasopressin-responsive water channel in the collecting ducts is aquaporin-2. These channels are stored in endosomes inside the cell and vasopressin causes their rapid translocation to the luminal membranes [53]. In addition, AVP enhances haemostasis by increasing factor VIII activity.

Cytokines

The concept that circulating factors, so-called 'wound hormones', released from the site of injury or trauma could be responsible for some of the metabolic changes associated with surgery has existed since the 1950s. Indeed, surgical patients have been described as 'a stew of pulsating cytokines' [54].

Cytokines are low molecular weight (<80 kDa), heterogeneous glycoproteins, which include interleukins, interferons, growth factors and tumour necrosis factor (TNF). They are synthesized by activated macrophages, neutrophils, lymphotcyes, fibroblasts, endothelial and glial cells in response to tissue injury from surgery or trauma [16]. Although they exert most of their effects locally (paracrine), they can also act systemically (endocrine). Cytokines have an important role in mediating immunity and inflammation by acting on surface receptors of target cells. The most important cytokine associated with surgery is IL-6. Increases occur 2–4 hours after the start of surgery, with peak values occurring after 12–24 hours. The size and duration of the IL-6 response reflects the severity of tissue damage [55]. Cytokine secretion cannot be modified by the use of neuronal blockade [56] but laparoscopic surgical techniques result in smaller increases in IL-6 than those following conventional open surgery [57]. Circulating TNF-α and IL-1β values do not change significantly unless there is malignancy or underlying chronic infection, but increases may be found locally at the site of tissue damage.

The immune and the neuroendocrine systems are closely interconnected. IL-1 and IL-6 have been shown to stimulate secretion from isolated pituitary cells [58]. In surgical patients, circulating cytokines may augment pituitary ACTH secretion and consequently increase the release of cortisol, sustaining the glucocorticoid response to injury for several days. A negative feedback system exists whereby glucocorticoids decrease cytokine production by inhibiting gene expression. Thus, the cortisol response to surgery limits the severity of the inflammatory response. It has been suggested that increased intracerebral IL-6 results in the enhanced cortisol secretion found after cerebral haemorrhage [58].

IL-6, and other cytokines, cause the acute phase response, which includes the production of acute phase proteins such as fibrinogen, C-reactive protein (CRP), complement proteins, amyloid P component, amyloid A and ceruloplasmin in the liver [59,60]. Their function is to promote haemostasis, limit tissue damage and enhance repair and regeneration. Synthesis of acute phase proteins occurs at the expense of decreased production of other key proteins such as albumin and transferrin. Concentrations of circulating cations such as zinc and iron decrease, partly as a result of changes in the production of transport proteins. Other important aspects of the acute phase response include fever, granulocytosis and lymphocyte differentiation (Table 21.2).

The acute phase response prevents further tissue damage, isolates and destroys infective organisms, activates the repair processes and is considered an integral part of wound healing and repair.

Metabolic consequences

Substrate mobilization, to provide fuel for oxidation, is an intrinsic aspect of the stress response to surgery or trauma.

Carbohydrate metabolism

Hyperglycaemia is a major feature of the metabolic response to surgery and results from an increase in glucose production and a reduction in peripheral

Table 21.2 The acute phase response.

Tissue injury → cytokine production, particularly IL-6

Acute phase protein synthesis in liver: C-reactive protein, serum amyloid A, serum amyloid P component, metal binding proteins, proteinase inhibitors, complement proteins, coagulation proteins

Hepatic sequestration of cations (e.g. iron and zinc)

Reduction in transport proteins (e.g. albumin, transferrin)

Pyrexia (fever of trauma)

Neutrophil leucocytosis

Increased muscle proteolysis

Increased vascular permeability

Activation of hypothalamic–pituitary axis (*in vitro*)

Lymphocyte differentiation

glucose utilization. This is facilitated by catecholamines and cortisol, which promote glycogenolysis and gluconeogenesis. The increase in blood glucose is proportional to the severity of surgery or injury and roughly parallels the increases in catecholamines in the early phases of injury. Cataract surgery under general anaesthesia causes a small increase of approximately 0.5–1 mmol/L [61], whereas cardiac surgery results in more marked hyperglycaemia and values greater than 10 mmol/L are not uncommon. The hyperglycaemic response is enhanced by the iatrogenic effects of administration of glucose infusions and blood products. The usual mechanisms that regulate glucose production and uptake are ineffective. Catabolic hormones promote glucose production and glucose utilization is impaired because of an initial failure of insulin secretion followed by insulin resistance. There is little evidence to suggest that growth hormone or glucagon have a significant role in perioperative hyperglycaemia. Glucose concentrations >12 mmol/L increase water and electrolyte loss and impair wound and anastomotic healing and increase infection rates [62,63]. There is also an increased risk of ischaemic damage to the nervous system and myocardium; prognosis after an acute myocardial infarction or cerebral event is worse in the presence of hyperglycaemia.

Protein metabolism

Initially, there is inhibition of protein anabolism, followed later, if the stress response is severe, by enhanced catabolism. Protein catabolism is stimulated by increased circulating cortisol and cytokine concentrations. The amount of protein degradation is influenced by the type of surgery and also by the nutritional status of the patient; following major abdominal surgery up to 0.5 kg/day of lean body mass can be lost resulting in significant muscle wasting and weight loss. Skeletal muscle protein is mainly affected but some visceral muscle protein may also be catabolized to release essential amino acids. Amino acids, particularly glutamine and alanine, are used for gluconeogenesis in the liver and renal cortex to maintain circulating blood glucose >3 mmol/L and also for synthesis of acute phase proteins in the liver. However, albumin production is reduced impairing the maintenance of the extracellular volume. The total amount of protein loss can be assessed indirectly by measuring nitrogen excretion in the form of urea in the urine; 3-methylhistidine excretion is a more precise estimate of skeletal muscle protein breakdown. The exact mechanisms responsible for muscle protein loss still have not been fully elucidated because catabolic hormones appear to have only a minor role. Prolonged infusions of catabolic hormones into volunteers have only minimal effects on nitrogen balance [64]. Attempts to prevent protein loss after surgery, by providing nutritional support — enteral and parenteral — have proved disappointing [65–67]. The availability of additional substrates has little effect in overcoming the inhibition of protein anabolism and preventing catabolism.

Fat metabolism

Interestingly, few changes occur in lipid mobilization following surgery, unless starvation becomes a major factor postoperatively. Plasma non-esterified fatty acids (NEFA) and ketone body concentrations do not change significantly. Increased catecholamine, cortisol and glucagon secretion, in combination with insulin deficiency, promote some lipolysis and ketone body production. Triglycerides are metabolized to fatty acids and glycerol; the latter is a gluconeogenic substrate. High glucagon and low insulin concentrations also promote oxidation of NEFAs to acyl CoA, which is converted in the liver to ketone bodies (β-hydroxybutyrate, acetoacetate and acetone). These serve as a useful water-soluble fuel source for many organs.

The most dramatic changes in lipid metabolism are seen during cardiac surgery. Heparinization activates lipoprotein lipase which acts on triacylglycerol to cause a dramatic increase in circulating NEFA concentrations. Circulating concentrations may exceed 2 mmol/L uring cardiopulmonary bypass, which may have toxic effects on cell membranes, in particular, promoting arrhythmias. The problem is less severe with the new 'cleaner' heparins.

Salt and water metabolism

AVP secretion results in water retention, concentrated urine and potassium loss and may continue for 3–5 days following surgery. Renin is secreted from the juxtaglomerular cells of the kidney secondary to sympathetic efferent activation. It converts angiotensin I to angiotensin II, which in turn releases aldosterone from the adrenal cortex promoting sodium and water retention from the collecting ducts. Under the influence of aldosterone, increased amounts of Na^+ are exchanged for K^+ and H^+, producing a K^+ diuresis and an increase in urine acidity.

Fatigue and behavioural changes

Although psychological changes such as increased anxiety and depression are common after major surgery, they usually resolve rapidly after the patient leaves hospital. However, feelings of malaise may persist for several months. These feelings of malaise are often referred to as postoperative fatigue and are commonly assumed to be a consequence of the physiological changes associated with surgery. This assumption led to the adoption of a simple stimulus–response model to explain the occurrence of postoperative fatigue. Minor surgery with small physiological changes would not result in fatigue, whereas major surgery with marked prolonged physiological responses would result inevitably in severe fatigue. It has been shown repeatedly that a simple physiological explanation for postoperative fatigue is untenable, as even in studies in which fatigue is a major occurrence it is absent in 30–40% of patients. It is likely that the pursuit of the physiological basis of fatigue has hindered progress in understanding the phenomenon. Currently, postoperative fatigue is poorly defined and inadequately measured. It is not inevitable even after major surgery, but the causes are still not known and there is essentially no specific treatment.

Recent research in this area has started to explore the psychological aspects of fatigue. It has been suggested that fatigue after surgery may be explained not as a pathological change, but as a component of motivational response. This notion is supported by studies showing that the severity of preoperative fatigue predicts postoperative fatigue, and that there is an association between fatigue and anxiety and depression or negative mood. The most obvious manifestation of fatigue is a reluctance to move. It is important to realize that immobility after surgery is common and originally served as a protective function in an injured animal. Rapid movement will impair healing. Movement is still possible if the external threat is sufficiently great and thus immobility can be considered a motivational response.

This new perspective on fatigue may explain some of the anomalous clinical findings. Postoperative fatigue is virtually absent after elective joint arthroplasty and yet is often severe and persistent after major abdominal surgery. However, the nature and severity of the physiological changes to surgery are similar. It is possible that psychological aspects of surgery may explain the differences in occurrence of postoperative fatigue. Joint arthroplasty is an operation that is often desired by the patient and expected to improve their quality of life, but major abdominal surgery is rarely life-enhancing and may even be life-threatening. The importance of the expectations of the patient and the staff in influencing the psychological changes after surgery in the patient are obvious. It is possible that in those 'integrated packages of care' designed to enhance recovery after major surgery, regional anaesthesia, laparoscopically assisted surgery, early oral feeding, vigorous rehabilitation, it is the altered expectations of the patient during the preoperative assessment that have a key role in ensuring early mobilization and minimal fatigue. It is important to note that patients tend to behave in ways that reflect the medical staff's expectations, so patient education will be ineffective unless the medical and nursing staff also advocate an early discharge policy.

At present, postoperative fatigue should be considered a component of the emotional rather than the physiological response to surgery.

Modifying the stress response

Although it is common practice to view the stress response as an inevitable consequence of surgical trauma, many approaches to decreasing the metabolic sequelae have been investigated. Kehlet [68] and others have suggested that the surgical stress response is an 'epiphenomenon' and decreasing the endocrine and metabolic changes that occur may reduce major perioperative morbidity.

Intravenous induction agents

Etomidate, an imidazole derivative, is a potent inhibitor of adrenal steroidogenesis and acts on the mitochondrial 11β-hydroxylase step and cholesterol cleavage part of the biosynthetic pathway. Fragen *et al.* [69] showed that a single induction dose of etomidate inhibited cortisol and aldosterone production for up to 8 hours after pelvic surgery. Etomidate is often used in sick patients with limited cardiovascular reserve without adverse effects, thereby raising the question of how much circulating cortisol is required in routine surgery for cardiovascular stability. The primate work by Udelsman *et al.* [70] inferred that only resting circulating values of cortisol were necessary to ensure a normal outcome after surgery. Both diazepam and midazolam have also been shown to inhibit cortisol production from isolated bovine adrenocortical cells *in vitro* [71]. Midazolam, which has an imidazole ring in addition to its benzodiazepine structure, was found to decrease the cortisol response to peripheral surgery [72] and major upper abdominal surgery [73] and may also have a direct effect on ACTH secretion [72].

Volatile anaesthetic agents

Volatile anaesthetic agents probably have little effect on the hypothalamic–pituitary–adrenal (HPA) axis at low concentrations. No difference was found between 2.1 and 1.2 MAC halothane in obtunding the pituitary hormone and sympathoadrenal responses to pelvic surgery [74]. It is likely that other volatile anaesthetic agents behave similarly at clinical concentrations.

High-dose opioid anaesthesia

The ability of morphine to inhibit the HPA axis has been known for many years [75], but it was only in the 1970s that the use of morphine to modify the metabolic and endocrine responses to surgery was first investigated [76]. However, large doses of morphine resulted in unacceptably prolonged recovery times. Fentanyl 50 µg/kg i.v. abolished the cortisol response to pelvic surgery [77] but 100 µg/kg was required in upper abdominal surgery [78]. The inhibitory effect of fentanyl on surgically induced secretion of pituitary hormones is mediated via the hypothalamus [79]. The inevitable penalty of this technique is profound respiratory depression for several hours postoperatively. Many studies have examined the effects of high-dose fentanyl and its congener, sufentanil, on the hormonal response to cardiac surgery [80]. In general, the majority of studies have shown that endocrine changes are attenuated only until the start of cardiopulmonary bypass.

Regional anaesthesia

It is well recognized that complete afferent blockade, both somatic and autonomic, is necessary to prevent stimulation of the HPA axis. Thus, an extensive T4–S5 block is necessary for pelvic surgery [81] and it has been known for over 30 years that it is very difficult to prevent cortisol secretion with regional anaesthesia in upper abdominal surgery [82]. Other operations, amenable to complete afferent blockade, are limb and eye surgery [83]. However, it is worth noting that cytokine-mediated responses, which occur as a consequence of tissue trauma, are not altered by afferent neuronal blockade [56].

Whether epidural anaesthesia and analgesia improve the outcome of major surgery is a long-running controversy. Proponents of the technique cite beneficial effects resulting from attenuation of the stress response, which in turn has advantages for postoperative hypercoagulability and cardiovascular, respiratory, gastrointestinal, metabolic and immune function [84,85]. Rodgers *et al.* [86] concluded that epidural or spinal anaesthesia results in a significant reduction in postoperative morbidity and mortality. However, this systematic review, which claimed a reduction in mortality of one-third that does not differ by surgical group, type of regional nerve blockade or use of general together with regional anaesthesia, has been the subject of intense controversy and many of its findings have been questioned. There is evidence that epidural analgesia provides better postoperative pain relief and shortens the intubation time and intensive care stay of patients undergoing specific procedures such as abdominal aortic surgery [87]. A recent randomized controlled trial found that in high-risk patients undergoing major abdominal surgery adverse morbid outcomes were not decreased by the use of

combined epidural and general anaesthesia and postoperative epidural analgesia [88]. The only significant benefit with the epidural regimen was a decreased occurrence of postoperative respiratory failure. Epidural analgesia following gastrointestinal surgery has been shown to be associated with improved pain control, a shorter duration of postoperative ileus and fewer pulmonary complications, but did not affect the incidence of anastomotic leakage, intraoperative blood loss, transfusion requirements, risk of thromboembolism or cardiac morbidity [89]. Epidural analgesia is an integral part of multimodal rehabilitation programmes that also include early nutrition, mobilization and avoidance of opiates. It is not possible to determine the precise role played by regional anaesthesia in these programmes [90–92].

At present there remains a need for large multicentre prospective randomized trials to assess definitively the impact of epidural anaesthesia and analgesia on morbidity and mortality [93].

Minimal access surgery

The introduction of endoscopic surgical techniques has drawn attention to the importance of the inflammatory aspects of surgery. Laparoscopic surgery causes less tissue damage than conventional procedures, so the increases in biochemical markers of inflammation, such as IL-6 and CRP are not as great. For individual surgeons, increasing the annual caseload of laparoscopic surgery results in shorter hospital stays for patients, although for laparoscopic cholecystectomy this has not affected postoperative mortality [94].

The classic neuroendocrine response (increases in cortisol, glucose and catecholamines) to abdominal surgery such as open cholecystectomy is not significantly altered by undertaking the operation using a laparoscopic technique. The anaesthetic technique has little effect on the cytokine response because it cannot influence tissue trauma [95,96]. Combined analgesic regimens, which included high-dose steroids (30 mg/kg prednisolone), cause a small decrease in IL-6 concentrations and the acute phase response. However, their use is precluded because of the risk of unwanted side-effects including wound dehiscence [97].

Table 21.3 Summary of the response to anaesthesia, surgery or trauma.

Surgery or trauma evoke a series of physiological and psychological changes commonly referred to as the stress response
There is increased secretion of hypothalamic–pituitary hormones and activation of the sympathetic nervous system
Increased catabolism mobilizes substrates that are then utilized to provide energy
Salt and water retention occur to maintain fluid volume and cardiovascular homoeostasis
Release of cytokines from damaged tissue mediates the metabolic, haematologic and immunological changes known collectively as the acute phase response
Psychological changes contribute to postoperative malaise and may delay functional recovery
Attempts have been made to modify the stress response following surgery with various anaesthetic techniques but the results are inconclusive at present

Endoscopic surgery results in a decreased acute phase response and preserves immune function compared with conventional open techniques [98]. It has been recommended as the treatment of choice, instead of laparotomy, for benign pelvic disease whenever feasible [99]. However, concerns have been expressed about its suitability for the treatment of malignant disease, particularly because of port-site recurrences when used in the treatment of colorectal cancer [100]. Recent studies have shown that laparoscopic resection of rectosigmoid carcinoma does not jeopardize survival and disease control of patients [101] and laparoscopically assisted colectomy is more effective than open colectomy in terms of morbidity, hospital stay, tumour recurrence and cancer-related survival [102]. The mechanism for this is unknown but it has been suggested that better immune function and reduced tumour manipulation may both contribute [102].

The effects of non-steroidal anti-inflammatory drugs (NSAIDs) on the inflammatory response to surgery depend on the timing of their administration. When given during and after surgery they are ineffective and must be used for 24 hours preoperatively in addition before any beneficial effects are found [103]. It has been suggested that cyclooxygenase-2 (COX-2) inhibitors would have a similar analgesic potency, but a better safety profile compared with older NSAIDs in terms of gastrointes-

tinal tract and platelet function [89], but this view has recently been challenged, particularly for patients with cardiovascular disease [104].

Conclusions

In summary, the stress response to surgery or trauma is characterized by a series of changes in the circulating levels of hormones and inflammatory mediators such as cytokines (Table 21.3). Psychological manifestations of the stress response, or postoperative fatigue, although not inevitable, may also occur. There have been several approaches to minimizing the stress response to surgery, including using regional anaesthesia or minimally invasive surgical techniques. Although some approaches have been successful, the effects of reducing, for example, IL-6 concentrations on overall morbidity and mortality are still not known.

References

1 Hall GM. The anaesthetic modification of the endocrine and metabolic response to surgery. *Ann R Coll Surg Engl* 1985; **67**: 25–9.
2 Salmon P, Hall GM. A theory of postoperative fatigue: an interaction of biological, psychological and social processes. *Pharmacol Biochem Behav* 1997; **56**: 623–8.

3 Singer M, De Santis V, Viale D, Jeffcoate W. Multiorgan failure is an adaptive, endocrine-mediated, metabolic response to overwhelming systemic inflammation. *Lancet* 2004; **364**: 545–8.

4 Kennedy BC, Hall GM. Neuroendocrine and inflammatory aspects of surgery; do they affect outcome? *Acta Anaesth Belg* 1999; **50**: 205–9.

5 Cuthbertson DP. Observations on the disturbance of metabolism produced by injury to the limbs. *Q J Med* 1932; **1**: 233–46.

6 Wilmore DW. From Cuthbertson to fast track surgery: 70 years of reducing stress in surgical patients. *Ann Surg* 2002; **236**: 643–8.

7 Mulholland JH, Co T, Wright A. Nitrogen metabolism, caloric intake and weight loss in postoperative convalescence: a study of eight patients undergoing partial gastrectomy for duodenal ulcers. *Ann Surg* 1943; **117**: 512–34.

8 Browne JSL, Schenker V, Stevenson JAF. Some metabolic aspects of damage and convalescence. *J Clin Invest* 1944; **23**: 932.

9 Howard JE. Protein metabolism during convalescence after trauma. *Arch Surg* 1945; **50**: 166–70.

10 Moore FD. Bodily changes in surgical convalescence: observations and interpretations. *Ann Surg* 1953; **137**: 289–315.

11 Hume DM. The neuro-endocrine response to injury: present status of the problem. *Ann Surg* 1953; **138**: 548–57.

12 Egdahl RH. Pituitary adrenal response following trauma to the isolated leg. *Surgery* 1959; **46**: 9–21.

13 von Euler US, Franksson C, Hellstrom J. Adrenaline and noradrenaline output in urine after unilateral and bilateral adrenalectomy in man. *Acta Physiol Scand* 1954; **31**: 1–5.

14 Franksson C, Gemzell CA, Von Euler US. Cortical and medullary adrenal activity in surgical and allied conditions. *J Clin Endocrinol Metab* 1954; **14**: 608–21.

15 Goodall M, Stone C, Haynes BW Jr. Urinary output of adrenaline and noradrenaline in severe thermal burns. *Ann Surg* 1957; **145**: 479–87.

16 Sheeran P, Hall GM. Cytokines in anaesthesia. *Br J Anaesth* 1997; **78**: 201–19.

17 Wallace A, Layug B, Tateo I, *et al.* Prophylactic atenolol reduces postoperative myocardial ischaemia. *Anesthesiol* 1998; **88**: 7–17.

18 Poldermans D, Boersma E, Bax JJ, *et al.* The effect of bisoprolol on perioperative mortality and myocardial infarction in high risk patients undergoing vascular surgery. *N Engl J Med* 1999; **341**: 1789–94.

19 Urban MK, Markowitz SM, Gordon M, Urquhart BL, Kligfield P. Postoperative prophylactic administration of β-adrenergic blockers in patients at risk for myocardial ischaemia. *Anesth Analg* 2000; **90**: 1257–61.

20 Oliver MF, Goldman L, Julian DG, Holme I. Effect of mivazerol on perioperative cardiac complications during non-cardiac surgery in patients with coronary heart disease: the European Mivazerol Trial (EMIT). *Anesthesiol* 1999; **91**: 951–61.

21 Talke P, Li J, Jain U, *et al.* Effects of perioperative dexmedetomidine infusion in patients undergoing vascular surgery. The Study of Perioperative Ischemia Research Group. *Anesthesiol* 1995; **82**: 620–33.

22 Stuhmeier KD, Mainzer B, Cierpka J, Sandmann W, Tarnow J. Small, oral dose of clonidine reduces the incidence of intraoperative myocardial ischemia in patients having vascular surgery. *Anesthesiol* 1996; **85**: 706–12.

23 Venn RM, Bryant A, Hall GM, Grounds RM. Effects of dexmeditomidine on adrenocortical function, and the cardiovascular, endocrine and inflammatory responses in post-operative patients needing sedation in the intensive care unit. *Br J Anaesth* 2001; **86**: 650–6.

24 Desborough JP. The stress response to trauma and surgery. *Br J Anaesth* 2000; **85**: 109–17.

25 Orth DN, Kovacs WJ, de Bold CR. The adrenal cortex. In: Wilson JD, Foster DW eds. *Williams Textbook of Endocrinology.* Philadelphia: WB Saunders, 1992: 489–621.

26 Hodges JR. The hypothalamo-pituitary-adrenocortical system. *Br J Anaesth* 1984; **56**: 701–10.

27 Thorén L. General metabolic response to trauma including pain influence. *Acta Anaesth Scand* 1974; **S55**: 9–14.

28 Chernow B, Alexander R, Smallridge RC, *et al.* Hormonal responses to graded surgical stress. *Arch Intern Med* 1987; **147**: 1273–8.

29 Traynor C, Hall GM. Endocrine and metabolic changes during surgery: anaesthetic implications. *Br J Anaesth* 1981; **53**: 153–61.

30 Hardy JD, Turner MD. Hydrocortisone secretion in man: studies of adrenal vein blood. *Surgery* 1957; **42**: 194–201.

31 Hume DM, Bell CC, Bartter FC. Direct measurement of adrenal secretion during operative trauma and convalescence. *Surgery* 1962; **52**: 174–87.

32 Hume DM, Nelson DH, Miller DW. Blood and urinary 17-hydrocorticosteroids in patients with severe burns. *Ann Surg* 1956; **143**: 316–29.

33 Kehlet H. A rational approach to dosage and preparation of parenteral glucocorticoid substitution therapy

during surgical procedures. *Acta Anaesth Scand* 1975; **19**: 260–4.

34 Kehlet H, Binder C. Alterations in distribution volume and biological half-life of cortisol during major surgery. *J Clin Endocrinol Metab* 1973; **36**: 330–3.

35 Desborough JP, Hall GM. Endocrine response to surgery. In: Kaufmann L, ed. *Anaesthesia Review*, Vol. 10. Edinburgh: Churchill Livingstone, 1993: 131–48.

36 Parrillo JE, Fauci AS. Mechanisms of glucocorticoid action on immune processes. *Ann Rev Pharmacol Toxicol* 1979; **19**: 179–201.

37 Balow JE, Rosenthal AS. Glucocorticoid suppression of macrophage migration inhibitory factor. *J Exp Med* 1973; **137**: 1031–9.

38 Blackwell GJ, Carnuccio R, DiRosa M, *et al.* Macrocortin: a polypeptide causing the antiphospholipase effects of glucocorticoids. *Nature* 1980; **287**: 147–9.

39 Jameson P, Desborough JP, Bryant AE, Hall GM. The effect of cortisol suppression on interleukin-6 and white blood cell response to surgery. *Acta Anaesth Scand* 1997; **41**: 304–8.

40 Chwals WJ, Bistrian BR. Role of exogenous growth hormone and insulin-like growth factor 1 in malnutrition and acute metabolic stress: a hypothesis. *Crit Care Med* 1991; **19**: 1317–22.

41 Ross RJM, Miell JP, Buchanan CR. Avoiding autocannibalism. *Br Med J* 1991; **303**: 1147–8.

42 Takala J, Ruokonen E, Webster NR, *et al.* Increased mortality associated with growth hormone treatment in critically ill adults. *N Engl J Med* 1999; **341**: 785–92.

43 Ljungqvist O, Nygren J, Thorell A. Insulin resistance and elective surgery. *Surgery* 2000; **128**: 757–60.

44 Frayn KN. Hormonal control of metabolism in trauma and sepsis. *Clin Endocrinol* 1986; **24**: 577–99.

45 Strommer L, Wickbom M, Wang F, *et al.* Early impairment of insulin secretion in rats after surgical trauma. *Eur J Endocrinol* 2002; **147**: 825–33.

46 van den Berghe G, Wouters P, Weekers F, *et al.* Intensive insulin therapy in critically ill patients. *N Engl J Med* 2001; **19**: 1359–67.

47 Byrne CR, Carlson GL. Can post-traumatic insulin resistance be attenuated by prior glucose loading? *Nutrition* 2001; **17**: 332–6.

48 Thorell A, Nygren J, Ljungqvist O. Insulin resistance: a marker of surgical stress. *Curr Opin Nutr Metab Care* 1999; **2**: 69–78.

49 Ljungqvist O, Thorell A, Dutniak M, Haggmark T, Efendic S. Glucose infusion instead of perioperative fasting reduces postoperative insulin resistance. *J Am Coll Surg* 1994; **178**: 329–33.

50 Edwards R. Thyroid and parathyroid disease. *Int Anesthesiol Clin* 1997; **35**: 63–83.

51 Woolf PD, Hamill RW, McDonald JV, *et al.* Transient hypogonadotrophic hypogonadism caused by critical illness. *J Clin Endocrinol Metab* 1985; **60**: 444–50.

52 Wang C, Chan V, Yeung RT. Effects of surgical stress on pituitary testicular function. *Clin Endocrinol* 1978; **9**: 255–66.

53 Tian Y, Serino R, Verbalis JG. Downregulation of renal vasopressin V2 receptor and aquaporin-2 expression parallels age-associated defects in urine concentration. *Am J Physiol Renal Physiol* 2004; **287**: 797–805.

54 Raeburn CD, Sheppard F, Barsness KA, Arya J, Harken AH. Cytokines for surgeons. *Am J Surg* 2002; **183**: 268–73.

55 Cruickshank AM, Fraser WD, Burns HJG, Van Damme J, Shenkin A. Response of serum interleukin-6 in patients undergoing elective surgery of varying severity. *Clin Sci* 1990; **79**: 161–5.

56 Moore CM, Desborough JP, Powell H, Burrin JM, Hall GM. The effects of extradural anaesthesia on the interleukin-6 and acute phase response to surgery. *Br J Anaesth* 1994; **72**: 272–9.

57 Joris J, Cigarini I, Legrand M, *et al.* Metabolic and respiratory changes after cholecystectomy performed via laparotomy or laparoscopy. *Br J Anaesth* 1992; **69**: 341–5.

58 Spangelo BL, Judd AM, Isakson PC, Macleod RM. Interleukin-6 stimulates anterior pituitary hormone release *in vitro*. *Endocrinol* 1989; **125**: 575–7.

59 Baumann H, Gauldie J. The acute phase response. *Immunol Today* 1994; **15**: 74–9.

60 Steel DM, Whitehead AS. The major acute phase reactants: C-reactive protein, serum amyloid P component and serum amyloid A protein. *Immunol Today* 1994; **15**: 81–8.

61 Barker JP, Vafidis GC, Robinson PN, Hall GM. Plasma catecholamine response to cataract surgery: a comparison between general and local anaesthesia. *Anaesthesia* 1991; **46**: 642–5.

62 Bessey PQ, Walters JM, Bier DM, Wilmore DW. Combined hormonal infusion stimulates the metabolic response to injury. *Ann Surg* 1984; **200**: 264–81.

63 Mossad SB, Serkey JM, Longworth DL, Gordon SM. Coagulase-negative staphylococcal sternal wound infections after open-heart operations. *Ann Thorac Surg* 1997; **63**: 395–401.

64 Verhofstad HJ, Hendriks T. Complete prevention of impaired anastomotic healing in diabetic rats requires

preoperative blood glucose control. *Br J Surg* 1996; **83**:1717–21.

65 Veterans Affairs Total Parenteral Nutrition Cooperative Study Group. Perioperative total parenteral nutrition in surgical patients. *N Engl J Med* 1991; **325**: 525–32.

66 Saunders C, Nishikawa R, Wolfe B. Surgical nutrition: a review. *J R Coll Surg Edinb* 1993; **38**: 195–204.

67 Kennedy BC, Hall GM. Metabolic support of critically ill patients: parenteral nutrition to immunonutrition. *Br J Anaesth* 2000; **85**: 185–8.

68 Kehlet H. The surgical stress response: should it be prevented? *Can J Surg* 1991; **34**: 565–7.

69 Fragen RJ, Shanks CA, Molteni A, Avram MJ. Effects of etomidate on hormonal responses to surgical stress. *Anesthesiol* 1984; **61**: 652–6.

70 Udelsman R, Ramp J, Gallucci WT *et al*. Adaptation during surgical stress: a re-evaluation of the role of glucocorticoids. *J Clin Invest* 1986; **77**: 1377–81.

71 Holloway CD, Kenyon CJ, Dowie LJ, *et al*. Effect of the benzodiazepines diazepam, des-N-methyldiazepam and midazolam on corticosteroid biosynthesis in bovine adrenocortical cells *in vitro*; location of site of action. *J Steroid Biochem* 1989; **33**: 219–25.

72 Crozier TA, Beck D, Schlaeger M, Wuttke W, Kettler D. Endocrinological changes following etomidate or methohexital for minor surgery. *Anesthesiol* 1987; **66**: 628–35.

73 Desborough JP, Hall GM, Hart GR, Burrin JM. Midazolam modifies pancreatic and anterior pituitary hormone secretion during upper abdominal surgery. *Br J Anaesth* 1991; **67**: 390–6.

74 Lacoumenta S, Paterson JL, Burrin J, *et al*. Effects of two differing halothane concentrations on the metabolic and endocrine responses to surgery. *Br J Anaesth* 1986; **58**: 844–50.

75 McDonald RK, Evans FT, Weise VK, Patrick RW. Effects of morphine and nalorphine on plasma hydrocortisone levels in man. *J Pharmacol Exp Ther* 1959; **125**: 241–52.

76 George JM, Reier CE, Lanese RR, Rower JM. Morphine anaesthesia blocks cortisol and growth hormone response to stress in humans. *J Clin Endocrinol Metab* 1974; **38**: 736–41.

77 Hall GM, Young C, Holdcroft A, Alaghband-Zadeh J. Substrate mobilisation during surgery: a comparison between halothane and fentanyl anaesthesia. *Anaesthesia* 1978; **33**: 924–30.

78 Klingstedt C, Giesecke K, Hamberger B, Järnberg P-O. High and low dose fentanyl anaesthesia, circulatory and plasma catecholamine responses during cholecystectomy. *Br J Anaesth* 1987; **59**: 184–8.

79 Hall GM, Lacoumenta S, Hart GR, Burrin JM. Site of action of fentanyl in inhibiting the pituitary-adrenal response to surgery in man. *Br J Anaesth* 1990; **65**: 251–3.

80 Desborough JP, Hall GM. Modification of the hormonal and metabolic response to surgery by narcotics and general anaesthesia. *Baillières Clin Anaesthesiol* 1989; **3**: 317–34.

81 Engquist A, Brandt MR, Fernandes A, Kehlet H. The blocking effect of epidural analgesia on the adrenocortical and hyperglycaemic responses to surgery. *Acta Anaesth Scand* 1977; **21**: 330–5.

82 Bromage PR, Shibata HR, Willoughby HW. Influence of prolonged epidural blockade on blood sugar and cortisol responses to operations on the upper part of the abdomen and thorax. *Surg Gynecol Obs* 1971; **132**: 1051–6.

83 Barker JP, Robinson PN, Vafidis GC, *et al*. Local analgesia prevents the cortisol and glycaemic responses to cataract surgery. *Br J Anaesth* 1990; **64**: 442–5.

84 Rigg JRA. Does regional blockade improve outcome after surgery? *Anaesth Int Care* 1991; **19**: 404–11.

85 Liu S, Carpenter RL, Neal JM. Epidural anaesthesia and analgesia: their role in postoperative outcome. *Anesthesiol* 1995; **82**: 1474–506.

86 Rodgers A, Walker S, Schug S, *et al*. Reduction of postoperative mortality and morbidity with epidural and spinal anaesthesia: results from overview of randomised trials. *Br Med J* 2000; **321**: 1493–7.

87 Park WY, Thompson JS, Lee KK. Effect of epidural anesthesia and analgesia on perioperative outcome; a randomized, controlled veterans affairs cooperative study. *Ann Surg* 2001; **234**: 560–71.

88 Rigg JRA, Jamrozik K, Myles PS, *et al*. Epidural anaesthesia and analgesia and outcome of major surgery: a randomised trial. *Lancet* 2002; **359**: 1276–82.

89 Fotiadis RJ, Badvie S, Weston MD, Allen-Mersh TG. Epidural analgesia in gastrointestinal surgery. *Br J Surg* 2004; **91**: 828–41.

90 Kehlet H, Wilmore DW. Mutimodal strategies to improve surgical outcome. *Am J Surg* 2002; **183**: 630–41.

91 Holte K, Kehlet H. Epidural anaesthesia and analgesia-effects on surgical stress responses and implications for postoperative nutrition. *Clin Nutr* 2002; **21**: 199–206.

92 Kehlet H, Dahl JB. Anaesthesia, surgery and challenges in postoperative recovery. *Lancet* 2003; **362**: 1921–8.

93 Grass JA. The role of epidural anaesthesia and analgesia in postoperative outcome. *Anaesthesiol Clin North Am* 2000; **18**: 407–28.

94 McMahon AJ, Fischbacher CM, Frame SH, MacLeod MCM. Impact of laparoscopic cholecystectomy: a population-based study. *Lancet* 2000; **356**: 1632–7.

95 Brix-Christensen V, Tonnesen E, Sorensen IJ, *et al*. Effects of anaesthesia based on high versus low doses of opioids on the cytokine and acute-phase protein responses in patients undergoing cardiac surgery. *Acta Anaesth Scand* 1998; **42**: 63–70.

96 Schneemilch CE, Schilling T. Effects of general anaesthesia on inflammation. *Best Pract Res Clin Anaesthesiol* 2004; **18**: 493–507.

97 Schulze S, Sommer P, Biggler D. Effect of combined prednisolone, epidural analgesia and indomethacin on the systemic response after colonic surgery. *Arch Surg* 1992; **127**: 325–31.

98 Buunen M, Gholghesaei M, Veldkamp R, *et al*. Stress response to laparoscopic surgery. *Surg Endosc* 2004; **18**: 1022–8.

99 Marano R, Margutti F, Catalanao GF, Marana E. Stress responses to endoscopic surgery. *Curr Opin Obstet Gynecol* 2000; **12**: 303–7.

100 Weiss EG, Wexner SD. Laparoscopic port site recurrences in oncological cancer: a review. *Ann Acad Med Singapore* 1996; **25**: 694–8.

101 Leung KL, Kwok SPY, Lam SCW, *et al*. Laparoscopic resection of rectosigmoid carcinoma: prospective randomised trial. *Lancet* 2004; **363**: 1187–92.

102 Lacy AM, Garcia-Valdecassas JC, Delgado S, *et al*. Laparoscopic-assisted colectomy versus open colectomy for treatment of non-metastatic colon cancer: a randomised trial. *Lancet* 2002; **359**: 2224–9.

103 Chambrier C, Chassard D, Bienvenu J, *et al*. Cytokine and hormonal changes after cholecystectomy: effect of ibuprofen pre-treatment. *Ann Surg* 1996; **224**: 178–82.

104 Topol EJ, Falk GW. A coxib a day won't keep the doctor away. *Lancet* 2004; **364**: 639–40.

CHAPTER 22

Temperature regulation

Anita Holdcroft

Introduction

Humans are homoeothermic, that is, they dynamically maintain their body temperature within narrow limits close to a set point, so that cellular systems can work effectively. There is almost always a gradient between surface and internal temperatures so that temperature varies from site to site and core temperature (head, chest and abdomen) differs from the shell. Physiological temperature regulation maintains core temperature at the expense of peripheral tissues through heat loss or heat gain mechanisms. Behavioural responses can also control heat gain and loss through conscious alterations in the environment, clothing and activity.

Regulation of body temperature

Body temperature is a theoretical concept [1] and can be calculated by a weighted formula:

Mean body temperature = 2/3 core temperature + 1/3 mean skin temperature

The body has a heat reservoir = specific gravity of body tissues × mean body temperature. Normal values for individual skin temperatures at room temperature are 31–35°C; mean skin temperature (T_{skin}) can be considered the mean of 15 or more sites or a weighted formula can be used. The four-site (nipple, upper arm, thigh, calf) weighted formula of Ramanathan has been validated for anaesthesia [2]:

$$\text{Mean } T_{skin} = 0.3 \, (T_{nipple} + T_{upper\,arm}) + 0.2 \, (T_{thigh} + T_{calf})$$

Body temperature is not constant, circadian rhythms result from variations in heat loss and gain controlled by the hypothalamic suprachiasmatic nuclei — the biological clock of the brain. Deviations from this cycle occur and have effects on physical and mental functions [3]. Core temperature is maximum in the late afternoon and minimum in the early morning. However, mean skin temperature is increased during the decline in core temperature. Core temperature ranges and their effects are demonstrated in Table 22.1. Between the core and skin temperatures there are intermediate temperatures (e.g. muscle or urine), with values approximately 1°C lower than core. Body temperature can be altered by many factors including the environment; physiological changes such as exercise or food ingestion; pathological factors such as thyroid disease or infection; and pharmacological effects [4]. These changes need to be sensed, processed and counteracted if necessary. Thus, thermoregulation can be conceptualized in three parts: the sensing afferent pathways, neuronal integration and control systems, and the effector pathways from the centre to peripheral structures.

Physical maintenance of temperature depends on the four factors governing heat loss and gain: heat is lost by radiation, conduction, convection and evaporation; heat is gained by increasing metabolic rate, radiation, convection and conduction (Table 22.2) [5]. The rate of heat loss depends on the temperature gradient between the body and the environment, the area exposed for this physical transfer and the thermal conductivity coefficients for each type of heat loss. The contribution of each of the four factors depends on the external temperature. When air temperature exceeds surface body temperature, evaporation is the only mechanism for heat loss, but its effectiveness depends on the relative humidity at the body surface and the available fluids and surface area (e.g. sweat, water, saliva, urine and the skin and respiratory system).

A fundamental control mechanism for temperature regulation is the flow of blood (convection and conduction) between different tissues at different temperatures within the body. Examples include the testis, where the organ is held at a different temperature than the core, and the brain, where temperature is controlled more precisely than the rest of the body.

Peripheral temperature regulation depends strongly on cardiovascular responses. Heat loss depends on the movement of heat from the core to the skin by vasodilatation and sweating. The skin is not a metabolic organ but it does act to control heat loss and gain (Fig. 22.1) [6,7]. The blood flow in the skin is organized to maintain homoeothermy. Cutaneous blood flow can be increased by vasodilatation by up to 6–8 L/min [8]. Sympathetic activity is reduced through central nervous system mechanisms and acetylcholine and vasoactive intestinal peptide are released from peripheral cholinergic sympathetic nerves to increase sweat production. Sweating is also under the control of circulating adrenaline (epinephrine) from the adrenal gland (Table 22.3). As skin temperature increases, and countercurrent heat exchange is reduced, local heat is lost by all four physical factors. However, although skin temperature governs the point at which sweating occurs, the intensity of this response depends on the temperature control in the brain. Interestingly, women respond to changes in temperature by altering blood flow in the extremities faster than men and this results in cooler fingers and toes.

Reduction in heat loss is controlled by vasoconstriction and, ineffectively in humans, by piloerection mediated by noradrenergic sympathetic stimulation of smooth muscle. Metabolic rate is increased by shivering and non-shivering thermogenesis. The point at which shivering occurs depends on skin temperature but its intensity is controlled by brain temperature. Thermogenesis is obligatory (basal metabolic rate) and thermoregulatory (e.g. increased metabolic rate, in the liver, muscles and intestine through stimulation by adrenaline, thyroxine, tri-iodothyronine, and noradrenaline [norepinephrine]), shivering, brown fat (in neonates; Table 22.4). Shivering can increase heat production by 2–5 times. The effectiveness of shivering is reduced because heat is moved into peripheral muscle tis-

Table 22.1 The effects of altering core body temperature in humans.

Core temperature (°C)	Effects
43	Upper limit of survival
40	Fever (hyperthermia)
37	Normal
35	Increased metabolism (hypothermia)
34	6% reduction in cerebral blood flow
33	Amnesia, shivering, cardiac dysrrhythmias
32	25% decrease in oxygen consumption
30	Cardiac output 60% normal Atrial fibrillation common Muscle rigidity, pupils dilated
28	50% decrease in oxygen consumption Unconscious, absent tendon reflexes
25	Spontaneous asystole
13–16	Lower limit of known survival

Table 22.3 Neurochemicals involved in thermoregulation.

Serotonin (5-HT, hydroxytryptamine)
Adrenaline (epinephrine)
Noradrenaline (norepinephrine)
Acetylcholine
Histamine
Dopamine
Cyclic nucleotides (cAMP, cGMP)
Nitric oxide
Vasoactive intestinal peptide
Interleukins (IL-1, IL-6)
Prostaglandins

Table 22.2 Principles of heat loss and gain through physical factors.

Radiation

Hot objects radiate much more than cold objects

Light colours have low emissivity so wearing light colours lowers radiation loss

Through the near infrared spectrum from the body to solid objects ($0.01-7 \times 10^{-5}$cm)

Only 85% of the naked body radiates heat

Conduction (solid to solid)

Depends on the material, material thickness, surface area and the temperature difference

Conduction has a role in heat loss when the skin is in contact with a cold surface

Fat conducts heat 1/3 as fast as other tissues

Females have more insulation than males

Cooling rate — depends on the exposure temperature as below

Exposure temperature (°C)	Change in core body temperature (°C/h)
20	0.5
15	1.5
10	2.5
5	4.0
0	0.6

Convection (fluid/gas to solid)

Convection differs from conduction in that the fluid or gas can be moving

Convection can be forced/active and depends on the speed of air flow

Evaporation

Only occurs if water evaporates from the skin — not if sweat is wiped off

1 g water needs 0.58 kcal or 2.4 kJ (latent heat of vaporization; 1 cal = 4.18 J)

Insensible heat loss is from skin and lungs

Evaporative heat loss varies widely between subjects

Normal sweat rate is maximal at night [5]

Evaporative heat loss is modulated by sleep

Elderly have decreased sweating response to thermal stimulation

External factors affecting evaporation: humidity, convection, clothing

Heat production [M (total energy production calculated from oxygen consumption) 0150 W (rate of external work (force × distance)] = heat loss [R + C + E + L + K + S].
R, radiation (60% if nude); C, conduction and convection = 15%; E, evaporation 15% heat loss from skin; L, loss from lungs (10% = 3% inhaled, 7% exhaled); K, direct conduction 3%; S, heat storage.

sues. Brown fat produces bursts of heat in response to a cold stress through a rich sympathetic nerve supply and uncoupling of oxidative phosphorylation and is strategically located in the neck and thorax close to major blood vessels and the kidneys [9].

Brown fat can double the basal metabolic rate. Neonates are unable to generate an effective shivering response to cold stimuli so this non-shivering mechanism acts as a heat generating blanket in a key location.

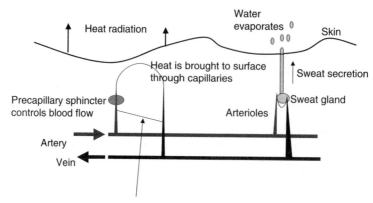

Figure 22.1 Temperature regulation at the skin. Neural control of skin arterioles is by a continuous discharge of stimuli along sympathetic fibres to maintain vasoconstriction through α_1-adrenergic receptors. An increase in body temperature will activate the hypothalamus generating a decrease in sympathetic activity leading to these vessels dilating and a rise in skin temperature. Other factors are also operating to dilate the blood vessels, including nitric oxide release [6]. In the extremities this leads to the opening up of arteriovenous anastomoses. At the same time an increase in blood flow to the eccrine sweat glands occurs to increase sweat production. At rest and in thermal neutrality, skin blood flow is controlled by sympathetic vasoconstriction which is under the control of rhythmic variations [7]. A decrease in body temperature will switch on, through the set point system, an increase in sympathetic activity, closing the anastomoses and cooling the skin. A cold environment will further stimulate the cold receptors and a spinal reflex occurs to further constrict the arterioles. In this cold environment the arterioles are more sensitive to circulating catecholamines. If blood volume is normal, blood pressure will tend to rise; the rate of rise depends on the effector system and is affected by age (e.g. slower in elderly). If other systems are not functioning (e.g. the blood volume is reduced), then these mechanisms may fail.

Table 22.4 Brown fat, its cellular characteristics and role in non-shivering thermogenesis and disease.

Brown adipocytes store lipids and contain large numbers of mitochondria packed with cristae

Brown adipocytes are innervated by sympathetic nerves, controlled centrally by the hypothalamic melanocortinergic system, that release noradrenaline to uncouple protein 1 (UCP1)

UCP1 is unique to brown fat and generates heat

Polymorphisms in UCP1 and the β_3-adrenergic receptor appear to be synergistic and are associated with obesity, possibly type 2 diabetes and lower basal metabolic rate in humans; in contrast to this synergism, UCP1 knockout mice are sensitive to cold but not obesity

UCP1 is found in the inner membrane of mitochondria where it uncouples oxidation from adenosine triphosphate (ATP) production

Brown adipocytes can be induced by cold or repressed by fasting and altered by hormones such as leptin, thyroid hormones and glucocorticoids (these compounds down-regulate UCP1 expression) which all modulate thermogenesis

Central control of temperature regulation depends on feedback mechanisms with effector controls that are limited and mainly dependent on the normal function of the cardiovascular, endocrine and nervous systems (Table 22.5) [10–12] and with central and peripheral sensors acting on a central controller. There are cutaneous, visceral (abdominal, vascular) and central nervous system (brain and spinal cord) temperature sensors [13]. In the central nervous system, arteries of considerable size are located in close proximity to thermosensitive neurones so that blood and brain temperatures are closely coupled. Cutaneous sensors respond to cold and heat through Aδ (these outnumber warm receptors by 3–10 times) and C fibres (slower to respond because they are deeper in the skin and unmyelinated), respectively. Their firing rate is dependent, not only on changes of temperature, but also on the static temperature of the skin. The sensitive range is 30–40°C. These sensors send afferent signals that converge via the dorsal horn (lamina 1) onto the contralateral anterior spinothalamic tracts, through the nucleus raphe magnus to the thalamus and hypothalamus. Relays occur to the sensory cortex to elicit behavioural responses.

The hypothalamus is organized for sensing and generates the efferent neuroendocrine responses but other integrative areas at different levels of the nervous system can control thermoregulatory responses [14]. In the pre-optic nucleus and anterior hypothalamus, warm sensors predominate over cold, and thermosensitivity is modulated by sleep. However, peripheral cold thermoreceptors also relay in this area and all contribute to the output into the posterior hypothalamus where the effectors origi-

nate into the autonomic nervous system [15]. The location of the normal upper and lower set point limits for thermoregulation is in the posterior hypothalamus. As shown in Figure 22.2, this type of thermostat provides a gain control and alters throughout the day and night, prior to ovulation in women, and in febrile conditions.

Heat production

Thermoregulatory responses progressively increase and are fully operational after puberty. Thermogenesis is obligatory and facultative. Facultative thermogenesis includes voluntary increases in activity, shivering and hormonal non-shivering thermogenesis. This is through the actions of sympathetically generated noradrenaline and brown fat heat production and adrenaline, glucagon, thyroid hormones, growth hormone and adrenocorticotrophic hormone [16,17]. Environmental pollutants such as dioxins show close structural similarity to thyroid hormones and may alter responses to heat [18]. Active tissues produce the most heat (e.g. liver, muscles; postural, exercise, shivering). At rest, percentage contributions are muscles 18%, brain 16% and internal organs, including liver, 56%. Local tissue differences in heat production have been observed in the brain such that heat may modulate synaptic events and could modulate signalling pathways through the mitochondrial uncoupling protein UCP2 [19].

Food ingestion and caffeine increase metabolic rate through substrate and catecholamine-induced thermic effects. Heat is produced through digestion,

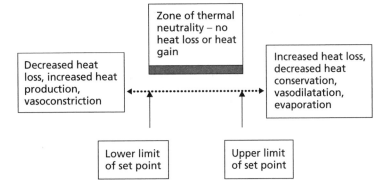

Figure 22.2 Limits of the set points and thermal neutrality in relation to effector responses with regard to increases and decreases in core body temperature (broken line). The set points vary in position, depending on the effector response and individual characteristics.

Zone of thermal neutrality – no heat loss or heat gain

Decreased heat loss, increased heat production, vasoconstriction

Increased heat loss, decreased heat conservation, vasodilatation, evaporation

Lower limit of set point

Upper limit of set point

Table 22.5 Physiological responses to temperature change.

Vasodilatation

Skin blood flow increases from 0.2 L/min or 10 mL/100 g/min at rest to 4 L/min or 200 mL/100 g/min

Blood flow to the skin can increase relatively more than that occurring in other organs

Renal blood flow and glomerular filtration rate decrease; urine becomes concentrated

Reduced systemic vascular resistance

Decrease in blood pressure

The greater the area for vasodilatation (e.g. longer limbs), the better the adaptation to heat loss; or in neonates where surface area/weight is higher than in adults unwanted heat loss occurs

Sweating (see Evaporation, Table 22.2)

Loss of blood volume

Urine voided first thing in the morning is concentrated because of evaporation at night

Increased blood viscosity

Increase heart rate

Decrease stroke volume

Sweat rate during exercise is highly variable between individuals and methods of assessment (continuous = 1 L/h; peak = 4 L/h; 4 L/h = acclimatization). Loss of salt (1% salt in 99% water). Lethal dehydration 15–25% body weight. Drinking water leads to cramps

Shivering

Disorganized muscle activity at about 10–12 Hz that can increase heat production up to 6 times

Coupled with piloerection to trap air close to skin to act as insulation

Men shiver more than women

Elderly shiver less because of a lower core temperature threshold [10], muscle mass is smaller and muscles contract less

Shivering increased oxygen consumption in the elderly by 38% and may be significant for oxygen delivery to tissues [11]

Opioid administration reduces shivering

Hormonal

Catecholamine (adrenaline, noradrenaline) induce glycogenolysis in muscle and liver cells

Thyroxine enhances the rate of most cellular reactions [12]

Skin cooling stimulates TRH which in turn induces the release of TSH

Metabolic rate increased by testosterone, GH, glucagons, insulin, ACTH

Chronic responses to cold — acclimatization

Increase in body fat/larger body structure to produce more heat from more cells/less efficient superficial heat loss

Changes in endocrine response (glucocorticoids, gluconeogenesis and protein breakdown, T3 and T4, catecholamine induced thermogenesis)

Development of non-shivering thermogenesis (e.g. brown fat) UCP2 and UCP3 mechanisms may be involved and white fat through adrenaline stimulation via β_3-adrenergic receptors

Females compared with males

Smaller blood volume

Smaller lean body mass and greater body fat

Greater surface area/body weight

Higher set point for vasodilatation and sweating

Greater resting vasoconstriction

Less sweat than men (men 50% more sweat than women)

Thinner extremities

Cyclical hormone changes (e.g. 0.5°C) lower during follicular than luteal phase; progesterone increases at ovulation and it raises the body temperature

Reproductive changes

ACTH, adrenocorticotrophic hormone; GH, growth hormone; TRH, thyroid-releasing hormone; TSH, thyroid-stimulating hormone.

absorption and assimilation, and is called the specific dynamic action of food. Protein ingestion increases the metabolic rate more than carbohydrates and fat. During exercise, muscle heat predominates.

Basal metabolic rate

The minimal level of heat produced by the body at rest in a thermoneutral environment is the basal metabolic rate (BMR). This ensures the maintenance of normal metabolic processes such as cellular activity. The BMR is less in women and in the elderly (Table 22.6) [20] and the thermoneutral environment also changes, such that people at the extremes of life feel more comfortable at higher temperatures. However, in the elderly, the range of core temperatures across which sweating and shivering effector responses are absent is twice as much (1.1°C) as in the young (0.4°C).

Acclimatization

Changes in the physiological regulation of temperature in response to hot or cold environments are described as acclimatization and are usually reversible. In a hot environment, the process occurs within 4–7 days and is complete in approximately 12–14 days. The changes that occur are an increase in sweat production and increased secretion of aldosterone.

In the cold, acclimatization is much slower. The mechanisms depend more on hormonal than cardiovascular changes. The hypothalamus increases the secretion of thyroid-stimulating releasing hormone which acts on the anterior pituitary cells to generate thyroid-stimulating hormone (TSH). The TSH increases the synthesis and release of thyroid hormones. In addition, release of noradrenaline and adrenaline release is stimulated. These catecholamines increase cellular metabolism and alter fat deposition. Other changes in the cold include cold vasodilatation to prevent frostbite.

Heat stress

If the rate of heat gain continues to be greater than heat loss, body temperature will rise, leading to heat stress and then heat stroke. In an unacclimatized subject, exercise can induce heat stress. Heat stroke begins with nausea, vomiting, generalized weakness, headache and the skin feels hot. If the exercise persists, circulatory collapse results from water and salt depletion, sweating is reduced, confusion and delirium supervene, with cerebral pathology (e.g. oedema), and renal and hepatic failure can result. Once body temperature increases to 42°C, cellular function deteriorates and this can be permanent. Management of heat stroke is to remove the subject from the heat, cool the skin and carefully administer fluids and electrolytes. Any system failure may require intensive care. The differences between the extremes of survival for heat loss and heat gain are dissimilar: Table 22.1 shows that a

Table 22.6 The average resting metabolic rate in young (20–33 years) and elderly (63–88 years) subjects at 22°C room temperature [18] (1 W = 1 J/s).

	Young male $n=29$	Young female $n=27$	Elderly male $n=32$	Elderly female $n=71$
Age (years)	27	23	73	72
Height (m²)	1.85	1.71	1.75	1.61
Weight (kg)	77	63	78	67
BMI (kg/m²)	23	22	25	26
Body fat (%)	14	28	30	39
Resting metabolic rate kJ/min (kJ/h/kg)	5.3 (4.1)	4.1 (3.9)	4.0 (3.1)	3.3 (3.0)

similar range of colder temperatures is better tolerated.

Less severe heat stress results in decreased efficiency and increases in pulse rate, thirst and a feeling of weariness. If the environment is warm with a high moisture content (high humidity), it is more difficult for physiological mechanisms to cope compared with less humid environments. Other clinical conditions that occur during heat exposure include heat rash, where sweat glands become plugged, retaining sweat, and heat cramps which are associated with the loss of salt.

Sweating

Sweat glands are found more frequently on the forehead than on the back of the arm. Sweat can be detected by using anhydrous cobalt chloride paper that goes pink when wet. Sweat is produced by acinar epithelial cells and has a final composition (compared with plasma) of 60 mmol (140) Na^+, 46 mmol (113) Cl^- and 8.8 mmol (5.0) K^+. As the sweat moves along the sweat ducts, sodium and chloride are reabsorbed provided there is time for this process. Thus, in excessive exercise without acclimatization there can be severe losses of salt. One mechanism acting to prevent this is the secretion of aldosterone from the zona glomerulosa of the adrenal cortex. Aldosterone acts not only on the distal convoluted tubules to enhance resorption of sodium ions, but also in the sweat ducts. The rate of sweating depends on both the core and skin temperatures. It occurs at a lower core temperature if the peripheral temperature is elevated.

Temporal changes: age and circadian modulation

Neonates lose heat faster than adults because of their larger surface area to body weight ratio and their lack of body fat. Heat production is not so well regulated, although brown fat mechanisms are protective, so that a higher thermoneutral temperature zone is needed to maintain body temperature, particularly in sick neonates, such as incubators or radiant heat warmers. In the second to third weeks after birth, the circadian rhythm of temperature regulation starts to develop and is complete at approximately 2 years of age.

As people age they become more vulnerable to hypothermia or hyperthermia because there is a progressive decrease in effector responses [21]. For example, older people do not shiver at the same intensity as younger subjects as the vasoconstrictor response to cold is less pronounced [22]. However, skin thermal receptors and their sensitivity may remain intact, as do thermal pain sensors, unless thresholds are increased as seen in neuropathic diseases such as diabetes. Other changes may contribute to a loss of skin temperature sensitivity, such as a loss of collagen, reduction and less compliance in the vascular supply, and lower thermal buffering capacity as a result of reduction in body water. It is the response to cold rather than to heat that is obtunded, leading to the potential for hypothermia. There is also a reduction in BMR related to the loss of fat-free heat producing tissue such as muscle. However, where activity is maintained these processes are protected and circadian rhythms are maintained. Food intake may be reduced so that its thermic effect may be lost. In addition, hormone levels change with ageing and the elderly are more vulnerable to decreased thyroid function.

Non-pharmacological and pharmacological events and temperature regulation

Cold shower

In a cool environment generated by cold water, peripheral vasoconstriction will occur and peripheral sensors activated. Movement of blood volume to the central compartment will lead to an increase in venous pressure, detected by pressure receptors in the atrium and stimulating the excretion of fluids through atrial natriuretic peptide. Heat production will increase with muscle activity and the overall changes will mainly relate to effectors in the cardiovascular system.

Anaesthesia

During anaesthesia, body heat is redistributed such that cold peripheral blood returns to the core. Set points may be altered through central nervous system effects. Physical factors in the operating theatre can further influence these effects, such as cold air, fluids and surfaces, dry gases, exposure of large areas of the body, especially if internal and wet, and lack of body movement. A greater awareness of these potential effects on body temperature has initiated active warming systems. The effects of cold as outlined below under hypothermia are always a danger to patients having prolonged surgery, but an added effect is that of poor organ function and the effect of other drugs.

In clinical research, factors that influence temperature regulation should be standardized (e.g. morbidity and age), and the results interpreted with normal ranges for that age. Blockade of sympathetic activity can inhibit vasoconstriction in the elderly, thus altering skin thermoregulation (e.g. during spinal anaesthesia) [23]. Patients with compromised cardiovascular systems can have significant morbidity if they become hypothermic [24].

Laparoscopic surgery
Loss of body heat during laparoscopic surgery illustrates the many factors that may reduce thermal capacity that occur during anaesthesia [25]. Conduction heat loss occurs from contact with objects at room temperature, convection from the flow of cold gases into the peritoneum, evaporation from the peritoneum to humidify the gases, and radiation from the body to other objects.

Pathological changes in temperature regulation

Fever
Fever is caused by exercise, heat stroke and anterior pituitary lesions as well as by disease. During a fever the brain is often at a higher temperature than the rest of the body [26]. An increase in the set point occurs so that for the same body temperature the sensation is one of cold, and the body responds by initiating heat conserving mechanisms such as shivering. Pyrogens are produced during the inflammatory response which act centrally on the hypothalamus through prostaglandin receptors (PGE_2) to modify membrane potential changes lead-ing to an alteration in the set point [27]. Such substances include interleukins (IL-1, IL-6) and tumour necrosis factor (TNF-α). Antipyretics such as acetyl salicylic acid (aspirin) inhibit the enzyme cyclo-oxygenase to prevent the synthesis of the pyrogenic prostaglandins and reverse the fever. Active warming in patients at risk of hyperthermia can lead to overheating and pyrexia [28].

Hyperthyroidism
A thyroid crisis may present with fever, tachycardia, atrial fibrillation, restlessness, confusion and coma. It can be precipitated by surgery and trauma, especially in the unprepared thyrotoxic patient. Intravenous fluids, β-adrenergic block, potassium iodide and carbimazole are first-line therapies.

Hypothermia
A reduction in body temperature can occur from various causes, including exposure (air, water), extremes of age, especially the elderly, in a cold climate, prolonged surgery and hypothyroidism [29].

Electrocardiographic changes
First a conduction defect occurs, with prolongation of PR and then QRS. However, an increase in muscle tone may obscure these effects. A J wave may be present at the junction of the QRS and ST segment and is usually seen at temperatures less than 32°C. It is not related to arterial blood pH but can be associated with myocardial ischaemia and sepsis.

Below 32°C, all types of dysrhythmias are common (Table 22.1). Ventricular fibrillation can result from re-entry pathways producing sporadic uncontrolled stimulation because conduction time is longer than the refractory period. It may be iatrogenic through hypovolaemia, hypoxia, increased blood viscosity and acid–base changes.

Respiratory effects
As body temperature is lowered, respiration is stimulated. Below 30°C, respiratory frequency will decrease and carbon dioxide production decreases by 50% for every 2°C reduction. Muscle stiffness reduces elasticity and thoracic compliance, secretions become more viscous and acute respiratory distress syndrome can develop.

Renal effects

Renal blood flow decreases by 50% at 30°C. An initial cold diuresis may occur because of peripheral shutdown and release of vasopressin in response to central increase in blood volume.

Blood

Variable local and central effects on coagulation occur that increase thromboembolism. Lowering the temperature shifts the oxygen dissociation curve to the left so that oxygen is more difficult to offload at the tissues. Thus, cellular hypoxia may be present with good oxygen saturation and oxygen saturation is no guide to adequate tissue oxygenation. However, the resultant tissue acidosis will tend to move the dissociation curve to the left and counterbalance the effects of temperature. There are major fluid shifts on cooling and the reverse occurs during re-warming. Lactated solutions are best avoided because the liver cannot metabolize the lactate. A condition of after drop is associated with movement of pockets of colder fluids into core tissues which lead to further reductions in core temperature.

Acute management of exposure hypothermia

Prevent further heat loss.
• Replace wet clothing with dry.
• Care with walking casualties, they can die from an after drop in temperature.
• Handle carefully to avoid fluid shifts and precipitation of dysrhythmias.
• Vital signs may not show a hypothermic picture if trauma has occurred.
• Warm inhaled gases and fluids.
• Begin cardiopulmonary resuscitation providing any injury is not lethal and signs of life are not present.
• Leave active rewarming until hospitalized [30].

Measuring temperature

The relationships between Celcius, Farenheit and Kelvin temperature scales are shown in Table 22.7. A temperature measuring device should be accurate, have an electronic output, be automated and easy to position alongside the patient. The laws of thermodynamics are relevant. If objects are in thermal equilibrium, no heat passes between them. If heat moves from one object to another, energy is transferred. If an object is heated the entropy (disorder) becomes greater, and if entropy is zero, temperature is zero (0°Kelvin). The Kelvin scale is an ideal scale, with a straight line relationship between zero and the triple point of water (273.15°K, when it is solid, liquid and vapour); there are 100 points in this practical scale between ice and steam. Electronic thermometers suitable for clinical use include thermistors, thermocouples, resistance thermometers and radiant heat.

Body sites for measuring temperature

The choice of body site used for measuring temperature depends on access, type of surgery and age (e.g. neonate). At these sites, one can measure skin, intermediate or core tissue temperature. For example, in neuroanaesthesia with cardiopulmonary bypass cooling, direct brain temperature corresponds to nasopharyngeal, oesophageal and pulmonary artery temperature but not to tympanic, rectal, axillary or bladder temperatures [31].

Oesophageal measures are suitable for unconscious patients and if the probe is positioned behind the heart a reasonable core temperature can be measured. The best site is at the junction of the first two-thirds and last third of the oesophagus. This position can be measured out on the surface of the body. If the probe is higher it will measure the temperature of gases entering the lungs. A nasopharyngeal temperature probe can be sited easily when the patient is asleep, at the back of the nasopharynx, where it is close to the brain. If an oral endotracheal tube is in place, interference from inhaled gases will be minimal and allow an adequate core temperature to be measured. The ear also allows a core temperature to be measured in active subjects, either with a tympanic probe or in the external auditory meatus, provided there is protection from draughts. Another invasive measure that records continuously but

Table 22.7 Temperature scales.

	Fahrenheit	Celsius	Kelvin
Absolute zero	−460	−273	0
Water freezes	32	0	273
Water boils	212	100	373

which can be used in awake patients in an intensive care unit is blood temperature via a pulmonary floatation catheter. The rectal temperature is not related to a core structure and interpretation of values obtained by this route are confounded by faecal impaction and fetal effects if pregnant. Urinary catheter temperatures have been used, but require a high basal urine production.

References

1 IUPS Thermal Commission 2001. Glossary of terms for thermal physiology. *Jpn J Physiol* 2001; **51**: 245–80.

2 Holdcroft A, Hall GM. Heat loss during anaesthesia. *Br J Anaesth* 1978; **50**: 157–64.

3 Van Someren EJW. More than a marker: interaction between the circadian regulation of temperature and sleep, age-related changes and treatment possibilities. *Chronobiol Int* 2000; **17**: 313–54.

4 Bulcao CF, Frank SM, Raja SN, Tran KM, Goldstein DS. Relative contribution of core and skin temperatures to thermal comfort in humans. *J Therm Biol* 2000; **25**: 147–50.

5 Wenger CB, Roberts MF, Stolwijk JA, Nadel ER. Nocturnal lowering of thresholds for sweating and vasodilation. *J Appl Physiol* 1976; **41**: 15.

6 Minson CT, Berry LT, Joyner MJ. Nitric oxide and neurally mediated regulation of skin blood flow during local heating. *J Appl Physiol* 2001; **91**: 1619–26.

7 Krauchi K, Wirz-Justice A. Circadian clues to sleep onset mechanisms. *Neuropsychopharmacol* 2001; **25**: S92–6.

8 Charkoudian N. Skin blod flow in adult human thermoregulation: how it works, when it does not, and why. *Mayo Clin Proc* 2003; **78**: 603–12.

9 Sell H, Deshaies Y, Richard D. The brown adipocyte: update on its metabolic role. *Int J Biochem Cell Biol* 2004; **36**: 2098–104.

10 Frank SM, Raja SN, Wu PK, el-Gamal N. α-Adrenergic mechanisms of thermoregulation in humans. *Ann N Y Acad Sci* 1997; **813**: 101–10.

11 Frank SM, Fleisher LA, Olson KF, *et al*. Multivariate determinants of early postoperative oxygen consumption in elderly patients. *Anesthesiology* 1995; **83**: 241–9.

12 Arancibia S, Rage F, Astier H, Tapia-Arancibia L. Neuroendocrine and autonomous mechanisms underlying thermoregulation in cold environment. *Neuroendocrinology* 1996; **64**: 257–67.

13 Berthoud HR, Neuhuber WL. Functional and chemical anatomy of the afferent vagal system. *Auton Neurosci* 2000; **85**: 1–17.

14 Mercer JB, Simon E. Lessons from the past: human and animal thermal physiology. *J Therm Biol* 2001; **26**: 249–53.

15 Tanaka M, Tonouchi M, Hosono T, *et al*. Hypothalamic region facilitating shivering in rats. *Jpn J Physiol* 2001; **51**: 625–9.

16 Jansky L. Humoral thermogenesis and its role in maintaining energy balance. *Physiol Rev* 1995; **75**: 237–59.

17 Jansky P, Jansky L. Sites and cellular mechanisms of human adrenergic thermogenesis: a review. *J Therm Biol* 2002; **27**: 269–77.

18 Gordon CJ, Miller DB. Thermoregulation in rats exposed perinatally to dioxin: core temperature stability to altered ambient temperature, behavioral thermoregulation, and febrile response to lipopolysaccharide. *J Toxicol Environ Health A* 1998; **54**: 647–62.

19 Horvath TL, Warden CH, Hajos M, *et al*. Brain uncoupling protein 2: uncoupled neuronal mitochondrial predict thermal synapses in homeostatic centres. *J Neurosci* 1999; **19**: 10417–27.

20 Visser M, Deurenberg P, van Staveren WA, Hautvast JGAJ. Resting metabolic rate and diet-induced thermogenesis in young and elderly subjects: relationship with body composition, fat distribution, and physical activity level. *Am J Clin Nutr* 1995; **61**: 72–8.

21 Anderson GS, Meneilly GS, Mekjavic. Passive temperature lability in the elderly. *Eur J Appl Physiol* 1996; **73**: 278–86.

22 Van Someren EJW, Raymann RJEM, Scherder EJA, Daanen HAM, Swaab DF. Circadian and age-related modulation of thermoreception and temperature regulation: mechanisms and functional implications. *Ageing Res Rev* 2002; **1**: 721–78.

23 Sessler DI. Perianaesthetic thermoregulation and heat balance in humans. *FASEB J* 1993; **7**: 638–44.

24 Frank SM, Fleisher LA, Breslow MJ, *et al*. Perioperative maintenance of normothermia reduces the incidence of morbid cardiac events: a randomized clinical trial. *JAMA* 1997; **277**: 1127–34.

25 Hazebroek EJ, Schreve MA, Visser P, *et al*. Impact of temperature and humidity of carbon dioxide pneumoperitoneum on body temperature and peritoneal morphology. *J Laparoendosc Adv Surg Tech A* 2002; **12**: 355–64.

26 Mariak Z. Intracranial temperature recordings in human subjects: the contribution of the neurosurgeon to thermal physiology. *J Therm Biol* 2002; **27**: 219–28.

27 Dinarello CA. Infection, fever and exogenous and endogenous pyrogens: some concepts have changed. *J Endotoxin Res* 2004; **10**: 201–22.

28 Deacock S, Holdcroft A. Heat retention using passive systems during anaesthesia: comparisons of two plastic wraps, one with reflective properties. *Br J Anaesth* 1997; **79**: 766–9.

29 Preston BR. Effect of hypothermia on systemic and organ system metabolism and function. *J Surg Res* 1976; **20**: 49.

30 Southwick FS, Dalglish PH. Recovery after prolonged hypothermia. *JAMA* 1980; **243**: 1250–3.

31 Stone JG, Young WL, Smith CR, *et al.* Do standard monitoring sites reflect true brain temperature when profound hypothermia is rapidly induced and reversed? *Anesthesiology* 1995; **82**: 344–51.

CHAPTER 23

Theories of pain

Lesley Colvin

Introduction

Theories of pain processing have changed dramatically over the years, with variable importance being placed on peripheral input versus central mechanisms. The separation of body from the mind (dualistic theory) is still in evidence today, although it is becoming increasingly clear that this simplistic approach is inadequate in defining the processes of pain perception. Aristotle (350 BC) defined pain as an emotion or sensation experienced in the heart, whereas Leonardo da Vinci (1452–1519) defined pain as a sensory experience mediated by touch nerves.

In 1664, Descartes described a hard-wired pain pathway that was modality specific and analogous to a 'bell rope'. Descartes used a mechanistic approach to pain, with the focus primarily on nociception and the assumption that there was a hard-wired and unbroken connection between pain receptors in the periphery and pain centres in the brain (Fig. 23.1).

It was only in the 1960s that peripheral nociceptors were identified and the influential Gate Theory of Pain was published. This theory focused on the importance of modulation at a spinal level, with continuous interaction between activity in small and large diameter afferents, local spinal neurones and descending systems from the brain [1]. The current view is of a dynamic system with marked neuroneal plasticity and interaction between the periphery, spinal cord and brain, with a neuromatrix within the brain involved in pain perception, modulating and interacting with both spinal and peripheral mechanisms.

It is important to remember the International Association for the Study of Pain definition of pain as 'an unpleasant sensory and emotional experience associated with actual or potential tissue damage or described in terms of such damage'. This chapter focuses on the sensory systems involved in pain perception (nociception) and how these may be altered in different pain states. It is important to remember that many other factors can have a significant role in the experience of pain, level of distress and functional disability.

Basic pain processing

Under normal conditions, acute pain serves a useful biological function, initiating a withdrawal response to remove and protect the threatened part from further injury, as well as immobilizing to allow wound healing. A basic outline of the anatomy of this nociceptive system is shown in Figure 23.2 and is discussed in more detail below. It must be emphasized that this is a dynamic system, dependent on input, tissue damage and other factors. Even in the acute situation (e.g. in the postoperative period), major changes may occur at all levels within the system.

Peripheral sensory processing

In the periphery, high intensity noxious stimuli are transduced by non-specialized free nerve endings, resulting in action potential generation in primary sensory neurones. Table 23.1 outlines the different types of peripheral sensory nerves and their role in nociception. It is predominantly unmyelinated C fibres and small myelinated Aδ fibres that are involved in transmission of nociceptive input. The cell bodies of these fibres are situated in the dorsal root ganglia, close to the spinal cord. This is where the nucleus lies and where all neurotransmitters necessary for sensory transduction are synthesized then transported peripherally or centrally. Specific receptors and channels have been identified in nociceptors involved in transducing particular types of noxious stimuli.

Noxious heat transduction

The vanilloid receptors, members of the transient re-

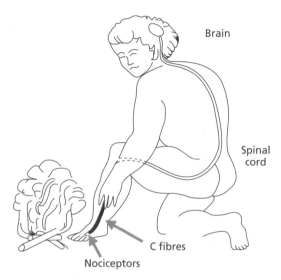

Figure 23.1 Descartes' picture of the 'pain pathway' (1664). The fire (noxious stimulus) generated minute rapidly moving particles that pulled on delicate threads attached to the spot on the skin that they touched. This instantly activated 'pores' in the brain, in the same way that pulling a bell rope instantly strikes a bell at the other end.

ceptor potential (TRP) family of ion channels, have been shown to be important in heat transduction. TRP channels of the vanilloid family (TRPV1–4) are excited by heat stimuli. The VR-1 (permeable to calcium ions) responds to moderate noxious heat and may be modulated by hydrogen ion concentrations. TRPV1 also responds to nociceptor-specific chemicals such as capsaicin or mustard oil. Sensitization of TRPV1 is an important mechanism for heat hyperalgesia whereas TRPM8 and ANKTM1 are cold responsive [2].

Noxious cold transduction

The mechanisms underlying transduction of cold information are less clear. A cold and menthol sensitive receptor (CMR1), of the TRP family of receptors, responds to cold in the 8–28°C temperature range and is expressed on small diameter sensory neurones. A related channel, TRPA1, has also been found which responds to lower temperatures [2].

Noxious chemical transduction

Changes in the local environment after tissue damage can result in activation of nociceptors secondary to release of chemical substances. These include extracellular protons, adenosine triphosphate (ATP), arachidonic acid and its metabolites, serotonin, bradykinin and nerve growth factor (NGF). In addition to this dramatic change in the local environment, nociceptors themselves may release neuropeptides when activated by noxious stimuli or

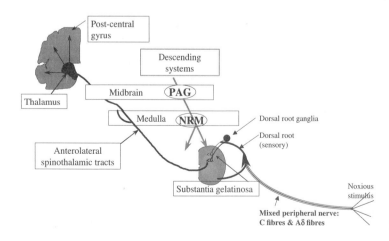

Figure 23.2 Nociceptive pathway. Peripheral noxious stimuli activate nociceptors with subsequent action potential generation that may eventually result in neuronal activity within the brain and pain perception. NRM, nucleus raphe magnus; PAG, periaqueductal grey matter.

Table 23.1 Classification of primary afferent neurones.

Fibre type	Diameter	Conduction velocity	Sensory modality	Spinal termination
Aβ: large, myelinated	6–15 μm	30–100 ms^{-1}	Light touch, proprioception	Laminae III/IV
Aδ: small, myelinated	2–6 μm	12–30 ms^{-1}	Noxious and innocuous sensory	Laminae I/II; V
C: unmyelinated	0.5–2 μm	0.5–2.0 ms^{-1}	Pain, temperature; also post-ganglionic autonomic	Laminae I/II

via antidromic activation of the peripheral nerve, which may also modulate the release of inflammatory mediators from surrounding tissues.

Changes in local hydrogen ion concentration are important whether indirectly, as by modifying the activity of other receptors such as the VR-1 receptor, or by a direct action on a family of cation channels termed the acid-sensing ion channel (ASIC) family. These are generally permeable to sodium, but are closed at physiological pH. Several subtypes of ATP receptor have been cloned and are localized on nociceptive afferents. There are several subtypes of the ionotropic form (P2X$_{1-7}$) as well as metabotropic forms (P2Y), which are linked to a number of processes including phospholipase C (PLC) activation [3].

Noxious mechanical transduction

Although no specific protein for transduction of mechanical stimuli has yet been found, a member of the mammalian degenerin (MDEG) ion channel family may be involved.

C fibres

Two main types of C fibres are detectable immunohistochemically. Approximately 40% of C fibres express tropomyosin-related kinase A (trk A) receptors for NGF, and most of these also express the neuropeptides substance P (SP) and calcitonin gene-related peptide (CGRP). The other group of C fibres express α-D-galactosyl-binding lectin (IB$_4$) and the P2X$_3$ ATP-gated ion channel [4].

The majority of nociceptors on C fibres are polymodal, responding in a non-specific manner to a va-

riety of noxious stimuli such as heat, mechanical and chemical, although some will only respond to specific noxious stimuli (e.g. cold). There are also 'silent' nociceptors, which do not normally respond to any form of stimulus until sensitized by tissue injury. There appear to be several different types of C fibres, such as those responsive to heat and mechanical stimuli (CMH units), mechano-insensitive units, which tend to respond to heat and have a slower conduction velocity (CH units) and some that are unresponsive to either heat or mechanical stimuli, but do respond to chemical stimuli [5].

As knowledge of the detailed molecular mechanisms underlying sensory transduction expands, it should be possible to classify subtype of nociceptors and sensory fibres by the transducer proteins they express. This may allow development of more targeted and peripherally acting analgesics.

Spinal processing

Primary afferent neurones synapse in the dorsal horn of the spinal cord with second-order neurones, in a precise somatotopic map of peripheral structures. The majority of C and Aδ fibres synapse in laminae I and II of the superficial dorsal horn, in the substantia gelatinosa. Some Aδ fibres synapse in lamina V deeper in the dorsal horn. The second-order neurones vary in their input specificity and how they respond to stimuli. Complex modulation of second-order activity can occur both via intrinsic spinal mechanisms and descending systems. The second-order projection neurones ascend to the brain in specific tracts [6].

Spinal cord anatomy

Nociceptive information is signalled by several anatomically distinct populations of primary afferents targeting different neuronal populations in the spinal cord. The neuronal grey matter forms a 'butterfly-shaped' arrangement around a central canal, surrounded by white matter. The grey matter has been divided into 10 laminae based on cytoarchitectonic characteristics. This makes up the dorsal and ventral horns (laminae I–IX), with lamina X surrounding the central canal. In all mammalian species, the dorsal horn consists of laminae I–V and receives all primary afferent input (see Fig. 23.3).

The majority of low-threshold mechanoreceptors (via large myelinated Aβ fibres) terminate in laminae III and IV, whereas high-threshold nociceptors terminate mainly in laminae I, II and V. C fibres terminate predominantly in lamina II, whereas Aδ fibres from the skin may terminate within superficial laminae, or deeper in lamina V. Visceral and muscle afferents project to mainly lamina V [6]. In addition to this laminar arrangement, the central terminals of primary afferent neurones also form an ordered somatotopic map of the skin surface in the dorsal horn of the spinal cord. Laminae I–III contain many small cells, with a few larger ones in laminae I and III. Many neurones in laminae I and III project to the brain, whereas most lamina II neurones arborize locally.

The thin outermost zone of the dorsal horn, lamina I, contains relatively few cells, many of which are projection neurones that join the spinothalamic tract (STT) and spinomesencephalic tract (SMT). Four main morphological cell types are found in lamina I: dendrites of fusiform, flattened and pyramidal cells remain within lamina I, whereas those of multipolar cells may enter lamina II or III. A population of large lamina I neurones receive input from SP-containing primary afferents and express neurokinin-1 (NK1) receptors. Their dendritic geometry and synaptic input suggests that these neurones may monitor the extent of injury rather than the specific localization of a discrete noxious stimulus [7].

Lamina II, the 'substantia gelatinosa', so-called because of its appearance under light microscope, lies ventral to lamina I. Its outer zone (lamina II_o) contains densely packed small cells ($5 \times 5\,\mu$m) with a less compact inner zone (lamina II_i). Two structural types of neurones are found within this lamina: islet cells (dendrites that spread rostrocaudally and axons that remain close to the cell body) and stalked cells (in lamina II_o, with dendrites that fan out ventrally and axons passing dorsally into lamina I) [8]. There is some evidence that stalked cells, receiving primary afferent input from glomerular synapses, are involved in processing of information on fine discrimination of the exact location of a noxious event [7].

Rapidly adapting mechanoreceptors, primary afferents from large hair follicles and pacinian corpuscles, terminate in lamina III, which contain larger and less tightly packed cells. Some of the second-order neurones send dendrites to laminae I and IV or join the spinocervical tract (SCT) and the postsynaptic dorsal column (PSDC) tract. Lamina IV is a thick layer containing large scattered cells, often with dendrites projecting into laminae I–III. This dendritic distribution means that lamina IV cells can receive both direct primary afferent input (from fibres entering the superficial layers) and indirect mediated inputs from other dorsal horn laminae. Many of the larger cells project to the SCT and PSDC. Lamina V forms the narrowest part of the dorsal horn. It con-

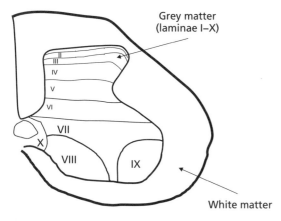

Figure 23.3 Section through spinal cord showing Rexed's laminae. The dorsal horn, where the sensory afferents terminate is mainly laminae I–VI. The substantia gelatinosa is where most of the C fibres and some of the Aδ fibres terminate, and consists of laminae I–II. It is so called because of its characteristic histological appearance.

tains the largest cells, many of which join the ascending STT.

Neurotransmitters within the dorsal horn

The wide range of neurotransmitters found in the dorsal horn has been studied extensively, as they present a potential site for analgesic action and show significant changes in chronic pain states. The main groups are amino acid neurotransmitters and neuropeptides each with specific inhibitory or excitatory effects.

Amino acids

Two main inhibitory amino acids found in the dorsal horn are γ-aminobutyric acid (GABA) and glycine. Although there is evidence that these neurotransmitters are co-released in the dorsal horn during development, with maturation and fine-tuning of nociceptive processing, this co-release does not appear to be found in the adult state. They do, however, still coexist in dorsal horn neurones. Most GABA-

containing cells are intrinsic to the dorsal horn, acting presynaptically on primary afferents to inhibit transmission, with a few GABAergic cells found in descending tracts. Glycine is also found in intrinsic neurones of the dorsal horn, again exerting presynaptic inhibitory effects on sensory input [9].

The main excitatory amino acid neurotransmitter is L-glutamate, acting at a variety of receptors (Table 23.2) and found within the majority of laminae I and II neurones. Of the ionotropic receptors, the non-*N*-methyl-D-aspartate (NMDA) receptors (α-amino-3-hydroxyl-5-methyl-4-isoxazole propionic acid [AMPA] and kainate) are thought to be important in fast synaptic transmission, while the NMDA receptor is involved in slower synaptic responses [10].

NMDA receptor

The NMDA receptor is an ionotropic glutamate receptor, permeable to calcium and sodium ions, found in both dorsal and ventral horns of the spinal cord. It

Table 23.2 Glutamate receptors.

Receptor class	Type	Subunits	
Ionotropic	AMPA	4 subunits: GluR-A-D subunits complete receptor Glu R1–4	Ca^{2+} permeable AMPARs: lamina I, outer lamina GluR2 subunit determines calcium permeability Widely distributed in CNS; GluR1 and GluR2: found mainly on neurones in superficial dorsal horn GluR3 and 4: lower levels in the superficial dorsal horn: GluR3 moderate levels laminae I–III; Glu–undetectable GluR3/4: ventral horn high levels in motor neurones
	Kainate		GluR5 subunit containing receptors: found on diameter primary afferent neurones GluR5 or GluR6 subunits: suppress or facilitate glutamatergic excitatory transmission in the dorsal horn
	NMDA	NR1; NR2 A-D	Functional unit: NR1 Channel characteristics: NR2 subunit; Permeable to calcium + sodium; Voltage-dependent magnesium block
Metabotropic	Three groups (I, II, III)	8 subunits	Gp I (mGluR1 and mGluR5): superficial dorsal Gp II (mGlu2 and 3): presynaptic; decrease glu release Gp III: varied roles: mGluR6: only in the retina amplifies visual inputs; mGluR4, 7 and 8: found at presynaptic sites

consists of a complex of proteins with various signalling and structural functions. The key functional unit is the NR1 subunit, which combines with the NR2 subunit (A–D). Thus, the NMDA receptor is a tetramer of NR1 and NR2A–D subunits. Specific subtype channel characteristics are conferred by the NR2 subunit. The intracellular C terminus end of the NR2 unit may interact with a family of proteins known as the membrane-associated guanylate kinase family (MAGUK), including protein complexes such as PSD-95/SAP90, which may have a significant role in chronic pain states [11].

NMDA receptors in the dorsal horn are largely inactive during acute nociceptive transmission, being blocked by magnesium ions in a voltage-dependent manner. However, with prolonged noxious stimuli, glutamate released from Aδ and C fibres may be sufficient to activate NMDA receptors in a process termed central sensitization or wind up (see below). If the dorsal horn neurone is sufficiently depolarized, or the receptor is phosphorylated via second messenger systems, NMDA receptor activation may occur. With NMDA receptor activation, by removal of the magnesium block, postsynaptic calcium flux increases as channel opening time is prolonged. Glutamate binding to the NMDA receptor may be modulated by a regulatory glycine-binding site. Glycine may act as a co-agonist, and Gly_{NMDA} site antagonists have been shown to suppress behavioural correlates of wind-up.

Non-NMDA receptors
Kainate receptors
Extensive study of these receptors has been limited by a lack of specific agonists and antagonists. Kainate receptors incorporating the GluR5 subunit are present at high levels on small diameter primary afferent neurones thought to mediate nociceptive inputs. GluR5 agonists may have a small effect in reducing C fibre-mediated reflexes in spinal cord preparations, but their analgesic effect *in vivo* is unclear [12,13].

AMPA receptors
AMPA receptors are involved in the fast transmission of sensory input — both noxious and innocuous stimuli. The majority of monosynaptic excitatory postsynaptic potentials (EPSP) in the dorsal horn evoked by C fibres are mediated via AMPA receptors and may culminate in action potential generation. The AMPA receptor is found in most areas of the central nervous system. The superficial dorsal horn contains significant numbers of AMPA receptors, with the GluR1 and GluR2 subunits. Although the majority of AMPARs are postsynaptic, some presynaptic AMPARs have been demonstrated in lamina II of the dorsal horn with an inhibitory role [12,13].

Metabotropic glutamate receptors
Metabotropic glutamate receptors (mGluRs) may also be involved in nociceptive processing. These are not ion channels, but are instead coupled to G-proteins, with glutamate binding producing intracellular changes in enzyme activation and calcium levels. All these functions lead to an increase cellular excitability and are likely to underlie the part group I metabotropic glutamate receptors are thought to play in various forms of synaptic plasticity, including long term potentiation in the hippocampus, wind-up and the development of chronic pain states. There is a family of eight subtypes, divided functionally into three groups. Group I metabotropic receptors (mGluR1 and mGluR5) are concentrated in the superficial dorsal horn of the spinal cord. Group II and III mGluRs are negatively coupled to adenylate cyclase via $G_{i/o}$ proteins, with presynaptic group II receptors (mGlu2 and 3) decreasing glutamate release. Group III mGluRs are involved in varied processes: mGluR6 is found only in the retina and has a role in the amplification of visual inputs. The remainder of group III receptors, mGluR4, 7 and 8, are also found at presynaptic sites [14].

Neuropeptides
A range of neuropeptides are found in primary afferent neurones, particularly unmyelinated or small myelinated fibres, although this changes in chronic pain states. Dorsal horn neurones themselves can also contain neuropeptides. A brief overview of some of the neuropeptides involved in sensory processing is given below and in Table 23.3.

Tachykinins
The tachykinins are a family of peptides derived

Table 23.3 Examples of neuropeptides involved in spinal sensory processing.

Group	Precursor molecules	Examples of peptides	Main spinal action
Tachykinins	PPT I	Substance P, neurokinin A (NK A), and neuropeptides K and γ	Excitatory
	PPT II	neurokinin B	
Opioids	Preprodynorphin (PPD)	Endorphin; dynorphin; Leuenkephalin	Inhibitory
	Preproenkephalin (PPE)	Enkephalins (Met- and Leu-enkephalin)	Inhibitory
Others		Galanin	Inhibitory
		Somatostatin	Inhibitory or excitatory
		Vasoactive intestinal peptide	Excitatory
		PACAP	Excitatory
		CCK	Excitatory
		CGRP	Excitatory

from the precursors preprotachykinin I and II (PPT I and II). Tachykinin immunopositive fibres have been demonstrated in laminae I–III, generally decreasing in number with increasing depth. Substance P has been identified in the dorsal horn, being released from primary afferents in response to noxious stimulation, acting at the postsynaptic NK1 receptor. NK1 receptor internalization secondary to activation by SP, combined with use of selective destruction of NK1-R expressing neurones, has revealed that the majority of lamina I neurones that project to higher centres express the NK1 receptor. Tachykinins have also been shown to co-localize with other neuropeptides such as CGRP, galanin and cholecystokinin (CCK) within the dorsal horn [15].

Opioid peptides
Endogenous opioid peptides are derived from several precursor molecules (see Table 23.2) and are found within nerve fibres in the superficial dorsal horn, largely within laminae I and II. The cell bodies of these fibres mostly lie within lamina II. The lamina I neurones that contain dynorphin and enkephalin have extensive local collateral connections, and are the main source of long ascending projections to the parabrachial nucleus in the rat. The pontine parabrachial nucleus, which has been implicated in nocicep-

tive as well as antinociceptive processes, expresses high levels of opioid receptors and is reciprocally connected with the spinal cord dorsal horn. In common with other neuropeptides, endogenous opioids are often coexpressed with other neurotransmitters in the dorsal horn such as somatostatin, SP and GABA.

Opioid receptors are found in high concentrations in the superficial dorsal horn, on primary sensory neurones and secondary interneurones, particularly in the substantia gelatinosa, where C fibres terminate. The majority of these are μ receptors, although δ and κ receptors are also found here [16].

There is currently some focus on peripheral opioid receptors, such as the μ receptor, where they may have an anti-inflammatory role. The endomorphins (EMs) are the most potent endogenous μ receptor ligands so far discovered, and it seems probable they are endogenous ligands for peripheral μ receptors. They are synthesized by nociceptive neurones and can be released from the peripheral nerve endings, as well as being produced by cells of the immune system in response to tissue damage and other stimuli [17]. An outline of opioid receptors is shown in Table 23.4.

Other neuropeptides
Other neuropeptides found in the dorsal horn and

Table 23.4 Opioid receptors.

Receptor	Molecular classification	Endogenous ligand	Site
μ	OP3	Beta-endorphin, Leu- and Met-enkephalin; Endomorphins	Pre- & postsynaptic neurones in spinal cord; brainstem (including PAG, NRM); thalamus, cortex; peripheral (inflammation)
κ	OP1	Dynorphins	Spinal cord, supraspinal, hypothalamus
δ	OP2	Enkephalins; beta-endorphin	Olfactory centres, motor integration areas in cortex, limited distribution in nociception areas
Orphan	ORL-1 (opioid-like receptor)	Nociceptin	Spinal cord

likely to be involved in sensory processing include the following.

1 *Galanin:* this is widely distributed in the central nervous system, with a high proportion of locus ceruleus neurones containing galanin and projecting to the spinal cord. Galanin is also found in intrinsic neurones in the spinal cord with highest levels in lumbar and sacral areas, being most abundant in laminae I, II and X [18]. It is thought to be predominantly inhibitory and levels change significantly in chronic pain states [19].

2 *Neuropeptide Y* (NPY)-containing terminals have been found in laminae I–II with lower levels deeper in the dorsal horn. Under normal conditions, it is found mainly in intrinsic neurones, where it may co-exist with galanin or GABA. The functional effects of NPY vary depending on the receptor activated, with some evidence for an inhibitory effect at a spinal level [20,21].

3 *Somatostatin:* a neuropeptide expressed by subpopulation small-diameter primary afferent neurones and in lamina II cells of the dorsal horn. Its role in nociception is not entirely clear, with evidence for both pro- and antinociceptive effects [22].

4 *Cholecystokinin:* may have a role in chronic pain and has been implicated in antagonizing the inhibitory effects of opioids [23].

5 *Vasoactive intestinal polypeptide* (VIP): has been found within laminae I and II, mainly in primary af-

ferent fibres, although a few VIP-containing cell bodies have been found that may extend to the midbrain [24].

6 *Pituitary adenylate cyclase-activating polypeptide* (PACAP): widely expressed within the central nervous system, with evidence that both VIP and PACAP modulate sensory input in the dorsal horn [25].

7 *CGRP:* another important mediator of nociceptive transmission, being found in both C and Aδ fibres. CGRP is often co-released with SP and may potentiate its effects by inhibiting SP endopeptidase [26].

Other neurotransmitters

Other neurotransmitters involved in sensory processing include the following.

1 *Cannabinoids:* two identified cannabinoid receptors, CB_1 and CB_2, have been identified in the superficial laminae of the spinal dorsal horn, with evidence for antinociceptive actions [27].

2 *Purines:* a range of purinergic receptors have been isolated, some of which are likely to important in nociceptive processing, particularly if there is any inflammation. ATP acts on $P2X_3$ and $P2X_{2/3}$ receptors, which are unique to nociceptive afferents [3].

Dorsal horn projection neurones and ascending spinal tracts

The exact cellular mechanisms by which nociceptive

information is transmitted to the brain and the nature of the interaction between higher centres and the spinal cord is not clearly understood. It is thought that projection neurones from the superficial dorsal horn have specific connections with brainstem descending systems, which in turn are closely involved in the regulation of tonic inhibition and excitation at a spinal level. These lamina I projection neurones (usually expressing NK1-R) also connect directly with the thalamus where information is relayed to somatosensory and insular cortices. As there are connections from the limbic system to the descending systems discussed below, the dorsal horn projection neurones may also be in a position to influence limbic system responses [15].

Ascending spinal tracts

Spinothalamic tract

The spinothalamic tract conveys sensory information from the contralateral dorsal horn to the thalamic nuclei, predominantly noxious mechanical information. This tract originates from cells in laminae I, II, IV and V. These excitatory pro-nociceptive neurones within lamina I also receive synapses from local inhibitory interneurones, as well as descending input from inhibitory fibre tracts.

Spinomesencephalic tract

The spinomesencephalic tract originates from cells in laminae I, V and VI to the mesencephalic tegmentum region including the periaqueductal grey area. It is likely that the contribution from lamina I cells is nocispecific.

Dorsal column pathways

The dorsal column pathways can be divided into the PSDC and the SCT. The PSDC originates in laminae III and IV, projecting ipsilaterally to the gracile and cuneate nuclei of the medulla via the dorsal funiculus. A variety of sensory modalities are conveyed by this tract, including pressure, cooling, pinch and hair movement as well as nociceptive information. The SCT originates from cells in laminae IV–VII, most of these projecting ipsilaterally to the lateral funiculus, although some fibres pass into the PSDC or cross the midline to run contralaterally in the ventral funiculus. Many neurones of the SCT are

multireceptive, and can respond to nociceptive stimulation [28].

Descending systems

Melzack and Wall's gate control theory introduced the concept of descending inhibitory pathways, or 'descending noxious inhibitory control' (DNIC). Local inhibitory mechanisms at a spinal level may be augmented by these descending inhibitory pathways from the brain, reducing nociceptive transmission [29].

The descending pathways involved originate in the brainstem from several areas. This includes the medullary nucleus raphe magnus (NRM) and adjacent structures of the rostral ventromedial medulla (RVM). The NRM provides a major descending serotonergic input to the dorsal horn laminae I, II and V. Stimulation of both this region, and the periaqueductal grey (PAG) in the midbrain, produces analgesia, probably via an opioid mechanism.

The locus ceruleus (LC) also has a role in modulating nociceptive transmission, via its actions on the parafascicular neurones of the thalamus. The LC exerts two opposing effects on nociceptive transmission. Descending noradrenergic fibres from the LC to the spinal cord have a predominantly inhibitory role, causing hyperpolarization of lamina II cells, thereby producing an antinociceptive effect [30]. It is clear from this overview that several regions in the brainstem have a key role in reducing nociceptive input.

More recently, there has been interest in the existence of both anti- and pro-nociceptive pathways from the RVM [31]. Stimulation around this area can enhance responses to noxious stimuli, via a mechanism that may involve the NMDA receptor. Persistent noxious input may increase activity of this system contributing to the increased excitability of the spinal cord. Additionally, there is evidence of an indirect connection of the RVM with the anterior cingulate cortex (ACC), an area of the brain known to be associated with pain perception, particularly the affective–motivational aspects. Thus, alterations in the balance of inhibition and facilitation from the brainstem, which may itself be modulated by higher centres, may alter inherent excitability at the level of the spinal cord (for review see Porreca et al. [32]).

Cortical processing

Pain perception is different from nociception, and it is at the cortical level that all the various components of pain perception are integrated (Fig. 23.4). Until recently, our understanding of detailed cortical processing of pain was limited, but brain imaging techniques, such as functional magnetic resonance imaging (fMRI), positron emission tomography (PET) scanning and magnetoencephalography (MEG), are allowing study of the wider aspects of pain perception. Although there is significant variability between studies of the brain areas involved in pain processing, several areas are fairly consistently activated. These include the second somatosensory cortex, insular regions and the ACC. The contralateral thalamus and primary somatosensory area are also often activated [33].

Activity within the ACC is fairly consistent and appears to reflect the subjective unpleasantness of the painful experience. Thus, it may have a role in endogenous modulation of pain. Cognitive modulation (e.g. using hypnotic techniques) can be used to reduce the perceived unpleasantness of a defined noxious stimulus and to significantly reduce activity in the ACC [34]. The limbic system, including the ACC, appears to be one of the sites where endogenous opioid peptides are involved in modulating both acute and sustained pain. Systemic

fentanyl can reduce pain-related activity in the ACC and other pain related cortical areas, as well as the thalamus [35].

The context of the painful experience is important as has been demonstrated by fMRI studies showing the role of varied attention to the painful stimuli on neuroneal activity within the brain. Using more focused imaging, it appears that activity within the PAG related to noxious stimuli can be modulated by attentional level, with subsequent effects on spinal activity. This emphasizes the importance of the degree of integration between cortical processes and nociceptive input. Mood can also alter pain processing, as has been shown using experimentally induced anxiety. The effect of attention on pain perception is the subject of much current research which is likely to lead to an improved understanding of the neuromatrix of pain and the modulation of spinal processing [36].

Response to tissue damage

There is a large amount of evidence of changes in nociceptive processing and pain perception as a result of tissue injury that can lead to the development of persistent pain states. This reflects the dynamic nature of the system as major alterations can be seen peripherally, within the spinal cord and at a cortical level. A summary of some of the main changes in

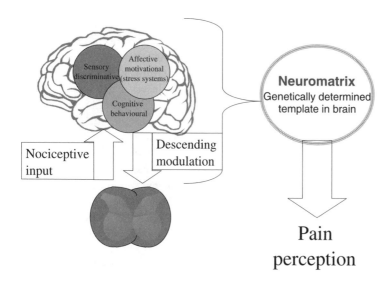

Figure 23.4 Pain perception. The importance of integration at a cortical level is only just beginning to be understood. There are important interactions between cortical centres, the brainstem and the spinal cord, resulting in perception of pain.

spinal neurotransmitters in different types of chronic pain states is shown in Table 23.5.

The effects of some of these changes is considered briefly below.

Inflammation

Inflammation may be either acute or chronic and is part of a complex response to injury or infection. Usually, acute inflammation resolves after the initiating stimulus has been removed and the damaged tissue has healed. If the inflammation does not resolve, or there is associated nerve damage, then the process may become chronic. This may occur with chronic infection (e.g. persisting trigger) or maladaptive response of the immune systems (e.g. autoimmune diseases). The classic signs of inflammation include pain (dolor: with nociceptor activation), redness (rubor: vasodilatation), heat (calor: increased metabolic activity and blood flow) and swelling (tumor: oedema resulting from plasma extravasation and increased capillary permeability) and consists of a complex array of innate non-immunological responses and specific immune system mechanisms. Changes may be initiated peripherally, but sensitization can be detected throughout the peripheral and central nervous systems [37].

Peripheral changes

Acutely, a wide variety of cells are involved, with release of a range of pro-inflammatory substances. Blood vessels (endothelium), cells of the immune system (e.g. lymphocytes, macophages, polymorphs, mononuclear cells and mast cells), cytokines and other mediators all interact at the site of tissue damage to produce peripheral sensitization (Fig. 23.5).

Cytokines are large peptides, which may be pro- or anti-inflammatory, such as tumour necrosis factor-α (TNF-α) and interleukins, as well as interferons,

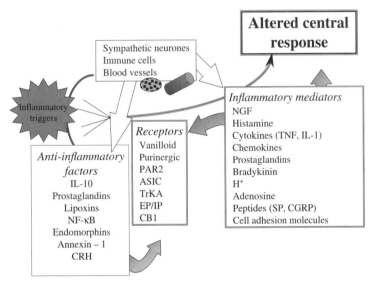

Figure 23.5 Peripheral sensitization. This shows some of the major factors involved in the peripheral inflammatory process. A range of inflammatory triggers such as tissue injury, infection or ischaemia initiates a series of events. Pro-inflammatory mediators are released from cells of the immune system, blood vessels and neurones (both primary afferent and sympathetic). These act on specific receptors to produce intracellular changes and result in a lowering of the activation threshold of nociceptors. There are also endogenous anti-inflammatory substances released that normally result in resolution of the inflammatory process. The particular receptors and mediators involved may vary. ASIC, acid sensing ion channel; CB, cannabinoid; CGRP, calcitoringene-related peptide; CRH, corticotrophin releasing hormone; EP, E type prostanoids receptor; IL-10, interleukin-10; IP, I type prostanoids receptor; NF-κB, nuclear factor kappa B; NGF, nerve growth factor; PAR2, protease-activated receptor; SP, substance P; TNF, tumour necrosis factor; TrKA, tyrosine kinase A.

Table 23.5 Neurochemical spinal changes in models of inflammation, nerve injury (partial and complete) and cancer pain. From Honore *et al.* Neuroscience 2000; **98** (3): 585–98., with permission.

	Inflammation (CFA)	Partial nerve injury (SNL)	Sciatic nerve transection	Cancer (sarcoma in bone)
Spinal cord				
SP lam I–II	↑	↓↓	↓↓	←→
CGRP lam I–II		↓↓	↓↓	←→
IB4 lam IIi		↓↓	↓↓	←→
Galanin lam I–II	←→	↑↑↑↑↑↑	↑↑↑↑↑↑	←→
SS lam I–II	←→	←→	←→	←→
NPY lam I–II	←→	↑↑	↑	←→
Dyn lam I–II	←→	←→	↑	←→
SPR lam I–II	↑	←→	←→	←→
PKCγ lam IIi	↑↑	↑↑	↑	←→
GAP-43 lam I–II	←→	↑↑↑	↑	←→
NeuN grey matter	←→	←→	←→	←→
Dyn lam III–VI	↑↑	←→	←→	↑↑↑
Glia				
GFAP grey matter	←→	↑↑↑	↑↑↑	↑↑↑↑↑↑
Ox 42 grey matter	←→	↑↑↑	←→	←→
Motor neurones				
NeuN motor neurones	←→	←→	↓↓↓	←→
Galanin motor neurones	←→	↑↑	↑↑	←→
NPY motor neurones	←→	↑↑↑	↑↑↑	←→

Results are summarized with arrows, with horizontal arrows (←→) showing no significant changes as compared to sham, whereas arrows going up (↑) or down (↓) (↑/↓: 25–50% increase/decrease; ↑↑/↓↓: 50–75% increase/decrease; ↑↑↑/↓↓↓: 75–100% increase/decrease; : ↑↑↑↑↑↑/↓↓↓↓↓↓ more than 150% increase) represent a significant increase or decrease in immunofluorescence levels (IF) or number of neurones (count) for neurochemical markers that are found in spinal cord (SP, CGRP, IB4, GAL, somatostatin, NPY, DYN, SPR, PKCg, GAP-43, NeuN, astrocyte marker (GFAP), and microglia marker (Ox-42)). Note that while increases in SP-IR and CGRP-IR were observed in inflammation, a decrease in these markers was observed in both SNL and nerve transection models. In addition, a strong increase in galanin-IR and NPY-IR was observed in both SNL and nerve transection models but these markers remained unchanged in inflammation. However, an increase in PKCg-IR was observed in models of inflammation, SNL, and nerve transection. Increase in glia markers (GFAP and Ox-42) and GAL-IR and NPY-IR in motor neurones were observed in both SNL and nerve transection models but not in the model of inflammatory pain. Finally, unique changes were observed in the model of bone cancer as an increase in dynorphin-IR and an increase in GFAP-IR, but no other changes were detected. Even if these two changes are common between cancer and inflammation for dynorphin-IR and cancer and neuropathy for GFAP-IR, the increases in these two markers were the most pronounced in the cancer model.

colony-stimulating factors and growth factors. Chemokines are a type of cytokine (e.g. interleukin-8) that act as chemoattractants for immune system cells to the damaged area. Cytokines act via kinase-linked receptors to alter gene expression at a cellular level. This can occur both peripherally and centrally, with post-translational, translational and transcriptional regulation. For example, mitogen-activated protein kinases (MAPK) such as extracellular signal-regulated protein kinase (ERK) and p38, are activated by inflammatory mediators in both primary sensory and secondary order dorsal horn neurones. They mediate intracellular signal transduction in response to a variety of stimuli and are involved in a range of other functions such as cell proliferation and differentiation and neuroneal plasticity, including long-term potentiation and memory. They may provide potential new pharmacological interventions in treating inflammatory pain [38].

Cytokines and other inflammatory mediators can also trigger the release of neuropeptides and other substances from nociceptor terminals, as well as causing depolarization of nociceptors. These can influence nearby cells in either a pro-inflammatory (e.g. SP, CGRP, ATP) or anti-inflammatory (endorphins) manner. Low-intensity stimulation, or locally acting mediators, may release substances from nerve terminals without evoking pain. This can cause graded changes in nearby membrane potentials ('axon reflex' or 'antidromic' conduction), recruiting the distal branches of other sensory nerve fibres, leading to a diffusion and amplification of the original localized stimulus. This local amplification of the inflammatory response by sensory neurones is termed neurogenic inflammation.

Kinins are another group of locally acting peptides. They are derived from the blood and are produced by the action of kallikrein enzymes, with broad effects mediated by two related G-protein-coupled receptors termed the bradykinin receptors. The endogenous kallikrein–kinin system promotes inflammation and pain and there is interest in pharmacological agents that will block this system and act as analgesics [39].

Several peripheral receptors also appear to play a significant part in the inflammatory process. For example, the vanilloid (capsaicin) receptor, transient receptor potential channel, vanilloid subfamily member 1 (TRPV1), is linked to intracellular signalling by various endogenous substances such as bradykinin and is up-regulated during inflammatory conditions [40]. There is another family of G-protein-coupled receptors activated by proteases, the protease-activated receptors (PARs) that appear to be involved in inflammatory processes, as well possibly in visceral pain mechanisms [41,42].

Relatively recently, the existence of a group of ion channels that are sensitive to extracellular pH changes, the ASICs, have been isolated. ASIC channels can induce action potential triggering on sensory neurones after a moderate extracellular pH decrease. Given that tissue acidosis is a dominant factor in inflammation, they are likely to be involved in peripheral sensitization, with evidence of transcriptional induction and post-translational regulation during inflammation [43].

Purines and some of their receptors are thought to be involved in inflammatory pain. P2X receptors are hetero-oligomeric ion channels, gated by extracellular ATP. In particular, the P2X3 subunit is found on a subset of sensory neurones involved in nociception, and ATP released during inflammation may activate this receptor, resulting in action potential generation. Some recent studies have also indicated a potential role for peripherally sited metabotropic glutamate receptors in inflammatory processes [44].

The end result of peripheral sensitization is a decrease in stimulus threshold required to activate nociceptors and an exaggerated response to a suprathreshold stimulus. This alteration in transduction sensitivity, responsiveness and activity of peripheral nociceptors along with recruitment of 'silent' nociceptors may manifest as primary hyperalgesia [45].

Central changes

Central sensitization can also occur in response to these peripheral changes, with hyperexcitability, involving wind-up of dorsal horn neurones (see below) and a range of neurotransmitters including glutamate, SP, neurokinin A, CGRP and prostaglandins. Other neurotransmitters may have an increased role in inflammatory processes with some evidence that spinal 5-hydroxytryptamine (5-HT) receptors may be of increased importance after inflammation [46]. MAPK pathways may have a peripheral role in inflammation, but there is also evidence for changes within the dorsal root ganglia (DRG) and dorsal horn, where ERK is phosphorylated in response to noxious peripheral stimulation contributing to persistent inflammatory processes, via transcriptional regulation of key gene products. On the other hand, peripheral inflammation and axotomy also induces p38 MAPK activation in DRG neurones.

In addition to changes at a spinal level, there may also be changes in cortical processing in the thalamus and somatosensory cortex in clinical models of hyperalgesia [35].

Nerve injury

Peripheral nerve injury can result in the development of neuropathic pain. Neuropathic pain is defined by the International Association for the Study of Pain (IASP) as pain initiated or caused by a primary lesion or dysfunction in the nervous system. While it is generally accepted that this can be a prolonged and chronic process, it often goes undiagnosed in the acute postoperative setting [47]. A remarkable range of changes occur in the peripheral and central nervous system in response to nerve injury, some of which are considered here.

Peripheral changes

Two major changes occur peripherally in sensory neurones after nerve injury:

1 Alterations in the electrical response properties
2 Alterations in the chemical nature of the neurones.

Electrical properties

The basic ion channels essential for neuronal conductivity and excitability are voltage-gated sodium channels (VGSCs), with changes in their conductance resulting in action potential generation. They are heteromeric protein complexes with a large pore-forming α subunit and two auxiliary β subunits. There are at least nine isoforms of the α subunit, widely distributed within the nervous system. Initially, sodium channels were characterized in terms of their pharmacological sensitivity to tetrodotoxin (TTX). The electrophysiological properties vary, with

the TTX-resistant (TTXr) being much slower than the TTX-sensitive (TTXs) sodium current, both in terms of time to peak and decay kinetics. Despite this, the TTXr current recovers from the inactivated state, or reprimes, more than 10 times faster than the TTXs current [48].

Spontaneous activity

Normally, a peripheral stimulus (e.g. pinprick) is required to activate peripheral nociceptors with subsequent action potential generation and propagation. After nerve injury, changes in neuroneal excitability result in 'pacemaker-like' potentials from which action potentials can arise spontaneously at sites distant from peripheral nociceptors, in the absence of peripheral stimulation. Both the injured neurone and surrounding non-injured neurones may be involved, with the phenomenon being more marked in A than C fibres [49]. These spontaneously arising action potentials, or 'ectopic discharges', can originate from the nerve injury site, and much more proximally, at the cell bodies themselves, in the DRG [50].

Several factors are important in the generation of these ectopic discharges. There is an up-regulation of VGSC. The particular subtypes of VCGS varies depending on sensory fibre type. Normally, TTXs $Na_v1.3$ is found at very low levels in the adult neurone and has been detected mainly in the embryonic nervous system. It is up-regulated rapidly after nerve injury, playing a part in ectopic impulse generation. Other sodium channels have also been implicated in sensory hypersensitivity and ectopic discharge generation, such as the TTXr $Na_v1.8$. Both animal models and clinical microneurographic work have shown that the rate of ectopic discharges may be related to the severity of spontaneous pain [51,52].

Down-regulation of potassium channels also occurs after nerve injury, as well as a decrease in the activation threshold of heat-sensitive channels, such that they may be activated at body temperature. This may account for spontaneous burning pain or thermal hypersensitivity [53].

Evoked activity

For action potential generation, a high-intensity peripheral stimulus is usually required to initiate action potentials in nociceptors that are propagated centrally along small myelinated Aδ fibres and unmyelinated C fibres. The initiation of action potentials stops when the stimulus has ceased and mechanical stimulation of the sensory axon distant from peripheral nociceptors does not generate action potentials. In contrast, after nerve injury, there may be continued action potential generation ('after discharges') and an altered pattern of action potential firing, with prolonged bursting discharges continuing after the stimulus has ceased [54].

Further impulses may be initiated at the nerve injury site, which becomes mechanosensitive after injury. The TTXr $Na_v1.8$ channel, usually found on small diameter sensory neurones in the DRG, is redistributed along the uninjured sensory axons after nerve injury, contributing to hypersensitivity. Interfering with the function of the $Na_v1.8$ channel in nerve injury may prevent the development of mechanical and thermal hyperalgesia [51]. As a result of peripheral nerve injury, action potential input to the spinal cord is altered and electrical input increased, losing the normally close links to stimulus-encoded input. This increase in primary afferent drive is likely to contribute towards the subsequent changes that occur in the spinal cord.

Chemical properties
After nerve injury there is a major change in the phenotype of primary sensory neurones (the characteristic pattern of neurotransmitters produced by primary afferent neurones). Normally, adult neurones are characterized by the expression of particular genes, enabling the cells to carry out their particular functions. These include those genes whose protein products regulate synaptic transmission and conduction, in addition to many cytoskeletal genes. After peripheral nerve injury, several hundred genes are either up- or down-regulated, altering the character of subsets of primary sensory neurones [55].

The exact trigger for this dramatic phenotypic change is unclear but, at least in part, alteration in the retrograde transport of peripherally synthesized substances, such as neurotrophins, by primary afferent fibres is likely to be important. Neurotrophins are a family of structurally related factors, which include

NGF, brain-derived neurotrophic factor (BDNF), neurotrophin-3 (NT-3) and NT-4/5. They regulate neuronal survival and multiple aspects of function via specific tyrosine kinase receptors [56].

Thus, for example, alterations in NGF derived from peripheral sources may be important in the subsequent central changes after nerve injury [57]. BDNF is normally expressed only in C fibres, but after peripheral nerve injury begins to be expressed in A fibre neurones. After peripheral nerve injury, the disrupted contact of cell bodies in the DRG with peripheral targets results in degeneration of primary sensory neurones. This may be because of loss of peripheral sources of neurotrophins essential for survival of these neurones, such as NGF. Glial cells (e.g. Schwann cells) may also be involved in this process, producing neurotrophins and other substances with alterations in particular pain states (see also Fig. 23.5).

Sympathetic nervous system
There has been much debate about the role of the sympathetic nervous system in neuropathic pain. Certainly, clinically it can have a major role, as demonstrated in complex regional pain syndromes [58].

In animal models of nerve injury there is evidence of sprouting of sympathetic fibres within the DRG, forming basket-like structures around primary afferent cell bodies [59]. Cross-talk between these sympathetic and sensory neurones may generate impulses in sensory fibres. Although the exact role of the sympathetic nervous system remains to be defined, it clearly is significant in some cases of neuropathic pain [60].

Central changes
Anatomical changes
Secondary to primary afferent neurone damage, central terminations in the spinal cord degenerate. Over a period of time, the injured neurones atrophy, with a decrease in cell body size and loss of central terminals in the dorsal horn, with eventual cell death, mainly of C fibres. This may be related to loss of retrogradely transported neurotrophins from the periphery, such as NGF and glial derived neurotrophic factor (GDNF). Trans-synaptic degeneration

may also occur with loss of second-order neurones, possibly related to factors at the time of nerve injury. Earlier studies have reported sprouting of Aβ fibres into the superficial dorsal horn after nerve injury, but there is considerable debate as to whether or not this may be an artefact resulting from immunohisto-chemical techniques [61–63].

Neurochemical changes

Neurotransmitter production, release and receptor activation change dramatically in response to peripheral injury. The neurochemical transmitter changes effect intracellular second and third messenger systems, with substances such as nitric oxide being implicated in altering gene expression. Immediate early genes, such as *c-fos* and *c-jun* may also have a role in maintaining chronic pain via alterations in protein synthesis. The major neurotransmitter changes are summarized in Figure 23.5.

Glial changes

Until relatively recently, glial cells in the central nervous system were thought to have no role in neuroneal regulation and activity. There is an emerging body of evidence that implicates spinal cord glia (microglia and astrocytes) in nociceptive processing, particularly in chronic pain states such as after nerve injury. Neuropeptides and excitatory amino acids may be released from glial cells. Glial cells may also be activated by changes in peripheral input, with spinal release of a range of compounds, including cytokines [64].

Amino acid changes

After peripheral nerve injury, the balance between excitation and inhibition is altered towards increased excitability at a spinal level (central sensitization). In this state of increased sensitivity of dorsal horn neurones, the threshold required for activation is reduced and responsiveness to synaptic inputs is increased, resulting in a general amplification of sensory input [65].

The main excitatory amino acid involved in pain processing is glutamate. After nerve injury, the types of glutamate receptors recruited changes, with increased activation in particular at the NMDA receptor. This receptor has been shown to have a key role

in 'wind-up', an activity-dependent form of central sensitization that can occur rapidly and may persist in chronic pain states. With repeated high-intensity noxious input, the NMDA receptor block by magnesium ions is lifted and wind-up occurs. The NMDA receptor–MAGUK interactions may be important in neuropathic pain. In addition, particular subunits of the NMDA receptor may have an increased role in neuropathic pain, with the potential for developing specific analgesics [11].

Metabotropic glutamate receptors may also be involved in nociceptive processing after nerve injury. These G-protein-coupled receptors alter intracellular enzyme activation and calcium levels and it has been postulated that this allows for a positive feedback between mGlu and NMDA receptors at an intracellular level [13,14].

The two main inhibitory amino acids found in dorsal horn neurones, GABA and glycine, are both altered after nerve injury. GABA or glycine antagonists within the dorsal horn produce pain behaviours, such as mechanical allodynia, similar to that of neuropathic pain with very prominent tactile allodynia [66]. GABA blockade may also recruit previously silent Aβ fibre inputs to cells in the superficial dorsal horn. After peripheral nerve injury, GABA levels in the dorsal horn are decreased bilaterally [67]. Glycine-containing inhibitory neurones in the dorsal horn may also be more susceptible to the massive neuroneal discharge occurring at the time of nerve injury, resulting in death of these neurones.

Neuropeptides

Many neuropeptides are involved in sensory processing, and there are dramatic alterations in their synthesis and release in response to peripheral injury. This is summarized in Figure 23.5.

Calcium channels

There are changes in calcium-channel activity after nerve injury that may offer therapeutic potential. There are many different isoforms of calcium channels, dependent on the specific subunit composition. The N-type calcium channel may be of particular relevance in neuropathic pain [68]. These are expressed mainly in the peripheral and central nervous system and there is clinical interest in ziconotide, a synthetic form of the marine snail toxin v-conopeptide MVIIA and specific channel antagonist [69].

Central sensitization

Dorsal horn neurones demonstrate increased responsiveness to synaptic inputs with a lowered activation threshold. This increased sensitivity has several components. After nerve injury, or a repeated noxious stimulus, magnesium block of the NMDA receptor is lifted and subsequent release of glutamate results in increased action potential generation, involving NMDA receptor activation, as outlined above. Rapid sensitization can occur with alterations in receptor activity and trafficking, most notably of the NMDA and AMPA glutamate receptors [13].

Brainstem modulation

Tonic spontaneous activity in the spinal cord increase after nerve injury. This may be related to a decrease in DNIC. The descending pathways involved originate in the brainstem, and normally exert a tonic inhibition on intrinsic spinal neurones by release of serotonin and norepinephrine with some evidence for a decrease in activity after peripheral nerve injury. After nerve injury, the relative role of both anti- and pro-nociceptive pathways from the RVM and other areas may change. Agents interfering with RVM activity can reduce behavioural signs of neuropathic pain. Additional cortical connections may be necessary to complete the neuroneal circuits utilized in regulating spinal input [32].

Cortical modulation

There is increasing evidence of the cortical areas involved in pain perception and how these may be modulated by cognitive and emotional factors. After nerve injury, major changes have been seen within the cortex. For example, it has been shown that there are rapid and persistent alterations in cortical responses after limb amputation [70].

The primary somatosensory area is located in the post central gyrus and is organized into a specific somatotopic map of the body. Following denervation, the cortical representation of a body part may expand into the cortex that previously supplied the deafferented area. Thus, in subjects with upper limb amputation, stimulation of areas of the face ipsilater-

al to the amputation consistently resulted in sensation in the phantom hand.

The magnitude of cortical remapping on the somatosensory cortex appears to correlate directly with the severity of phantom pain. The underlying mechanism for this may vary between patients, as local anaesthetic block of primary afferent input resulted in reversal of cortical remapping and alleviation of phantom pain in only half of the subjects studied [71]. Potential mechanisms include unmasking of silent synapses and neuronal sprouting from the thalamus and within the sensory cortex itself. There is some evidence for cortical and thalamic changes in primates that would support the work from brain imaging studies in the clinical setting [72].

In addition to cortical changes in phantom limb pain, other neuropathic conditions such as complex regional pain syndrome have also shown alterations in cortical responses and it seems likely that further studies in this area will demonstrate additional changes in cortical responses in neuropathic pain conditions [73].

Conclusions

To manage pain effectively in the clinical setting, whether it is acute or chronic, we need to understand the essential pathophysiological factors involved in order to refine our current therapies. By improved understanding of underlying mechanisms, it may be possible to target treatment appropriately to either peripheral or central changes [55,74].

As we begin to understand the basic pain pathways and how they respond to tissue injury — whether it be inflammatory, neuropathic or cancer related — we may be able to link signs and symptoms with mechanisms and to direct treatment appropriately in individual patients [75–77]. Further information on pain perception from clinical studies will help to link basic science and clinical research, allowing more rapid development of appropriate therapies, whether they be pharmacological or psychological [78].

References

1 Melzack R, Wall PD. Pain mechanisms: a new theory. *Science* 1965; **150**: 971–9.

2 Lin SY, Corey DP. TRP channels in mechanosensation. *Curr Opin Neurobiol* 2005; **15**: 350–7.

3 Burnstock G, Wood JN. Purinergic receptors: their role in nociception and primary afferent neurotransmission. *Curr Opin Neurobiol* 1996; **6**: 526–32.

4 Julius D, Basbaum AI. Molecular mechanisms of nociception. *Nature* 2001; **413**: 203–10.

5 Wang H, Woolf CJ. Pain TRPs. *Neurone* 2005; **46**: 9–12.

6 Willis WD, Coggeshall RE. *Sensory Mechanisms of the Spinal Cord*, 2nd edn. New York, London: Plenum Press, 1991.

7 Morris R, Cheunsuang O, Stewart A, Maxwell D. Spinal dorsal horn neurone targets for nociceptive primary afferents: do single neurone morphological characteristics suggest how nociceptive information is processed at the spinal level. *Brain Res Brain Res Rev* 2004; **46**: 173–90.

8 Todd AJ. Electron-microscope study of golgi-stained cells in lamina-II of the rat spinal dorsal horn. *J Comp Neurol* 1988; **275**: 145–57.

9 Todd AJ. GABA and glycine in synaptic glomeruli of the rat spinal dorsal horn. *Eur J Neurosci* 1996; **8**: 2492–8.

10 Wilcox GL. Excitatory neurotransmitters and pain. In: Bond MR, Charlton JE, Woolf CJ, eds. *Proceedings of the VIth World Congress on Pain*. Elsevier Science, 1991: 97–117.

11 Garry EM, Fleetwood-Walker SM. Organizing pains. *Trends Neurosci* 2004; **27**: 292–4.

12 Bleakman D, Lodge D. Neuropharmacology of AMPA and kainate receptors. *Neuropharmacology* 1998; **37**: 1187–204.

13 Garry EM, Fleetwood-Walker SM. A new view on how AMPA receptors and their interacting proteins mediate neuropathic pain. *Pain* 2004; **109**: 210–3.

14 Pin JP, Acher F. The metabotropic glutamate receptors: structure, activation mechanism and pharmacology. *Curr Drug Targets CNS Neurol Disord* 2002; **1**: 297–317.

15 Mantyh PW, Hunt SP. Setting the tone: superficial dorsal horn projection neurones regulate pain sensitivity. *Trends Neurosci* 2004; **27**: 582–4.

16 Janecka A, Fichna J, Janecki T. Opioid receptors and their ligands. *Curr Top Med Chem* 2004; **4**: 1–17.

17 Stein C, Schafer M, Machelska H. Attacking pain at its source: new perspectives on opioids. *Nat Med* 2003; **9**: 1003–8.

18 Zhang X, Nicholas AP, Hokfelt T. Ultrastructural studies on peptides in the dorsal horn of the rat spinal cord: II. Co-existence of galanin with other peptides in local neurones. *Neuroscience* 1995; **64**: 875–91.

19 Liu HX, Hokfelt T. The participation of galanin in pain processing at the spinal level. *Trends Pharmacol Sci* 2002; **23**: 468–74.

20 Silva AP, Cavadas C, Grouzmann E. Neuropeptide Y and its receptors as potential therapeutic drug targets. *Clin Chim Acta* 2002; **326**: 3–25.

21 Colmers WF, Bleakman D. Effects of neuropeptide Y on the electrical properties of neurones. *Trends Neurosci* 1994; **17**: 373–9.

22 Hannon JP, Nunn C, Stolz B, *et al.* Drug design at peptide receptors: somatostatin receptor ligands. *J Mol Neurosci* 2002; **18**: 15–27.

23 Wiesenfeld-Hallin Z, Xu XJ, Hokfelt T. The role of spinal cholecystokinin in chronic pain states. *Pharmacol Toxicol* 2002; **91**: 398–403.

24 Leah J, Menetrey D, Depommery J. Neuropeptides in long ascending spinal tracts in the rat: evidence for parallel processing of ascending information. *Neuroscience* 1988; **24**: 195–207.

25 Dickinson T, Fleetwood Walker SM, Mitchell R, Lutz EM. Evidence for roles of vasoactive intestinal polypeptide (VIP) and pituitary adenylate cyclase activating polypeptide (PACAP) receptors in modulating the responses of rat dorsal horn neurones to sensory inputs. *Neuropeptides* 1997; **31**: 175–85.

26 Durham PL. CGRP receptor antagonists: a new choice for acute treatment of migraine? *Curr Opin Investig Drugs* 2004; **5**: 731–5.

27 Malan TP, Ibrahim MM, Lai J, *et al.* CB2 cannabinoid receptor agonists: pain relief without psychoactive effects? *Curr Opin Pharmacol* 2003; **3**: 62–7.

28 Ossipov MH, Lai J, Malan P, Porreca F. Spinal and supraspinal mechanisms of neuropathic pain. *New Med Drug Abuse* 2000; **909**: 12–24.

29 Dickenson AH. Gate control theory of pain stands the test of time. *Br J Anaesth* 2002; **88**: 755–7.

30 Sonohata M, Katafuchi T, Yasaka T, *et al.* Actions of noradrenaline on substantia gelatinosa neurones in the rat spinal cord revealed by *in vivo* patch recording. *J Physiol* 2004; **555**: 515–26.

31 Suzuki R, Rahman W, Hunt SP, Dickenson AH. Descending facilitatory control of mechanically evoked responses is enhanced in deep dorsal horn neurones following peripheral nerve injury. *Brain Res* 2004; **1019**: 68–76.

32 Porreca F, Ossipov MH, Gebhart GF. Chronic pain and medullary descending facilitation. *Trends Neurosci* 2002; **25**: 319–25.

33 Peyron R, Laurent B, Garcia-Larrea L. Functional imaging of brain responses to pain: a review and meta-analysis. *Clin Neurophysiol* 2000; **30**: 263–88.

34 Bao QYH, Rainville P. Emotional modulation of experimental pain under hypnosis. *J Dental Res* 2002; **81**: 3721.

35 Borsook D, Becerra L. Pain imaging: future applications to integrative clinical and basic neurobiology. *Adv Drug Deliv Rev* 2003; **55**: 967–86.

36 Eccleston C, Crombez G. Attention and pain: merging behavioural and neuroscience investigations. *Pain* 2005; **113**: 7–8.

37 Kidd BL, Urban LA. Mechanisms of inflammatory pain. *Br J Anaesth* 2001; **87**: 3–11.

38 Ji RR. Mitogen-activated protein kinases as potential targets for pain killers. *Curr Opin Investig Drugs* 2004; **5**: 71–5.

39 Marceau F, Regoli D. Bradykinin receptor ligands: therapeutic perspectives. *Nat Rev* 2004; **3**: 845–52.

40 Cortright DN, Szallasi A. Biochemical pharmacology of the vanilloid receptor TRPV1: an update. *Eur J Biochem* 2004; **271**: 1814–9.

41 Vergnolle N, Ferazzini M, D'Andrea MR, Buddenkotte J, Steinhoff M. Proteinase-activated receptors: novel signals for peripheral nerves. *Trends Neurosci* 2003; **26**: 496–500.

42 Noorbakhsh F, Vergnolle N, Hollenberg MD, Power C. Proteinase-activated receptors in the nervous system. *Nat Rev Neurosci* 2003; **4**: 981–90.

43 Voilley N. Acid-sensing ion channels (ASICs): new targets for the analgesic effects of non-steroid anti-inflammatory drugs (NSAIDs). *Curr Drug Targets Inflamm Allergy* 2004; **3**: 71–9.

44 Neugebauer V. Peripheral metabotropic glutamate receptors: fight the pain where it hurts. *Trends Neurosci* 2001; **24**: 550–2.

45 Millan MJ. The induction of pain: an integrative review. *Prog Neurobiol* 1999; **57**: 1–164.

46 Riering K, Rewerts C, Zieglgansberger W. Analgesic effects of 5-HT3 receptor antagonists. *Scand J Rheumatol Suppl* 2004; **119**: 19–23.

47 Wilson JA, Colvin LA, Power I. Acute neuropathic pain after surgery. *R Coll Anaesthetists Bull* 2002; **15**: 739–43.

48 Catterall WA. From ionic currents to molecular mechanisms: the structure and function of voltage-gated sodium channels. *Neurone* 2000; **26**: 13–25.

49 Liu CN, Wall PD, Ben Dor E, *et al.* Tactile allodynia in the absence of C-fiber activation: altered firing properties of DRG neurones following spinal nerve injury. *Pain* 2000; **85**: 503–21.

50 Kajander KC, Wakisaka S, Bennett GJ. Spontaneous discharge originates in the dorsal root ganglion at the onset of a painful peripheral neuropathy in the rat. *Neurosci Lett* 1992; **138**: 225–8.

51 Lai J, Porreca F, Hunter JC, Gold MS. Voltage-gated sodium channels and hyperalgesia. *Ann Rev Pharmacol Toxicol* 2004; **44**: 371–97.

52 Nystrom B, Hagbarth KE. Microelectrode recordings from transected nerves in amputees with phantom limb pain. *Neurosci Lett* 1981; **27**: 211–6.

53 Caterina MJ, Rosen TA, Tominaga M, Brake AJ, Julius D. A capsaicin-receptor homologue with a high threshold for noxious heat. *Nature* 1999; **398**: 436–42.

54 Sotgiu ML, Biella G, Riva L. Poststimulus afterdischarges of spinal WDR and NS units in rats with chronic nerve constriction. *Neuroreport* 1995; **6**: 1021–4.

55 Costigan M, Woolf CJ. No DREAM, no pain. Closing the spinal gate. *Cell* 2002; **108**: 297–300.

56 Kirstein M, Farinas I. Sensing life: regulation of sensory neurone survival by neurotrophins. *Cell Mol Life Sci* 2002; **59**: 1787–802.

57 Ramer MS, Kawaja MD, Henderson JT, Roder JC, Bisby MA. Glial overexpression of NGF enhances neuropathic pain and adrenergic sprouting into DRG following chronic sciatic constriction in mice. *Neurosci Lett* 1998; **251**: 53–6.

58 Bruehl S, Harden RN, Galer BS, *et al.* Complex regional pain syndrome: are there distinct subtypes and sequential stages of the syndrome? *Pain* 2002; **95**: 119–24.

59 McLachlan EM, Janig W, Devor M, Michaelis M. Peripheral nerve injury triggers noradrenergic sprouting within dorsal root ganglia. *Nature* 1993; **363**: 543–5.

60 Urban LA. Sympathetic component of neuropathic pain: animal models and clinical diagnosis. *Behav Brain Sci* 1997; **20**: 468.

61 Coggeshall RE, Lekan HA, Doubell TP, Allchorne A, Woolf CJ. Central changes in primary afferent fibers following peripheral nerve lesions. *Neuroscience* 1997; **77**: 1115–22.

62 Doubell TP, Woolf CJ. Growth-associated protein 43 immunoreactivity in the superficial dorsal horn of the rat spinal cord is localized in atrophic C-fiber, and not in sprouted a-fiber, central terminals after peripheral nerve injury. *J Comp Neurol* 1997; **386**: 111–8.

63 Tong YG, Wang HF, Ju G, *et al.* Increased uptake and transport of cholera toxin B-subunit in dorsal root ganglion neurones after peripheral axotomy: possible implications for sensory sprouting. *J Comp Neurol* 1999; **404**: 143–58.

64 Watkins LR, Milligan ED, Maier SF. Glial activation: a driving force for pathological pain. *Trends Neurosci* 2001; **24**: 450–5.

65 Woolf CJ, Salter MW. Neuroneal plasticity-increasing the gain in pain. *Science* 2000; **288**: 1765–8.

66 Sivilotti L, Woolf CJ. The contribution of GABAa and glycine receptors to central sensitization: disinhibition and touch-evoked allodynia in the spinal cord. *J Neurophys* 1994; **72**: 169–79.

67 Moore KA, Kohno T, Karchewski LA, *et al.* Partial peripheral nerve injury promotes a selective loss of GABAergic inhibition in the superficial dorsal horn of the spinal cord. *J Neurosci* 2002; **22**: 6724–31.

68 Miller RJ. Rocking and rolling with Ca^{2+} channels. *Trends Neurosci* 2001; **24**: 445–9.

69 Murakami M, Nakagawasai O, Suzuki T, *et al.* Antinociceptive effect of different types of calcium channel inhibitors and the distribution of various calcium channel alpha 1 subunits in the dorsal horn of spinal cord in mice. *Brain Res* 2004; **1024**: 122–9.

70 Flor H. Phantom-limb pain: characteristics, causes, and treatment. *Lancet Neurol* 2002; **1**: 182–9.

71 Birbaumer N, Lutzenberger W, Montoya P, *et al.* Effects of regional anesthesia on phantom limb pain are mirrored in changes in cortical reorganization. *J Neurosci* 1997; **17**: 5503–8.

72 Florence SL, Taub HB, Kaas JH. Large-scale sprouting of cortical connections after peripheral injury in adult macaque monkeys. *Science* 1998; **282**: 1117–21.

73 Eisenberg E, Chistyakov AV, Yudashkin M, *et al.* Evidence for cortical hyperexcitability of the affected limb representation area in CRPS: a psychophysical and transcranial magnetic stimulation study. *Pain* 2005; **113**: 99–105.

74 Woolf CJ. Dissecting out mechanisms responsible for peripheral neuropathic pain: implications for diagnosis and therapy. *Life Sci* 2004; **74**: 2605–10.

75 Hunt SP, Mantyh PW. The molecular dynamics of pain control. *Nat Rev Neurosci* 2001; **2**: 83–91.

76 Mantyh PW, Clohisy DR, Koltzenburg M, Hunt SP. Molecular mechanisms of cancer pain. *Nat Rev Cancer* 2002; **2**: 201–9.

77 Jensen TS, Baron R. Translation of symptoms and signs into mechanisms in neuropathic pain. *Pain* 2003; **102**: 1–8.

78 Craig AD. A new view of pain as a homeostatic emotion. *Trends Neurosci* 2003; **26**: 303–7.

CHAPTER 24

Neuromuscular transmission and function

Andrew D. Axon and Jennifer M. Hunter

Introduction

Neuromuscular physiology has been extensively studied and is well understood. Bernard [1], in 1856, identified the gap between nerve and muscle, and Dale *et al.* [2] demonstrated that acetylcholine was the transmitter at the neuromuscular junction in 1936. Our understanding has been greatly aided by the availability of the large, and therefore easily studied, electric organ of electric fish which, despite millions of years of evolution, has remarkable similarity to the human neuromuscular junction.

The lower motor neurone

The cell bodies of the motor neurones, containing their solitary nucleus, lie in the grey matter of the anterior horn of the spinal cord or, in the case of the cranial nerves, within their midbrain nuclei. As motor neurones are mononuclear, all the genetic material of the neurone and therefore its ability to construct proteins and organelles, resides in the cell body. The cell body synapses with other neurones, either directly or through any number of fine processes, known as dendrites [3–9].

A single efferent axon leaves the cell body to form a unicellular link from the central nervous system to the muscle; this may involve a distance of 1 m. The motor axon diameter is large, in the range 10–20 μm, and the conduction velocity is fast at 50–120 m/s (fast axonal conduction). The Schwann cell sheath of the axon is up to 100 membrane-layers thick, but deficient intermittently at the nodes of Ranvier. These areas, approximately 0.5–1 μm in length, are rich in sodium channels, although lacking in rectifier potassium channels, to allow the rapid saltatory conduction of the nerve action potential. The perinodal region contains rectifier potassium channels, which may be important in rapidly repeated neuronal firing. The internodal axon membrane does not contain sodium channels.

The axon may divide at a node of Ranvier into a variable number of terminal branches, each supplying an individual muscle fibre (Fig. 24.1). As the terminal branch approaches the muscle fibre, the myelin sheath is lost and it branches into shorter and finer telodendria, which are less than 100 μm in length. These unmyelinated processes come to lie in the junctional or synaptic clefts, thus forming the presynaptic part of the neuromuscular junction.

The telodendria are deficient in sodium channels; the action potential is propagated passively over this remaining short distance. The lack of sodium channels is thought to prevent the reflection and repropagation of the neurone action potential. Voltage-gated potassium channels are present and these repolarize the membrane potential to its resting value; they prevent excessive and cytotoxic influx of calcium into the nerve terminal.

Depolarization of the nerve terminal membrane by the arriving action potential causes the opening of voltage-gated calcium channels and, in turn, the release of acetylcholine. Magnesium is a physiological antagonist to calcium at the nerve terminal.

The motor unit

The group of muscle fibres innervated by a single motor neurone is described as a motor unit. The size of the motor unit varies from as few as 5 fibres in the extraocular lateral rectus muscle to as many as 2000 in the medial gastrocnemius in the leg, and varies as a function of the fineness and force of the movements generated by the innervated muscle [10].

The majority of human muscle fibres are thought to be focally innervated; that is, they are innervated at a single point on their surface by a single axon. The point of innervation is usually near the midpoint of the muscle fibre. Some muscles are multifocally innervated, and this innervation may be polyneuronal; these tend to be muscles with a mixture of long parallel and short, serially connected fibres (i.e. connected end-to-end). Examples of multifocal innervation can be found in the extraocular, intrinsic laryngeal, middle ear and facial muscles. Multifocal polyneuronal innervation has also been demonstrated in human brachioradialis muscle. However, the significance or function of such an arrangement has not been explained [11].

Nerve terminals at multifocally innervated muscle fibres are described as 'en grappe', a descriptive term for the appearance of the terminal axon. 'En plaque' is a term used to describe the raised plaque appearance of the nerve terminal of the focally innervated, fast, pale muscle fibre [5].

The neuromuscular junction

The neuromuscular junction comprises a nerve terminal and the sole plate, or motor endplate, formed in the muscle fibre cell membrane. The nerve terminal is oval-shaped, with a corresponding depression in the muscle fibre surface, and its dimensions are estimated to be in the range 15–30 × 20–50 nm. The nerve and muscle are not in contact, but are separated by the synaptic or junctional cleft, the distance between the two being 50–60 nm (Fig. 24.2). The synapse is completely enclosed, the terminal

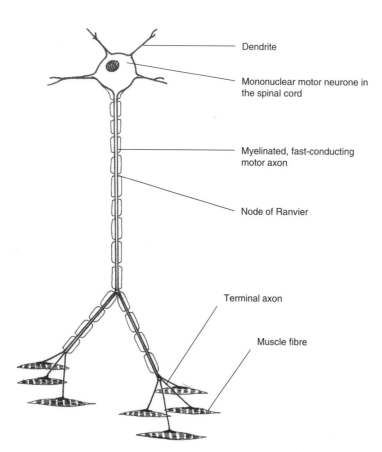

Dendrite

Mononuclear motor neurone in the spinal cord

Myelinated, fast-conducting motor axon

Node of Ranvier

Terminal axon

Muscle fibre

Figure 24.1 The motor unit. The majority of muscle fibres have mononeuronal, unifocal innervation. A single motor neurone may supply thousands of muscle fibres.

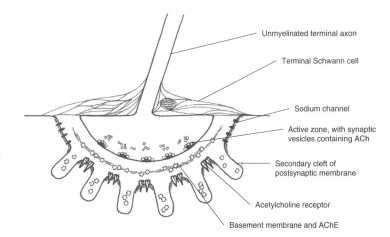

Figure 24.2 The neuromuscular junction. The terminal Schwann cell encloses the junctional cleft; across the junctional cleft, the active zones of the presynaptic membrane are closely aligned with clusters of acetylcholine receptors. ACh, acetylcholine; AChE, acetylcholinesterase.

Schwann cells forming teloglia, or lids, which help maintain the structure of the neuromuscular junction and act as a diffusion barrier. In addition, the terminal Schwann cells provide a reservoir of calcium, which becomes available during repetitive neuronal firing; calcium release is mediated by G-protein-coupled receptors [12]. The junctional cleft contains basement membrane, rich in polysaccharides, laminin and collagen, and is abundant in the enzyme acetylcholinesterase (Fig. 24.2).

The postjunctional muscle fibre membrane is folded into secondary clefts, which increases the surface area of the postsynaptic membrane. The crests of these secondary clefts contain a huge density of acetylcholine receptors (nAChR), lined up precisely opposite the release sites for acetylcholine (ACh; Fig. 24.2). This alignment is maintained, regardless of how stretched the muscle fibre becomes, in part because the neuromuscular junction is quite rigid; because of the presence of the basement membrane, and also because the postjunctional membrane can accommodate a degree of stretch by unfolding of the secondary clefts.

Acetylcholine

Synthesis of acetylcholine

Choline + acetyl coenzyme A $\rightleftarrows$ acetylcholine + coenzyme A

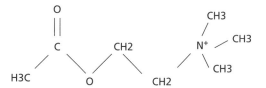

Figure 24.3 The acetylcholine molecule, 2-acetyloxy-N, N, N-triethylammonium, an ester group attached to acetic acid and choline.

This reaction requires the soluble enzyme choline acetyltransferase, which is synthesized in the motor neurone cell body and is concentrated largely in the axoplasm, although a smaller amount may be found in the synaptic vesicle membrane. Acetyl coenzyme A is thought to derive from mitochondrial pyruvate, a product of glucose metabolism, and requires an intermediate carrier in order to pass through the mitochondrial membrane into the axoplasm.

Up to 50% of the choline liberated by the hydrolysis of acetylcholine is recycled to make new acetylcholine. The remainder is sourced from the extracellular fluid of the junctional cleft, where the concentration is approximately $10\,\mu mol/L$. The majority of choline is obtained from the diet, with a small amount synthesized in the liver. Uptake of choline into the nerve terminal is by active sodium-dependent transport (choline is a cation, unable to cross the phospholipid cell membrane by simple diffusion). All cells have low-affinity transporters which collect choline to make membrane phosphatidyl choline; cholinergic nerve endings have, in addition, a high-affinity choline transporter. Release of acetylcholine may increase its synthesis by two mechanisms: an increase in axoplasmic sodium concentration, favouring choline uptake; and increasing activity of the high-affinity carrier. The postjunctional muscle fibre membrane has relatively high choline turnover through membrane phosphatidyl choline; the significance of this is not known.

Storage of acetylcholine

The majority of ACh in the nerve terminal is stored in small clear vesicles; approximately 20% is axoplasmic. Each vesicle contains a quantum of ACh, estimated at between 5000 and 10 000 molecules. The interior of the vesicle is very hypertonic in relation to the axoplasm, 300 µmol compared with 0.3 mmol/L, and the vesicles also contain adenosine triphosphate (ATP), magnesium and calcium. The external diameter of the vesicle is approximately 45 nm, the wall is 5 nm thick and the volume is $5.4 \times 10^4 \, nm^3$.

The vesicles are synthesized in the cell body; the exact mechanism is not well understood. The vesicles are then moved along the entire length of the axon to the nerve terminal, by fast antegrade axonal transport at 1–3 µm/s; this compares with the transport of soluble proteins at somewhat less than 10 mm/day.

A microtubule network has been demonstrated in some types of axon, and is assumed to occur in others, including the motor axon. The micotubules are orientated with a plus-end pointing towards the synapse and a minus-end pointing towards the cell body, this arrangement allowing organized and unidirectional transport. The motive force is provided by the kinesins and dyneins, families of motor proteins associated with the microtubules. The kinesins appear to be predominantly plus-end directed, while the dyneins appear minus-end directed; thus, fast antegrade conduction is likely to be kinesin-driven, although an actin-anchored myosin-driven mechanism may also be important. Microtubules may be important in neuronal migration [13–15].

Work in Torpedo fish, which are the electric rays, suggests that the small clear vesicles are delivered empty to the nerve terminal, to be loaded with ACh by a magnesium-dependent ATP-ase, the ACh being co-transported with protons. Approximately 1% of the ACh vesicles are clustered around the thickened electron-dense areas of the presynaptic membrane that form the active zones. These are the immediately releasable store. They are held in close relation to each other, and to the adjacent presynaptic membrane and calcium channels by cytoskeletal proteins (Fig. 24.2). These proteins mediate the complex interactions that occur following calcium entry into the nerve terminal, leading to exocytosis of the contents of the synaptic vesicle. The vesicles of the active zone are lined up to directly oppose the greatest density of ACh receptors, on the crests of the secondary postsynaptic clefts.

There exists a considerable reserve pool of vesicles, which can be mobilized into the active zones under conditions of heavy demand. These vesicles are normally bound to the actin cytoskeleton of the nerve terminal by synapsin I. The synapsins are a family of neuronal phosphoproteins; the tail of the molecule attaches to the synaptic vesicle and the head to the actin molecule (Fig. 24.4).

Acetylcholine release by vesicular exocytosis

Acetylcholine release is triggered by influx of calcium into the nerve terminal. Exocytosis requires very complex interactions of calcium ions and cellular proteins, which are not fully understood. It is helpful to consider a cycle of synaptic vesicle exocytosis and endocytosis, well described in his comprehensive review by Naguib *et al.* [16].

Calcium channels

The calcium channels at the nerve terminal are voltage gated, opening when the nerve action potential depolarizes the presynaptic nerve terminal. They are tightly packed into parallel double rows and highly concentrated at the active zones, thus enabling the local calcium concentration to rapidly rise, perhaps to as much as 1000 µmol. Not all of the calcium channels open on arrival of an action potential, because their opening time constant (≥1.3 ms) is greater than the duration of the action potential (≤1 ms). Increasing the extracellular calcium concentration, or the duration of calcium channel opening, will increase the amount of ACh released. Calcium accumulates

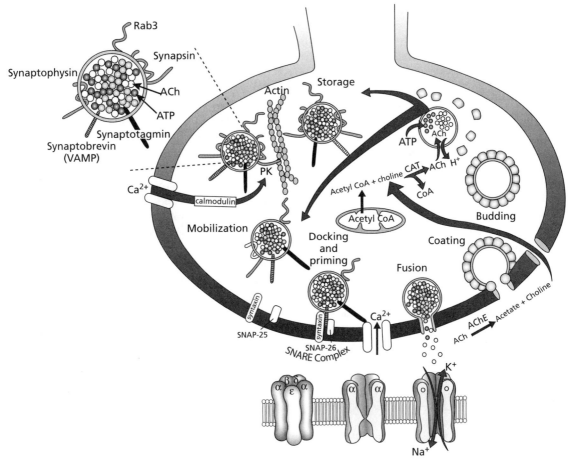

Figure 24.4 Acetylcholine release by vesicular exocytosis. The combination of a motor axon action potential and calcium influx activates a chain of events, mediated by intracellular proteins, and resulting in the quantal release of acetylcholine. PK = protein kinase. (Reproduced with permission of Lippincott Williams and Wilkins, Inc. from Naguib M, Flood P, McArdle JJ and Brenner HR in *Anesthesiology* 2002; **96**: 20–31.) ACh, acetylcholine; AChE, acetylcholinesterase; ATP, adenosine triphosphate; CoA, coenzyme A; CAT, choline acetyl transferase; PK, protein kinase; SNAP, synaptosome associated membrane protein; VAMP, vesicle associated membrane protein.

in the nerve ending during post-tetanic potentiation.

Nerve terminal calcium channels are of the P/Q type, quite different to the L type found in cardiac tissue. Therefore they are not affected by therapeutic doses of calcium-channel blocking drugs in health. Membrane potential is rectified by outward flow of potassium; potassium-blocking drugs, such as tetraethyl ammonium, will increase nerve terminal calcium and, in turn, ACh release.

Other calcium channel types have been identified, in animal models, at the neuromuscular junction. Calcium channels have subunits: α_1, α_2/δ, γ and β. The large α_1 subunit forms the ion channel and volt-age gate and is varied genetically, resulting in the different isoforms: P/Q, L, N and R types [17]. L and N types are present at the neuromuscular junction; however, their function in health is not known. In mice, L-type channels have been shown to be important during reinnervation [18]. Removal of presynaptic N-type channels in *Drosophila* reduces synaptic growth, possibly because of a reduction in downstream calcium-dependent growth factors [19].

Knockout mice, where the gene expressing the P/Q channels has been removed, depend on R- and N-type calcium channels for neuromuscular transmission [20–22]. Lambert–Eaton myasthenic syndrome is caused by autoantibodies directed at the P/Q-type calcium channel [23]; in clinical practice, this is often a paraneoplastic syndrome. These patients may be vulnerable to postoperative weakness, or have increased sensitivity to neuromuscular blocking drugs when (L type) calcium channel antagonists are used (e.g. verapamil, diltiazem and nicardipine) [24,25].

Reserve pool mobilization

Influx of calcium into the nerve terminal triggers the phosphorylation of synapsin I at three different sites, by three separate processes: cyclic adenosine monophosphate (cAMP) dependent protein kinase and calcium-calmodulin dependent protein kinase I and II. Calmodulin is found closely associated with the synaptic vesicle membrane. The phosphorylation of synapsin frees it from the cytoskeleton, allowing it to move to the active site, to which the reserve pool vesicles are linked by fodrin.

Docking and priming

Integral vesicle membrane proteins control docking of the synaptic vesicle into the active zone: these are the synaptotagmins, synaptophysin and synaptobrevin (also named vesicle associated membrane protein, VAMP; Fig. 24.4). Synaptotagmin I is thought to both locate the vesicle within the active zone, and to bind calcium.

The process of binding the synaptic vesicle to the junctional membrane, and its subsequent exocytosis, is not fully understood. A proposed mechanism attributes this function to the SNARE complex; other protein complexes may be involved. The SNARE complex comprises three proteins: two plasma membrane proteins, SNAP 25 (synaptosome associated membrane protein of 25 kDa), and syntaxin I; and the vesicle membrane protein, synaptobrevin.

Priming describes the process by which a docked vesicle becomes readily releasable; this is mediated by Rabs, which are guanine nucleotide-binding proteins.

Fusion

Any number of interactions involving calcium, and vesicle and nerve terminal membrane proteins may be important. Synaptotagmin may be the calcium receptor promoting fusion and Rab3 may oppose this action, thereby regulating the number of synaptic

vesicles that are exocytosed. Fusion of the synaptic vesicle membrane with the axon terminal membrane requires ATP and is magnesium dependent. How the repulsive electrical and hydrostatic forces that must exist between these two membranes are overcome is not known. However, it would appear that the two membranes become temporarily fused.

Each synaptic vesicle contains a quantum of ACh molecules. In all species investigated, including humans, spontaneous fusion of single synaptic vesicles occurs randomly, perhaps at a rate of one per second. This process is calcium dependent, and occurs more frequently at higher concentrations of intracellular calcium. It even continues after denervation, when the terminal Schwann cell becomes the source of ACh. The release of a single quantum of ACh results in a miniature endplate potential (mepp), of amplitude 0.5–1 mV, which is insufficient to generate an action potential in the muscle fibre membrane. The role of the mepp is not known.

The number of quanta required to generate an endplate potential is quoted as 20–300 per single nerve stimulus. This represents less than 0.2% of the total amount of ACh present at the nerve terminal, yet greatly exceeds what is required to cause adequate depolarization of the postsynaptic membrane; enough ACh is released following a nerve stimulus to create an endplate potential of peak amplitude +20 to +30 mV — sufficient to propagate a muscle action potential.

Non-quantal release of ACh also occurs, accounting for more than 99% of spontaneous ACh release, by continuous calcium-independent leakage. This produces an ACh concentration of 800 nmol/L in the synaptic cleft, the function of which is not known.

Endocytosis

The synaptic vesicle membrane, including its attendant specific proteins, is recovered into the nerve terminal. As with exocytosis, this is protein mediated. A number of hypotheses have been proposed but the exact process remains obscure.

Co-transmitters and other receptors

Torpedo synaptic vesicles have been shown to release substances other than ACh. Those identified include calcium, which may represent the excess entering the synaptic vesicle during exocytosis, proteins, a proteoglycan and ATP. ATP potentiates the effects of ACh at the nicotinic receptor and ATP receptors occur in skeletal muscle. ATP is broken down into adenosine, which may be inhibitory on calcium channels, an A1 receptor effect. In contrast, an A2 receptor effect of adenosine may be excitatory, increasing ACh production. The actual role of co-transmitters at the neuromuscular junction in humans remains to be elucidated [26].

Presynaptic nerve terminals contain a number of receptors, including opioid and adrenergic receptors; their function is not understood. Acetylcholine receptors have been demonstrated, of both nicotinic [27,28] and muscarinic [29] types, in animal models, in the presynaptic nerve terminal. Prejunctional nicotinic receptors differ structurally from the postjunctional receptor, in that the α_7 isoform of the α subunit is present. The postjunctional α subunit is designated α_1; muscle has the genetic code for only the α_1 (and β_1) subtype, in contrast to neural tissue, which has code for a number of α and β subtypes. The presence of the α_7 subunit alters the pharmacology of the nAChR; for example, α-bungarotoxin binds reversibly at the prejunctional receptor and irreversibly at the postjunctional receptor.

Activation of the prejunctional nAChR facilitates neuromuscular transmission — positive feedback. In contrast, activation of the prejunctional muscarinic AChR inhibits further acetylcholine release — negative feedback [30].

Acetylcholinesterase

Each acetylcholine molecule exists only for enough time to bind to a single acetylcholine receptor (nAChR); half of the acetylcholine released is hydrolysed before even reaching the postjunctional membrane by asymmetrical forms of the enzyme acetylcholinesterase (AChE), which are heavily concentrated in the basement membrane of the synaptic cleft. Globular forms of AChE also occur pre- and postsynaptically in the plasma membranes and, in a less hydrophobic form, in the axoplasm. Functionally, the different forms of the enzyme are very

similar; the structural differences determine their different locations. AChE production may be controlled, in part, by the release of calcitonin gene-related peptide from the motor neurone [31].

Every molecule of AChE has, potentially, six active sites, where acetylcholine may be bound and hydrolysed. The number of available sites, in total, seems to be quite similar to the number of nAChR. The amount of AChE present seems related to muscle activity, being greatest in fast muscle and much diminished in denervated muscle.

Each active site of the enzyme has two domains: a negatively charged anionic site, which binds the substrate at its positively charged head, the $N(CH_3)_3^+$ group; and an esteratic site, at which hydrolysis occurs. The first step in hydrolysis is the cleaving of the choline molecule, much of which is recycled in the nerve terminal. The acetylated esteratic site is then further hydrolysed, by water, to release acetate and regenerate the enzyme.

Acetylcholinesterase inhibitors

Neostigmine and pyridostigmine are oxydiaphoretic inhibitors; a carbamate group is transferred to the enzyme, forming a covalent bond, which is only slowly hydrolysed, resulting in inactive enzyme. Edrophonium is a prosthetic inhibitor; a hydrogen bond forms at the esteratic site, resulting in competitive inhibition of the enzyme.

The postjunctional receptor

Dale described nicotinic and muscarinic acetylcholine receptors as long ago as 1914. The availability of the large nAChR of the electric eels and rays has enabled this receptor to be very well characterized. Recent rapid advances in molecular biology, molecular genetics and molecular imaging, with resolutions greater than 1 nm now possible, have enabled the direct observation of individual ion channels. This may refine or even challenge our understanding of the nAChR.

Postjunctional receptors are of the nicotinic type, and are heavily concentrated on the crests of the postjunctional folds, being in excess of $10\,000\,\mu m^{-2}$. They are synthesized in the muscle cell and inserted into the cell membrane by an ATP-dependent process. The nAChR seems to be preserved by nerve activity; away from the neuromuscular junction, these receptors are evanescent and scarce.

The receptor is a pentamer of approximately 250 kDa, made up of five protein subunits, each of 200–300 amino acids, which surround a central ion channel. Each of the subunit proteins has four transmembrane spans; these anchor the receptor in the lipid bilayer. One face of the M2 span of each subunit lines the inner aspect of the ion channel (Fig. 24.5). The channel is closed, and impermeable to ions, under resting conditions. The nAChR lumen is funnel-shaped, with the receptor sites lying inside the outer cone-shaped part. They are estimated to be separated by a minimum of 2–3 nm and a maximum of 5 nm (Fig. 24.6) and have two subsites: an anionic site to attach the positively charged methonium head of acetylcholine, and a hydrogen binding site [32–36].

There are two α subunits and one each of β, δ and ε. Each subunit has a positive and a negative face; the positive face of one subunit lies alongside the negative face of the next. They are arranged clockwise, viewed from the synaptic side: αεαδβ (Fig. 24.5). The ligand binding domains for acetylcholine occur at the αε and αδ junctions, rather than purely on the α subunits as previously described. Two acetylcholine molecules must bind to open the channel (while a competitive antagonist need occupy only one). Binding of two acetylcholine molecules results in a change in the structural conformation of the subunits, thus opening the channel, the minimum diameter of which is ≤0.7 nm. This is adequate to allow free passage of ions; sodium and calcium enter the cell and potassium exits. The channel is open for

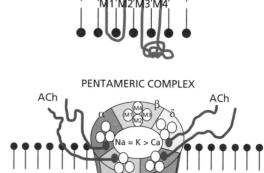

Figure 24.5 Subunit conformation of the nicotinic acetylcholine receptor. The N termini of two adjacent subunits form the acetylcholine binding site. (Reproduced with permission of Lippincott Williams and Wilkins, Inc. from Naguib M, Flood P, McArdle JJ and Brenner HR in *Anesthesiology* 2002; **96**: 202–31.)

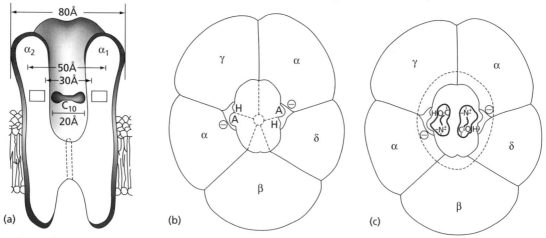

Figure 24.6 (a) Dimensions of the nicotinic acetylcholine receptor, (b) cross section at the level of the binding site, and (c) opening of the ion channel by the cooperative binding of two acetylcholine molecules. The fetal receptor is shown. A = anionic binding site, B = hydrogen bond donor site. 1 Angstrom = 0.1 nm. (Reproduced with permission of Oxford University Press from Lee, C in *British Journal of Anaesthesia* 2001; **87**: 755–69.)

approximately 1 ms, during which time 10^4 ions might flow, the majority of which are sodium and potassium, by virtue of their steep concentration gradients. The simultaneous opening of up to 500 000 channels ensures that the muscle fibre membrane is sufficiently depolarized to generate a muscle action potential.

The mammalian ε subunit replaces the γ subunit found in the electric fish. However, in mammals, including humans, the γ subunit is present in the fetus, and appears to be completely replaced, within a few weeks of birth, by ε. The purpose of this change is not known, but mutations of the ε subunit in humans results in a congenital form of myasthenia gravis; in knockout mice, its absence is lethal.

Endplate response

The resting membrane potential of the muscle cell is −70 to −90 mV. The endplate and surrounding perijunctional zone are rich in sodium channels. In contrast to the nAChR, these consist of only one type of protein subunit and have rather limited conductance for other ions; they are voltage-gated and open in response to the partial depolarization resulting from the opening of the nAChR ion channels. Opening of increasing numbers of sodium channels completes the depolarization of the membrane, resulting in the propagation of an action potential along the muscle fibre.

Any acetylcholine in the junctional cleft is hydrolysed before the end of the muscle refractory period. Rectification of the endplate membrane is a result of increased permeability to potassium, occurring later than the increase in permeability to sodium, suggesting the involvement of a different channel.

Development

Migration of the motor axon to an individual muscle fibre is not a random process, but specifically directed from the central nervous system in a stepwise manner by local chemotactic factors [37,38]. This miracle of human physiology is not well understood.

Muscle fibre cells are multinucleated, with each nucleus containing a full set of genetic information to produce both types of nicotinic acetylcholine receptors. In the embryonic myotube, 'fetal' type nAChR are expressed, containing the γ subunit, instead of ε. As the leading edge of an approaching axon reaches the myotube, acetylcholine is released, and this is sufficient to open the ion channel of the fetal receptors; a myotube action potential is generated. This electrical activity at the natent synapse causes the subsynaptic muscle cell nuclei to express the 'adult' type nAChR, $\alpha_2\beta\varepsilon\delta$. Electrical activity also promotes survival of the synaptic nAChR — their half-lives are approximately 10 days, compared with less than 1 day away from the postjunctional area. Calcium influx through L-type calcium channels may also be important for receptor survival. Initially, a myotube is innervated by several axons. A process of synaptic elimination results in the mononeuronal unifocal innervation of the adult neuromuscular junction. Synaptic maturation is a gradual process, occurring over the first 2 years of life in humans. Why one synapse is selected over the others is not fully understood.

Several proteins are also important in the formation of neuromuscular synapses; knowledge in this area is rapidly expanding. Agrin and neuregulin are signalling proteins released by the nerve; both bind to the basal lamina of the muscle fibre. Agrin leads to nAChR clustering through an interaction with MuSK (muscle-specific kinase). Both are required to form a neuromuscular junction; if either is absent, neuromuscular junctions are not formed. Neuregulin may be important in activating gene expression in the subsynaptic nuclei, such that the elements of the specialized postjunctional membrane are constructed. Another protein, rapsyn, is also important in clustering of nAChR and assembling the cytoskeletal elements of the postjunctional receptor. If rapsyn is absent, neuromuscular junctions will form, but without clustering [39–41].

Extrajunctional receptors and denervation

Acetylcholine receptors of the fetal immature type, containing the ε subunit, occur across the whole surface of the muscle membrane, being more common in the area of the tendon. They are greatly outnumbered by the mature receptor type at the neuromuscular junction. In normal innervated muscle, their density on the muscle fibre surface is less than $10\,\mu m^{-2}$, compared with the mature receptor density at the motor endplate of greater than $10\,000\,\mu m^{-2}$. They are evanescent, surviving only 20 hours on average. Their physiology differs from that of the postjunctional receptor: their opening time is longer, by as much as 10 times, and their ion conductance is less.

While these extrajunctional receptors are present in innervated muscle, their production is suppressed. Following denervation, they rapidly proliferate across the whole of the muscle fibre membrane; a density of approximately $1000\,\mu m^{-2}$ may be achieved. This is similar to the density in fetal muscle, but the denervated state is not strictly equivalent to the fetal state, in that receptor density remains greatest at the postjunctional folds of the motor endplate, and adult-type receptors continue to be expressed here by the subsynaptic nuclei.

The pharmacodynamic response of the extrajunctional receptor is also different, in that it is more sensitive to agonists, including acetylcholine and suxamethonium. Large numbers of receptor ion channels are opened simultaneously, and direct activation of muscle contraction occurs, transmitted through the T-tubule system from the receptor, without the need for a muscle action potential. The result is an initial contraction, followed by a prolonged contracture. Sudden opening of vast numbers of ion channels results in a massive efflux of potassium and hyperkalaemia. This effect may occur within 24 hours of denervation, and lead to cardiac arrest.

Fetal-type receptors in denervated muscle are resistant to non-depolarizing muscle relaxants. Clinically, this effect is most marked with the long-acting agents, such as pancuronium and tubocurarine. In the hemiplegic patient, the non-paresed side may also have reduced sensitivity to neuromuscular blocking drugs. The effect on the muscles of the airway and diaphragm in these patients is not known. However, apparent recovery from neuromuscular blockade, monitored in a denervated muscle, may mask residual curarization in normally innervated muscle, causing respiratory compromise in the postoperative patient [42–44].

Age and the neuromuscular junction

The nervous system degenerates with age, resulting in decreased muscle mass, less generation of force during contraction, reduced force control and slower fine movements. These changes are more marked from the seventh decade [45–47].

Lower motor neurone numbers in the anterior horn decrease; this change has been shown to be uniform in humans through the segments L1–S3 [48]. The number and diameter of large myelinated axons both decrease, while smaller motor fibres appear relatively preserved. The myelin sheath degenerates and conduction velocity in myelinated nerves is reduced. At the neuromuscular junction, the terminal axons branch more and the endplate elongates and is more folded. The amount of synaptic vesicles, acetylcholine and nicotinic receptors also change, the direction of change depending on the animal model studied. It is likely that the safety margin of neuromuscular transmission is maintained, and that the changes at the neuromuscular junction might be compensatory for the surrounding degeneration.

Muscle fibres atrophy and are replaced by connective tissue and fat; the proportion of body weight that is fat increases with age. The size of the type 2 (fast twitch) fibres is reduced and, overall, there is a reduction in muscle fibre numbers. Some workers have proposed selective loss of type 2 fibres, but this is controversial. Fibre types group together, reflecting a constant cycle of denervation and reinnervation; relatively, there is more denervation, and this causes muscle degeneration.

There is very little evidence for altered sensitivity of the aged neuromuscular junction to neuromuscular blocking drugs. Any clinical effects are a result of altered pharmacokinetics; in particular, decreased renal and hepatic function [49]. The diaphragm is affected by age-related degeneration, and the work of breathing may be increased.

Critical illness and the neuromuscular junction

Sir William Osler [50] is widely cited as being the first to describe a myopathy associated with sepsis in 1892. Other workers have subsequently described the association of a myopathy or neuropathy with a range of severe illnesses (e.g. burns and coma [51]). However, it was not until 1983 that the syndrome of critical illness polyneuropathy became recognized as a discrete entity [52]. To suggest that there exists a unified syndrome of features, caused by a single pathophysiological process is false: both may vary considerably.

The significant clinical feature is failure to wean from mechanical ventilation; other clinical findings include distal greater than proximal weakness and depressed or absent tendon reflexes, with relative sparing of the cranial nerves. The absence of the latter does not preclude critical illness polyneuropathy as the cause of failure to wean; nerve conduction studies or electromyography are more reliable indicators. The common finding is of reduced compound action potential amplitude, with a normal conduction velocity (i.e. there is no demyelination) [53,54]. The exact criteria for diagnosis have not been agreed.

Three types of polyneuropathy are described: a sensory axonal neuropathy (least common), a motor axonal neuropathy, and a mixed motor and sensory axonal neuropathy (most common) [55]. The motor neuropathy seems to primarily affect the distal part of the motor axon. This has been demonstrated by single fibre electromogram (EMG) [56]; that recovery is frequently rapid suggests that only a short length of the axon is affected. There is evidence of denervation; fibrillation potentials and positive sharp waves are seen. The precise location of the lesion is not known, but the neuromuscular junction and/or motor endplate may be involved.

Critically ill patients may have an acute myopathy; the incidence of this may be greater than that of polyneuropathy [57]. Here, the muscle membrane has been shown to be inexcitable [58], and this has been proposed to discriminate myopathy from neuropathy, in which the denervated muscle membrane is excitable by direct stimulation. In clinical practice, it is likely that a neuropathy and myopathy frequently coexist, and that electrophysiological studies are affected by the presence of tissue oedema, which could make nerve action potentials appear spuriously low, and by the use of muscle relaxants. A consensus in the nomenclature and diagnosis of weakness in the intensive care patient is overdue.

The pathophysiology is not understood. Bolton [59] has suggested a number of possible mechanisms including distal axonal or neuromuscular junction hypoxia resulting from tissue oedema; a direct toxic effect of the cytokines released in sepsis on the nerve or muscle; and the neurotoxic effects of certain drugs, such as the aminoglycosides.

The major overriding risk factor for critical illness polyneuropathy is the systemic inflammatory response syndrome (SIRS). Indeed, the polyneuropathy might be considered as part of the multiorgan dysfunction syndrome (MODS) seen in this group of patients. Aminoglycosides, use of parenteral nutrition, poor glycaemic control, use of vasopressors for >72 h and low Glasgow Coma Score are independent risk factors. The evidence for the non-depolarizing muscle relaxants as an independent risk is, perhaps surprisingly, not conclusive, except in the case of thick filament myopathy; this syndrome affects asthmatics treated concurrently with neuromuscular blocking drugs and large doses of corticosteroids [60].

References

1 Bernard C. Physiological analysis of the properties of the muscular and nervous systems by means of curare. *C R Acad Sci* 1856; **43**: 825–9.

2 Dale HH, Feldberg W, Vogt M. Release of acetylcholine at voluntary nerve endings. *J Physiol* 1936; **86**: 353–80.

3 Brown G, Dale HH, Feldberg W. Reactions of the normal mammalian muscle to acetylcholine and eserine. *J Physiol* 1936; **87**: 394–424.

4 Bowman WC. Prejunctional mechanisms involved in neuromuscular transmission. In: Booij LHDJ, ed. *Neuromuscular Transmission*. London: BMJ Publishing Group, 1996: 1–27.

5 Bowman WC. *Pharmacology of Neuromuscular Function*. London: Wright, 1990: 1–125.

6 Bevan DR, Bevan JC, Donati FD. *Muscle Relaxants in Clinical Anaesthesia*. Chicago: Year Book Medical Publishers, 1988: 13–34.

7 King JM, Hunter JM. Physiology of the neuromuscular junction. *BJA CEPD Rev* 2002; **2**: 129–33.

8 Standaert FG. Neuromuscular physiology and pharmacology. In: Miller RD, ed. *Anesthesia*, 5th edn. New York: Churchill Livingston, 2000: 735–51.

9 Ruff RL. Neurophysiology of the neuromuscular junction: overview. *Ann N Y Acad Sci* 2003; **998**: 1–10.

10 Enoka RM, Fuglevand FJ. Motor unit physiology: some unresolved issues. *Muscle Nerve* 2001; **24**: 4–17.

11 Lateva ZC, McGill KC, Johanson ME. Electrophysiological evidence of adult human skeletal muscle fibres with multiple endplates and polyneuronal innervation. *J Physiol* 2002; **544**: 549–65.

12 Colomar A, Robitaille R. Glial modification of synaptic transmission at the neuromuscular junction. *Glia* 2004; **47**: 284–9.

13 Goldstein LSB, Yang Z. Microtubule based transport systems in neurons: the roles of kinesins and dyneins. *Annu Rev Neurosci* 2000; **23**: 39–71.

14 Trimble WS, Linial M, Scheller RH. Cellular and molecular biology of the presynaptic nerve terminal. *Annu Rev Neurosci* 1991; **14**: 93–122.

15 Augustine GJ, Burns ME, DeBello WM, *et al.* Proteins involved in synaptic vesicle trafficking. *J Physiol* 1999; **520**: 33–41.

16 Naguib M, Flood P, McArdle JJ, Brenner HR. Advances in neurobiology of the neuromuscular junction. *Anesthesiology* 2002; **96**: 202–31.

17 Kleopa KA, Barchi RL. Genetic disorders of neuromuscular ion channels. *Muscle Nerve* 2002; **26**: 299–325.

18 Katz E, Ferro PA, Weisz G, Uchitel OD. Calcium channels involved in synaptic transmission at the mature and regenerating mouse neuromuscular junction. *J Physiol* 1996; **497**: 687–97.

19 Riekhof GE, Yoshihara M, Guan Z, Littleton JT. Presynaptic N-type calcium channels regulate synaptic growth. *J Biol Chem* 2003; **278**: 41099–108.

20 Urbano FJ, Piedras-Renteria ES, Jun K, *et al.* Altered properties of quantal neurotransmitter release at endplates of mice lacking P/Q type calcium channels. *Proc Natl Acad Sci U S A* 2003; **100**: 3491–6.

21 Nudler S, Piriz J, Urbano FJ, *et al.* Calcium channels and synaptic transmission at the adult, neonatal and P/Q-type deficient neuromuscular junction. *Ann N Y Acad Sci* 2003; **998**: 11–7.

22 Pagani R, Song M, McEnery M, *et al.* Differential expression of alpha 1 and beta subunits of voltage dependent calcium channels at the neuromuscular junction of normal and P/Q calcium channel knockout mouse. *Neuroscience* 2004; **123**: 75–85.

23 Lang B, Vincent A. Autoantibodies to ion channels at the neuromuscular junction. *Autoimmun Rev* 2003; **2**: 94–100.

24 Hiroi Y, Nakao T, Tsuchiya N. Exacerbation of Lambert–Eaton myasthenic syndrome caused by an L-type calcium channel antagonist. *Jpn Heart J* 2003; **44**: 139–44.

25 Swash M, Ingram D. Adverse effect of verapamil in myasthenia gravis. *Muscle Nerve* 1992; **15**: 396–8.

26 De Lorenzo S, Veggetti M, Muchnik S, Losavio A. Presynaptic inhibition of spontaneous acetylcholine release by adenosine at the mouse neuromuscular junction. *Br J Pharmacol* 2004; **142**: 113–24.

27 Singh S, Prior C. Prejunctional effects of the nicotinic ACh receptor agonist dimethylphenylpiperazinium at the rat neuromuscular junction. *J Physiol* 1998; **511**: 451–60.

28 Coggan S, Paysan J, Conroy WG, Berg DK. Direct recording of nicotinic responses in presynaptic nerve terminals. *J Neurosci* 1997; **17**: 5798–806.

29 D'Agostino G, Bolognesi ML, Lucchelli A, *et al.* Prejunctional muscarinic inhibitory control of acetylcholine in the human isolated detrusor: involvement of the M4 receptor. *Br J Pharmacol* 2000; **129**: 493–500.

30 Vizi ES, Somogyi GT. Prejunctional modulation of acetylcholine release from the skeletal neuromuscular junction: link between positive (nicotinic)- and negative (muscarinic)-feedback modulation. *Br J Pharmacol* 1989; **97**: 65–70.

31 Rossi G, Dickerson IM, Rotundo RL. Localization of the calcitonin gene-related peptide receptor complex at the vertebrate neuromuscular junction and its role in regulating acetylcholinesterase expression. *J Biol Chem* 2003; **278**: 24994–5000.

32 Lee C. Conformation, action and mechanism of action of neuromuscular blocking muscle relaxants. *Pharmacol Ther* 2003; **98**: 143–69.

33 Lee C. Structure, conformation and action of neuromuscular blocking drugs. *Br J Anaesth* 2001; **85**: 755–69.

34 Prince RJ, Sine SM. The ligand binding domains of the nicotinic acetylcholine receptor. In: Barrantes FJ, ed. *The Nicotinic Acetylcholine Receptor, Current Views and Future Trends.* Berlin: Springer, 1998: 31–59.

35 Sine SM. The nicotinic receptor ligand binding domain. *J Neurobiol* 2002; **53**: 431–46.

36 Taylor P, Abramson SN, Johnson DA, Valenzuela CF, Herz J. Distinctions in ligand binding sites on the nicotinic acetylcholine receptor. *Ann N Y Acad Sci* 1991; **625**: 568–87.

37 de Rouvroit CL, Goffinet AM. Neuronal migration. *Mech Dev* 2001; **105**: 47–56.

38 Schneider VA, Granato M. Motor axon migration: a long way to go. *Dev Biol* 2003; **263**: 1–11.

39 Burden SJ. Building the vertebrate neuromuscular synapse. *J Neurobiol* 2002; **53**: 501–11.

40 Meier T, Hauser DM, Chiquet M, *et al.* Neural agrin induces ectopic postsynaptic specializations in innervated muscle fibres. *J Neurosci* 1997; **17**: 6534–44.

41 Glass DJ, Bowen DC, Stitt TN, *et al*. Agrin acts via a MuSK receptor complex. *Cell* 1996; **85**: 513–23.

42 Graham DH. Monitoring neuromuscular block may be unreliable in patients with upper-motor-neuron lesions. *Anesthesiology* 1980; **52**: 74–5.

43 Shayevitz JR, Matteo RS. Decreased sensitivity to metocurine in patients with upper motor neurone disease. *Anesth Analg* 1985; **64**: 767–72.

44 Iwasaki H, Namiki A, Omote K, Omote T, Takahashi T. Response differences of paretic and healthy extremities to pancuronium and neostigmine in hemiplegic patients. *Anesth Analg* 1985; **64**: 864–6.

45 Lexell J. Evidence for nervous system degeneration with advancing age. *J Nutr* 1997; **127**: 1011S–3S.

46 Roos R, Rice CL, Vandervoort AA. Age-related changes in motor unit function. *Muscle Nerve* 1997; **20**: 679–90.

47 Larsson L, Ansved T. Effects of ageing on the motor unit. *Prog Neurobiol* 1995; **45**: 397–458.

48 Tomlinson BE, Irving D. The numbers of limb motor neurones in the human lumbosacral cord throughout life. *J Neurol Sci* 1977; **34**: 213–9.

49 Cope TM, Hunter JM. Selecting neuromuscular blocking drugs for elderly patients. *Drugs Aging* 2003; **20**: 125–40.

50 Osler W. *The Principles and Practice of Medicine, Designed for the Use of Practitioners and Students of Medicine*. New York: Appleton, 1892: 114–8.

51 Oslen C. Lesions of peripheral nerves developing during coma. *JAMA* 1956; **160**: 39–41.

52 Bolton CF, Brown JD, Sibbald WA. The electrophysiologic investigation of respiratory paralysis in critically ill patients. *Neurology* 1983; **33**(S2): 186.

53 Hund EF, Fogel W, Krieger D, DeGeorgia M, Hacke W. Critical illness polyneuropathy: clinical findings and outcomes of a frequent cause of neuromuscular weaning failure. *Crit Care Med* 1996; **24**: 1328–33.

54 van Mook WNKA, Hulsewe-Evers RPMG. Critical illness polyneuropathy. *Curr Opin Crit Care* 2002; **8**: 302–10.

55 Coakley JH, Nagendran K, Yarwood GD, Honavar M, Hinds CJ. Patterns of neurophysiological abnormality in prolonged critical illness. *Intensive Care Med* 1998; **24**: 801–7.

56 Schwarz J, Planck J, Briegel J, Straube A. Single-fibre electromyography, nerve conduction studies and conventional electromyography in patients with critical illness polyneuropathy: evidence for a lesion of terminal motor axons. *Muscle Nerve* 1997; **20**: 696–70.

57 Lacomis D, Petrella JT, Giuliani MJ. Causes of neuromuscular weakness in the ICU: a study of ninety-two patients. *Muscle Nerve* 1998; **21**: 610–7.

58 Rich MM, Bird SJ, Raps EC, McCluskey LF, Teener JW. Direct muscle stimulation in acute quadriplegic myopathy. *Muscle Nerve* 1997; **20**: 665–73.

59 Bolton CF. Sepsis and the systemic inflammatory response syndrome: neuromuscular manifestations. *Crit Care Med* 1996; **24**: 1408–16.

60 Barohn RJ, Jackson CE, Rogers SJ, Ridings LW. Prolonged paralysis due to non-depolarizing neuromuscular blocking agents and corticosteroids. *Muscle Nerve* 1994; **17**: 647–54.

PART 3

Clinical measurement

CHAPTER 25
Magnetic resonance imaging

Fiona J. Gilbert and Thomas W. Redpath

Introduction

Nuclear magnetic resonance (NMR) was discovered in the late 1940s, the discovery arising from the interest of physicists in fundamental properties of the atomic nucleus. In the 1950s and 1960s, NMR became a powerful tool in chemical research, as the NMR signal revealed much about the atomic and molecular environment surrounding the nucleus. The use of NMR to form images was proposed in 1973, by Paul Lauterbur, a physicist working in the USA. Following early pioneering work in the UK from the mid 1970s to the early 1980s, magnetic resonance imaging (MRI) became a practical method of producing medical images. Since then it has become increasingly used in hospital radiology departments worldwide [1].

Nuclear magnetism and spin

Atoms consist of a tiny, positively charged nucleus surrounded by a relatively large cloud of negatively charged electrons circulating around it. Some nuclei can be thought of as spinning around their axis. However, not all nuclei have this property. A spinning nucleus generates a magnetic field in the same way that a current circulating round a loop will generate a magnetic field. The magnetic field it generates is similar to that produced by a tiny bar magnet.

Normally, nuclear magnets, which we now refer to as nuclear 'spins', do not have any preferred direction of alignment. However, if they are placed in a strong magnetic field, B_0, they will tend to align with it, in much the same way as a set of compass needles will align with the Earth's magnetic field. If a sample of water were to be placed in a strong magnetic field,

the hydrogen nuclei in the water molecules (H_2O) would be very slightly magnetized as a result of this effect. Similarly, if the human body is placed in a powerful magnetic field, the aqueous hydrogen nuclei in the soft tissue is also magnetized, and this is what makes MRI possible.

Magnetic resonance images are normally formed from hydrogen nuclei (^1H) as they are so abundant in the body, because the body is approximately 75% water. Body fat contains lipids and therefore hydrogen atoms and hydrogen nuclei, so that body fat is also visible on MR images. Other nuclei that have a nuclear spin and that could be used for MRI are far less abundant (e.g. sodium [^{23}Na] and phosphorus [^{31}P]), so that the effect is too small to be useful, thus making MRI a much more difficult proposition.

Nuclear precession and the Larmor frequency

The gyroscope or spinning top is a good analogy to the behaviour of nuclear magnetization (Fig. 25.1). If the top is perturbed from its initial alignment with the Earth's gravitational field, then it precesses around a vertical axis through its point of contact with the table. The precession in revolutions per second is much slower than the spin of the top around its own axis. Similarly, if nuclear spins are perturbed from their alignment with the magnetic field (B_0), they precess around it. The direction of the magnetic field is called the z-axis. In NMR, the precession frequency f_0 is often referred to as the Larmor frequency. It is directly proportional to field strength. Hydrogen nuclei are protons and precess at 42.6 MHz in a magnetic field of strength 1 tesla, at 63.9 MHz at 1.5 tesla, and so on. Other nuclei have very different values for f_0 at a given field strength. For instance phosphorus nuclei (^{31}P) have a Larmor frequency of 17.2 MHz in a field of 1 tesla.

Whereas the spinning top can be pushed from the vertical by a tap of the finger, nuclear spins have to be

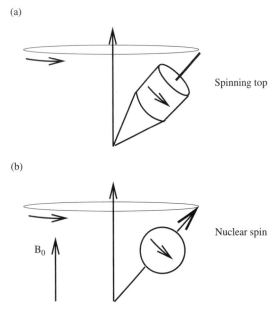

(a)

(b)

B_0

Spinning top

Nuclear spin

Figure 25.1 The physics of a spinning top. (a) Precessing around the vertical Earth's gravitational field is a good analogy to the Larmor precession of a nuclear spin around an applied magnetic field B_0 (b).

pushed away from their alignment with the magnetic field by short pulses of radio waves. The frequency must match the Larmor precession frequency precisely. The radiofrequency (RF) pulse is applied by a coil surrounding the patient's body or head, with power supplied by an RF power amplifier. An RF pulse that rotates the nuclear spins through 90° from their initial position along z is called a 90° pulse. Although most of the energy of the RF pulse is absorbed by the patient as heat, a tiny fraction of the energy is absorbed by the nuclear spins.

Relaxation in nuclear magnetic resonance

If the nuclear spins are rotated away from their natural alignment with the magnetic field B_0 by applying an RF pulse, they will begin to realign with z as soon as the RF pulse is switched off (Fig. 25.2). The nuclear spins do this by giving out the energy they have absorbed from the RF pulse. The realignment follows an exponential recovery with a time constant T1, the 'longitudinal relaxation' time. The longer T1, the longer it takes for the nuclear spins to realign along z. For historical reasons T1 is sometimes called the spin-lattice relaxation time.

During a 90° RF pulse, nuclear spins are rotated into the 'transverse' plane, at right angles to the magnetic field. As outlined above, they precess around the z-axis at the Larmor frequency. Initially, they all

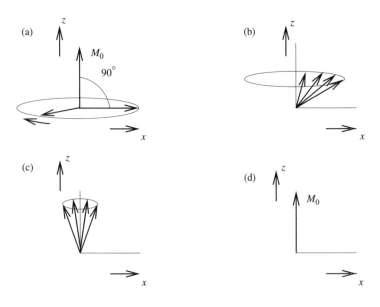

(a)

M_0

90°

x

(b)

z

x

(c)

z

x

(d)

z

M_0

x

Figure 25.2 Following a 90° pulse, magnetization initially along the z-axis precesses in the transverse plane. As time progresses the nuclear spins dephase, so that their magnetism fans out into a cone. At the same time the nuclear spins progressively recover their alignment with the main magnetic field B_0, so that the cone folds upwards as shown. The dephasing effect occurs with a time constant T2, while the recovery toward alignment with B_0 occurs with a time constant T1.

precess in phase with each other, but in time they begin to lose synchronicity (Fig. 25.2). This happens because the spins are in very slightly different molecular and atomic environments owing to Brownian motion of atoms and molecules in cells and interstitial spaces between cells. The magnetic effects of these neighbouring atoms change the local strength of the magnetic field very slightly and hence also change the Larmor precession frequencies of the nuclear spins. As the spins spread out in the transverse plane, the effective sum of these magnetic vectors is reduced exponentially as time goes on. The time constant of this process is T2, or the transverse relaxation time. For historical reasons, it is sometimes called the spin–spin relaxation time. In pure water, T2 equals the longitudinal relaxation time T1. Note that T2 is always less than or equal to T1, because no transverse magnetization remains when the magnetization has realigned with the magnetic field.

NMR signal

A coil of wire surrounding the patient is used to apply a 90° RF pulse. This coil can also be used to pick up the tiny NMR signal (see below). Initially, the nuclear spins are aligned along z, the direction of the magnetic field. After the RF pulse, the nuclear spins precess rapidly in the transverse plane. The magnetic field associated with the nuclei is now rapidly rotating, and this induces a voltage in the coil. The voltage (the NMR signal) induced in the coil alternates at the same frequency as the precession frequency, so that the coil picks up an RF signal at the Larmor frequency. The size of the NMR signal declines exponentially with time constant T2 as the nuclear spins diphase, as described above.

Principles of magnetic resonance imaging

Using magnetic field gradients to form images

The basis of MRI is that the Larmor precession frequency is used to mark the position of an object within the scanned volume. The precession frequency f_0, and hence the frequency of the NMR signal, is directly proportional to the strength of the static magnetic field B_0. A magnetic field gradient coil can modify the strength of the magnetic field, denoted by B_0, and hence the Larmor frequency, depending on position (x) within the scanner. A graph of the modified static field strength B_0 versus x would look like Figure 25.3, when a steady electrical current is driven through the x gradient coil. The size of the gradient G_x is directly proportional to the current flowing through the gradient coil, and its direction can be reversed by reversing the direction of current flow.

The process of image formation is not straightforward. There are three dimensions to be determined, and yet only one dimension can be encoded at any one time. MRI scanners are fitted with three separate magnetic field gradient coils, which can be independently controlled, one each for the x, y and z directions. The imaging process therefore encodes each direction sequentially, with the x, y and z gradients switched on and off in turn. The details are too complex to be described in this short chapter (see Further Reading at the end of the chapter for details).

Tissue contrast in MRI

If MRI were only capable of producing images of water or proton density, it would be of little value as a clinical imaging tool, as most soft tissues have similar water content, which is little changed by disease. In MRI, however, the influence of T1 and T2 relaxation times can greatly modify NMR signal strength, and therefore the intensity of different tissues in the displayed image. Not only are relaxation times markedly different between various tissues, but disease

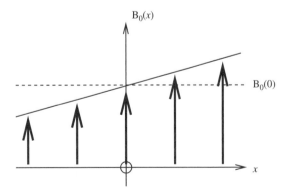

Figure 25.3 The magnitude of the magnetic field B_0 varies linearly with position x in the presence of a magnetic field gradient G_x, which determines the steepness of the slope.

can also alter them. Table 25.1 gives examples of normal T1 and T2 values for some soft tissues. Note that T1 tends to increase with magnetic field strength.

T1 is approximately 3 s for protons in pure water, or for tissues with a very high water content, such as cerebrospinal fluid (CSF). Water protons which are bound into soft tissues have a much shorter T1 value. Table 25.1 gives typical *in vivo* T1 values of various tissues at 0.5, 1.0 and 1.5 tesla [2,3]. Body fluids tend to have the longest T1 relaxation times, this being a consequence of the relatively weak magnetic interaction of their ^1H nuclei with neighbouring atoms and nuclei. Similar arguments apply to transverse relaxation, so that fluids also have long T2 values. Although it is possible to measure the T1 and T2 values of tissue *in vivo*, and present the results as maps with T1 or T2 values in milliseconds, this is seldom carried out. Instead, the differences in T1 and T2 values between tissues are used to give contrast in T1- and T2-weighted images, as outlined below.

A large number of signals are needed to form an image. Thus, a number of RF pulses have to be applied to the tissue being imaged, as usually only one signal is produced for each 90° RF pulse. The time between each 90° RF pulse is called the 'time for repetition' (TR). We can choose TR to be long or short, compared with the tissue T1 value. A T1-weighted image is formed by imaging relatively rapidly, with a

TR value that is of the same order as, or shorter than the T1 values of the tissues being imaged. Tissues with long T1 values tend therefore to give a low signal, as the nuclear spins tend not to recover their alignment along the magnetic field between the successive RF pulses. Therefore, there is less nuclear magnetism to be rotated into the transverse plane by the RF pulse and a weak signal results.

The TE value of a sequence is the time delay between the 90° RF pulse, which rotates the nuclear spins into the transverse plane, and the time at which signal is measured. In a T1-weighted image, the influence of transverse relaxation has to be removed. For T1-weighted images TE is therefore chosen to be short, so that only a small degree of transverse relaxation can occur before the signal is measured. In other words, TE must be much shorter than the tissue T2 values. Thus, in a T1-weighted MR image, signal intensity depends primarily on tissue T1, and of course on proton density. Typical TR values for T1-weighted images are approximately 500 ms, and have TE values of approximately 10–20 ms. In T1-weighted images, fluids tend to appear dark, owing to their long T1 values.

For T2-weighted imaging, it is necessary to remove the influence of T1. This is done by extending TR such that most tissues have enough time for the nuclear spins to realign with the magnetic field before the next 90° RF pulse is applied. A typical choice of TR is approximately 2500 ms. Having reduced the T1-weighting by extending TR, T2-weighting is introduced by extending TE, typically to approximately 100 ms. This allows time for the effect of differences in transverse relaxation times T2 to come into play before the signal is measured. In a T2-weighted image, tissues with a long T2, such as fluids, will therefore appear to be bright areas of high signal.

Proton density weighted images are obtained with long TR (typically 2500 ms) and short TE (typically 10–20 ms). From the arguments above, the TR and TE values are chosen to minimize the effects of T1 and T2 relaxation effects. It is convenient to acquire them simultaneously with T2-weighted images. This is achieved by collecting two NMR signals after each 90° RF pulse: one at a short TE for the proton-density image, the other at the longer TE needed for the T2-weighted image. This is called a 'double-echo'

Table 25.1 Proton T1 relaxation times for some important tissues at 0.5, 1.0 and 1.5 T. T2 is also given and does not vary greatly with Larmor frequency.

Tissue	T1 (0.5 T) (ms)	T1 (1.0 T) (ms)	T1 (1.5 T) (ms)	T2 (ms)
Grey brain matter	–	1040	1140	100
White brain matter	450	660	720	90
Muscle	560	–	1160	35
CSF	4000	4000	4000	2000
Liver	360	–	720	60

sequence. 'Echo' is a term often used for the NMR signal.

Gradient-echo and spin-echo pulse sequences

Before measuring the signal, a complicated sequence of RF pulses and magnetic field gradients have to be gone through. This chapter is too short to go into this in any great detail. However, it is important to distinguish between two main types of sequence. The simplest type of sequence uses only gradient pulses after the initial 90° RF pulse and is therefore called a 'gradient-echo' sequence. More complicated sequences use a pair of 90° and 180° RF pulses, combined with magnetic field gradients, before the echo signal is measured. This type of sequence is called a 'spin-echo' sequence.

Spin-echo sequences have the important advantage over gradient-echo sequences; they inherently compensate for the unwanted effects of imperfect magnet designs. A perfect magnet would produce a perfectly homogeneous magnetic field, so that all nuclear spins would precess at exactly the same Larmor frequency and any dephasing as they precess would be caused only by microscopic fluctuations in the local magnetic fields near the nuclear spins, arising from the Brownian motion of atoms and molecules. In reality, magnets are not perfect and magnetic field strength can vary with position, albeit by tiny amounts. It is therefore necessary to compensate for the unwanted effect of an imperfect magnet by using a spin-echo sequence when using the relatively long TE needed for T2-weighted imaging. As a result, the observed T2 relaxation time with a gradient-echo sequence is less than that observed with a spin-echo sequence. The shorter T2 relaxation time seen in gradient-echo sequences is termed T2*. The T2* time can be reduced by the presence of venous blood, as deoxyhaemoglogin is paramagnetic, or by magnetic resonance contrast agents.

Suppressing the signal from fat

Fat usually has high signal intensity on T1- and T2-weighted images unless steps are taken to suppress it. Bright fat can sometimes hinder image interpretation and can cause artefacts. Two main methods are used to suppress the fat signal: the short TI inversion recovery (STIR) sequence; or chemical shift saturation. The methods are outlined below.

An inversion-recovery (IR) sequence uses a 180° RF pulse to rotate the nuclear spins from alignment along the magnetic field so that they are 'inverted' to point in the opposite direction. This produces no signal because no magnetization is rotated into the transverse plane. At a time TI later, the 'time from inversion', a 90° RF pulse tips the spins into the transverse plane to generate an NMR signal. The nuclear spins then regain their alignment along their preferred direction parallel to the magnetic field with a time constant T1. As they do this, their average magnetism is changing from negative (antiparallel to the magnetic field) to positive (parallel to the magnetic field), passing through zero at a time approximately equal to 70% of the relaxation time T1. It is important to realize that as the nuclear spins realign with the applied magnetic field, no NMR signal occurs during the interval TI, as there is no nuclear spin magnetism in the transverse plane.

The T1 of fat is shorter than most other tissues. Therefore, TI can be chosen so that the 90° RF pulse is applied just at that time when the nuclear spin magnetism of the hydrogen nuclei in fat has recovered to its zero value, as shown in Figure 25.4. Fat will therefore be dark on the MR image as it will produce no NMR signal. This special case of IR sequence is called a STIR sequence.

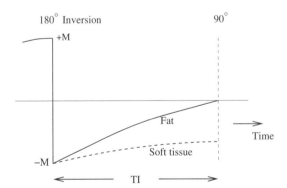

Figure 25.4 In a STIR sequence, TI is chosen such that the nuclear magnetism of fat is zero when the 90° RF pulse is applied. Therefore fat gives no signal and appears dark in a STIR image.

The fat or lipid signal can also be suppressed using methods based on the very small difference in the Larmor frequency of lipid protons compared with water protons. The difference in resonant frequency f_0 is termed a chemical shift, as it arises from the different molecular environment of the hydrogen protons. The effective magnetic field 'seen' by water protons, and hence their Larmor frequency, differs very slightly from that seen by lipid protons. It is therefore possible to apply a 90° RF pulse tuned to the lipid molecules, but not the water molecules. This is possible because RF pulses only work if they are applied at precisely the correct frequency. This special 90° RF 'chemical shift fat suppression' pulse is performed shortly before each 90° RF pulse in an imaging sequence. Although an NMR signal is produced by the saturation pulse, it is not measured. The purpose of this step is to leave no nuclear magnetism in the fatty tissue protons which can be used by the imaging pulse sequence that follows. The effect of the fat suppression pulse is to remove the signal from lipid protons in the image so that fat appears dark as an area of low signal.

Practical multislice imaging

MRI is a digital imaging modality. An image is broken up into a large number of small picture elements (pixels), each represented by a number. The numbers lie with a range (e.g. from 0 to 255). The computer displays the image by showing pixels with value zero as a black dot or square, and pixels with value 255 as white. Each pixel corresponds to a particular tiny rectangular volume of tissue called a volume cell (voxel). A typical MR image consists of 256 × 256 pixels and represents the signals obtained from a thin slice through the body, as does X-ray computed tomography (CT). As originally proposed, MRI needed at least 256 separate signals to form a 256 × 256 pixel image — today there are a number of methods of speeding this up. However, from the arguments above, it is obvious that MR image acquisition can be time consuming. For instance, the time needed to acquire a 256 × 256 T1-weighted image with a typical TR of 500 ms will be 256 times TR, or approximately 2 minutes. The time needed for a T2-weighted image with a TR of 2000 ms will be 8 minutes. This would be unacceptable if this was the time to produce a single image, as it would take hours to complete an MRI head scan for example. Fortunately, the process can be made more efficient by scanning many slices (up to 20 or 30) at once. This is possible because, having applied a 90° RF pulse to a particular slice and measured the NMR signal at a time TE later, there is a time (TR-TE) remaining before the process is repeated for that slice. TE is much shorter than the repetition time TR, so that instead of doing nothing having measured the signal, the scanner uses the time (TR-TE) to collect signals from other slices. Thus, although the imaging time is relatively long compared with an X-ray procedure, efficiency is improved by imaging many slices in that time.

Contrast agents in MRI

Initially, it was thought that intravenous contrast agents would not be needed to improve the conspicuity of lesions upon MRI, as the inherent soft tissue contrast is, in many cases, excellent. However, the value of gadolinium in highlighting brain tumours was first demonstrated in 1984 [4], and since then the usage and applications of MRI contrast agents have greatly increased. The gadolinium (Gd) atom, when ionized, has a relatively strong magnetic effect arising from the configuration of its atomic electrons. It therefore interacts with neighbouring hydrogen nuclei in tissue water, modifying their MRI signal strength. The effect arises because the T1 and T2 relaxation times of the tissue water are greatly shortened by the proximity of Gd ions. Because gadolinium is a toxic element, it must be incorporated into a non-toxic molecule. The most common example of this is gadolinium diethylene triamine penta-acetic acid (Gd-DTPA). Following intravenous injection, it distributes throughout the blood plasma space, and diffuses into the extravascular space, excluding the brain, because it does not cross the intact blood–brain barrier. Thus, in brain tumours, it crosses into the extravascular space, shortening the T1 value of water molecules in this space, so that the tumour exhibits a substantially increased signal intensity on a T1-weighted image. Gd-DTPA is rapidly cleared from the body by glomerular filtration in the kidneys.

Other types of MRI contrast agent use tiny particles of magnetized iron. An example of this is the use of superparamagnetic iron oxide nanoparticles

(SPIO) to highlight liver tumours. Following intravenous injection, these particles are taken up by the phagocytic action of Kupffer cells in the liver. This greatly reduces the T2 relaxation time of healthy liver tissue. However, in tumours, where there is a reduced Kupffer cell density, this effect is much less marked. Therefore, on a T2-weighted spin-echo image taken at an appropriate delay after an injection of SPIO particles, the tumour will appear bright against a dark background of normally functioning liver tissue.

Advances in MRI technology and applications

MRI has advanced rapidly since the first practical whole-body MR imager was used to image a patient in Aberdeen in August 1980 [5]. The field strength of that scanner was 400 G (0.04 tesla) and it used a water-cooled four-coil electromagnet. Since then, superconducting magnets have become the most commonly used magnet type, and a field strength of 30 000 G (3.0 tesla) is the new benchmark for MR brain imaging.

Hardware

The major hardware systems in MRI scanners are the magnet, the RF transmitter and receiver, the gradient coils and amplifiers and the computing system.

Magnet designs have advanced, in that very high field strengths are now possible, which use superconducting technology, with excellent magnetic field homogeneity. Previously, such magnets would have made a large area dangerous for public access, by virtue of their large 'stray' field. Modern self-shielded designs minimize the spill-over of the field into surrounding rooms, greatly reducing the problems related to scanner installation. Superconducting magnets have completely replaced the simple air-cored electromagnets used in the very early scanners. Permanent magnets can also be used if low capital cost, and low maintenance and running costs are important. A compromise is the use of electromagnets with iron cores, which allows a lower power to be used to achieve a given field strength. C-shaped iron-cored magnets are used in 'open' designs where the patient is not confined in a long narrow tube, as in most superconducting designs, thus reducing the possibility of claustrophobia.

Gradient coils now allow much larger gradient strengths to be achieved. Early whole-body scanners, such as the Aberdeen 0.04 tesla design, used gradients of the order of 2 milliteslas per metre, which could be switched on or off in a time of a millisecond or so. Modern designs, with their associated powerful amplifiers, can achieve gradients of 50 milliteslas per metre, with a switching time of 0.25 ms. A major advance is that of the 'self-shielded' gradient coil, which confines the magnetic fields generated by the coil within the cylinder on which it is wound. This allows gradients to be switched off and on very rapidly without unwanted interactions with the surrounding metal in the magnet.

Modern RF receiving coils or 'phased arrays' consist of multiple elements, and are considerably more complex and sophisticated than the simple single element designs used in the early scanners. They provide considerably higher sensitivity (i.e. signal : noise ratio; SNR) than early designs and can also be used to speed up image acquisition by using the different spatial sensitivities of each element to reduce the number of spatial encoding steps needed to form images.

Modern computing systems offer faster image reconstruction, advanced image processing and display capabilities and, as a result of modern icon-driven software, are simple to use, despite the multiplicity of modern imaging methods.

Applications

High-speed gradient systems, novel image reconstruction methods harnessed to multicoil phased array coils, and the high signal : noise ratio available from high field magnets have revolutionized the possibilities of MR imaging. Modern fast and ultra-fast gradient-echo and spin-echo imaging methods allow images to be collected in a few seconds or even faster if needed, albeit with reduced image SNR and spatial resolution. High-quality fast spin-echo imaging allows T2-weighted images to be collected in 1–2 minutes, where imaging times of 15 minutes were common in the early days of clinical MRI.

Functional brain MRI (fMRI) uses high-speed imaging to obtain images of the whole brain every 1 or

2 s, while visual, cognitive or other stimuli are presented during scanning. By using an MRI sequence sensitive to blood oxygenation, the response of different parts of the brain to the stimuli can be monitored, so that different brain functions can be mapped in three dimensions. This is a major new tool in understanding brain function.

MR contrast agents allow brain, tumour and cardiac perfusion to be mapped. Cardiac wall motion can be seen by synchronizing MR data acquisition to patients' ECG signal. New types of MR contrast agent are allowing molecular processes to be imaged.

MR hardware and methodology and its applications continue to advance rapidly: MRI is not yet a mature technology.

MRI safety

Because of the strong magnetic field, the scan room is a potentially hazardous environment. Patients with pacemakers, neurostimulators and metal foreign bodies, including many aneurysm clips, should not undergo MRI. Powerful magnets are usually shielded and so the magnetic field outwith the scan room is usually less than 5 G. This does not have any harmful effects. However, all staff should be warned about taking metallic objects into the MR scan room. There is normally a controlled area surrounding the scanner where metal chairs and trolleys, oxygen cylinders, etc., are required to be exchanged for 'MR safe' equipment. Horrific accidents have occurred as a result of unsuspecting staff taking ferromagnetic oxygen cylinders and even industrial cleaning equipment into the magnet room, which act as projectiles [6]. Non-ferrous MR-compatible monitoring equipment must be used in the MR room to avoid accidents and are widely available. While it is possible to image patients who are intubated or under heavy sedation, visual inspection of the patient is difficult. A nominated consultant should be responsible for anaesthesia services in MR units. The Association of Anaesthetists has guidelines specific to MRI [7].

Although no adverse effects have been reported, current recommendations state that MR imaging in the first trimester of pregnancy should be avoided [6]. During imaging, energy deposition occurs in the tissues, causing heating effects. This effect is not no-

ticeable but specific absorption rates can be calculated from the imaging sequences being undertaken, and machines are set so that these cannot be exceeded. Time-varying magnetic field gradients can induce electric currents in the body that can result in peripheral nerve stimulation or cause the sensation of flashes of light, 'the magnetic phosphenes' that are the result of the retina being stimulated by the MR induced current [8].

Clinical applications

Neuroimaging
The first clinical whole body MR examination was performed in Aberdeen in August 1980, where the technique was used to demonstrate liver metastases in a patient with oesophageal cancer [5]. However, imaging in the body was difficult because of movement of organs from respiration, pulsation from the aorta and bowel peristalsis. Movement caused considerable degradation of the images and so early clinical applications were only used for the brain and spine. The excellent anatomical detail revealed good differentiation between grey and white matter and allowed identification of brain structures, exceeding the quality attained by CT examination. The success in neuroimaging resulted in MR equipment being installed primarily for this purpose in the 1980s and 1990s. In 2005, more than 50% of the MR workload was neuroimaging, with the majority of examinations being undertaken to identify or exclude primary or more commonly secondary brain tumours; in addition, acoustic neuromas, demyelination, stroke, ischaemia, heterotopia or scarring as a cause of epilepsy. The lumbar spine is imaged next most frequently, to identify the causes of low back pain or sciatica, and the cervical spine to ascertain if any disc disease or foraminal compression of nerve roots is present.

Brain imaging
Standard spin-echo sequences are used, which are usually sagittal T1-weighted, axial proton-density and T2-weighted double-echo, and coronal T1-weighted. Fluid-attenuated inversion recovery (FLAIR) imaging is used if demyelination is suspected as this technique is extremely sensitive to fluid, and recent plaques of demyelination are more

readily identified using this sequence. FLAIR suppresses the signal from cerebrospinal fluid in the ventricles in a similar manner to STIR suppressing the fat signal (see above) and makes the visualization of periventricular lesions more obvious [9]. Signs of multiple sclerosis (MS) are oval-shaped periventricular flares horizontal to the lateral ventricles together with plaques of different ages in the deep white matter (Fig. 25.5a,b). MRI is not only much more sensitive than CT for identifying MS plaques, but it can also be used to quantify the number and location of lesions. This non-invasive test means disease progression and novel treatment effects can be monitored. Characteristically, multiple punctuate white matter lesions usually less than 1 cm in size are seen. Lesions are typically central adjacent to the ventricular margins with their long axis parallel to the white matter fibres in the corona radiate [9]. Corpus callosum lesions are most likely to be MS plaques, as ischaemic events are much less common there because of the vascular supply from the numerous short perforating vessels direct from the pericallosal artery [10].

Differentiation of demyelination from ischaemic disease can be difficult in the over-40 age group as white matter disease is often seen. White matter changes in the periventricular region and deep to the cortex are seen in ischaemia, together with some brain shrinkage or atrophy, and can be regarded as normal in the ageing brain [11,12].

Infarcts are readily identifiable using brain MRI and also CT, but it may take up to 24 hours for the features of an infarct to become evident. Haemorrhagic infarcts account for 10–15% of all cerebrovascular infarcts and CT is the best method of demonstrating this, as fresh blood can sometimes be difficult to image and has a variety of MR appearances depending on the amount and age of the accumulated blood. Where there is a requirement to make a very early diagnosis of a thromboembolic occlusion of the cerebral circulation, dynamic susceptibility contrast-enhanced MRI is the best approach [13].

Ischaemia is seen in approximately 85% of strokes and leads to early changes in the water content of the affected brain so that MRI can detect abnormalities within 1 hour of onset [14]. Once cerebral perfusion

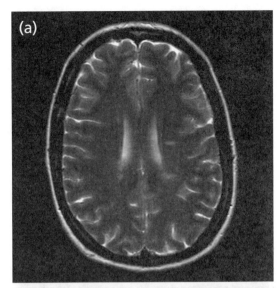

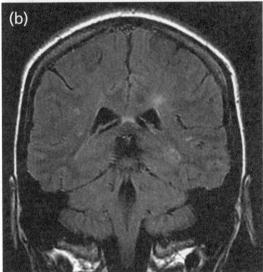

Fig. 25.5 (a) T2W axial image through lateral ventricles demonstrating an ovoid high signal area perpendicular to the lateral ventricle. This is typical of a plaque of demyelination found in multiple sclerosis. (b) Same patient. Coronal FLAIR image through posterior horns of lateral ventricles showing areas of high signal representing further areas of demyelination.

drops below a critical level (10–22 mL/100 g/min), ischaemia occurs [15]. Cells start to swell within an hour (cytotoxic oedema), followed by loss of vascular endothelial integrity, leading to leakage of fluid (vasogenic oedema) after 6 hours [10]. FLAIR images are very sensitive to oedema in the early stages of ischaemia [16]. Intravenous contrast shows arterial enhancement as an early sign — within minutes — due to slow flow. Meningeal enhancement, caused by leptomeningeal collaterals, are seen with large cerebral infarcts usually observed at 1–3 days. Mass effect resulting from oedema in the infarcted tissue is maximum at 3–7 days. Eventually, gliosis results in a low signal area on the MRI.

Magnetic resonance angiography is able to demonstrate thrombosis in the circle of Willis and cerebral arteries and also significant stenosis of the carotid and vertebral arteries. Similarly, MR venography has been shown to be an accurate non-invasive method for the evaluation of dural sinus thrombosis (Fig. 25.6) [16].

Diffusion-weighted images have been shown to be superior to T2-weighted images for detecting early ischaemic change (Fig. 25.7) [17]. Protons in moving water molecules alter their magnetization in the presence of a magnetic field and the greater (faster) the diffusion, then the more the signal attenuates. Increasing the magnetic fields results in increased sensitivity of the MR signal to diffusion. By applying diffusion sensitizing gradients, an apparent diffusion coefficient (ADC) can be calculated. In ischaemic areas, the ADC drops within 45 min of the event, reflecting reduced water diffusion. This is thought to be a result of cell swelling (cytotoxic oedema) so there is less water movement in the extracellular compartment. However, there are a number of early tissue changes that may be contributing, such as changes in osmolality, temperature or loss of tissue pulsation [16]. Perfusion imaging uses ultrafast MR techniques to measure the T2* shortening effect caused by the initial vascular transit of a bolus of contrast. Dynamic ultrafast imaging allows a semi-quantitative measure to be made so that regional cerebral blood volume and regional blood flow can be calculated (Fig. 25.7c,d) [13]. The combination of the above MR techniques makes the characterization of pathophysiological processes possible, allowing treatment of potentially reversible ischaemic areas [17].

MR is a useful examination in infections of the brain, as normally there is breach of the blood–brain barrier and brain oedema. It is particularly useful in viral encephalitis as CT can appear normal, or only show mild brain swelling, which can be overlooked.

Brain tumours, both primary and the more common secondary tumours resulting from metastases, can be clearly delineated, with mixed signal intensity and surrounding oedema in the more aggressive

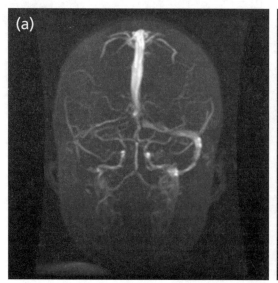 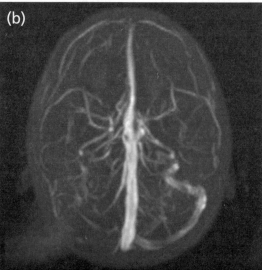

Figure 25.6 Magnetic resonance venography demonstrating contrast in the superior sagittal sinus and left transverse sinus but an absence of contrast in the right transverse sinus indicating a venous thrombosis on these (a) coronal and (b) axial images.

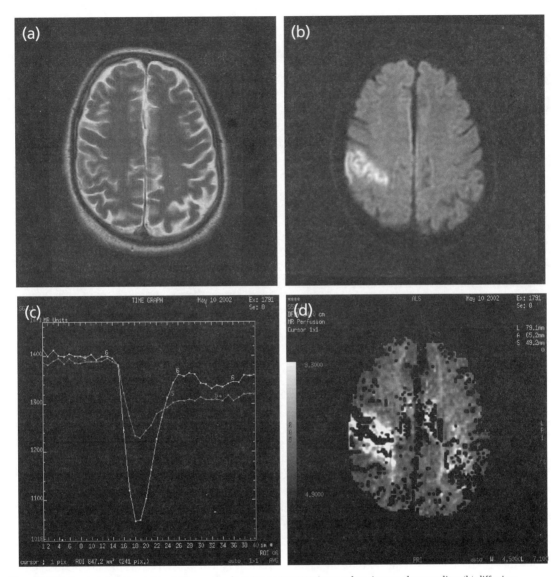

Figure 25.7 Acute infarct in right middle cerebral territory; (a) T2W image showing no abnormality; (b) diffusion weighted image showing high signal in infarct; (c) bolus tracking curves from T2* sequences showing less signal drop (purple) in ischaemic brain compared with normal; and (d) perfusion map with no perfusion in infarct and surrounding luxury perfusion (white).

lesions. Acoustic neuromas are best seen on MRI using a T2-weighted sequence (Fig. 25.8).

Meningeal deposits are difficult to visualize on both CT and MR, but contrast enhancement of the meninges will often give a clue to the diagnosis. The multiplanar capability and high tissue contrast, together with the ability of contrast to alter signal as a result of disruption of the blood–brain barrier, make

MRI extremely useful in diagnosis and management of brain tumours. Localization of the tumour can be determined accurately and the images used to guide brain biopsy and to target radiotherapy. Monitoring of treatment effects is possible because of the reproducibility and non-invasive nature of the technique. Complications of brain tumours can be diagnosed; for example, secondary haemorrhage,

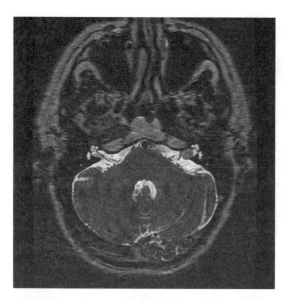

Figure 25.8 T2W axial section through internal auditory meati and cerebellum. Normal 8th nerve on right and acoustic neuroma on left measuring 1 cm in diameter.

hydrocephalus and recurrence following treatment can be differentiated.

MRI is extremely helpful when pituitary abnormalities are suspected; for example, in patients presenting with bi-temporal hemianopia or with abnormalties of the pituitary hormones. Pituitary adenomas are the most common primary neoplasm in the sellar region. Macroadenomas greater than 10 mm in size are usually non-functioning. However, microadenomas are more commonly functioning. They normally have low signal on T1-weighted images and variable signal on T2-weighted images. Intravenous contrast results in the normal pituitary, infundibulum and cavernous sinuses intensely increasing in signal, but within microadenomas the tissue enhances moderately.

The spine

Cervical and lumbar disc herniations are well demonstrated on MR, with sagittal T1- and T2-weighted and axial T2-weighted spin-echo sequences commonly used to demonstrate the level and size of the herniation and any involvement of the adjacent nerve roots. Discitis is best seen on MR, and contrast is given to confirm the diagnosis. MR can show any

extension into the epidural space as well as the degree of collapse of adjacent vertebral bodies. While isotope bone scanning is the most frequently used investigation for identifying metastatic bone disease, MR can be helpful in equivocal examinations [18]. Comparisons of whole body MRI with isotope bone scan has shown that MRI was more sensitive and specific in the detection of metastases [19]. Low back pain is a common condition, which resolves spontaneously in most patients (approximately 90%). The remaining 10% are referred to secondary care and may require imaging investigations. MRI is indicated in sciatica where an intervention is proposed, to determine the level of the abnormality, which is usually a disc herniation. However, imaging in low back pain does not itself alter patient management or outcome, although in a randomized trial there was a small but significant improvement in patients' well-being [20]. Patients with 'red flags' (over 50 years of age, raised erythrocyte sedimentation rate, a history of tumour or infection) do merit imaging [21]; however, arguably MRI is more cost effective than plain radiographs because of the greater sensitivity for the detection of disease [22].

Spinal cord compression is one of the few indications for an emergency MR investigation [21]. The level and degree of the compression can be clearly shown and often the cause can be identified from the examination. MR has replaced myelography and contrast CT examinations. Spinal cord tumours are shown as fusiform swellings either centrally or eccentrically, depending on the cell type from which the tumour has arisen. Neuromas and schwannomas on nerve roots can be seen. Post-traumatic lesions such as brachial plexus tears or post-traumatic syrinxes are shown as high signal on T2-weighted spin-echo sequences.

A normal MR examination can be very reassuring because of the high sensitivity of the examination to oedema, which usually accompanies most pathology. This is often used to reassure the clinician and patient in cases where there are non-specific neurological features.

Musculoskeletal applications

The excellent anatomical information obtained has made MR very useful in the examination of joints, and contrast arthrography has largely been replaced. The most commonly imaged joint is the knee, where tears of the menisci and cruciate ligaments can be demonstrated with over 90% accuracy [23,24]. The collateral ligaments can be clearly seen and associated bone bruising demonstrated in many cases, following an acute injury. Similarly, shoulder joints can be examined and tears of the rotator cuff displayed as gaps within the tendon and inflammation as abnormally high signal. Infective changes are clearly seen, as large effusions are often present within the joint, along with bone oedema and adjacent diffuse oedematous change within the soft tissues. MR can be particularly useful in non-specific joint pain where radiographs are normal, as early infective changes can be demonstrated, or other causes such as avascular necrosis or transient osteoporosis can be seen [25].

Abdominal imaging

CT and ultrasound are still used most commonly for diagnosis, staging and treatment monitoring of the abdomen. Abdominal imaging is more challenging

as any motion from respiration or bowel peristalsis can degrade MR image quality. However, the more modern rapid imaging sequences has meant MR of the abdomen is now used more commonly. In particular, magnetic resonance cholangio-pancreatography (MRCP) is now an attractive alternative to endoscopic imaging techniques of the bile and pancreatic ducts, as there is no radiation dose and no risk of inducing pancreatitis [26]. MRCP uses a very strongly T2-weighted ultrafast spin-echo sequence to minimize motion artefact and highlight the fluid content of the bile ducts (Fig. 25.9). The diagnostic accuracy is equivalent [27] although endoscopic retrograde cholangiopancreatography (ERCP) is required if gallstones need to be removed endoscopically. Liver imaging is undertaken with either Gd-DTPA or liver-specific MR contrast agents (see above), which can improve the conspicuity of liver abnormalities. Renal examinations are performed to examine morphology and also the renal arteries so a 'one-stop' examination can be performed to demonstrate renal artery stenosis and renal function (Fig. 25.10). Pancreatic imaging is of similar quality to CT. As both hardware and software improvements occur

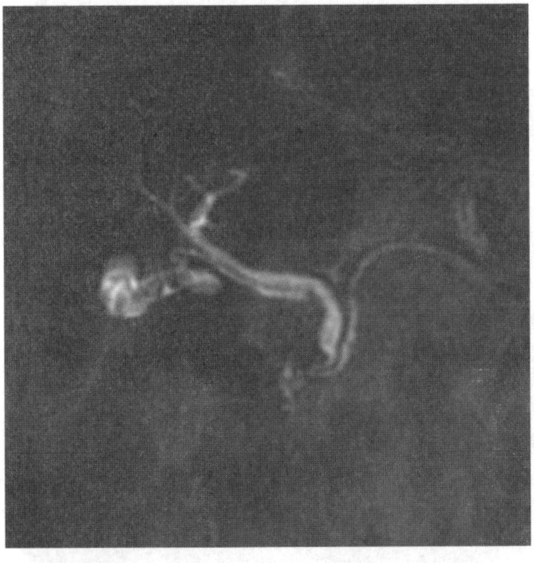

Figure 25.9 Magnetic resonance cholangio-pancreatography – thick slab T2W technique, demonstrating gallstones as filling defects in the gall bladder, slightly dilated common bile duct and a normal pancreatic duct.

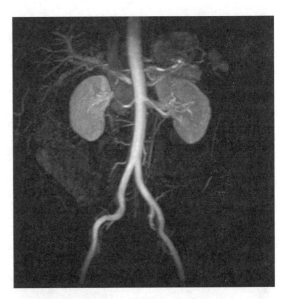

Figure 25.10 Magnetic resonance angiography demonstrating normal aorta and bifurcation. There is a significant renal artery stenosis on the right with a smaller right kidney.

in both CT and MR, it is likely that both modalities will continue to be used in abdominal imaging.

Pelvic imaging, however, appears slightly better on MR than CT for cervical, ovarian and rectal cancer staging, particularly for establishing local spread [28]. It is the multiplanar capacity that aids diagnosis, particularly when ascertaining whether there is

spread through the wall to contiguous organs or if there is lymph node involvement. Contrast agents specific for lymph nodes have been developed: ultrasmall superparamagnetic iron oxide particles are infused into the blood stream and normal nodes take up the particles, causing a drop in signal. Abnormal nodes full of tumour cannot take up the iron

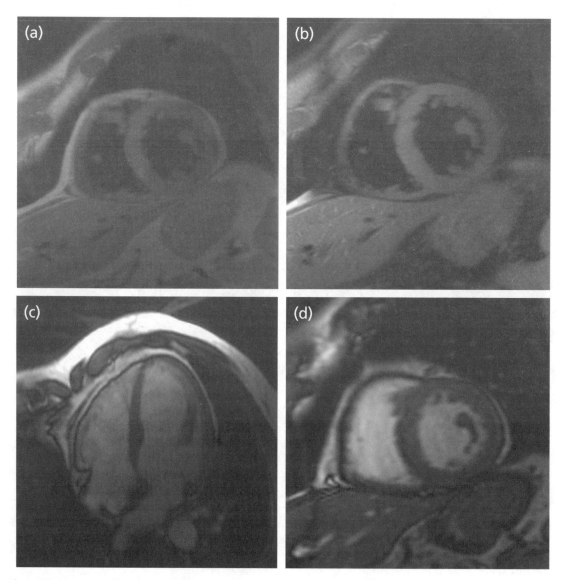

Figure 25.11 (a) T1W double inversion recovery, black blood short axis view of right and left ventricles. (b) T1W fat suppressed, black blood image through both ventricles. (c) FIESTA long axis view showing four chambers of the heart. (d) FIESTA short axis view of both ventricles following IV contrast.

oxide particles and there is no signal change [29]. However, while this method appears promising, it is not yet in widespread use.

In patients who are acutely unwell, the more rapid CT examination or bedside ultrasound examination is more often used, because MR takes longer and the patient is relatively inaccessible during the examination.

Vascular

The advent of paramagnetic contrast agents has allowed imaging of the vasculature in a similar fashion to CT and angiography. The multiplanar and three-dimensional acquisition technique allows images to be displayed in a variety of ways. However, by altering flip angles and acquisition parameters, blood can be made to appear dark or bright. This is particularly useful in cardiac imaging (Fig. 25.11). A moving table technique now means that the legs can be examined relatively easily with an image quality approaching that of angiography. The size of an aortic aneurysm can be monitored with this technique (Fig. 25.12).

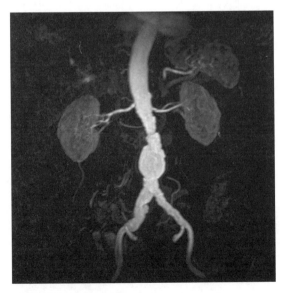

Figure 25.12 Magnetic resonance angiography demonstrating an ectatic aorta and aneurysm above the bifurcation. Both kidneys are also seen with renal arteries.

MR in anaesthesia

MRI offers a non-invasive method of imaging organ blood flow and function during anaesthesia and is therefore a powerful research tool. To date its potential has yet to be fully exploited. Recent studies have been carried out to measure the cerebral metabolic oxygen in rats anaesthetized by isoflurane [30]; cerebral blood flow and vasoreactivity in volunteers following administration of esmolol [31]; and to image brain function in adult volunteers anaesthetized by propofol [32]. These studies are based on the T2* contrast available from the small magnetic difference in haemoglobin as it changes from the oxy- to the deoxy-form, the so-called blood oxygen level dependent (BOLD) contrast mechanism. The study of brain function using the BOLD contrast mechanism is often called fMRI. fMRI has also been used to investigate the occurrence of very low-frequency brain activation in the occipital cortices of anaesthetized children [33]. A similar study has been carried out to investigate very low frequency brain activity in the motor cortices of adult volunteers undergoing servoflurane anaesthesia [34]. In addition to studies of brain function, MRI has been used to image the spread of a local anaesthetic solution in patients undergoing eye surgery [35].

The increasing availability of human and animal MRI systems to research groups, the continuing refinement of quantitative MRI techniques of measuring perfusion and blood flow, in addition to fMRI methods of probing brain activity, will yield new insights into the physiological function of anaesthetic agents.

References

1 Redpath TW. MRI developments in perspective. *Br J Radiol* 1997; **70**: S70.

2 Henriksen O, de Certaines JD, Spisni A, *et al. In vivo* field dependence of proton relaxation times in human brain, liver and skeletal muscle: a multicenter study. *Magn Reson Imaging* 1993; **11**: 851–6.

3 Hopkins AL, Yeung HN, Bratton CB. Multiple field strength *in vivo* T1 and T2 for cerebrospinal fluid protons. *Magn Reson Med* 1986; **3**: 303–11.

4 Carr DH, Brown J, Bydder GM, *et al.* Intravenous chelated gadolinium as a contrast agent in NMR imaging of cerebral tumours. *Lancet* 1984; **i**: 484–6.

5 Smith FW, Hutchison JM, Mallard JR, *et al.* Oesophageal carcinoma demonstrated by whole-body nuclear magnetic resonance imaging. *Br Med J* 1981; **282**: 510–2.

6 Medical Devices Agency. *Guidelines for Magnetic Resonance Equipment in Clinical Use*. 2002.

7 Association of Anaesthetists of Great Britain and Ireland. *Provision of Anaesthetic Services in Magnetic Resonance Units*. 2002.

8 Shellock FG. *Magnetic Resonance Procedures: Health Effects and Safety*. CRC Press, 2001.

9 Pretorius PM, Quaghebeur G. The role of MRI in the diagnosis of MS. *Clin Radiol* 2003; **58**: 434–48.

10 Gean-Marton AD, Vezina LG, Marton KI, *et al.* Abnormal corpus callosum: a sensitive and specific indicator of multiple sclerosis. *Radiology* 1991; **180**: 215–21.

11 Leaper SA, Murray AD, Lemmon HA, *et al.* Neuropsychologic correlates of brain white matter lesions depicted on MR images: 1921 Aberdeen Birth Cohort. *Radiology* 2001; **221**: 51–5.

12 Staff RT, Murray AD, Deary IJ, Whalley LJ. What provides cerebral reserve? *Brain* 2004; **127**: 1191–9.

13 Keston P, Murray AD, Jackson A. Cerebral perfusion imaging using contrast-enhanced MRI. *Clin Radiol* 2003; **58**: 505–13.

14 Brant-Zawadzki M, Pereira B, Weinstein P, *et al.* MR imaging of acute experimental ischemia in cats. *Am J Neuroradiol* 1986; **7**: 7–11.

15 Camarata PJ, Heros RC, Latchaw RE. 'Brain attack': the rationale for treating stroke as a medical emergency. *Neurosurgery* 1994; **34**: 144–57.

16 Jensen MC, Brant-Zawadski MN, Jacobs BC. Ischaemia. In: Stark DD, Bradley WG, eds. *Magnetic Resonance Imaging*, 3rd edn. Mosby, 1999.

17 Mintorovitch J, Moseley ME, Chileuitt L, *et al.* Comparison of diffusion- and T2-weighted MRI for the early detection of cerebral ischemia and reperfusion in rats. *Magn Reson Med Official* 1991; **18**: 39–50.

18 Aitchison FA, Poon FW, Hadley MD, Gray HW, Forrester AW. Vertebral metastases and an equivocal bone scan: value of magnetic resonance imaging. *Nucl Med Commun* 1992; **13**: 429–31.

19 Engelhard K, Hollenbach HP, Wohlfart K, von Imhoff E, Fellner FA. Comparison of whole-body MRI with automatic moving table technique and bone scintigraphy for screening for bone metastases in patients with breast cancer. *Eur Radiol* 2004; **14**: 99–105.

20 Gilbert FJ, Grant AM, Gillan MG, *et al.* Low back pain: influence of early MR imaging or CT on treatment and outcome: multicenter randomized trial. *Radiology* 2004; **231**: 343–51.

21 Royal College of Radiologists. *Making the best use of a department of clinical radiology*. 2003.

22 McNally EG, Wilson DJ, Ostlere SJ. Limited magnetic resonance imaging in low back pain instead of plain radiographs: experience with first 1000 cases. *Clin Radiol* 2001; **56**: 922–5.

23 Kaplan PA, Dussault RG. Magnetic resonance imaging of the knee: menisci, ligaments, tendons. *Top Magn Reson Imaging* 1993; **5**: 228–48.

24 Thornton DD, Rubin DA. Magnetic resonance imaging of the knee menisci. *Semin Roentgenol* 2000; **35**: 217–30.

25 Ratcliffe MA, Gilbert FJ, Dawson AA, Bennett B. Diagnosis of avascular necrosis of the femoral head in patients treated for lymphoma. *Hematol Oncol* 1995; **13**: 131–7.

26 Bearcroft PW, Gimson A, Lomas DJ. Non-invasive cholangio-pancreatography by breath-hold magnetic resonance imaging: preliminary results. *Clin Radiol* 1997; **52**: 345–50.

27 Mougenel JL, Hudziak H, Ernst O, *et al.* Evaluation of a new sequence of magnetic resonance cholangio-pancreatography in thick cut and one shot acquisition. *Gastroenterol Clin Biol* 2000; **24**: 888–95.

28 Husband JES, Reznek RH. *Imaging in Oncology*. Oxford: ISIS Medical Media, 1998.

29 Stets C, Brandt S, Wallis F, *et al.* Axillary lymph node metastases: a statistical analysis of various parameters in MRI with USPIO. *J Magn Reson Imaging* 2002; **16**: 60–8.

30 Liu ZM, Schmidt KF, Sicard KM, Duong TQ. Imaging oxygen consumption in forepaw somatosensory stimulation in rats under isoflurane anesthesia. *Magn Reson Med* 2004; **52**: 277–85.

31 Heinke W, Zysset S, Hund-Georgiadis M, Olthoff D, von Cramon DY. The effect of esmolol on cerebral blood flow, cerebral vasoreactivity, and cognitive performance: a functional magnetic resonance imaging study. *Anesthesiology* 2005; **102**: 41–50.

32 Heinke W, Kenntner R, Gunter TC, *et al.* Sequential effects of increasing propofol sedation on frontal and temporal cortices as indexed by auditory event-related potentials. *Anesthesiology* 2004; **100**: 617–25.

33 Kiviniemi V, Ruohonen J, Tervonen O. Separation of physiological very low frequency fluctuation from aliasing by switched sampling interval fMRI scans. *Magn Reson Imaging* 2005; **23**: 41–6.

34 Peltier SJ, Kerssens C, Hamann SB, *et al.* Functional connectivity changes with concentration of sevoflurane anesthesia. *Neuroreport* 2005; **16**: 285–8.

35 Niemi-Murola L, Krootila K, Kivisaari R, *et al.* Localization of local anesthetic solution by magnetic resonance imaging. *Ophthalmology* 2004; **111**: 342–7.

Further reading

Stark DD, Bradley WG Jr. *Magnetic Resonance Imaging*, 3rd edn. St Louis: Mosby, 1999.

Medical Devices Agency. *Guidelines for Magnetic Resonance Equipment in Clinical Use*. 2002.

CHAPTER 26
Nanotechnology

The Nanotechnology Study Group, University of Aberdeen
Members of the group: K. Al-Tarrah, L. Balchin, T. Gilbertson, Y. Gourtsoyannis,
F. Khiard, J. Partridge, R. Sidhu, N.R. Webster and J. Weir-McCall

Introduction

Nanotechnology is fast emerging as the future of modern medicine. It is revolutionizing the way in which we image the body and diagnose a variety of conditions. It allows scanning at the molecular level which can be used to build personalized models of an individual's body system to determine susceptibility to disease and disease pathogenesis.

Through nanotechnology, science fiction is fast becoming science fact, as *ex vivo* nanomedical applications are predicted to be widely available as soon as 2010, with *in vivo* applications following soon after. The exponential development of this technology brings advances into areas such as tissue repair and early diagnosis and treatment of diseases such as cancer. It also opens new doors in methods of drug delivery and distribution. Nanotechnology is a field under development and although still far from being used in routine practice, it has the potential to take medicine into a whole new era.

Imaging and disease diagnosis

Cellular bioscanning is being developed for the non-invasive non-destructive examination of the human cell *in vivo*. The nanosensors being developed should be able to provide detailed information about cell membranes and structures and the molecular activities taking place within the cell. This information could then be used in disease diagnosis [1].

There are a number of different sensory techniques that are being developed and evaluated to fulfil these objectives:
- Cellular topography
- Near-field optical nanoimaging
- Cell volume sensing
- Microscopy techniques.

Cellular topography

Current technology allows the *ex vivo* examination of a live cell by atomic force microscopy (AFM) in which a 20–40 nm radius tip is used to scan around 50 nm across the top 10 nm of a cell. In cellular topography, a similar technique would be used to acquire, *in vivo*, a live cell scan using a nanodevice fitted with a tactile scanning probe which will acquire comparable results to AFM. The nanodevice first travels to its target cell where it anchors itself securely to the surface. The scanning probe can then image a variety of cell structures at a high resolution quickly; for example, 0.1% of the plasma membrane in 2 s or an entire mitochondrial surface in 100 s [1].

In addition, using a variation of the same technology, membrane dysfunction could be detected using chemical nanosensors to monitor the passage of molecules [2]. Special scanning tips and techniques could also be developed to allow adhesiveness and magnetic, chemical, electrical and other properties to be measured [3].

Near-field optical imaging

Certain behaviour characteristics of electromagnetic fields dominate at one distance from a radiating source, while a completely different behaviour can dominate at another location. Electrical engineers define boundary regions to categorize behaviour characteristics of electromagnetic fields as a function of distance from the radiating source. These regions are the near-field, transition zone and far-field.

The regional boundaries are usually measured as a function of the wavelength, with near-field effects predominating at up to two wavelengths from the source. Near-field optical imaging (NFOI) concerns itself with the near-field component of optical wavelength electromagnetic waves. Conventional techniques in use in medicine today use only the far-field component in imaging (e.g. X-rays), but this does not give as detailed an image and would be unpractical for use in nanomedicine *in vivo* as the short wave X-rays would damage living cells [1].

Near-field optical microscopes (NFOM) have already been developed and can produce extremely detailed images. They are able to detect the orientation and depth of a molecule within 30 nm of the scanned area and optical images of individual dye molecules added to cells have already been demonstrated [1]. By attaching a NFOM-like device to a nanoprobe it is thought that it will be possible to scan cell surfaces and organelles to <1 nm resolution optically, as well as mapping their topographical characteristics to within tens of nanometers [1].

Cell volume sensing

Unlike the other methods so far described, cell volume sensing can monitor a living cell *in vivo* without directly imaging it. It involves an intracellular nanodevice being used to indirectly measure cell volume by one of two methods:

1 *Mechanical deformation:* the plasma membrane, stretch receptor channels, cytoskeleton and other structures are all highly sensitive to a change in cell volume. By developing a nanodevice to monitor the changes of one or more of these factors, cell volume could be determined.

2 *Molecular level:* concentration and dilatation changes brought about by shifting cell volumes activate a variety of volume regulating responses. A nanodevice could monitor one or more of any of these responses using chemical nanosensors (e.g. phosphoinositide turnover, eicosanoid turnover, kinase/phosphatase systems, p38 activity or G-protein activity).

As all the above applications for nanotechnology in imaging and monitoring are envisaged being used *in vivo* and will give results in a matter of seconds

without the need for a separate sampling and laboratory analysis, real-time monitoring of disease progression and therapeutic efficiency will be possible [4]. By using a large number of nanodevices, constantly monitoring the health of patients, earlier warnings of the appearance of pathological processes will be available allowing earlier and perhaps more effective treatment to be given [2]. These devices should also be able to give information on the effectiveness of treatment and allow for more sensitive adjustment, perhaps even becoming semi-automatic in the future by administering treatment in response to a biological change (e.g. insulin administration in diabetics, when chemical nanosensors detect a rise above an optimal glucose concentration).

As with all things in nanotechnology, the information gathered from any imaging or monitoring nanodevice is for an extremely small area. However, the size and predicted low cost of nanodevices will allow the use of thousands at any one time for routine diagnosis, giving multiple pieces of highly detailed information about different parts of the biological system. Putting all this information together will require powerful computer technology [5]. Being able to image full biological processes *in vivo* at a molecular level will allow us to develop an understanding of the whole living system and how one biological process affects another, a concept known as *systems biology* — a newly developing science that is intimately related to developments in nanotechnology [4].

Enthusiasts believe the benefits of nanotechnology imaging and monitoring are endless. It is suggested that by being able to directly detect a pathological process, a reliable trustworthy diagnosis can be made with no uncertainty [4].

Scanning probe microscopy

Scanning probe microscopy allows mapping of a surface to almost atomic resolution. It relies on the interaction between the very fine tip of a probe (ideally only one atom thick) and the atoms of the surface [6]. A variety of different techniques are now available and are currently being developed for *in vivo* use. Scanning tunnelling microscopy uses the quantum effect of tunnelling whereby a particle has a probability of crossing a barrier, which would be forbidden in classic physics. In the case of scanning tunnelling microscopy, the particle is an electron, and the barrier is a gap of approximately 1 nm between the conductive probe tip and the surface of the sample. The resultant tunnelling current can be measured and used to gain an impression of the peaks and troughs of the surface below the probe. In atomic force microscopy, the surface is mechanically probed and forces between the atoms produce slight vertical movements of the probe, which again can be used to map the surface on an atomic scale. Atomic force microscopy has also been used to physically manipulate individual atoms.

Examples of the use of nanotechnology in disease diagnosis

Cancer diagnosis

Several methods are being researched and developed with a view to making possible the diagnosis of cancer at the level of DNA mutations [7,8].

• Arrays of nanoscale cantilevers (bars anchored at one end) to which specific proteins or altered DNA sequences bind. This binding bends the cantilevers, applying a stress force to the cantilever. If the stress on the cantilevers is monitored, it is then possible to ascertain the presence or absence of the particular molecule being tested.

• Bulky marker molecules are attached to mutated sections of DNA and the molecule scanned using atomic force microscopy, which is able to detect the presence of these markers.

• Efficient DNA sequencing using nanotechnology may allow rapid assessment of gene abnormalities. Nanopores can now be engineered that allow one strand of DNA to pass through at a time and coated wires are now in development to sequence these individual strands of DNA.

• Quantum dots, crystals as small as 1 nm in diameter, emit light of a wavelength specific to their size when irradiated with ultraviolet light. These crystals can be seeded onto microscopic beads in certain quantities so that they emit a unique spectrum. These microbeads are engineered to bind to specific DNA sequences and then by observing the emitted spectra it is possible to identify which sequences are present,

and therefore find out if mutations are present [9,10].

Blood tests

In addition, nanotechnology devices may allow faster, more efficient *ex vivo* blood testing to be performed. For example, a device already at the prototype stage is a silicon chip coated with an array of antibodies for several different viruses. When dipped in a blood sample, any viruses present will bind to a specific antibody. This binding creates a ridge detectable by atomic force microscopy, and thus allows the rapid identification of any virus present [11].

Therapeutic applications

Tissue regeneration, repair and replacement

The use of nanotechnology for the regeneration, repair or replacement of tissues or organs has a promising future and is much needed as current technologies and medicines are sorely lacking. At present, apart from the body's own responses, organ transplant remains the only method of curing badly damaged organs and tissue grafting is still the main treatment of severe damage to tissues. Both of these techniques are limited by a lack of donors and restrict the patient to a lifetime of immunosuppressive treatment.

Electrospun nanofibrous scaffolds

The main development in this area concerns the use of electrospun nanofibrous scaffolding as both a growth template and a source of growth and differentiation factors. The nanofibrous scaffold mimics the extracellular matrix, providing a template for growth. Cells grown on the scaffold maintain their phenotypic shape and tend to grow in the orientation of the nanofibres [12]. As well as providing a template for growth, DNA plasmids can be bound to the scaffold, these can code for growth factors specific to individual tissues and are released into the surrounding tissue. These plasmids are capable of cell transfection and have bioactivity [13]. Currently, skin and cartilage replacement are the main targets of such therapy as it is their mechanical properties that the scaffold most closely resembles, but it is envisaged that the material of the electrospun nanofibres will eventually develop so that it can mimic the characteristics of other tissue types [12].

Microspheres

Another approach is the use of sustained release bioerodible microspheres to direct tissue remodelling *in vivo* [14]. For example, the sustained release of perivascular elastase has been proven to redirect smooth muscle migration away from the intima, limiting the development of pathological neointima following injury to the arterial wall [15].

Implant immunoisolation

Organ transplant rejection resulting from antibody reactions and complement fixation has stimulated research to try to prevent its initiation. One way currently being studied is to encapsulate transplanted cells or tissues with size-selective membranes, which allow the free diffusion of oxygen and other nutrients while inhibiting the passage of larger molecules such as antibodies — acting as an immunoprotective semi-permeable shield.

The essential requirements for such a capsule include well-controlled pore size, stability, non-biodegradability and biocompatibility [16]. Because of its mechanical strength and inertness, silicon and its oxides are used and provide capsules with well-controlled membranes and mechanical and chemical stability. Despite the advantages of silicon, research has shown that fibroblast and other inflammatory cells adhere to its surface and polyethylene glycol (PEG) modified microfabricated silicon is used to minimize this problem (Fig. 26.1).

PEG is a water soluble, non-toxic and non-immunogenic polymer and has been shown to decrease both protein and cell adsorption on several biomaterials [16]. Recent research has compared the effects of unmodified silicon and PEG-modified silicon biocapsules *in vivo*. A rich network of blood vessels were visible in the proximity of the PEG-modified capsules while few vessels surround the control. In histological examination, the modified samples had no signs of infiltration and the tissue had a characteristic structure and composition of the tissue at the site of implantation (Fig. 26.2) [17].

Another advantage of microfabricated capsule membranes is that they can be tailor-made to a specific pore size and have uniform distribution. Thus, they can be made for attaining desired imunoglobulin G (IgG) diffusion kinetics even to the extent of complete deselection of IgG. It has been demonstrated that IgG diffusion in 18 nm pores over 150 hours was only 2% and this low rate indicates superior immunoprotection over methods currently available [18].

Bioartificial organs

The development of bioartificial organs would abolish the need for transplantation of organs but will require several major developments in nanotechnology. The use of molecularly manipulated nanostructured biomimetic materials (biomimicry) involves replicating the cell surface morphology, its microenvironment and mechanical properties (e.g. elasticity in heart and skeletal muscle or high tensile strength as in bone). Secondly, a sensing and control system will need to be developed which will require microelectronic and nanoelectronic interfaces to be produced. Third, some application of drug delivery and medical nanosystems will be required to replace the lost function of the specific organ [19].

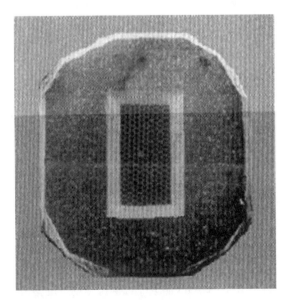

Figure 26.1 Microfabricated membrane.

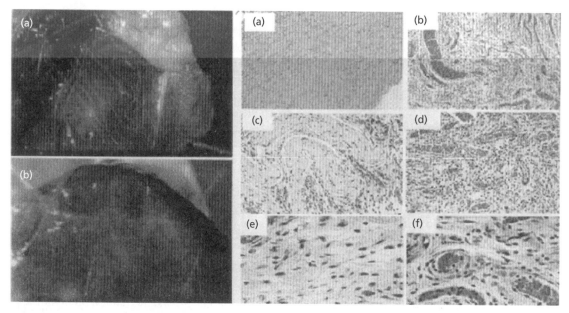

Figure 26.2 Left: gross appearance of tissue surrounding: (a) unmodified silicon membrane; and (b) polyethylene glycol (PEG) modified silicon membrane 17 days post-implantation [36]. Right: Histological sample of tissues surrounding modified silicon implants [36].

Drug delivery systems

One of the most important areas in medicine in which nanotechnology is currently being applied is in the field of drug delivery systems. Nanoparticles can be used to target drugs to specific cells or tissues, to delay drug metabolism and clearance, and to increase the bioavailability of the drug. Their submicron size allows them to penetrate tissues via capillaries and pass through fenestrae in the cellular endothelial lining enabling efficient uptake of the therapeutic agent. A variety of techniques for drug delivery are being developed.

Nanospheres and nanocapsules

Nanoparticles either trap the drug within or attach it to the matrix of the particle. Nanocapsules enclose the drug-containing cavity in a polymer membrane while nanospheres have the drug evenly distributed throughout their matrix. The nanocapsule/sphere polymers are usually either polylactides (PLA) or D,L-lactide-co-glycolide (PLGA). They can be hydrolysed to form substances that can be metabolized and removed from the body by the tricarboxy-

lic acid cycle. The drug is released at a constant rate by diffusion through the matrix and degradation of the PLGA matrix. It is possible to vary the rate of degradation, and hence the rate of drug release by altering the composition of the PLA/PLGA polymer [20].

Targeted delivery

Targeting increases the bioavailability of a drug at the site of action. This reduces the dose needed and potentially harmful side-effects. Active targeting involves the conjugation of the carrier system to a tissue- or cell-specific ligand or antibodies. Passive targeting involves targeting the reticuloendothelial system so that the therapeutic agents, coupled to a macromolecule, reach the target passively. The nanoparticles enter the cell by endocytosis, and once inside the cell the surface charge on the endolysosome can be altered to push the nanoparticle into the cytoplasm. Nanoparticles can also cross biological barriers, such as the blood–brain barrier, where they have been used to administer antitumour and anti-HIV drugs [20].

Ceramic nanoparticles

Ceramic nanoparticles are made from biologically compatible substances such as silica, aluminia and titania. The tiny size of ceramic nanoparticles allows them to avoid the reticuloendothelial system. They protect the drug from pH and temperature changes. They are often used with the anticancer drug, 2-devinyl-2-(1-hexyloxyethyl) phyropheophorbide which is water insoluble and photosensitizing. The tumour cells take up the particles and when the drug is irradiated oxygen-derived free radicals are released which damage the tumour cells [21].

Polymeric micelles

In polymeric micelles, the drug is trapped in the hydrophobic core while the outer surface of the micelle is hydrophilic. These micelles are very thermodynamically stable compared with normal micelles. They are used to treat certain cancers because of the increased permeability of vascular tissues in the tumour and impaired lymphatic drainage. There is an accumulation of colloid drug carriers in the tumour tissue [21].

Liposomes

Liposomes are made of phospholipids and cholesterol which make them ideal for drug delivery because of their size, biocompatibility and hydrophobic/hydrophilic properties. They are classed according to their number of bilayers and size. Saturation of their component phospholipids lends them a more rigid, impermeable character (stable), whereas polyunsaturated bilayers make them more permeable (unstable). They can also be given a surface charge by adding positively or negatively charged lipids. The attachment of a PEG unit to liposomes increases the amount of time they circulate within the body. It is also possible to conjugate liposomes with antibodies or ligands for specific targeting to receptors and thus tissues [21].

Dendrimers

Dendrimers have an inner core (a small molecule or linear polymer) surrounded by a number of polymer branches. By altering the terminal groups of the polymer it is possible to switch the hydrophobic/hydrophilic character of the interior and exterior surfaces, thus changing the way they interact with the environment [21].

Fullerenes

Fullerenes are frameworks of carbon atoms, the simplest of which are buckminsterfullerenes, C_{60} balls, nicknamed 'bucky balls'. These bucky balls and 'bucky tubes' are extremely adept at crossing the cell membrane as their structure mimics that of clathrin which promotes endocytosis. In theory, drugs could be attached to bucky balls and bucky tubes and transported directly and rapidly into cells [22].

Infection and vaccination

Biodegradeable nanoparticles offer a sustained release mechanism for antigen. It has been shown that co-injecting tetanus toxoid-loaded nanoparticles with usual tetanus toxoid-alum causes a synergistic immune response. Also, tetanus toxoid loaded nanoparticles induce a better immune response than conventional delivery but can also be successfully delivered by different routes (e.g. the intranasal route) [18,21].

Nanotechnology in cancer treatment

Researchers are currently investigating nanotechnology for developing ways to destroy cancer cells without injuring neighbouring healthy cells. The aim of researchers is to produce nanomaterials that can both identify cancer and subsequently deliver treatment. The following are a few examples of the approaches being evaluated.

Nanomaterials aiding drug delivery

This involves using a dendrimer to which a molecule that detects cancer cells has been attached. This dendrimer also carries a signal to induce apoptotic cell death of the tumour cell and can also carry a caner chemotherapeutic agent. This therapeutic agent is only released in the presence of certain molecules associated with particular cancer cells.

Medibots

Medibots are miniature 'robots' that can physically enter cells and scan the chemicals inside, they will then destroy the cell if it is cancerous using the principle that cancer cells contain different chemicals to that of normal cells [23].

Nanoshells

Nanoshells are beads coated with gold that have been manipulated to absorb certain wavelengths of light. The absorption of light by the nanoshells generates heat in sufficient quantity to be fatal to cells. These are still in development, but at present antibodies have been attached to nanoshells so that they are able to detect cancer cells. The ultimate goal will be for nanoshells to find tumour cells, and then to destroy them by exposing them to infrared light. In laboratory cell culture experiments, the heat generated by the light-absorbing nanoshells has successfully killed tumour cells while leaving neighbouring cells intact [7].

In theory, nanoshells could also be filled with a drug-containing polymer [24]. Heating the shell changes the polymer shape and releasing the drug allows much higher local tissue concentrations of drug to be delivered. The use of nanoshells is especially appealing in treating cancers that are in more accessible sites such as the prostate gland.

AC magnetic field induced excitation of biocompatible supermagnetic nanoparticles

Cancerous cells could be enriched with many nanoparticles, which are activated by a specific signal such as a magnetic field, killing all particle containing cells when the induced magnetic field is applied [25].

Facilitation of laser surgery by nanocapsules

Laser surgery can be facilitated using nanocapsules containing nanoparticles with a magnetic core of gadolinium compounds or iron oxide, plus a photocatalyst [26]. The nanocapsules consist of an outer layer of PEG linked to target molecules which permit the nanocapsules to adhere onto cancerous cells. The structure of the nanocapsule centre is such that it is visible to magnetic resonance imaging (MRI). The technique has the potential to make very small tumours visible, including those too small to treat by laser surgery. However, with these nanoparticles, laser light hitting the MRI target will activate the photocatalyst releasing oxygen-derived free radicals.

This approach may be particularly successful for the treatment of brain tumours, both because of the possibility of direct exposure to laser light and also because the cancer makes the blood–brain barrier more permeable, therefore nanocapsules only pass across when brain tumours are present.

Several pharmaceutical companies are actively working in nanotechnology for drug delivery for cancer (Table 26.1) [27–29].

Future applications

Metabolic control

Nanotechnology can be used in treatment of a variety of metabolic conditions ranging from chronic diabetes to Addisonian crises. Nanomachines can be injected into the blood, reach the target cell and affect its metabolism in a variety of ways. First, such machines could reduce its metabolism, repair the cell if damaged and then restart metabolism after repair, thus restoring the normal functions of the cell. Secondly, they could modify stimulatory and inhibitory actions affecting the cell at both external and internal levels. For example, they can act as a surface receptor for a cell, thus controlling the binding of an effector hormone and thereby altering the degree of

Table 26.1 Two companies actively involved in nanotechnology research in cancer therapy.

Company	Product description
ALZA (Mountain View, CA)	Doxil: nanoparticles used for the treatment of refractory ovarian cancer and AIDS-related Kaposi's sarcoma
Advectus Life Science (West Vancouver, CA)	Nanotechnology for the delivery of cancer fighting drugs across the blood–brain barrier for the treatment of brain tumours

stimulation or inhibition of the cell's metabolism. Thirdly, they could completely shut off the metabolism of the cell, either by depriving it of resources or by inhibiting steps in its metabolism. Examples include diabetes where such techniques can be used to maintain secretion of insulin at an optimal level following measurement of the prevailing glucose concentration.

Cell replacement and the artificial red blood cell — the respirocyte

In the future, nanotechnology could be used to replace the functions of entire cells. In particular, a replacement for the red blood cell, the respirocyte, has already been conceived and several detailed designs produced (Fig. 26.3). Some of the chemicals required are already in Phase I trials. Respirocytes could bind oxygen and carbon dioxide like a normal red blood cell, or, in the most promising design, they could act as tiny containers storing the gases at high pressure.

(a)

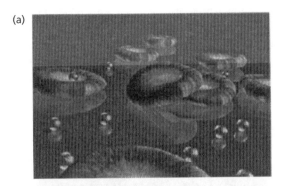

(b)

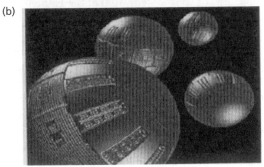

Figure 26.3 (a) Computer generated image of the small respirocytes next to red blood cells. (b) Image of what four respirocytes could look like [29].

Just like normal erythrocytes, respirocytes could use blood glucose as an abundant source of energy for collecting, compressing, storing and releasing the gases and powering the cell [30].

Preventing disease

Most of the possible medical implementations of nanotechnology would contribute toward a disease prophylactic effect, and also overall life extension. Specific examples of prophylactic measures include treating atheromatous plaques, removing or breaking down tar in the lungs, dealing with infection, strengthening parts of the body, rapidly responding after trauma and monitoring (e.g. the onset of thrombotic or haemorrhagic events). To treat atheromatous plaques, nanoprobes could allow non-invasive detection of plaques in high-risk patients. They could then release drugs locally or could stabilize plaques by mechanically removing components (e.g. oxidized low density lipoprotein (LDL)) [14,31].

Life extension and anti-ageing

The body is normally in a state of homoeostasis, and nanotechnology could help to maintain this; however, sometimes the body's homoeostatic mechanisms can cause detrimental effects. Moreover, it seems that the human body is designed for a different lifestyle than the type we now live. Nanotechnology techniques could be used to correct or optimize some of these mechanisms. It could be used to keep certain parts of the body intentionally out of synchronization with each other, in so-called heterostasis. Certain factors (e.g. chemical concentrations and chemoreceptors) could be altered at a local level. Attempting to change and rebalance the body's natural regulatory systems would require much research prior to implementation. In the most radical form of heterostasis, most intersystem signalling could be stopped and the systems regulated indirectly, which could be of use during extensive dysfunction [32].

DNA damage

As cells divide, many of them gradually decrease a length of DNA known as the telomere, and die when it runs out. Nanotechnology could replace the telomere, which may extend the life of the body.

Nanobots could also mop up DNA-damaging chemicals and encourage the cell's self-repair. They could also directly repair or alter the DNA themselves.

Chemical clearance

Nanobots could be used to remove harmful chemicals, particularly ones the body cannot deal with or remove itself, notably prions.

Infection

Nanobots would be immune to damage by invading natural pathogens, and could be more intelligent than specific immune cells. They could be trained to additionally detect new bacteria and viruses as they evolve and are detected worldwide.

Accidents

Nanobots and technology kept in the body permanently could greatly increase the ability of the body to withstand accidents and trauma, and to repair itself properly and quickly as soon as damage occurs. For example, they could strengthen the body, repair tears and wounds (better as well as quicker), cushion the brain, provide oxygen for several minutes, reduce the oxygen consumption of tissues without killing them, and buy a lot of time for emergency services to transport individuals to hospital — or even perhaps the local nanotechnology repair centre.

Artificial mitochondria

In cells that have been deprived of oxygen, the mitochondria may be damaged and the cell therefore unable to use oxygen. Nanotechnology could be used to support such cells by making and releasing ATP into the cells [33].

Cryonics

Cryonics involves freezing someone who has just died, in the hope of being able to revive them in the future when the required technology may exist. One presently insurmountable problem in this area is that freezing cells irretrievably damages them. Nanotechnology could be used to repair, or even replace the damaged cells when attempting to revive the patient, and may also provide ways of curing them [34].

Common problems

Nanobot manufacture requires ultraclean conditions, where the number of particles in the production space must be minimal. In silicon chip manufacture, the minimum standard is 10 per cubic metre, but even more stringent precautions may be required as even the tiniest particle compared with the scale of the nanobot may be sufficiently large to pose a problem [35].

The reliability of software that is used to program the nanobot should also be considered. This would be a factor in determining cost of treatment and production (e.g. how many of the nanomachines produced would actually be viable to be used for treatment). Lifespan and half-life of the nanomachines would also have to be considered. Will the nanobots be designed to be dormant and act only if the need arises or will they be designed more like conventional drugs at present with considerations like clearance and volume of distribution and the need for top-up doses?

Nanomachines can be much more power hungry than human cells, thereby using more energy than their biological counterparts. Hence, nanomachines to be implanted in the body will be limited by a power budget and possibly waste heat in excess — both factors may require design compromises [32].

Systems biology and complex systems

The science of complex systems involves precise modelling of body systems so that the pathology of disease and modes of drug function can be worked out on a computer-simulated model. Nanotechnology machines facilitate more detailed measurement of function, chemical change and other factors thereby enabling the production of a model very similar to the actual disease process or mode of action of drug.

The approach of systems biology can be classed under three headings [36]:

1 *Predictive medicine:* the human genome project and nanotechnology together under the context of systems biology and modelling would enable better recognition of an individual's genetic susceptibility or predisposition to diseases and hence pave the way

for preventative measures, more timely therapy and counselling.

2 *Preventative medicine:* this follows on from predictive medicine in terms of therapeutic options that would be made available. The agents for preventative medicine include drugs, embryonic stem cell therapy, engineered proteins, genetically engineered cells and many others.

3 *Personalized medicine:* each of us differ by approximately 6 million DNA variations; this would mean that the drug efficacy and uptake, for example, would vary. Personalized models depending on the predisposing factors such as changes in DNA would determine how best therapy could be personalized for each patient in order to bring about the best outcome.

It is envisaged that predictive, preventative and personalized medicine may extend the average lifespan by 10–30 years. It would require profound changes in the training of physicians and the education of the lay public about medicine and hence would directly impact diagnosis and therapy in the evolving world of modern medicine.

Conclusions

In conclusion, nanotechnology opens up new possibilities in medicine and could without doubt fundamentally alter the way in which patients are diagnosed, managed and treated. Obviously, some predictions will remain in the realms of science fiction, but with current rapid growth in research it is difficult to tell what direction advancements will take.

References

1 Freitas RA Jr. *Nanomedicine*, Volume 1. *Basic Capabilities*. Landes Bioscience, 1999.

2 United States Department of Health and Human Services. Testimony. Available at: http://www.hhs.gov/asl/testify/t030507a.html

3 Drexler KE. Engines of creation. Available at: http://www.foresight.org/EOC/EOC_chapter_7.html

4 News and events. Available at: http://www.crnano.org/news.htm#releases

5 Zyvex. Assembling tomorrow. Available at: http://www.zyvex.com

6 Gross M. *Travels to the Nanoworld: Miniature Machinery in Nature and Technology*. Plenum, 1999.

7 National Institutes of Health. Nanotechnology and cancer. Available at: http://cancerweb.ncl.ac.uk/cancernet/400388.html

8 Arntz Y, Seelig JD, Lang HP, *et al.* Label-free protein assay based on a nanomechanical cantilever array. *Nanotechnology* 2003; **14**: 86–90.

9 Arlington V. Color-coded quantum dots for fast DNA testing. Available at: http://www.whitaker.org/news/nie.html

10 Gorman J. NanoLights! Camera! Action!. Available at: http://www.sciencenews.org/20030215/bob10.asp

11 Coghlan A. Nanoparticles to pinpoint viruses in body scans. Available at: http://www.newscientist.com/hottopics/tech/article.jsp?id=99994076&sub=Nanotechnology

12 Li WJ, Laurencin CT, Caterson EJ, Tuan RS, Ko FK. Electrospun nanofibrous structure: a novel scaffold for tissue engineering. *J Biomed Mater Res* 2002; **60**: 613–21.

13 Luu YK, Kim K, Hsiao BS, Chu B, Hadjiargyrou M. Development of a nanostructured DNA delivery scaffold via electrospinning of PLGA and PLA-PEG block copolymers. *J Control Release* 2003; **89**: 341–53.

14 Buxton DB, Lee SC, Wickline SA, Ferrari M, National Heart, Lung, and Blood Institute Nanotechnology Working Group. Recommendations of the National Heart, Lung, and Blood Institute Nanotechnology Working Group. *Circulation* 2003; **108**: 2737–42.

15 Wong AH, Waugh JM, Amabile PG, Yuksel E, Dake MD. *In vivo* vascular engineering: directed migration of smooth muscle cells to limit neointima. *Tissue Eng* 2002; **8**: 189–99.

16 Desai TA. Micro- and nanoscale structures for tissue engineering constructs. *Med Eng Phys* 2000; **22**: 595–606.

17 Leoni L, Desai TA. Micromachined biocapsules for cell based reusing and delivery. *Adv Drug Deliv Rev* 2004; **56**: 211–29.

18 Siegel RA, Ziaie B. Biosensing and drug delivery at the microscale. *Adv Drug Deliv Rev* 2004; **56:** 121–3.

19 Prokop A. Bioartificial organs in the twenty-first century: nanobiological devices. *Ann N Y Acad Sci* 2001; **944:** 472–90.

20 Panyam J, Labhasetwar V. Biodegradable nanoparticles for drug and gene delivery to cells and tissue. *Adv Drug Deliv Rev* 2003; **55**: 329–47.

21 Sahoo SK, Labhasetwar V. Nanotech approaches to drug delivery and imaging. *Drug Discov Today* 2003; **8**: 1112–20.

22 Foley S, Crowley C, Smaihi M, *et al*. Cellular localization of a water-soluble fullerene derivative. *Biochem Biophys Res Commun* 2002; **294**: 116–9.

23 Phoenix C. Molecular Nanotechnology and Medicine. Available at: http://cpheonix.best.vwh.net/tandy. html#cancer

24 Sutton A. Researchers Explore Possible Applications of Nanotechnology in Cancer Treatment. Available at: http://www2.mdanderson.org/depts/oncolog/ articles/03/7-8-julaug/7-8-03-1.html

25 Jordan A, Scholz R, Wust P, Fahling H, Felix R. Magnetic fluid hyperthermia (MFH): cancer treatment with AC magnetic field induced excitation of biocompatible superparamagnetic nanoparticles. *J Magn Magn Mater* 1998; **201**: 413–9.

26 Stephenson J. Nanotechnology may facilitate laser surgery for brain tumours. *Lancet Oncol* 2001; **2**: 651.

27 Orive G, Hernandez RM, Gascon AR, Dominguez-Gil A, Pedraz JL. Drug delivery in biotechnology: present and future. *Curr Opin Biotechnol* 2003; **14**: 659–64.

28 Brigger I, Dubernet C, Couvreur P. Nanoparticles in cancer therapy and diagnosis. *Adv Drug Deliv Rev* 2002; **54**: 631–51.

29 US Department of Health and Human Services. Nanotechnology and cancer. Available at http://otir.nci.nih. gov/brochure.pdf

30 Freitas RA Jr. Respirocytes: a mechanical artificial red cell: exploratory design in medical nanotechnology. Available at: http://www.xenophilia.org/nano_life_ extension.html

31 Rubinstein L. A practical nanorobot for treatment of various medical problems. Available at: http:// www.foresight.org/Conferences/MNT8/Papers/ Rubinstein/

32 Phoenix C. nanotechnology and life extension. Available at: http://www.xenophilia.org/nano_life_ extension.html

33 Merkle RC. Nanotechnology and medicine. Available at: http://www.zyvex.com/nanotech/nanotechAnd-Medicine.html

34 Merkle RC. The molecular repair of the brain. Available at: http://www.merkle.com/cryo/techFeas. html

35 Merkle RC, Warren J. Nanotechnology in the future. Available at: http://www.witn.psu.edu/articles/print. phtml?article_id=41

36 Institute for systems biology. Predictive, preventive and personalized medicine. Available at: http://www. systemsbiology.org/Default.aspx?pagename= predictiveandpreventive

CHAPTER 27

Assessment of the cardiovascular system

Charles S. Reilly

Introduction

In the healthy heart, the blood returning in the major veins (inferior and superior vena cava [IVC and SVC]) enters the right atrium (RA), passes into the right ventricle (RV) where it is ejected into the pulmonary artery (PA), as shown in Figure 27.1. After passing through the pulmonary circulation, the blood returns in the pulmonary vein to the left atrium (LA) then to the left ventricle (LV) and is ejected into the aorta. This simple progression occurs in two phases: diastole when the heart muscle is relaxed; and systole when the muscle contracts. This is dependent on a normal conduction system and normal mechanical function.

Assessment of the cardiovascular system is an essential element of anaesthetic practice. A clear understanding of the various inter-relationships between the structural and functional components of the cardiovascular system is therefore required. A starting point for this can be a simple model in which the cardiovascular system is arranged as three components. Central to this is the heart (pump), which is primed by the venous return (preload) and its output pressure is determined by the peripheral resistance (afterload). This simple model can be expanded to demonstrate the various components and interactions involved in the function and control of the cardiovascular system (Fig. 27.2). This model forms the basis of this chapter and addresses these three components before bringing them together as a structure for assessment. It is clear that the sympathetic and parasympathetic components of the autonomic nervous system have a major role in the control and responses of the cardiovascular system.

The heart

Conduction system

The cardiac impulse arises in the sinoatrial (SA) node, which is located near the junction of the SVC and RA. The SA node contains pacemaker cells which display rhythmic depolarization (Fig. 27.3). This arises from an unstable diastolic membrane potential which gradually depolarizes from a resting value of −60 mV to a threshold firing value of −40 mV. The origin of this is an increased permeability to calcium ions which enter after potassium channel closure. The inherent rate of discharge in the SA node is 100–110/min, but this is influenced by vagal and sympathetic neural inputs, which alter the rate (slope) of depolarization, by temperature and by drugs. Pacemaker cells are also normally found in the atrioventricular (AV) node and Purkinje system which have inherent rhythms of 40–60/min and 20–40/min, respectively, as a result of slower rates (slopes) of spontaneous discharge. Therefore, because of its higher rate, the SA node normally acts as the pacemaker for the heart rate. There are a number of potential mechanisms that can influence the pacemaker rate. For example, an increase in the rate of SA node discharge can be brought about by increasing the slope of Phase 4; lowering the threshold potential (more negative); or by raising the resting potential (less negative). The impulse from the SA node spreads radially through the atrium at a rate of approximately 1 m/s resulting in atrial contraction and reaches the AV node in less than 0.1 s.

Conduction at the AV node is slower (0.05 m/s), causing a delay of approximately 0.1 s. This delay has two beneficial effects. It allows atrial systole to increase the volume of blood in the ventricle before it,

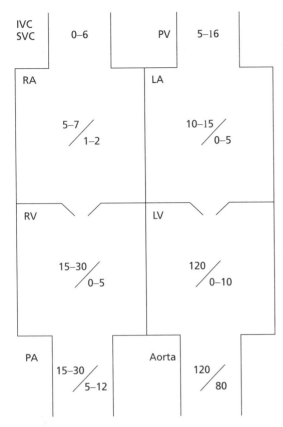

Figure 27.1 Pressures in the chambers of the heart (systolic/diastolic, mmHg). IVC, inferior vena cava; PA, pulmonary artery; PV, pulmonary vein; SVC, superior vena cava.

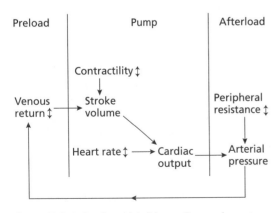

Figure 27.2 A simple model of the cardiovascular system. ↕ Site where the autonomic nervous system can exert direct stimulatory and inhibitory effects.

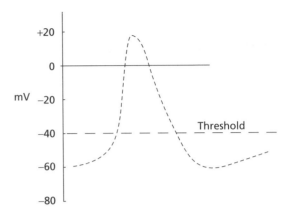

Figure 27.3 Action potential of an atrial pacemaker cell.

in turn, contracts. The delay also minimizes the risk of additional atrial impulses being conducted to the ventricle with the risk of arrhythmias. As with the SA node, vagal and sympathetic inputs attenuate the speed of conduction through the AV node.

The impulse then travels (1 m/s) down the right and left branches of the bundle of His which run in the interventricular septum to link with the Purkinje fibres. The Purkinje fibres are a rapidly conducting (4 m/s) network on the endocardial surface of both ventricles. The speed of conduction allows the impulse to reach all parts of the ventricle in <0.1 s and leads to a synchronized contraction which moves from endocardium to epicardium and spreads from the septum to the apex, then along the ventricular walls to the AV junction. The rapid conduction means that the impulse returns to the conducting system during the refractory period, over the normal range of heart rates. However, at very slow ventricular rates, this is a possible source of arrhythmia.

In response to the spreading impulse, the cardiac muscle cell action potential is triggered. These fibres differ from the pacemaker cells in both resting membrane potential and action potential generated. The resting membrane potential is approximately −80 mV and does not exhibit rhythmic depolarization. The action potential generated is described classically in five phases, labelled 0–4 (Fig. 27.4). Phase 4 is at resting membrane potential. A partial depolarization to −60 mV allows rapid influx of sodium ions (Phase 0) resulting in full depolarization to +20 mV. Sodium

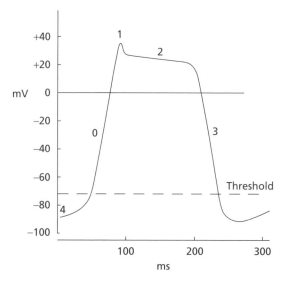

Figure 27.4 Action potential of myocardial cells showing the phases 0–4 (see text).

channels then start to close and the potential falls (Phase 1). However, a slower influx of calcium, resulting from increased permeability, maintains a plateau around 0 mV (Phase 2), before potassium permeability increases and efflux of potassium (Phase 3) restores the resting membrane potential (Phase 4).

The action potential has a duration of 200–300 ms. Sodium influx is rapid (similar to nerve action potential) and is complete in <10 ms. The bulk of sodium efflux (90%) occurs rapidly and immediately but, as calcium influx peaks, sodium efflux plateaus until the repolarization phase. Calcium influx starts immediately but proceeds more slowly than that of sodium, reaching a peak at approximately 30 ms. Efflux then follows a similar initial rate, but levels out at approximately 90 ms until the repolarization phase. Potassium efflux starts as calcium influx peaks and is rapid. Potassium influx then occurs slowly up to the late repolarization phase.

Electrocardiography

As the body is a good conductor, the electrical activity described above can be recorded on the body surface and provides us with useful information about the rate, rhythm and function of the heart.

The classic description of three bipolar leads on the upper limbs and left leg with the heart at the centre — Einthoven's triangle — gives rise to the bipolar leads used in current electrocardiograph (ECG) recording. These leads — I, right arm negative, left arm positive; II, right arm negative, left leg positive; III, left arm negative, left leg positive — measure the electrical potential between the two electrodes and record the direction of current flow. Current flowing towards the positive electrode results in upward deflection, and away a downward deflection. The use of unipolar leads, which measure the potential from a positive electrode relative to a reference electrode at the centre of the heart, provide further information. The reference electrode is formed from connecting the three limb leads. This gives us the six chest leads (V1–V6) and the augmented limb leads, which record the potential between one limb and the other two, giving a greater amplitude. The ECG displacement at these electrodes is similar to the bipolar with flow towards the electrode producing an upward displacement. This is best illustrated by comparing chest lead V1, which is over the right side of the heart, and lead V6, which lies lateral to the left side of the heart. The conducted impulse spreads initially to the LV, which, in addition, has a much larger muscle mass. The flow recorded initially in V6 will therefore be mainly towards the electrode, resulting in an upward displacement during ventricular contraction. In contrast, measurement at V1 will show the flow towards it, in the right ventricular muscle mass, will be swamped by the larger flow away from it resulting from left ventricular contraction and the initial displacement will be mainly negative (Fig. 27.5).

The ECG waveform corresponds to the changes described in the previous sections and an understanding of this relationship is important in interpretation of the normal and abnormal preoperative ECG (Fig. 27.6). The P wave is produced by atrial depolarization, and the QRS complex and T wave by ventricular depolarization and repolarization, respectively. The ECG waveform also provides evidence of the integrity of the conduction system through analysis of the timescale of the complex. The PR interval, measured from the start of the P wave to the start of the QRS, corresponds to atrial

V₁   V₆

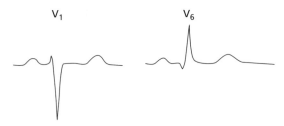

Figure 27.5 The electrocardiograph (ECG) trace for V1 and V6.

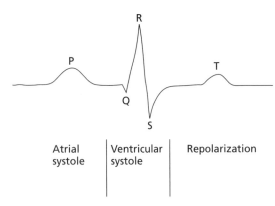

Figure 27.6 A normal electrocardiograph (ECG) trace. Normal values: P wave 0.06–0.10 s; PR interval 0.12–0.20 s; QRS wave 0.08–0.12 s; QT interval 0.35–0.45 s.

depolarization and conduction through the AV node, and is normally in the range of 0.12–0.2 s. The QRS reflects ventricular depolarization and lasts up to 0.1 s. The QT interval covers depolarization and repolarization and lasts up to 0.43 s.

Abnormalities in the conduction system at the AV node produce heart block. This can be graded as: first degree (incomplete), where all atrial impulses are conducted but slowed resulting in a longer PR interval; second degree, where some but not all impulses are conducted (e.g. every second giving 2 : 1 block); or a situation in which the PR interval progressively lengthens until a ventricular beat is missed (Wenckebach); and third degree (complete heart block) in which no atrial impulses are conducted and the atrial and ventricular rates are independent (atrial usually >110 b/min and ventricular <45 b/min, Fig. 27.7). Interruption in conduction through the bundle of His results in right or left bundle branch block (BBB). In left BBB for example, the impulse reaches the ventricles only through the right bundle, resulting in depolarization occurring first in the RV (in contrast to the normal pattern) which then spreads to the left. This produces a distinctive change in the ECG trace with V1 having no or smaller initial upstroke (LV) and the lateral leads having a broader, notched QRS

First degree

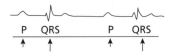

P   QRS   P   QRS

Second degree

2 : 1 block

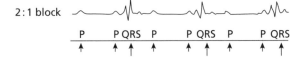

P   P QRS   P   P QRS   P   P QRS

Wenkebach

P QRS   P   QRS   P   QRS   P   P

Third degree

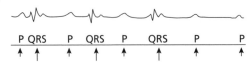

QRS P   P   P QRS P   P   P QRS

Figure 27.7 Electrocardiograph (ECG) trace in heart block.

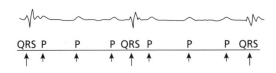

as the RV depolarizes first and then spreads to the LV.

Impairment of, or permanent damage to cardiac muscle also produces changes in the ECG trace. An inadequate blood supply to an area of myocardium results in ischaemic cells with impaired function. Ischaemia causes more rapid opening of the potassium channels leading to a quicker repolarization. The ECG detects this as a flow out of the infarcted area early in repolarization. As outward flow is shown as positive, this appears as elevation of the ST segment. The altered repolarization phase means that ischaemia can produce changes in the T wave, such as inversion or a biphasic trace. Continuing ischaemia will lead to cell death and myocardial infarction. The detection of ST segment elevation localizes the site of the occluded vessel as these end-arteries supply discrete areas of the myocardium and altered conductivity will appear as changes in specific ECG leads. Occlusion of the left anterior descending coronary artery will produce an anterior infarction with changes in the anteroseptal (V1–V3) and/or anterolateral (V4–V6) leads. Infarction in the area supplied by the circumflex coronary artery (lateral part of ventricle) produces changes in leads I, aVL and V6. Right coronary occlusion produces an inferior infarct with changes in leads II, III and aVF.

Mechanical function

To describe the sequence in greater detail it is best to start in late diastole. During diastole, blood returning to the atria from the systemic or pulmonary circulation passes passively down a pressure gradient into the ventricles through the open tricuspid and mitral valves. The rate of filling slows in late diastole as the ventricle distends and the pressure rises towards that of the atria, but the passive filling accounts for approximately 70% of ventricular volume.

The first event of systole is atrial contraction, which forces some additional blood into the ventricles producing a small increase in intraventricular pressure (Fig. 27.8). Ventricular contraction consists of two phases: isovolumetric contraction and ejection. The initial effect of ventricular muscle contraction is an increase in intraventricular pressure which causes the mitral (and tricuspid) valves to close (Fig. 27.8). The muscle continues to contract with no change in volume and an abrupt increase in pressure (isovolumetric contraction) because all four heart valves are closed. When the left ventricular pressure exceeds that in the aorta (usually approximately 80 mmHg), the aortic valve opens and ejection occurs, with contraction continuing to a peak intraventricular pressure of approximately 120 mmHg. With a normal contraction, 70–90 mL

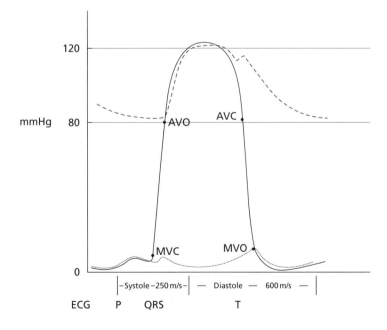

Figure 27.8 Left ventricle (LV; solid line), left atrial (LA; dotted line) and aortic (dashed line) pressure curves during 1 cardiac cycle. AVC, aortic valve closes; AVO, aortic valve opens; MVC, mitral valve closes; MVO, mitral valve opens. The period MVC to AVO represents isovolumetric contraction, and AVC to MVO isovolumetric relaxation.

blood is ejected and aortic pressure briefly exceeds ventricular pressure. On the right side of the heart, a similar sequence occurs, with the pulmonary valve opening at approximately 12 mmHg and achieving a peak pressure of approximately 25 mmHg. Contraction on the right side starts after that on the left, but ejection occurs slightly earlier as a lower pressure is required.

At the end of systole, intraventricular pressure falls rapidly and the aortic (pulmonary) valve closes, maintaining aortic pressure and starting a period of isovolumetric relaxation. At this time, all four valves are again closed and the ventricular muscle is relaxing round a fixed end-systolic volume of blood (usually approximately 50 mL). This continues until atrial pressure exceeds that of the ventricle (approximately 4 mmHg) and the mitral (tricuspid) valve opens and passive filling restarts.

Cardiac muscle

In contrast to skeletal muscle, which has large polynucleate cells, cardiac muscle cells are small, with only one or two nuclei but with similar striations from the regular arrangement of sarcomeres. The cells are often described as X- or Y-shaped as they interlink with several neighbouring cells, an arrangement that may spread mechanical stress more equally. The electrical impulse is conducted directly from cell to cell, without a motor endplate. As each cell contracts with every beat, the recruitment and summation mechanisms that regulate skeletal muscles do not apply. Mechanical tension is transmitted between cells by intercalated discs. Cardiac muscle can achieve the highest sustained metabolic rate of all the tissues in the human body. Cardiac myocytes are specialized for energy production and mechanical work, with up to 40% of the cell volume occupied by mitochondria and most of the remainder by contractile fibrils. This continuous high energy demand can only be met by aerobic metabolism and, in normal circumstances, <1% of the total energy comes from anaerobic metabolism. In a period of hypoxia, this could increase to 10%, but the capacity to generate adenosine triphosphate (ATP) by anaerobic glycolysis is severely limited, and will soon fail to support normal contractile or electrical activity. Glucose entry into cardiac cells is insulin-dependent, and

under normal circumstances approximately 60% of the energy comes from free fatty acids, ketone bodies and lactate, all of which are completely oxidized to carbon dioxide and water. This high energy system, therefore, requires a continuous and high oxygen supply. The heart is capable of varying oxygen extraction to meet the demand. For example, at rest with a heart rate of 70 b/min and a cardiac output of just over 5 L/min, the oxygen demand of 250 mL/min is met by extracting approximately 5 mL oxygen per decilitre of blood (measured as AV difference in oxygen content). This can be compared with the situation in severe exercise in an athlete where the oxygen demand could be as high as 3000 mL/min. This is achieved with a cardiac output of 20 L/min and the oxygen extraction is increased to nearly 15 mL/dL. The importance of this for our assessment is the dependence of normal function on supply; that is, a continuous adequate level of blood oxygenation, and coronary vessels which are capable of supplying blood flow over a wide range of values. Therefore, in a patient with a constriction in a proximal coronary vessel, the rate-limiting step will be the inability to increase blood flow to meet demand (the relationship of pressure, flow and resistance is discussed below), but in a patient with primarily lung disease (e.g. chronic obstructive airways disease [COPD]), the limiting factor will be the amount of oxygen in the blood supplying the heart.

Left ventricular function

The LV is obviously the prime chamber of the heart, the normal functioning of which determines key aspects of cardiovascular function. However, LV function is dependent on the function of the other chambers. For example, the output of the LV, cardiac output, must be matched by the output of the RV.

The cardiac output is determined by two factors: heart rate and stroke volume. Stroke volume (SV) is the volume of blood ejected with each ventricular contraction. At the end of diastole, the ventricle will normally contain approximately 140 mL blood (left ventricle end-diastolic volume, LVEDV). A contraction will normally eject some 70–90 mL (SV), resulting in an ejection fraction (SV/LVEDV) of 50–70%. Inotropic input, such as exercise, will increase LVEDV to maximum of over 300 mL, and may also increase ejection fraction, resulting in an SV of up to 180 mL.

There is a close relationship between ventricular volume and pressure. The relationship between LVEDV and LV muscle function can be described using pressure–volume loops (Fig. 27.9). These are essentially an expression of the length–tension (Frank–Starling) mechanism which relates initial muscle fibre length (LVEDV) to tension achieved by the subsequent contraction (LV pressure). From this it can be seen that with increasing initial length, a greater tension will be achieved up to a maximum

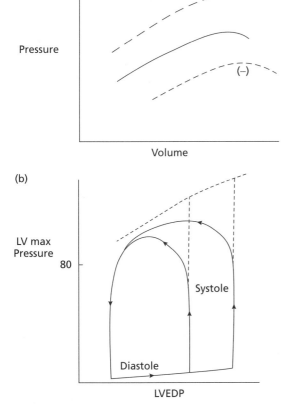

(a)

Pressure

(+)

(−)

Volume

(b)

LV max Pressure

80

Systole

Diastole

LVEDP

Figure 27.9 Pressure–volume relationship for the left ventricle (LV). (a) The relationship between initial fibre length (volume) and tension (pressure) achieved and the effect of positive (+) and negative (−) inotropy. (b) Pressure–volume loops for two different left ventricle end-diastolic volume (LVEDV) values and LV pressure. The theoretical pressure (dashed line) is not reached because of opening of the aortic valve.

tension above which further increase in length results in lower tension being reached. A positive inotropic effect will move this curve upwards and to the left (Fig. 27.9a). That is, for a given initial length (volume), a higher pressure will be achieved. Likewise, a negative inotropic effect will move it down and to the right. This relationship holds for LVEDV and LV pressure. The pressure equivalent to the active tension line is never achieved, as this represents an isovolumetric pressure and, in the LV, the aortic valve opens when LV pressure exceeds aortic pressure (Fig. 27.9b). However, for an intact heart, progressively increasing LVEDV (length) will generate a larger LV pressure and SV. Similarly, increasing volume beyond a certain value will result in a progressive fall in LV pressure achieved (i.e. a failing heart). The volume at which this will occur depends on the initial state of the myocardium. For example, it can occur, rarely, in young fit individuals in severe exercise or with overenthusiastic fluid resuscitation, but in an older person after myocardial infarction (MI) even minor changes in cardiac work or fluid load may precipitate failure. In the clinical setting, this can be seen in situations where the heart is damaged or has an increased workload.

Examples of this would include:
• Where LVEDV is increased because of a damaged (infarcted) area of ventricular wall, which will bulge out rather than contract during systole such that the remaining muscle has to generate a higher pressure to achieve the same output
• Mitral valve incompetence, where blood will be forced into the RA through the leaking valve, dissipating the LV pressure
• In aortic stenosis, when high pressures are required to force blood through a narrowed orifice.

Heart rate

The atrial pacemakers have an inherent rate of approximately 110 b/min and the ventricles a rate of 30–40 b/min. The heart rate is modulated by neural, humoral and physical inputs.

Neural control is through the parasympathetic and sympathetic systems. The parasympathetic component is carried in the vagus nerves (right and left) which send branches to the SA node. Both have similar effects but the right is thought to have the greater role. Vagal stimulation results in acetylcholine release to muscarinic receptors which cause an increased loss of potassium from the pacemaker cells. This has the effect of hyperpolarizing the membrane and slowing spontaneous depolarization as more calcium then has to enter the cell to reach the depolarization threshold. As well as slowing the heart rate, vagal stimulation also slows atrial and AV node conduction and reduces atrial, but not ventricular, contractility.

Sympathetic innervation comes from the first four thoracic nerve roots (T1–T4) on both sides. The nerves arising from the right side appear to have more effect on heart rate (chronotropic) and those from the left have more effect on contractility (inotropic). At the SA node, sympathetic stimulation causes release of noradrenaline (norepinephrine) which facilitates calcium entry, thus increasing the rate of spontaneous depolarization. Sympathetic stimulation also speeds the rate of conduction in the atria, AV node and ventricles and has a positive inotropic effect on atrial and ventricular contraction. Catecholamines reaching the heart in the circulation have a similar effect.

The resting heart rate is normally approximately 70 b/min. As the rate for unopposed vagal activity would be approximately 40 b/min, and for unopposed sympathetic activity 110 b/min, this shows that, at rest, vagal tone predominates. The maximum heart rate attainable is approximately 200 b/min and this decreases with age (220 minus age in years). Above a rate of 150 b/min, cardiac output may fall as stroke volume decreases, as a result of the short diastolic filling time. At a heart rate of 60 b/min (1 beat per second), systole lasts just under 0.3 s, giving a diastolic filling time of just over 0.7 s. If the rate is doubled to 120 b/min (1 beat per 0.5 s), systolic time can be reduced, but only to approximately 0.2 s, reducing diastole to 0.3 s. At the other end of the scale, a heart rate below 45 b/min may result in a decrease in cardiac output as the relatively long diastole will result in maximal filling of the LV and stroke output cannot be increased.

Measurement of cardiac output

A number of theoretical and practical methods have been used for measurement of cardiac output. All the methods have some limitations with respect to practicality or accuracy and the majority (indeed, all in clinical use) rely on indirect or inferential measurements.

The Fick principle relates the flow through an organ to the amount of a substance taken up per unit time and the inflow–outflow difference in concentration of the substance. This can be applied to the heart using oxygen uptake. To do this requires knowing the oxygen uptake over 1 min (Vo_2) and the mixed venous and arterial oxygen content (Cvo_2 and Cao_2). Thus:

$$\text{Cardiac output} = Vo_2 / (Cao_2 - Cvo_2)$$

The practicalities of maintaining a steady state during these measurements make this of limited use.

Measuring the profile of change in the concentration of an indicator dye, such as indocyanine green, has been used to quantify cardiac output. However, it is not a quick or regularly repeatable technique as the dye, despite having a rapid clearance, tends to accumulate. This has been replaced by thermodilution, which is a development of the same principle. Injection of a bolus of fluid, of known volume and temperature, results in a transient temperature change downstream. The profile of this temperature change can be detected by a thermistor distal to the site of injection. The area under the curve of this change can be calculated 'on-line' (integrated) and is inversely proportional to cardiac output. This technique is used widely with a PA catheter where cold saline is injected through a proximal port in the RA and the change is detected by a thermistor placed near the tip of the catheter (10 cm distal) in the PA and connected to a computer, which calculates cardiac output based on the relationship described above. A more recently introduced variation on this method is a catheter with a small heating filament. The filament is positioned on a PA catheter so that it lies within the RV. A pulsed current produces a rapid local heating which can be continuously detected as temperature change distally. This has been used to give a 'continuous' measure of cardiac output by regular (e.g. 30 s) measurement and averaging. This has been shown to give fairly accurate and reproducible measurements in clinical practice.

Other methods of measuring cardiac output, including echocardiography, radionucleotides, Doppler and pulse pressure are discussed below.

Afterload

The function of the arterial system is to ensure a continuous and adaptive supply of oxygen and nutrients to all body tissues. Its structure reflects these requirements. The aorta and main arteries have to cope with high pressure and high flow. Their structure allows them to withstand large pressure changes and also to deliver blood to the tissues at an appropriate flow rate and perfusion pressure. The vessel wall is relatively thick and not readily distensible which minimizes the loss of energy from ventricular ejection and thus maintains systolic and diastolic pressures. In the larger arteries that conduct blood to the periphery, the middle layer of the arterial wall contains more elastic tissue than smooth muscle tissue. This elasticity has the effect of dampening out peaks and troughs in the pressure waveform. That is, the systolic peak pressure is lower, and diastolic higher, than would occur in a rigid system. This effect can be seen in elderly patients with arteriosclerosis where a larger pulse pressure (systolic minus diastolic) is found, and the opposite in children, where the more elastic vessels result in a lower pulse pressure. The net effect of this is that blood arrives at the start of the arterioles with a pulsatile pressure of approximately 90–70 mmHg and a mean flow rate of approximately 25 cm/s. Flow in the arteries is usually laminar which minimizes the energy lost. Turbulence can occur in areas of high flow velocity or distal to an area on narrowing in a vessel. Turbulence causes energy loss to the vessel wall which can be recognized by palpation or auscultation. Clinical examples of this would be the systolic murmur and thrill accompanying a stenotic aortic valve and the bruit heard over a severely narrowed carotid artery. These meet both the conditions of high flow and narrowing. The Korotkoff sounds delected by auscultation are also an effect of turbulent flow occurring as blood flow restarts beyond the compressed segment of artery.

Vessels with a diameter <500 μm, down to a size of around 20 μm, are classified as arterioles. Like arteries, they have a thick wall, but the middle layer is predominantly smooth muscle. The muscle layer has a key role in regulating tissue blood flow and maintaining systemic pressure (see below). The arterioles are responsible for the delivery of oxygen to the actual tissues within an organ or system. They sequentially bifurcate, getting smaller and smaller until they become the capillary bed. While the individual vessels are getting smaller, there is a huge increase in the number of vessels, resulting in a marked increase in cross-sectional area. This has two effects: the rate of flow slows (to <1 cm/s at the capillaries) and the pulsatile pressure waveform smoothes out to a steady pressure of 30–40 mmHg. Thus, in normal circumstances, blood is delivered to the tissues at a consistent rate with an adequate perfusion pressure. Although the resistance to flow in an individual capillary is obviously greater than in a single arteriole, total resistance falls. This can be explained by the large number of capillaries arising from an arteriole, which form a set of resistances in parallel. In a system of parallel resistances, total resistance is the sum of the reciprocals of the individual resistances (in contrast to resistances in series where total resistance is the sum of the individual resistances). In a parallel system, the conductance (reciprocal of resistance) is therefore summatively increased. This results in a low resistance, high conductance system.

The term microcirculation is used to describe the complex of arterioles, capillaries and venules that are involved in tissue perfusion. The arterioles undergo sequential bifurcation, becoming thinner walled until they merge into the capillary system, which in turn divides into a mesh of vessels (capillary bed) within a small area of tissue. At the distal side of a capillary bed the reverse process occurs, with the capillaries merging to form venules. Control of flow in the microcirculation is complex with neural, humoral and local factors all able to contribute. The proximal arterioles have dense sympathetic innervation which serves to regulate flow to a tissue bed. At the level of precapillary arterioles the innervation is much less dense and humoral (e.g. catecholamines) and local (e.g. cytokines) factors exert the major influence. Other circulating factors, in addition to catecholamines, that produce constriction in the microcirculation include angiotensin II and vasopressin, and those that produce dilatation include acetylcholine, artial natriuretic peptide (ANP), adenosine, kinins and prostaglandins. Local factors influencing vessel tone and diameter include metabolically and locally released substances. Metabolic influences include P_{O_2}, P_{CO_2}, pH, lactate, calcium and potassium. For example, local hypoxic conditions ($\downarrow P_{O_2}$, $\uparrow P_{CO_2}$, $\downarrow$ pH and $\uparrow$ lactate) will cause vasodilatation, producing a strong enough stimulus to override opposing neural or circulating input. Locally released factors that produce vasodilatation include adenosine, nitric oxide and histamine, while endothelin produces vasoconstriction.

Blood pressure

The relationship between blood pressure and cardiac output can be explained on the basis of Ohm's law, which in its usual form states that:

Voltage = current × resistance

but this can be adapted to:

Arterial pressure = cardiac output (CO) × peripheral resistance (PR)

Stated simply, this means that changes in arterial pressure can be brought about by changes in rate of flow of blood from the heart (cardiac output) or changes in the diameter of arterial vessels (peripheral resistance). In practice, the two factors have a dynamic interaction which involves related changes in both. For example, in acute haemorrhage the arterial pressure is maintained initially, despite a fall in cardiac output, by peripheral vasoconstriction (increased resistance).

The key element in peripheral resistance is the arterioles (or precapillary resistance vessels) which are 15–100 µm in diameter. From Poiseuille's law:

$$Q = \pi (P_1 - P_2)\, r^4 / 8 \acute{\eta} L$$

where Q is flow, $P_1 - P_2$ is the pressure difference over the system, r is the radius of vessel, r is viscosity and L is length of vessel.

While the viscosity and length are obviously important elements of this, they will not vary much with flow. Thus, the equation can be developed to show that:

$$\text{Resistance} = 8 \acute{\eta} L / \pi r^4$$

This means that resistance is inversely proportional to the radius^4, which means that small changes in radius have a major effect on resistance. For example, halving the radius (with pressure, viscosity and length unchanged) would result in flow decreasing to 1/16th. Intuitively, this would appear to suggest that arterial pressure would increase as blood moved to the periphery. However, the result of the numerous branchings of the arteries is a huge increase in cross-sectional area. The aorta has a diameter of approximately 2.5 cm and a cross-sectional area of approximately 4.5 cm^2, the main arteries of a diameter of approximately 0.4 cm have a total area of approximately 20 cm^2 and the arterioles an area of approximately 400 cm^2. This means that, in the presence of a normal cardiac output, pressure is reasonably well maintained from the aorta to the arteries but declines across the arteriolar bed from a pulsatile 90–70 mmHg to a virtually non-pulsatile 40 mmHg.

The units used for quantifying peripheral resistance are dynes/s/cm^5. This is arrived at from resistance being pressure (mmHg)/flow (mL/min). Pressure can be expressed as dynes/cm^2 and flow as cm^3/s. Putting these units into the pressure–flow equation resolves to dynes/s/cm^5. The normal range for systemic vascular resistance is 700–1500 dynes/s/cm^5, which is much greater than the pulmonary vascular resistance (80–300 dynes/s/cm^5).

To bring together the structural elements of the arterial system and effect on peripheral resistance, it is worth reviewing the distribution of blood flow (cardiac output) to the various tissues and organs. At rest, with a cardiac output of 5 L/min, the vital organs will receive approximately 70% of the total flow (brain approximately 750 mL/min, the kidneys and gut/liver approximately 1200 mL/min each and coronary flow of 250 mL/min). Of the remainder, total muscle blood flow may be approximately 1000 mL/min and skin receives approximately 200 mL/min. The distribution of blood flow adapts to various physiological and clinical changes. In exercise, the arteriolar beds of the muscles open up to meet the increased metabolic requirement of the muscle cells and changes including increased heart rate, increased cardiac output and diversion of blood flow away from tissues such as the gut occur to maintain the perfusion pressure.

Control of blood pressure

The control of arterial pressure demonstrates a classic feedback loop with sensors, integrating centre and effectors. The principal sensors involved in control of arterial pressure are the baroreceptors located in the carotid sinus and aortic arch. These are stretch receptors whose rate of discharge increases with increasing arterial pressure (Fig. 27.10). Additional inputs come from other stretch receptors in the heart and pulmonary circulation which respond to changes in blood volume, thus are activated by events like haemorrhage, and also from chemoreceptors in the pulmonary and systemic circulation which, while primarily responding to changes in oxygen and carbon dioxide content, are active in response to hypotension. The impulses are carried in the glossopharyngeal and vagus nerves to the vasomotor and cardioinhibitory centres in the medulla, ventral to the fourth ventricle. The latter appears to have specific inhibitory and stimulatory areas. The medullary centres have connections, in both directions, with the hypothalamus and cerebral cortex, which appear to be involved in integrating responses. These centres modulate a feedback loop with the afferent (sensor) input from the baroreceptors altering the efferent (effector) output. The efferent output goes mainly to the autonomic nervous system but also involves neurohumoral responses. The autonomic responses involve both the sympathetic and parasympathetic divisions and are immediate, but the neurohumoral response tends to be slower. For example, haemorrhage leading to a sudden decrease in arterial pressure will cause decreased afferent impulses which result in a stimulation of vasoconstrictor activity and an inhibition of the cardioinhibitory centre. This produces an increase in heart rate, vasoconstriction and a rise in arterial pressure which increases the afferent input. The change in intravascular volume will also have been sensed and the neurohumoral responses involving the renin–angiotensin–aldosterone system and atrial natriuretic peptide will be activated to restore blood volume.

Preload
Blood volume and distribution

In adults, total blood volume (TBV) is approximately 70 mL/kg but in young children this is nearer 80 mL/kg. This gives a TBV of around 5 L in a 70-kg adult. The distribution of the blood around the body will obviously vary with activity, position (e.g. Trendelenburg) and disease state (e.g. sepsis). At rest, approximately 12% of TBV is contained in the heart, 18% in the pulmonary circulation, 11% in the systemic arterial vessels, 5% in capillaries and the remaining 54% in the venous system. This clearly demonstrates the functions of the arterial and venous systems, with the latter containing nearly five times the volume of the supply vessels, showing its role as a capacitance reserve for changes in demand.

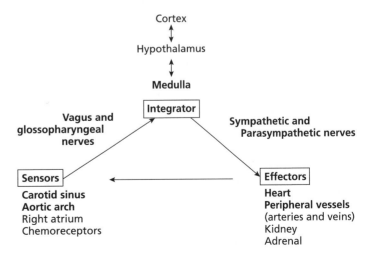

Figure 27.10 Control of arterial pressure. The primary components of the feedback loop and the most important parts of each are shown in bold type.

There are a number of methods for measuring TBV. The simplest involve injection of a dye, such as Evans blue, which is bound to plasma proteins and does not immediately go into tissues, or radiolabelled (iodine-125) albumin and measuring the resultant concentration following mixing. As these indicators are plasma protein bound and do not readily enter red cells, this allows calculation of plasma volume (dose/measured concentration). Measurement of the haematocrit then allows calculation of TBV:

$$TBV = plasma\ volume \times 1/1 - haematocrit$$

For example, a measured plasma volume of 3.6 L and haematocrit of 0.4 would give a TBV of 6 L ($3.6 \times 1/0.6 = 3.6 \times 1.66 = 5.98$).

Venous return

The pressure at the venous end of a capillary bed is approximately 10 mmHg. As normal central venous pressure is 0–4 mmHg, this does not result in a large pressure gradient for flow back to the heart. The effect of gravity has also to be taken into account. In a supine position, the venous pressure in the feet and head will be a few mmHg greater than the central venous pressure. However, abruptly moving to an upright position will increase the pressure in the foot by the weight of the column of blood above it and decrease the pressure in the head. This would cause pressure equivalents of +90 mmHg in the feet and –30 mmHg in the head, resulting in pooling of the blood in the feet. This does not occur, as the lower limb veins constrict in response to the distension and this maintains venous return.

A number of mechanisms ensure that venous return is maintained both at rest and in exercise; skeletal muscle contractions force blood out of the adjacent veins and valves ensuring unidirectional flow (muscle pump), sympathetic neural input varies the capacity of the venous system by adjusting vessel diameter (venous tone), and the negative intrathoracic pressure generated by inspiration increases venous flow into the thoracic veins (thoracic pump). These effects can be illustrated by exercise, where increased muscle pumping, increased sympathetic tone and increased respiratory effort result in an increased venous return required for the increased car-

diac output. In contrast, a 'vasovagal' faint can occur with prolonged quiet standing, because of decreased muscle and thoracic pumping and lowered venous tone.

Assessment of function

An understanding of the scientific basis of cardiovascular function is essential in anaesthesia to allow appropriate assessment of patients. This applies to preoperative assessment of elective surgical patients, to trauma patients, to severely ill patients in the intensive care unit (ICU) and to patients with postoperative problems. The ability to relate the history and examination findings to likely physiological mechanisms will lead to appropriate investigation and treatment. Indeed, awareness of the simple relationships stated above (CO = HR × SV and BP = CO × PR) acts as a good starting point.

History

The initial assessment of cardiovascular function will involve an accurate history. It is important to understand the physiological basis of common cardiovascular symptoms. For example, limitation of exercise capability of cardiovascular origin, manifest by shortness of breath after walking 100 m on the flat or climbing one flight of stairs, demonstrates that the heart is incapable of sustaining the required output to supply peripheral tissues with oxygen. This essentially means that the heart is incapable of increasing cardiac output to match requirements and has therefore been unable to increase heart rate (HR) and/or SV. Further questioning may help to determine whether this is related to the HR (e.g. rhythm disorder such as heart block), SV (e.g. left ventricular failure) or outlet obstruction from aortic valve stenosis.

A further important element of assessment is a drug history. The 'pharmacological' action of a drug acting on the cardiovascular system results in a 'physiological' change, the effect of which can be measured. For example, β-adrenergic blockade will result in a lowering of raised arterial pressure. This is achieved by a number of mechanisms including decreased contractility, decreased HR and decreased peripheral resistance. The effects of commonly used

Table 27.1 The effect of commonly used cardiovascular drugs on preload, contractility, afterload and heart rate. After Ross [1].

	Preload	Contractility	Afterload	Rate
Cardiac glycosides	↓	↑↑	↓	↓↓
PDE inhibitors	–	↑↑	↓↓	–
Thiazide diuretics	↓↓	–	↓	–
Loop diuretics	↓↓↓	–	–	–
Acetazolamide	↓	–	–	–
Adenosine	–	↑/– Local regulation	↓	↓↓
Ia Quinidine	–	↓	↓	↓↓
Ib Lidocaine	–	–	–	↓↓
Ic Flecainide	–	↓↓	–	↓↓
II β-Blocker	–	↓↓	–	↓↓
III Amiodarone	–	–/↓	–	↓↓
IV Ca channel block	–/↓	↓↓(V) ↓(N)	(V)↓/↓↓(N)	↓
K⁺ channel block	↓↓	↓	↓↓	–
ACE inhibitors	↓↓	↑	↓↓	–
Angiotensin-II antagonist (losartan)	↓↓	–	↓↓	–
Direct vasodilators (hydralazine)	–	–	↓↓	–
Central vasodilators (clonidine)	↓↓	–	↓↓	↓
Nitrates	↓↓↓	↑ Regional perfusion	↓↓ Higher doses	–
α-Blockers	↓↓	–	↓↓	–
α-Agonists	↑↑	–	↑↑↑	–
β₁-Agonists	–	↑↑	–	↑↑
β₂-Agonists	↓↓	–	↓↓	↑↑

↓ Mild; ↓↓ moderate; ↓↓↓ marked decrease (↑ increase).
ACE, angiotensin-converting enzyme; N, nifedipine; PDE, phosphodiesterase; V, verapamil.

cardiovascular drugs on the key elements of cardiovascular function are summarized in Table 27.1.

Examination

The findings on examination of the cardiovascular system, as well as being discrete measures of function, can also be combined into the structure of preload–pump–afterload discussed above. For example, in the examination of a trauma patient in whom ongoing haemorrhage is suspected — HR and BP (pump), peripheral perfusion, pallor (afterload), venous return (preload) — or identifying the site of the lesion in a patient with significant valvular disease.

Investigations

Electrocardiography

As well as the basic data on heart rate and rhythm, the 12-lead ECG can provide information on conduction defects, ventricular hypertrophy, previous ischaemic damage and ongoing myocardial ischaemia. Further information on functional reserve can be gained from an exercise ECG. This involves the patient walking on a treadmill set at a fixed protocol of increasing severity with continuous ECG recording. The outcome measures will include the amount of the programme the patient can complete, the maximum HR achieved, the time for HR to return to baseline value after exercise and evidence of myocardial ischaemia. Thus, a patient with a normal exercise ECG would complete the full programme, achieve an appropriate maximum heart rate, which returns promptly to baseline after finishing, and show no evidence of ischaemia at any stage. Abnormal results are essentially a marker of pump failure and would include inability to complete the test because of breathlessness, angina or ECG changes; failure to achieve an expected maximum HR response; overshooting the maximum HR; prolonged recovery time for the HR; and significant changes in rhythm. In a patient physically unable to manage a standard exercise test (e.g. after amputation for peripheral vascular disease), a pharmacological stress test using either a vasodilator, such as dipyridamole, or an inotrope, such as dobutamine, can be used to assess the integrity and capacity of the cardiovascular responses.

Arterial pressure

Measurement of arterial pressure using a sphygmomanometer and Riva–Rocci cuff detects systolic and diastolic pressure from the sounds produced by turbulent flow. As the cuff pressure decreases below systolic pressure, some blood is able to pass through the narrowed artery. The narrowing of the vessel results in a faster flow/unit pressure (Ohm's law — see above) and the speed of flow exceeds critical velocity, producing turbulent flow which can be heard by auscultation. When the cuff pressure is below systolic but above diastolic pressure, flow is interrupted during each pulsation giving a distinct sound on auscultation. Below diastolic pressure the flow

may still be turbulent but is continuous, thus sounding muffled. Automated cuff systems use various methods to detect the turbulent flow and identify systolic and diastolic pressure. Direct measurement of arterial pressure with a cannula placed in an artery is used intraoperatively and in intensive care. The transducer is placed at the estimated level of the RA. Placement above this level would lead to an underestimation of pressure, and below to an overestimation.

Cardiac output

A number of other investigations are used to provide information on cardiac function as part of an assessment.

Radionucleotides

Intravenous injection of a radionucleotide, such as technetium-99, can be used to quantify ventricular volume and ejection fraction (ventriculography) by gated X-ray scanning. This is an accurate method but it requires specialized radiology facilities and is not appropriate for repeated measurements because of the radiation exposure required. Injection of the nucleotide thallium can be used to identify areas of myocardium that are infarcted or have borderline perfusion. Thallium is taken up by myocardial cells. It is given after a dose of dipyridamole, a coronary vasodilator that can precipitate myocardial ischaemia. The heart is scanned to detect areas in which uptake has not occurred: a perfusion defect. The scan is repeated 4 hours later when the vasodilator is no longer effective. The scans are compared to show perfusion defects that are present in both and are therefore irreversible and represent infarcted tissue, and those that are not present on the second scan and are, thus, reversible, indicating ischaemic tissue.

Echocardiography

Ultrasonic examination of the heart and major vessels can give useful information on cardiac function, either as preoperative assessment or intraoperative monitoring. The probe can either be placed external to the chest wall (transthoracic) or in the oesophagus (transoesophageal). The penetration of ultrasonic waves decreases with increasing frequency but higher frequency gives better definition. Therefore, transthoracic ultrasound uses frequencies of 1–7 MHz, as the chest wall has to be crossed, but the transoesophageal probe uses 3.5–7 MHz as there is less tissue to cross, and can give higher definition. The two-dimensional images can give both structural and functional assessments. The valves can be visualized to identify damage or evidence of retrograde flow (e.g. mitral incompetence) and the chamber wall, particularly LV, for abnormalities in motion (e.g. an ischaemic or infarcted area will not show contraction during systole and may move in the opposite direction to adjacent contracting muscle). Measurement of the images can help to quantify ventricular function by calculating LVEDV and ejection fraction. Intraoperatively, images of LV filling give an estimate of preload, thus guiding fluid therapy and the use of inotropes. The use of a calculated SV and concurrent HR gives an estimate of cardiac output.

Transoesophageal Doppler

An image of the descending aorta can be obtained by placing an ultrasound probe in the oesophagus. Using a Doppler technique, the pattern of reflection of the ultrasound beam can be used to calculate the velocity of flow. The diameter of the aorta can either be assumed, on the basis of age, height and weight, or measured with the ultrasound at the start. It follows that measuring the profile of flow velocity per contraction through a known cross-sectional area will allow estimation of cardiac output and stroke volume. Plotting the flow velocity against time results in a triangular profile with a steep upward slope to a peak and a more gently sloped tail. The upward slope and peak value reflect contractility and the area under the curve relates to volume. The trace can therefore give an indication of cardiac function and volume status. Thus, the trace in hypovolaemia will be narrower and more peaked; in cardiogenic shock, the peak would be lower and the profile more rounded; and in a hyperdynamic state, the peak will be higher and the tail wider and longer. This technique has been used to direct fluid therapy and inotrope infusion in major surgery and in the intensive care setting.

Pulse pressure and cardiac output

There has been long-standing interest in using a peripherally measured pulse as a measure of stroke volume and cardiac output. It is logical to assume that the magnitude of a detected pulse will be related to the volume of blood generating that pulse (SV). There are a number of problems inherent to this concept: the compliance of the arterial system, in particular the large vessels, is non-linear; the profile of the waveform will vary with the size of vessel the measurement is taken in; interference from peripherally reflected waves will alter the profile; and damping can occur in the vessels and in a measuring system. However, a number of techniques have been used to overcome these problems, including pulse-contour analysis and pulse-power analysis. These systems require an initial calibration of cardiac output (e.g. lithium dilution) and have an in-built algorithm taking into account compliance, waveform and vessel site and size. These systems use a peripheral arterial line and the measured SV and cardiac output have been shown to correlate well with that measured with more invasive methods.

Conclusions

Assessment of the cardiovascular system requires integration of a series of potentially complex interactions. Starting with a simple model, it is possible to develop an understanding of the structure and function of each unit. With this knowledge, the clinician is then able to explore the relationship between these units and their interactions. This is perhaps best illustrated in assessing the cardiovascular status of a patient following haemorrhage, where the responses of each unit are definable but are also clearly interdependent. It is important, when faced with increasingly complicated and sophisticated information available from monitors and investigative methods, that the clinician has a clear understanding of the basic principles governing the function of the cardiovascular system, in order to apply this information correctly.

References

1 Ross JJ. A systematic approach to cardiovascular pharmacology. *Br J Anaesth CEPD Rev* 2001; **1**: 1–6.

Further reading

Brown JM. Use of echocardiography for haemodynamic monitoring. *Crit Care Med* 2002; **30**: 1361–4.

Burchell SA, Yu M, Takiguchi SA, Ohta RM, Myers SA. Evaluation of a continuous cardiac output and mixed venous oxygen saturation catheter in critically ill surgical patients. *Crit Care Med* 1997; **25**: 383–91.

Colreavy FB, Donovan K, Lee KY, Weekes J. Transoesphageal echocardiography in critically ill patients. *Crit Care Med* 2002; **30**: 989–96.

Galley HF, Webster NR. Physiology of the endothelium. *Br J Anaesth* 2004; **93**: 105–13.

Gomez CM, Palazzo MG. Pulmonary artery catheterisation in anaesthesia and intensive care. *Br J Anaesth* 1998; **81**: 945–56.

Mihaljevic T, von Segesser LK, Tonz M, *et al.* Continuous versus bolus thermodilution cardiac output measurements: a comparative study. *Crit Care Med* 1995; **23**: 944–9.

Poldermans D, Fioretti PM, Forster T, *et al.* Dobutamine stress-echocardiography for assessment of perioperative cardiac risk in patients undergoing major vascular surgery. *Circulation* 1993; **87**: 1506–12.

Stephan F, Flahaut A, Dieudonne N, *et al.* Clinical evaluation of circulating blood volume in critically ill patients. *Br J Anaesth* 2001; **86**: 754–62.

Tyberg JV. How changes in venous capacitance modulate cardiac output. *Eur J Physiol* 2002; **445**: 10–7.

Young JD. The heart and circulation in severe sepsis. *Br J Anaesth* 2004; **93**: 114–20.

CHAPTER 28

Assessment of respiratory function

Stuart Murdoch

Introduction

The aim of assessment in the context of anaesthesia and the preoperative evaluation of a patient is in part to predict the likelihood of complications following the planned surgery. This information may also be used to influence the decision to proceed to surgery: some surgery may be inappropriate in view of a large perioperative risk, although some high-risk surgery is still appropriate when the consequences of leaving the disease untreated are known. It is also used in the decision as to what anaesthetic technique to employ, if a patient needs high dependency or intensive care afterwards, and to inform the patient as part of the consent process.

Respiratory complications are a major cause of morbidity and mortality after surgery. Some studies have recorded them to be the most common postoperative complication encountered, with a greater incidence than those affecting the cardiovascular system. However, although several scoring systems have been developed for cardiac complications, little work exists predicting the development of respiratory problems. The Goldman cardiac-risk index, however, can be used to predict pulmonary as well as cardiac complications [1]. Much of the work that has been carried out examining risk in relation to pulmonary complications has focused on small numbers of patients undergoing thoracotomy or lung resection. This chapter mainly deals with the far greater number of patients undergoing non-thoracic surgery, which includes a significant number of patients with co-existent lung disease.

There are a large number of potential complications affecting the respiratory system postoperatively; these can vary greatly both in their significance and their severity. Complications encountered include pneumonia, respiratory failure and the need for respiratory support, atelectasis, hypoxia and the exacerbation of any underlying respiratory disease. Any one problem can vary greatly in the extent to which it affects a patient. Pneumonia can be such that the patient has minimal problems but has a productive cough, to the patient who is severely affected and needs artificial ventilatory support, developing sepsis and requiring support for multiorgan failure. Similarly, hypoxia can be transient and easily resolved resulting in the need for physiotherapy or minimal respiratory support such as continuous positive airway pressure (CPAP), or be significant and unresponsive to simple measures and again result in a need for ventilatory support for a period of time. The difficulty in defining respiratory complications makes comparison of studies difficult; studies also differ in the time at which they assess respiratory complications, with some studies only assessing complications up to 24 hours postoperatively, while others examine complications up to 72 hours or even the full length of stay of the patient. In patients undergoing major non-thoracic surgery, it has been reported that 10–30% of patients have postoperative respiratory problems. Very few studies define how anaesthetic management of a patient is altered following preoperative assessment, or if some patients have had their surgery altered or cancelled. The development of respiratory problems can lead to a prolongation of hospital stay as well as an increase in mortality.

The most important part of any preoperative assessment is the history and examination of the patient. This will identify the majority of patients at risk of complications, and only then should specialized test and investigations be considered. The studies that have been performed using laboratory testing of pulmonary function to predict pulmonary complications have generally failed to demonstrate superior sensitivity or specificity compared with simple history and examination of the patient in predicting the risk of respiratory complications in non-thoracic surgery [2].

History

Chronic obstructive pulmonary disease

Chronic obstructive pulmonary disease (COPD) is a syndrome of progressive airflow limitation caused by chronic inflammation of the airways and lung parenchyma [3]. It typically presents in smokers and may not present until substantial deterioration in respiratory function has occurred. It results in a decrease in forced expiratory volume in 1 second (FEV_1), an increase in functional residual capacity (FRC), hyperinflation of the chest, hypoxia and a decrease in exercise tolerance. Before embarking on surgery, the medical management of the patient should be optimized where possible. This may involve the use of steroids, antibiotics, physiotherapy and bronchodilators. Several studies have examined the relationship between pre-existing COPD and postoperative pulmonary complications. They uniformly report an increase in the incidence of such complications.

In a study by Wong *et al.* [4] of patients with severe COPD ($FEV_1 < 1.2l$) undergoing surgery, of whom 95% had duration of surgery longer than 2 hours, 37% had major pulmonary complications. Overall 2-year survival in this group of patients was less than 50%, similar to that of patients with severe cardiac disease. The factor most predictive of outcome, however, was the American Society of Anesthesiologists (ASA) classification. This probably reflects the multifactorial cause of pulmonary complications and the fact that one of the major causes of respiratory disease and COPD, smoking, also has a significant impact on the cardiovascular system.

In a similar group of patients ($FEV_1 < 50\%$ of predicted), Kroenke *et al.* [5] demonstrated similar results, with 29% of patients having significant postoperative pulmonary problems. The major predictors of pulmonary complications were type and duration of operation, as well as the patient's ASA classification. Mortality in this study was strongly associated with patients undergoing cardiac surgery.

Smoking

Smoking is a major risk factor for postoperative pulmonary complications. Studies consistently demonstrate a significant increase in pulmonary complications in smokers following surgery compared with non-smokers. A sixfold increase in pulmonary complications in smokers after abdominal surgery compared with non-smokers has been reported [6–8]. It is difficult to separate a pure smoking effect in studies from that resulting from end-organ damage brought about by smoking, although in practice this is of little practical importance. However, an increase in postoperative pulmonary complications in smokers without chronic lung disease has been demonstrated [9].

Smoking results in decreased cilia function and increased mucus production, leading to a failure to clear secretions, airway plugging and collapse, leading to postoperative complications. Stopping smoking prior to surgery is associated with a short-term increase in pulmonary complications compared with smokers but a return to a normal rate of complications over time. The time period over which an increase in complications occurs may be 2 months or longer, and the increase in risk of complications is greatest in those patients who reduce smoking closest to surgery. In cardiac surgical patients, a fourfold increase in pulmonary complications has been observed in those giving up smoking within 2 months of surgery compared with non-smokers [10]. The reason for the increase in pulmonary complications following a reduction in smoking prior to anaesthesia is hypothesized to be an increase in sputum production following the reduction in smoking [11]. An alternative hypothesis is that the observation is a result of selection bias, with those people reducing cigarette consumption prior to surgery being more unwell.

Asthma

Asthma is among the most common respiratory diseases, affecting a wide age range of patients and presenting a broad spectrum of disease severity. Early studies reported a high incidence of pulmonary perioperative complications, with over one-quarter of patients affected [12,13].

A more recent review of the medical records of 706 patients with asthma undergoing surgical procedures, looking at the frequency of bronchospasm and laryngospasm, documented only 12 cases (1.7%) of bronchospasm and two cases of laryngospasm. These complications were associated with higher ASA status, recent use of anti-asthmatic drugs, recent asthma symptoms and recent medical admission for asthma [14]. This study, together with other more recent studies, seems to indicate that patients with active disease are more at risk of pulmonary complications than those patients with the disease but with no recent symptoms; this latter group have an incidence of pulmonary problems close to that of the general population.

In a prospective study of perioperative outcomes which included 486 patients, 1.7% experienced a severe respiratory problem, including 0.81% who had bronchospasm [15]. In the non-asthmatic group, 0.94% experienced severe pulmonary problems and 0.13% bronchospasm. However, after statistical analysis of the data the authors claimed that asthma was not predictive of severe pulmonary complications or bronchospasm. Examination of the ASA closed claims project database revealed 88 cases of bronchospasm resulting in patient injury [16]. Of these claims, 28 patients (32%) had a history of asthma. This is in the context of a reported 4% incidence of asthma in the general population of the USA.

In conclusion, asthma is a predisposing factor for bronchospasm in patients undergoing anaesthesia. In the general population with a label of asthma or inactive asthma, there is probably a small increase in the risk of postoperative pulmonary complications. In patients with active disease, the risk of complications is significantly increased and it is this that is used to justify the routine use of preoperative bronchodilators and steroids. Indeed, it may be that the routine use of these drugs has resulted in a decrease in morbidity in the asthmatic population undergoing anaesthesia.

Obesity

There is little evidence to support the assumption that obesity is a major risk factor for postoperative pulmonary complications [17]. Most studies have failed to demonstrate any significant difference in the incidence of pulmonary complications between obese and non-obese patients [18,19]. However, the incidence of sleep apnoea is significantly increased in the morbidly obese [20] and care must be taken in the use of opiates in this group of patients, who must also be carefully monitored postoperatively in case of apnoea.

Examination

Examination of the respiratory system should have a structured approach. This usually begins with a general examination of the patient and then proceeds to focus specifically on the respiratory system. Important information of relevance to the anaesthetist includes the patient's breathing pattern, the presence of cyanosis and signs in the chest indicative of infection or chronic obstructive pulmonary disease.

Chest X-ray

Chest X-rays are often performed prior to elective surgery, and a large number of studies have investigated their use [21–23]. These studies have reported a relatively small number of positive results (abnormalities seen on chest X-ray) and a smaller number of changes in anaesthetic management based on the results of the X-ray. In 1992, the Royal College of Radiologists described criteria to help decide which patients should receive a chest X-ray prior to surgery [24]:

- Those with acute respiratory symptoms
- Those with possible metastases
- Those with suspected or established cardiorespiratory disease who have not had chest radiography in the past 12 months.

The recommendations by the National Institute for Clinical Excellence (NICE), who recently reviewed all preoperative investigations prior to elective surgery, suggest that a chest X-ray should only be routine in patients prior to cardiovascular surgery, and in patients about to undergo major surgery who are over the age of 60 years and have significant cardiovascular disease. This is similar to the most recent recommendations by the Royal College of Radiologists.

Pulmonary function testing

Studies examining the use of pulmonary function preoperatively in patients undergoing non-thoracic surgery have found conflicting results. Older studies give a high predictive value to the use of spirometry over that of history and examination to predict complications and has led to a recommendation by the American College of Physicians advocating their more widespread use [25]. More recent studies have failed to demonstrate such an equivocal predictive value, especially when clinical descriptive data is taken into account, and many of the abnormal values obtained from spirometry could be predicted by the patient's known underlying disease.

In a study of 361 patients undergoing laparotomy, Barisone *et al.* [26] recorded a history from patients, and performed a pulmonary physiological evaluation to record all standard respiratory variables. A standard anaesthetic technique was employed and the patients were followed for evidence of serious respiratory complications. Fourteen per cent of patients had severe respiratory complications and of these three patients died as a result of such complications. Analysis was performed on the data collected to identify predictive variables for respiratory complications. The presence of mucous hypersecretion (mucous production for 3 or more months of the year) and dyspnoea were most significantly associated with complications. When all variables were analysed simultaneously, mucous hypersecretion in conjunction with a raised residual volume was found most likely to predict complications. The analysis showed, to a lesser extent, that low values of FEV_1 and single breath transfer factor (TlCOsb) were also predictive of respiratory complications. This is in keeping with the observed increased risk for patients with obstructive respiratory disease.

In a study of 60 patients undergoing abdominal surgery, Kocabas *et al.* [27] showed that the incidence of pulmonary complications was higher in patients with abnormal preoperative spirometry. However, no advantage was shown in using spirometry to predict complications than the presence of abnormal physical findings on examination. In concurrence with other studies, age, smoking, length and site of operation and higher ASA classification were predictive of the development of pulmonary complications.

NICE reviewed the use of pulmonary function testing prior to elective surgery in their assessment of preoperative testing [28]. Ten studies were identified over a 35-year period. There were criticisms of all the studies in terms of their design, and none of the papers reported any change in clinical management of patients based on the results of pulmonary function testing. The final recommendations with regard to the use of pulmonary function testing in patients was that it should be considered for patients only with morbidity from respiratory disease who were undergoing major surgery.

One area in which spirometry and pulmonary function testing may be more useful is in identifying the extent of known existing respiratory disease and monitoring its response to therapy prior to surgery.

Arterial blood gases

Baseline blood gases are generally not believed to help in identifying the patient at risk of respiratory complications over the use of history taking [29]. Older studies identified a raised P_{CO_2} above 45 mmHg as a risk factor for complications, although in all patients so identified, significant respiratory disease was present [30]. As with pulmonary function testing, the published studies do not state how the management of patients was changed by abnormal results.

Pulmonary risk index

Several attempts have been made to develop a respiratory risk index to predict postoperative respiratory complications in a similar way to how the Goldman index predicts cardiac complications [31,32]. These attempts are often limited to certain patient populations, based on small numbers and are not validated. One of the largest studies examined data collected prospectively by the Veterans Affairs National Surgical Quality Improvement Program (NSQIP) to determine factors associated with the development of postoperative pneumonia using a standard definition of nosocomial pneumonia [33]. It did not look at other pulmonary complications. The study examined data on over 160 000 patients and was validated with a different dataset. The scoring system was similar to that used for the Goldman cardiac risk index, although in this instance the most important factors were advanced age, site of operation and functional status. Until scoring systems become more generalized it is unlikely they will gain widespread acceptance.

Exercise testing

The use of exercise testing has been used to select patients suitable for thoracic surgery [34] and it has also been investigated as a means of predicting postoperative pulmonary complications. A simple way to assess exercise capacity is the ability to climb stairs. In a study in which patients were asked to walk up stairs until limited by exhaustion, dyspnoea, leg fatigue or chest pain, the height climbed by patients was predictive of complications [35]. The lower the height climbed, the more likely postoperative complications were to occur. Other studies have also used the ability to climb stairs as a predictor of outcome, with an inability to climb three flights of stairs predicting those most likely to develop pulmonary complications [36]. Invasive and more formal respiratory function testing has also been used in patients undergoing lung resection; patients with a reduced ability to increase their maximal oxygen have been shown to have an increased risk of pulmonary complications or are judged unsuitable for surgery [37].

The risk of developing pulmonary complications following surgery is related not only to the patient's preoperative condition but also to the nature and site of surgery, with a greater number of complications in patients undergoing upper abdominal or thoracic procedures compared with peripheral surgery. Atelectasis develops in nearly all patients following the induction of anaesthesia within a short period of time [38]. The pattern of breathing is altered because of the anaesthetic drugs used as well as the surgical positioning of the patient. Movement of the chest may also be impaired by the incision and traction by the surgical instruments or a pneumo-peritoneum in the case of laparoscopic surgery [39]. In the postoperative period, breathing is altered by a number of mechanisms, including pain from the site of incision causing the patient to limit their respiratory movement — this is greater in patients having surgery near the diaphragm. The residual effects of anaesthetic drugs and the respiratory depressant effect of drugs employed to control pain also contribute to postoperative respiratory impairment. The reduced respiratory movement is believed to contribute to a decreased FRC and vital capacity, which together with atelectasis is believed to contribute to the development of pneumonia in some patients. The management of patients in the postoperative period should aim to reduce the incidence of pulmonary complications. Methods employed include adequate analgesia, early mobilization and appropriate physiotherapy, which may begin preoperatively. It is believed that epidural analgesia has some benefits over the use of opiate-based regimens [40], although randomized studies have not always been supportive of this. Prolonged duration of anaesthesia and advanced age has also been shown to be associated with an increased risk of respiratory complications following surgery.

Conclusions

Postoperative pulmonary complications are very common. Many studies have repeatedly shown an increased incidence of respiratory complications in those with a higher ASA classification, smokers and in those patients undergoing prolonged surgery close to the diaphragm. The vast majority of patients can be assessed solely by careful history and examination. The use of chest X-rays should be limited to patients fitting into clearly defined groups. Specialist investigations such as arterial blood gases and spirometry may also identify patients at risk but appears to add little further information and cannot be recommended for routine use.

References

1 Lawrence VA, Dhanda R, Hilsenbeck SG, Page CP. Risk of pulmonary complications after elective abdominal surgery. *Chest* 1996; **110**: 744–50.

2 Rock P, Rich PB. Postoperative pulmonary complications. *Curr Opin Anaesthesiol* 2003; **16**: 123–32.

3 Sutherland ER, Cherniack RM. Current concepts: management of chronic obstructive pulmonary disease. *N Engl J Med* 2004; **350**: 2689–97.

4 Wong DH, Weber EC, Schell MJ, *et al*. Factors associated with postoperative pulmonary complications in patients with severe chronic obstructive pulmonary disease. *Anesth Analg* 1995; **80**: 276–84.

5 Kroenke K, Lawrence VA, Theroux JF, Tuley MR. Operative risk in patients with severe obstructive pulmonary disease. *Arch Intern Med* 1992; **152**: 967–71.

6 Morton HJV. Tobacco smoking and pulmonary complications after operation. *Lancet* 1944; **1**: 368–70.

7 Bluman LG, Mosca L, Newman N, Simon DG. Preoperative smoking habits and postoperative pulmonary complications. *Chest* 1998; **113**: 883–9.

8 McAlister FA, Khan NA, Straus S, *et al*. Accuracy of the preoperative assessment in predicting pulmonary risk after nonthoracic surgery. *Am J Respir Crit Care Med* 2003; **167**: 741–4.

9 Wightman JA. A prospective study of the incidence of postoperative pulmonary complications. *Br J Surg* 1968; **55**: 85–91.

10 Warner MA, Offord KP, Warner ME, *et al*. Role of preoperative cessation of smoking and other factors in postoperative pulmonary complications: a blinded prospective study of coronary artery bypass patients. *Mayo Clin Proc* 1989; **64**: 609–16.

11 Pearce AC, Jones RM. Smoking and anaesthesia: preoperative abstinance and perioperative morbidity. *Anesthesiology* 1984; **61**: 576–84.

12 Gold MI, Helrich M. A study of the complications related to anaesthesia in asthmatic patients. *Anesth Analg* 1963; **42**: 282–93.

13 Schnider SM, Papper EM. Anaesthesia for the asthmatic patient. *Anesthesiology* 1961; **22**: 886–92.

14 Warner DO, Warner MA, Barnes RD, *et al*. Perioperative respiratory complications in patients with asthma. *Anesthesiology* 1996; **85**: 460–7.

15 Forrest JB, Rehder K, Cahalan MK, Goldsmith CH. Multicenter study of general anesthesia. III Predictors of severe perioperative adverse outcomes. *Anesthesiology* 1992; **76**: 3–15.

16 Cheney FW, Posner KL, Caplan RA. Adverse respiratory events infrequently leading to malpractice suits: a closed claims analysis. *Anesthesiology* 1991; **75**: 932–9.

17 McAlister FA, Khan NA, Straus SE, *et al*. Accuracy of the preoperative assessment in predicting pulmonary risk after nonthoracic surgery. *Am J Respir Crit Care Med* 2003; **167**: 741–74.

18 Phillips EH, Carroll BJ, Fallas MJ, Pearlstein AR. Comparison of laparoscopic cholecystectomy in obese and non-obese patients. *Am Surg* 1994; **60**: 316–21.

19 Licker M, Spiliopoulos A, Frey J, *et al*. Risk factors for early mortality and major complications following

pneumonectomy for non-small cell carcinoma of the lung. *Chest* 2002; **121**:1890–7.

20 Adam JP, Murphy GP. Obesity in anaesthesia and intensive care. *Br J Anaesth* 2000; **85**: 91–108.

21 Royal College of Radiologists. Pre-operative chest radiology: a national study by the Royal College of Radiologists. *Lancet* 1979; **ii**: 83–6.

22 Walker D, Williams P, Tawn J. Audit of requests for preoperative chest radiography. *Br Med J* 1994; **309**: 772–3.

23 National Institute of Clinical Excellence. *Preoperative Tests: The Use of Routine Preoperative Tests for Elective Surgery*. 2003.

24 Royal College of Radiologists Working Party. *Making the Best Use of a Department of Clinical Radiology Guidelines for Doctors*, 2nd edn. 1992.

25 American College of Physicians. Preoperative pulmonary function testing. *Ann Intern Med* 1990; **112**: 793–4.

26 Barisone G, Rovida S, Gazzaniga GM, Fontana L. Upper abdominal surgery: does a lung function test exist to predict early severe postoperative respiratory complication. *Eur Respir J* 1997; **10**: 1301–8.

27 Kocabas A, Kara K, Ozgur G, Sonmez H, Burget R. Value of preoperative spirometry to predict postoperative pulmonary complications. *Respir Med* 1996; **90**: 25–33.

28 National Institute of Clinical Excellence. *Preoperative Tests: Appendices: Guidelines & Information*. 2003.

29 Rock P, Rich PB. Postoperative pulmonary complications. *Curr Opin Anaesthesiol* 2003, **16**: 123–32.

30 Milledge JS, Nunn JF. Criteria of fitness for anaesthesia in patients with chronic obstructive lung disease. *Br Med J* 1975; **3**: 670–3.

31 Lawrence VA, Dhanda R, Hilsenbeck SG, Page CP. Risk of pulmonary complications after elective abdominal surgery. *Chest* 1996; **110**: 744–50.

32 Brooks-Brunn JA. Validation of a predictive model for postoperative pulmonary complications. *Heart Lung* 1998; **27**:151–8.

33 Arozullah AM, Khuri SF, Henderson WG, Daley J. Development and validation of a multifactorial risk index for predicting postoperative pneumonia after major noncardiac surgery. *Ann Intern Med* 2001; **135**: 847–57.

34 Soders CR. Clinical evaluation of the patient for thoracic surgery. *Surg Clin North Am* 1961; **41**: 545–56.

35 Bruneli A, Al Refai M, Monteverde M, *et al*. Stair climbing test predicts cardiopulmonary complications after lung resection. *Chest* 2002; **121**: 1106–10.

36 Holden DA, Rice TW, Stelmach K, Meeker DP. Exercise testing, 6-min walk, and stair climb in the evaluation of patients at high risk for pulmonary resection. *Chest* 1992; **102**: 1774–9.

37 Reilly JJ. Evidence-based preoperative evaluation of candidates for thoracotomy. *Chest* 1999; **116**: 474S–6S.

38 Tokics L, Hedenstierna G, Strandberg A, *et al*. Lung collapse and gas exchange during general anesthesia: effects of spontaneous breathing, muscle paralysis and positive end-expiratory pressure. *Anesthesiology* 1987: **66**: 157–67.

39 Warner DO. Preventing postoperative pulmonary complications: the role of the anesthesiologist. *Anesthesiology* 2000; **94**: 1467–72.

40 Rigg JR, Jamrozik K, Myles PS, *et al*. Epidural anaesthesia and analgesia and outcome of major surgery: a randomised trial. *Lancet* 2002; **359**: 1276–82.

CHAPTER 29

Monitoring the depth of anaesthesia

Praveen Kalia

Introduction

Balanced anaesthesia consists of analgesia, amnesia, anaesthesia, muscle relaxation and lack of reflex movements. An adequate depth of anaesthesia is essential for preventing awareness, defined as spontaneous recall of events occurring during anaesthesia. Soon after the introduction of ether anaesthesia, it became clear that increasing the concentration of the inhalation agent would progressively depress the central nervous system, eventually leading to respiratory or cardiac arrest. Various classifications of stages of anaesthesia were proposed in order to ensure the correct depth of anaesthesia without subjecting the patient to such adverse events. In 1847, Snow described five stages of anaesthesia, with only the fourth degree providing adequate depth of anaesthesia and allowing safe conduct of surgery (Table 29.1) [1]. However, it was not until 1937 that Guedel described the classic stages of anaesthesia in patients breathing ether, based on reflexes, muscle tone, pupillary size and respiratory pattern. Before the introduction of muscle relaxants in the 1940s, muscle relaxation was achieved by increasing the depth of anaesthesia. Use of muscle relaxants abolished these important clinical signs which had been relied on previously to monitor the depth of anaesthesia.

Even today, a higher incidence of awareness was reported when muscle relaxants were used compared with anaesthesia without muscle relaxants (0.18% versus 0.11%) [2]. Sebel *et al.* [3] reported a 0.13% incidence of awareness in a recently published study in adults and Davidson *et al.* [4] reported a 0.8% incidence of awareness during anaesthesia in children. Awareness during anaesthesia is extremely distressing for patients and can result in neurological and psychological problems seen as post-traumatic stress disorder. In addition, medical litigation may follow. Ensuring adequate depth of anaesthesia is therefore essential.

Memory

Memory is not a single entity but comprises several specific types. It can be described as short- or long-term memory. Long-term memory can be further divided into implicit or explicit memory (Table 29.2). Awareness is retention of events in the form of memory because of inadequate depth of anaesthesia.

Prior experiences can affect behaviour automatically without conscious awareness (non-declarative) or through the mediating experience of conscious memory (declarative). Of most clinical relevance is explicit recall, often used synonymously with the term 'awareness' and entailing a conscious spontaneous recollection of undesired events during surgery.

Stages of awareness are described in Table 29.3 [5]. Explicit recall is usually revealed by structured questioning in the postoperative period. In contrast, implicit recall does not require conscious recognition and manifests as subtle changes in behaviour or performance. Detection of implicit awareness is more complex and requires expert psychological testing.

Explicit recall

The incidence of explicit recall during surgery has been estimated to be 0.01% [6,7]. However, the reported incidence depends upon the type of anaesthesia and the nature of the surgical procedure. Higher incidences have been documented during emergency obstetric surgery, high-risk cardiac surgery and major trauma cases. Patients experiencing intraoperative awareness report feelings of fear, anxiety

Table 29.1 Classic stages of anaesthesia.

Stage	Manifestation	Signs
Stage 1	Analgesia	Ends with loss of eyelash reflex and unconsciousness
Stage 2	Excitement	Irregular breathing, struggling, dilated pupils. Susceptible to vomiting, coughing, laryngospasm. Ends with onset of automatic breathing and loss of eyelid reflex
Stage 3	Surgical anaesthesia	
Plane I		Until eyes central with loss of conjunctival reflex, pupils normal/small, lacrimation increased
Plane II		Until onset of intercostal paralysis, deep regular breathing, loss of corneal reflex, pupils larger
Plane III		Until complete intercostal paralysis, shallow breathing, laryngeal reflexes and lacrimation depressed
Plane IV		Until diaphragmatic paralysis, lacrimal reflexes depressed
Stage 4	Overdose	Apnoea and dilated pupils

Table 29.2 Types of memory.

Short-term memory
Long-term memory
Implicit (non-declarative)
Procedural
Priming
Conditioning
Explicit (declarative)
Somatic
Episodic

Table 29.3 Stages of awareness.

Conscious awareness (perception) with explicit recall (memory)
Conscious awareness (perception) with no explicit recall (memory)
Dreaming
Subconscious awareness (perception) with implicit recall (memory)
No awareness (perception) or implicit recall (memory)

and impending death. They recollect auditory, visual and tactile perception suggesting a high level of cognitive performance. The psychological sequelae vary from temporary sleep disturbance, anxiety and nightmares to longer term post-traumatic stress disorders. Irrespective of the severity, an empathetic approach with offer of psychological support should be adopted.

Some patients have explicit memories of some intraoperative events but experience no pain. Such patients are undistressed by their experiences and may not have recall of events in the immediate postoperative period. Structured interviews at a later date are required to appreciate these events.

Implicit recall

This is a much more tenuous concept. Numerous behavioural techniques have been used to test for implicit memory formation during anaesthesia, with conflicting results. Examples of implicit memory include reduced patient controlled analgesia (PCA) usage when patients have been played recordings during their operation suggesting that they will feel comfortable after surgery. The characteristic of implicit memory is that the patients cannot remember hearing these recordings. Because anaesthesia is mainly directed at preventing cortical awareness, subcortical learning could theoretically be preserved. Further work is necessary to elucidate the clinical relevance of implicit learning.

Recommendations have been proposed by Griffith and Jones [5] as to the correct course of action following a complaint of awareness by a patient after anaesthesia:

1 Visit the patient as soon as possible, along with a witness (preferably a consultant)
2 Take a full history and document the patient's exact memory of events
3 Attempt to confirm the validity of the account
4 Keep your own copy of this account
5 Give a full explanation to the patient
6 Offer the patient follow-up, including psychological support, and document that this has been offered
7 Reassure the patient that they can safely have further general anaesthetics, with minimal risk of a further episode of awareness
8 If the cause is not known, try to determine it
9 Notify your medical defence organization
10 Notify your hospital administration
11 Notify the patient's GP.

Awareness duing anaesthesia is particularly distressing and understanding of awareness and its proper management by medical personnel has been reported to be poor or totally lacking [6,7].

Methods to monitor the depth of anaesthesia

Achieving an adequate depth of anaesthesia is fundamental to good clinical practice. It is achieved when concentrations of anaesthetic agents are sufficient to suppress conscious perception of surgical stimulus. While deep anaesthesia may cause cardiovascular depression and prolonged recovery times, light anaesthesia may lead to profound psychological sequelae for the patient.

Prevention of awareness relies on meticulous anaesthetic technique. This involves delivery of an uninterrupted supply of an appropriate quantity of anaesthetic agent using functional equipment by a competent practitioner with suitable monitoring. With increasing diversity of anaesthetic techniques (newer volatile agents, total intravenous anaesthesia and potent opiate analgesia), there is an impetus

towards using subjective methods of monitoring with more objective techniques, particularly those analysing neurophysiological parameters. Features of the ideal monitor are summarized in Table 29.4. Unfortunately, there is no absolute unit of anaesthetic depth that can be used universally in all patients.

Various methods have been used to monitor the depth of anaesthesia but the ideal monitor has not yet been developed.

Clinical signs

Historically, clinical signs indicating an autonomic response to a light plane of anaesthesia — tachycardia, hypertension, sweating, lachrimation and pupillary dilatation — have all been used to monitor the depth of anaesthesia. A scoring system was devised by Evans in 1987 called the pressure, rate, sweat, tears score (PRST), based on a patient's response to surgical stimulus [8]. It was found to be unpredictable, as patients reported awareness even when the PRST score indicated adequate depth, whereas patients showing signs of light anaesthesia did not complain of awareness. Many of the PRST signs can also be caused by hypovolaemia, inadequate analgesia, hypoxia or hypercapnia.

Lower oesophageal segment motility

Inflation of a balloon placed in the lower oesophagus provokes secondary contractions. The amplitude of these contractions decreases with increasing depth of anaesthesia. Good correlation was reported between oesophageal motility and depth of anaesthesia during inhalation anaesthesia but not during opioid-based anaesthesia. This method is no longer used in clinical practice.

Table 29.4 Features of an ideal 'depth of anaesthesia' monitor.

Safe, non-invasive and reliable
Easy to interpret
Suitable for both intravenous and inhalation anaesthesia
Accurately reflects depth of anaesthesia
Sensitive to various stimuli (e.g. intubation and incision)

Isolated forearm technique

Administration of a muscle relaxant after inflation of a tourniquet applied to the arm results in sparing of muscles of the arm from neuromuscular paralysis. Movement of the arm in response to spoken words under anaesthesia indicates an inadequate depth of anaesthesia and hence potential awareness. The technique had limitations, as reflexes operating at spinal levels could result in movement. Many patients could not recall any of the intraoperative events, even when movement was observed during conduct of anaesthesia. The technique had the disadvantage that it could not be used in prolonged procedures because of the danger of ischaemia to muscles.

Electroencephalography

The electroencephalogram (EEG) can be obtained by a standard 19-electrode technique which detects voltages of $1-50\mu V$. The resulting waveforms comprise α, β, δ and θ waves. With increasing depth of anaesthesia, there is a progressive increase in signal amplitude with reduced frequency (burst suppression). Clearly, interpretation of complex waveforms is time consuming and requires specialised training. This limits the clinical utility of the raw EEG. A processed EEG is far more valuable. Fast Fourier transformation can be used to separate the raw EEG into a number of component sine waves. EEG is essentially summation of many sine waves of different frequency and amplitude. The '0' crossing method measures time between adjacent points where signal crosses the 0 baseline. The derived parameters, spectral edge frequency and median frequency describe the entire EEG as a single value. Spectral edge frequency (SEF) represents the frequency below which 95% of EEG power is obtained. The median frequency (MF) is the point at which 50% of EEG power lies above and below this value. Both SEF and MF values correlate with clinical measures of depth of anaesthesia but changes in values are not consistent for all anaesthetic agents. General limitations of EEG-based techniques are given in Table 29.5 and specific limitations of different EEG-based techniques are given in Table 29.6.

Processed or derived EEG techniques
Compressed spectral array

The compressed spectral array (CSA) is a processed EEG that provides a simplified analysis of brain activity. Separate time segments of EEG activity are recorded and the power contained within different frequencies calculated and displayed in a series of peaks and troughs. During deep anaesthesia, the peaks of the CSA shift from high frequencies to low frequency activity. The converse is true during recovery. Although CSA is more compact than raw data, it is still a complex display which takes time to interpret. Agent-dependent changes also limit its use.

SNAP™ and patient state index

SNAP™ is a processed EEG monitoring device. SNAP™ index is derived by analysing both the low (0–40 Hz) and high (80–320 Hz) frequency segments of EEG. Rapid analysis of both ends of the frequency spectrum can be useful during inductance and emergence. SNAP™ index correlated with propofol induced loss of conciousness in a recent study [9].

The patient state index (PSI), provides an objective assessment of depth of anaesthesia derived by quantitative analysis of the EEG (QEEG). The index is derived from retrospective analysis of multivariate changes in brain activity observed from loss to return of consciousness. In a study involving 176 surgical patients, PSI was obtained from QEEG, analysed

Table 29.5 General limitations of electroencephalography (EEG) based monitoring techniques.

Electrical interference from mains, diathermy, facial EMG
High electrode impedance
Excitatory anaesthetic agents (ketamine)
Inaccuracies with nitrous oxide based anaesthesia
EEG altered by pathophysiological events such as hypotension, hypoxia and hypercarbia
Pre-existing neuropathology (epilepsy, brain injury)

EMG, electromyography.

Table 29.6 Specific limitations of different electroencephalography (EEG) based monitoring techniques.

Technique	Methodology	Limitations
EEG	Monitors suppression of cerebral activity in response to anaesthesia	Time consuming Bulky Requires expert interpretation
Compressed spectral array	Bifrontal electrodes Fourier analysis of electrical signals	Changes in amplitude and frequency is agent specific
Bispectral index	Quantifies the phase relations of the EEG with power and frequency information to calculate a single numerical value	No evidence of a reduction in awareness with its use Poor predictor of movement response particularly when opiates used
Auditory evoked responses	Monitors EEG activity in response to acoustic stimuli via headphones	Confounding artefacts can alter evoked potentials Interpatient variability

from a 19-channel EEG recording [10]. After intravenous induction, anaesthesia was maintained with inhalation agents or narcotic/total intravenous anaesthesia (TIVA). The difference in the PSI values in different anaesthetic states was highly significant. The study showed that PSI can significantly predict the level of arousal in varying stages of anaesthetic delivery.

Bispectral index

Bispectral index (BIS) analysis combines power spectral analysis of phase relationships with the component sine waves. BIS was developed by recording EEG data for healthy adults who underwent repeated transitions between consciousness and unconsciousness using a variety of anaesthetic regimes. The EEG features that best correlated with clinical depth of sedation and anaesthesia were then fitted to a model. The resulting algorithm generates a bispectral index. BIS demonstrates a dose-dependent relationship with inhalation and hypnotic intravenous agents and correlates with clinical assessments of level of consciousness. This is agent independent.

The BIS monitor (Fig. 29.1) displays a real-time EEG trace acquired from a frontotemporal montage and generates a value on a continuous scale of 1–100. A value of 100 represents normal cortical electrical activity and 0 indicates cortical electrical silence. The

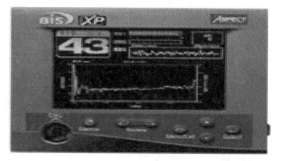

Figure 29.1 Bispectral index (BIS) monitor.

display also shows a signal quality index and an indicator of electromyographic (EMG) activity. The probability of postoperative recall is very low if the intraoperative BIS value is <60. However, BIS values vary considerably between patients. A value of 75 may be recorded in one patient who is unresponsive to command while the same value can be recorded in a patient who remains responsive.

The major drawback of using BIS to assess the depth of balanced anaesthesia is that it does not fully reflect the synergistic effect of opioids with hypnotic agents. Baseline BIS values are not reduced by nitrous oxide (inspired concentrations up to 50%). The addition of nitrous oxide to established anaesthesia has little effect on BIS in the absence of surgical stimulation. Ketamine causes EEG activation, complicating BIS interpretation. BIS is not able to predict movement in response to surgical stimulation because the generation of reflexes is likely to be at spinal cord rather than cortical level. Studies comparing BIS-titrated anaesthesia with clinical judgement of anaesthetic depth show reduced anaesthetic use and more rapid wakening using BIS. The inference is the use of excessively deep anesthesia in an attempt to avoid awareness. However, the concern is that emphasis is placed upon maintaining a target BIS value with a potential for increasing the risk of awareness.

Evoked responses

Evoked responses are derived from the EEG in response to auditory (audible clicks in auditory canal), somatosensory (tibial or peroneal nerve stimulation) and visual stimuli (flashes of light). There is increase in latency and decrease in amplitude of mid-latency auditory evoked responses (MLAER) as transition response to various types of stimuli which forms the basis of monitoring the evoked responses. Following the stimulus, EEG over the representing area (auditory, somatosensory or occipital cortex) is recorded. Averaging of the signal results in cancellation of random background noise and clear waveform of EEG can be recorded. Successful eliciting of an evoked response confirms presence of intact nervous pathways between receptors and cortex.

Recording and analysis of evoked responses

Bipolar electrodes are used with an active electrode placed on the scalp overlying the auditory, visual or somatosensory cortex. The electric potential difference between an inactive electrode placed on the centre of the scalp and an active electrode is recorded to analyse the evoked response.

Auditory, visual and somatosensory evoked responses

Increasing the depth of anaesthesia affects a specific segment of all types of evoked responses. Clearly, visual evoked responses cannot be used during anaesthesia as these need an awake patient to focus on a board. Visual flashes can be used in a sleeping patient but the method is not very accurate. Somato-

sensory evoked responses recorded in the cortex are affected by analgesic agents and not by increasing depth of anaesthesia with propofol and hence are not very reliable for monitoring depth of anaesthesia.

Auditory evoked responses

Most research with respect to depth of anaesthesia has been undertaken using auditory evoked responses (AER). Because of the small size of the signal it is necessary to average multiple individual signals over a period of 30–120 s and then extract the evoked response from the background spontaneous EEG (noise). The auditory evoked response can be subdivided into brainstem, early or middle latency and delayed cortical responses (Figs 29.2 and 29.3) and these reflect the electrical activity at various points of auditory pathway between cochlea and auditory cortex (Table 29.7). Goldstein and Rodman labelled the waves in the AER as No, Po, Na, Pa and Nb, occurring at latencies of 8–10, 10–13, 16–30, 30–45 and 45–60 msec respectively [11] (Table 29.7).

Brainstem evoked responses are not affected by intravenous anaesthetic agents and late cortical responses are too sensitive and can be abolished by sedative and anaesthetic agents; hence none of these can be used to monitor the depth of anaesthesia. Early cortical responses take place between the awake state and increasing depth of anaesthesia. Thornton et al. [12] confirmed a reduction of amplitude of cortical responses in patients under thiopentone, halothane and nitrous oxide anaesthesia. An increase in amplitude of N_b and P_b/P_c waves was observed following surgical stimulation. The study confirmed the role of AER in monitoring the depth of anaesthesia.

Auditory evoked potential index

This mathematical derivative is calculated by recording the difference between two segments of an auditory evoked response curve. Difficulty in analysing the auditory evoked responses in clinical settings led to evaluation of the auditory evoked potential (AEP) index to monitor the depth of anaesthesia. Gajraj et al. [13] compared BIS, AEP index, 95% SEF and MF for monitoring depth of anaesthesia in surgical patients under propofol anaesthesia. Mean values during conscious and unconscious state were 60.8 and 37.6 (AEP index), 85.1 and 66.8 (BIS), 24.2 and

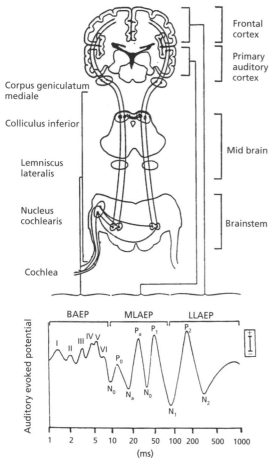

Figure 29.2 Auditory pathways and auditory evoked potentials. From Schwender *et al.* [19] with permission. BAEP, brainstem auditory evoked potential; LLAEP, long latency auditory evoked potential; MLAEP, mid-latency auditory evoked potential.

Table 29.7 Interpretation of Bispectral index (BIS) values.

BIS values	Condition
100	Awake
65–85	Sedation
45–65	General anaesthesia
<40	Burst suppression
0	No electrical activity

18.7 (SEF) and 10.9 and 9.8 (MF), respectively. AEP index was best in detecting transition from unconsciousness to consciousness.

In the case of AER, brainstem responses are recorded as five positive peaks labelled in roman numerals and cortical responses are recorded as a series of positive (P_o, P_a, P_1, P_2) and negative (N_o, N_a, N_b, N_1, N_2) peaks (Fig. 29.2). The AER peaks generated from the brainstem (<10 ms) are followed by mid-latency potentials (10–50 s) and then the late cortical response. The brainstem responses are relatively insensitive to general anaesthesia. Delayed cortical responses are abolished by sleep, sedation and deep anaesthesia and hence are not ideal for monitoring the depth of anaesthesia. However, MLAER are depressed during anaesthesia. The amplitudes of the peaks decrease and the latencies of the peaks are prolonged in a dose-dependent manner. During anaesthesia, persistent MLAER with latency of N_b wave less than 40 ms may indicate insufficient blockade of auditory processing with the risk of intraoperative awareness. Various factors can affect AER independently of anaesthesia (Table 29.8).

Agreement between EEG-based techniques

Various methods have been used to monitor the depth of anaesthesia. An ideal monitor should be able to predict spontaneous movement before the procedure in the presence of inadequate depth of anaesthesia. In one study, a laryngeal mask airway (LMA) was inserted after commencing a target controlled infusion comprising propofol and alfentanil [14]. The effectiveness of AEP index, BIS, 95% SEF and MF was assessed to predict spontaneous movement in response to insertion of the LMA. Values were analysed 30 s before LMA insertion. The AEP index was the most reliable predictor of movement (prediction probability 0.872) in response to LMA insertion.

Another study compared AEP index and BIS in assessing depth of anaesthesia and emergence from anaesthesia in spontaneously breathing surgical patients [15]. Measurements were recorded while patients were both conscious and unconscious following computer-controlled propofol

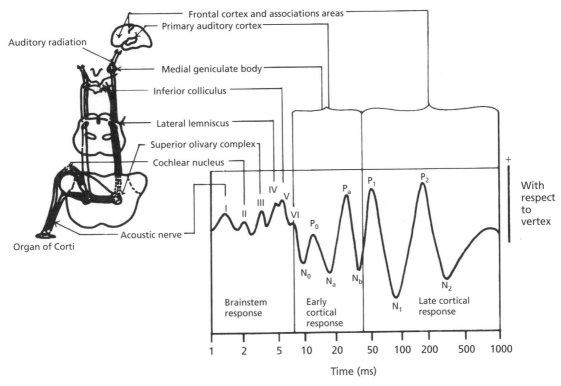

Figure 29.3 Anatomy of auditory pathway and auditory evoked responses (AER). From Thornton [20] with permission.

Table 29.8 Auditory evoked responses (AE) [11].

Components of AER	Anatomical site of origin	Waveform	Latency (ms)	IV or inhalation agents	Monitor depth of anaesthesia?
Brainstem responses	Cochlear nerve Cochlear nucleus Superior olivary Complex lateral/ leminiscus Inferior colliculus	I II III IV & V	Up to 10	Not affected by propofol Increased latency with isoflurane and enflurane	No
Early cortical or middle latency responses	Medial geniculate body Primary auditory cortex	N_o P_o N_a P_a N_b	8–10 10–13 16–30 30–45 40–60	Dose-dependent increase in latency and reduction in amplitude with propofol, isoflurane and enflurane	Latency and amplitude of P_a and N_b wave used to monitor depth of anaesthesia
Late cortical responses	Frontal cortex and associated areas	P_1, N_1 P_2, N_2	50–1000	Can be abolished by anaesthetic agents	No

Table 29.8 Factors that may influence auditory evoked response (AER).

Variable	Example
Physiological variables	Hypothermia
	Hyperthermia
Psychophysiological factors	Habituation
	Vigilance
	Attention
Pathophysiological factors	Conductive and sensory hearing disorders
	Demyelinating diseases
	Ischaemia
	Coma
	Tumours

anaesthesia. The mean AEP index recorded during the conscious and unconscious state were 74.5 (standard deviation 14.7) and 36.7 (SD 7.1), respectively. BIS was 89.5 (SD 4.6) and 48.8 (SD 16.4), respectively. Obviously, values were greater in conscious state but, compared with BIS, the average awake values of the AEP index were significantly higher than average values during unconsciousness. Transition from the unconscious to conscious state was detected better by AEP index. BIS value increased gradually during emergence from anaesthesia in this study.

Propofol and remifentanil anaesthesia was administered in 19 female patients who were undergoing minor gynaecological surgery. Prediction probability was used to analyse the ability of the above-mentioned parameters to differentiate different depth of anaesthesia, awake versus loss of response, awake versus anaesthesia, anaesthesia versus first reaction and anaesthesia versus extubation. The SNAP™ index and BIS were superior to mean arterial blood pressure and heart rate and SEF in distinguishing between different steps of anaesthesia [16].

Respiratory sinus arrhythmia and heart rate variability

Heart rate varies with phases of respiration and this forms the principle of use of this parameter for monitoring the depth of anaesthesia through continuous recording of high-resolution electrocardiography (ECG) and the respiratory cycle. Respiratory sinus arrhythmia (RSA) increases or decreases with light and deep anaesthesia respectively and can be distinguished from pathological arrhythmias on a breath-to-breath analysis. It was concluded [17] that measurements of RSA could form the basis of a useful index of anaesthetic depth during isoflurane anaesthesia.

Minimum alveolar concentration

End-tidal concentration is an essential part of monitoring while administering low flow inhalation anaesthesia. Concentrations of inhalation anaesthetic agents correlates very closely with alveolar concentration. Minimal alveolar concentration (MAC) of an inhalation agent required to produce immobility in 50% of subjects in response to a noxious stimulus enables us to compare the potency of different agents. An adequate depth of anaesthesia prevents sympathetic stimulation and prevents awareness. MACbar is the minimum alveolar concentration of the agent required to prevent an adrenergic response in 50% of the subjects in response to standard noxious stimulus.

Although these indices guide us in setting up an adequate end-tidal concentration of inhalation agents, the ideal concentration can vary from patient to patient. Various factors such as age, hypothermia, use of nitrous oxide, sedatives and hypothyroidism can reduce the anaesthetic requirement. Use of TIVA is popular for several reasons (e.g. a low incidence of postoperative nausea and vomiting). Unlike the end-tidal concentration monitored during an inhalation technique, target concentrations recommended with use of a TIVA technique are not very reliable. There is significant pharmacokinetic and pharmacodynamic variability between patients, making it difficult to fix a single target concentration for all patients. Wide variation in the plasma concentration of propofol from the set target concentration has been reported [18].

Conclusions

There is no ideal monitor for depth of anaesthesia. Fortunately, awareness under anaesthesia is very

Table 29.9 Causes of awareness.

Cause	Example	Explanation
Faulty technique	Light anaesthesia	Patients with poor cardiac reserve Caesarean section
	Increased anaesthetic requirements	Age Tobacco smoking Regular use of cocaine, alcohol or amphetamines
Faulty apparatus	Equipment malfunction or misuse	Empty vaporizer Intravenous pump malfunction Delivery tubing disconnection

rare. The probability of awareness is higher in certain procedures and sequence induction. Decreases in the delivery of anaesthetic agents and provision of 100% oxygen in patients with unanticipated difficult airway can result in awareness (Table 29.9). In the absence of a perfect monitor for the depth of anaesthesia, simple steps such as adequate premedication, equipment and vaporizer check, adequate induction dose and maintenance of optimum end-tidal concentration of inhalation agents are vital. The use of benzodiazepines and ear plugs in high risk patients should be considered. In addition to causing emotional trauma to the patient, awareness can be very stressful to the anaesthetist because of the medicolegal implications. Detailed and accurate documentation of clinical signs and events during anaesthesia is extremely important [6,7].

References

1 Eke Z, Bell K. Depth of anaesthesia. *CPD Anaesth* 2004; **6**: 140–2.
2 Sandin RH, Enlund G, Samuelsson P, Lenmarken C. Awareness during anaesthesia: a prospective study. *Lancet* 2000; **355**: 707–11.
3 Sebel PS, Bowdle TA, Ghoneim MM, *et al.* The incidence of awareness during anaesthesia. *Anesth Analg* 2004; **99**: 833–9.
4 Davidson AJ, Huang GH, Czarnecki C, *et al.* Awareness during anesthesia in children. *Anesth Analg* 2005; **100**: 653–61.
5 Griffith D, Jones JB. Awareness and memory in anaesthetized patients. *Br J Anaesth* 1990; **65**: 603–7.
6 Cobcroft MD, Forsdick C. Awareness under anaesthesia: the patient's point of view. *Anaesth Intensive Care* 1993; **21**: 837–43.
7 Liu WH, Thorp TA, Graham SG, Aitkenhead AR. Incidence of awareness with recall during anaesthesia. *Anaesthesia* 1991: **46**: 435–7.
8 Evans JM. Pain and awareness during general anaesthesia. *Lancet* 1987; **2**: 1033.
9 Wong CA, Fragen RJ, Fitzgerald PC, McCarthy RJ. The association between propofol induced loss of consciousness and SNAP index. *Anesth Analg* 2005; **100**: 141–8.
10 Prichep LS, Gugino LD, John ER, *et al* The Patient State Index as an indicator of the level of hypnosis under general anaesthesia. *Br J Anaesth* 2004; **92**: 393–9.
11 Goldstein R, Rodinan LB. Early components of averaged evoked responses to rapidly repeated auditory stimuli. *J Speech Hear Res* 1967; **10**: 697–705.
12 Thornton C, Sharpe RM. Evoked responses in anaesthesia. *Br J Anaesth* 1998; **81**: 771–81.
13 Gajraj RJ, Doi M, Mantzaridis H, Kenny GNC. Analysis of the EEG bispectrum, auditory evoked potentials and the EEG power spectrum during repeated transition from consciousness to unconsciousness. *Br J Anaesth* 1998; **80**: 46–52.
14 Doi M, Gajraj RJ, Mantzaridis H, Kenny GNC. Prediction of movement at laryngeal mask airway insertion: comparison of auditory evoked potential index, bispectral index, spectral edge frequency and median frequency. *Br J Anaesth* 1999; **82**: 203–7.
15 Gajraj RJ, Doi M, Mantzaridis H, Kenny GNC. Comparison of bispectral EEG analysis and auditory evoked potentials for monitoring depth of anaesthesia during propofol anaesthesia. *Br J Anaesth* 1999; **82**: 672–8.

16 Schmidt GN, Bischoff P, Standl T, *et al*. SNAP index and Bispectral index during different states of propofol/remifentanil anaesthesia. *Anaesthesia* 2005; **60**: 228–34.

17 Pomfrett CJ, Sneyd JR, Barrie JR, Healy TE. Respiratory sinus arrythmia: comparison with EEG indices during isoflurane anaesthesia at 0.65 and 1.2 MAC. *Br J Anaesth* 1994; **72**: 397–402.

18 Hoymork SC, Raeder J, Grimsmo B, Steen PA. Bispectral index, serum drug concentration and emergence associated with individually adjusted target controlled infusions of remifentanil and propofol for laparoscopic surgery. *Br J Anaesth* 2003; **91**: 773–80.

19 Schwender D, Klasing S, Madler C, Poppel E, Peter K. Midlatency auditory evoked potentials and cognitive function during general anesthesia. *Int Anesthesiol Clin* 1993; **31**: 89–106.

20 Thornton C. Evoked potential in anaesthesia. *Eur J Anaesthesiol* 1991; **8**: 89–107.

CHAPTER 30
Research study design

John Robert Sneyd

Introduction

This chapter summarizes the key stages in conception, planning, organization, implementation, analysis and reporting of a research study. It is not intended to provide a 'recipe' but to offer general guidance and perhaps a checklist for inexperienced researchers.

Getting started

The idea

All research starts with an idea, which can arise from a clinical experience, a research publication or simply a comment made during a discussion. Critical to each is the genuine interest of the investigator. Ask yourself whether the question you are addressing is important. Investing time and effort into addressing questions that are in themselves essentially trivial is unfair on patients and proposals of this type may well be rejected by an ethical committee. An excellent example of clinical research beyond importance is the proliferation of studies describing different and in some cases bizarre techniques for attenuating or preventing pain on injection of propofol (Table 30.1) [1]. Pain on injection of propofol is easily modifiable by the addition of lidocaine [2] and it seems likely that the proliferation of clinical studies reflects their easy conduct rather than the actual importance of the topic.

Discussion

Take every opportunity to discuss your idea with your colleagues. Conferences and research meetings are excellent places to formulate research ideas in discussion with others who are active in the field and against a background of the latest developments. Although a novice researcher might feel anxious that their research idea will be used by someone else with whom they discuss it, in reality most researchers are delighted to find someone else interested in their own area and will commonly give constructive advice and encouragement. Remember that clinical studies often require significant numbers of patients and may be impracticable without collaboration between different centres — this may be your opportunity to find someone who can help you to recruit patients. Patients, their families and carers often have a completely different perspective on clinical matters from that held by doctors and scientists. Ethical committees and funding bodies are now very interested in the broader 'community' and will expect you to have considered this as well. At the simplest level, you could ask some patients what they think of your ideas; larger and more sophisticated schemes may involve focus groups or patient representatives. It is important to get this right if researchers are to deliver projects that matter to society as a whole. Bear in mind that charities and funding bodies commonly include patients and other lay representatives who will be looking for evidence that you have thought this through properly.

Literature search

A comprehensive literature search is vital, using more than just Medline; remember, there are broader databases such as EMBASE and possibly some nursing databases. Unless you are already an expert at computer searches, this is a good point at which to get help from your librarian. Getting the best out of a computer search takes time and experience [3]. Experienced researchers and colleagues are often a valuable source of information and someone who is an expert in the field or a related area may be

Table 30.1 Methods to alleviate or modify pain on injection with propofol which have been evaluated in randomized controlled trials. From Sneyd and the *British Journal of Anaesthesia* [1] with permission.

Local anaesthetics	Analgesics
Lidocaine	Fentanyl
EMLA cream	Ketorolac
Prilocaine	Tramadol
Lidocaine tape	Nafamostat mesilate
Lidocaine iontophoresis	Alfentanil
Technique modifications	Anaesthetic agents
5-μm filter	Nitrous oxide
Carrier fluid	Thiopental
Large vein	Ketamine
Speed of injection	
Aspiration of blood	Other drugs
	Ephedrine
Antiemetics	Magnesium sulphate
Metoclopramide	Neostigmine
Granisetron	Clonidine
Dolasetron	Nitroglycerin
Ondansetron	

aware of other unpublished (or sometimes published) information that is not easily found.

Hypothesis

All research must test a hypothesis. For example, one does not just 'try out remifentanil on neurosurgical patients', rather, we evaluate the hypothesis that 'remifentanil offers superior haemodynamic stability and faster recovery than another (specified) technique'. Your project must be described in terms of a hypothesis.

Endpoints

The measure you will use to test your hypothesis must be considered. Increasingly, we look to researchers to provide information about outcomes rather than surrogate measures. For example, myocardial infarction, stroke and a death are important outcomes. Haemodynamic response to laryngoscopy, intraoperative blood pressure and heart rate are surrogates whose relevance to the important

outcomes is uncertain. Those considering your proposal for funding or ethical approval will want convincing that your endpoints are meaningful [4]. Consider the patient/consumer perspective. Will you be considering patient satisfaction or other endpoints that may seem unimportant to doctors but are valued highly by patients?

The protocol

When you are clear what your hypothesis is and have organized your thoughts about how you are going to test it, it is time to write a protocol. This is a critical point in the life of a project as it forces you to think clearly about the practicalities. The most comprehensive protocols are those used by the pharmaceutical industry in commercial clinical trials. Start with one of these and write your own, using the headings as appropriate and omitting those that are not relevant. Section headings that you can use when writing a protocol are listed in Table 30.2.

Patients

Clinical research requires adequate numbers of patients. The size of your treatment groups will be determined by a power calculation. Although it is possible to make a power calculation yourself using resources available within statistical packages or from Internet sites, it is generally sensible to discuss your project with a statistician. He or she will want to know what is the most important endpoint (i.e. the endpoint against which you want the sample size and study power to be calculated). For this endpoint, they will require a measure of variability, typically a standard deviation (if the data are normally distributed) from a previous patient population. Thus, if a study concerns change in blood pressure after a clinical intervention, then the statistician would want to know the standard deviation of systolic arterial pressure before intervention and an estimate of a change that would be considered important. Thus, the estimated standard deviation might be 20 mmHg and the clinically important change may be 25 mmHg. Finally, they will ask for the acceptable α and β errors. These are the probability of avoiding false positive and false negative results and are typically 0.05 and 0.08, respectively, although commercial

Table 30.2 Headings list for writing a clinical trial protocol.

Study personnel	Who is doing the work and how can they be contacted?
Timescale and locations	When and where is the study to happen?
Protocol summary	
Introduction and rationale for the study	Background to the study, why it is being done?
Study objectives	Objectives (primary and secondary)
Regulatory and ethical aspects	Regulatory authority approval, ethics committee approval and patient consent
Study design	Number of patients, type of study: randomized controlled trial, cross-over, etc.
Study population	Patient enrolment, inclusion and exclusion criteria, provision for men and women, young and elderly, non-English speakers, special groups, etc.
Study treatment	Medication, packaging and labelling, dosage regimen, treatment assignments and preparation of study drug
Study procedures	Description of study phases, assessments, withdrawal of patients
Action to be taken in emergencies	
Statistics	General comments: sample size and power calculation, provision for interim analysis, background demographics, primary and secondary outcome measures, safety
Study monitoring procedures and quality assurance	How is the study to be monitored and by whom?
Termination of study	
Investigations obligations	Details of study staff, data recording, deviations from protocol and adverse event reporting
Procedure for breaking randomization code	
Storage and tracking of study supplies	
Disclosure of data	Data protection, confidentiality, regulatory authority, publications and intellectual property, study records and storage
Indemnity/study sponsor	Compensation for negligent and non-negligent harm, who is funding the study and who has overall responsibility?
Publication	Who has access to the data and who will write papers, etc? Agreements about authorship
Protocol amendments	

contract research commonly uses a more rigorous β error. Realistic consideration of whether this number of patients can be recruited in the timeframe proposed must be made. Operating room records or audit data will enable an estimation of numbers and hence feasibility. Where necessary, collaboration involving other centres may be used to increase patient recruitment. Finally, it is worth seeking opinions from the patients themselves and large research studies now include patient representatives in the planning process to achieve this.

Study design

Prospective double-blind randomized controlled trials are generally considered the most robust form of investigation. However, this methodology is not always appropriate. Sometimes an individual patient may undergo a particular treatment repeatedly (e.g. electroconvulsive therapy [ECT]). In these circumstances, a patient may receive a particular treatment on one occasion and a different treatment the next time. Thus, the patient undergoing ECT might participate in a cross-over trial between propofol and etomidate as the principal anaesthetic agent. Individual patients could be randomized as to which treatment they receive first and then receive the other treatment for their second anaesthetic. In cross-over studies where one treatment follows shortly after another (e.g. comparing different antihypertensive treatments), a washout period may be necessary and the effect of the first treatment may persist beyond the end of the period during which it was administered. These types of study require statistical manipulation and invariably merit input from a statistician. Sometimes the therapeutic intervention cannot be contained within a single patient; thus, an investigation to determine the effect of a dedicated acute pain nurse visiting patients after surgery could not simply randomize individual patients to this intervention or not. Were that done, then patients in adjacent beds could be randomized to opposite regimes and it is possible that some effect of the nurse visit to the 'active' treatment group might influence the outcome of the 'control' patient. Cluster randomization allocates patients in larger groups to fit with the operational realities of the clinical environment. In the circumstance described above, the cluster might comprise a whole surgical ward or perhaps a single bay within it. An alternative approach to cluster randomization is to give 15–20 consecutive patients the same intervention, then to have a washout period when the particular ward has no nurse visit, and then for the alternative treatment to be allocated for 15–20 patients.

Randomization

In a randomized trial, patients are distributed between alternative treatments by chance. This process, if properly conducted, avoids bias by the investigating team deciding how an individual patient is to be treated. Successful randomization strategies ensure that the patient's treatment allocation is made at the last possible moment, is independent of the allocation of previous patients and that there is an identifiable audit trail allowing confirmation that the treatment assigned is that which was originally intended. Random allocations of individual patients are summarized in a randomization table which is prepared before the start of the trial. The table is maintained in a secure environment and withheld from the investigators. At the time that each treatment allocation is made, there should be no access to details of subsequent allocations.

Randomization is a key principle of most clinical trials and was first used in the Medical Research Council (MRC) streptomycin study published in 1948 [5]. In a properly randomized study, the allocation of a patient's treatment is entirely determined by chance. Allocation of patients to treatments according to the initial letters of their surname, days of the week or giving particular treatments to consecutive or individual patients are not random and are subject to bias. The simplest method of randomization is to toss a coin and allocate 'heads' to one treatment and 'tails' to another. Apart from the weariness of repeated coin tossing for a large clinical trial, this method of randomization does not guarantee that group sizes will be equal; indeed, it is unlikely that they will be. Drawing from a bag of equal numbers of coloured beads will give two equal-sized treatment groups but it is possible that all the patients receiving one treatment might precede all those receiving the other or (more likely) that the treatments are relatively unevenly distributed throughout the period of the study. If there is some possibility that a study might be terminated early or there are doubts about the total number of patients that may be recruited, then additional measures can keep the treatment groups relatively symmetrical while maintaining secrecy. If random allocations are made in blocks of N, where N is a multiple of the number of treatment groups, then each time a block of N patients has been entered into the trial, the treatment groups will be of equal size. If the block size was to be 2, then after each individual treatment allocation it would be possible to guess which one came next. In practice, larger blocks (10–20 patients) are used and the block size is not necessarily known by the investigator. Sometimes a study compares a new with a well-established treatment, and in addition to hypothesis testing between the two treatments it is also considered desirable to obtain experience with the new treatment. This is commonly the case with new pharmaceuticals, and in such cases the treatment groups may be deliberately made unequal with (perhaps) twice as many patients receiving the new treatment as the comparator. Although this reduces the statistical power of the study, it yields important safety data to support the licensing of a new compound.

Blinding

Ideally, the staff giving care or treatment, the patient and staff making assessments or measurements should be unaware of which treatment a patient has received but this is sometimes easier said than done. Blinding increases study costs by involving more staff and necessitating special arrangements for the preparation of drugs, etc. Whereas a single bolus injection of a clear intravenous drug may easily be blinded against a saline placebo, the situation is much more difficult for other types of treatment. Few tablets are identical and comparing two oral medications therefore requires specially prepared placebos. In addition, modern pharmaceutical practice may involve special physical formulation such as slow release where even if a placebo is involved, it is impossible to disguise another compound to look the same and still maintain its original performance. In these circumstances, a design known as double-blind,

double-dummy can be used in which each active treatment has a matched placebo and patients receive two 'treatments' at once, one being active and the other being the placebo version of the other group.

Physical differences between treatments may be extreme. Consider a study comparing propofol and sevoflurane; while it is possible to have the sevoflurane vaporizer concealed from the clinician and to use a lipid emulsion to mimic propofol, there are still difficulties around end-tidal gas analysis or target controlled infusion systems. In addition, the application of double-blind, double-dummy techniques in a complex clinical environment such as the outpatient room adds layers of complexity and might, in certain circumstances, compromise patient safety. If the treatments themselves cannot be safely blinded, then an appropriate compromise may be to conceal the treatments from the patient and to ensure that, wherever possible, staff making assessments do so using rigorous measures and preferably without knowledge of the treatment allocations. Thus, in the propofol/sevoflurane study described above, assessments of postoperative nausea and vomiting might be undertaken by a research nurse unaware of which treatment a patient had received.

An excellent example of rigorous methodology applied to an important clinical question tackled the question of epidural regional anaesthesia with local anaesthetic versus systemic opioids administered by patient controlled analgesia. A double-blind, double-dummy design used two pumps for each patient with one infusing into the epidural space and the other administering an intravenous solution. This allowed full blinding of the study, which addressed outcomes from elective aortic surgery. However, consideration of this trial design shows that the double-blind, double-dummy design offered at least some opportunity for serious patient harm should the local anaesthetic solution have been inadvertently administered intravenously. Note also that the addition of blinding will not salvage a study whose design is otherwise flawed (e.g. underpowered) or simply a wrong design.

Research pharmacists can give good information on drug blinding and will commonly prepare identical solutions for perioperative drug administration.

While offering the highest level of service, these arrangements are time consuming and costly and the pharmacy will often require a substantial period of notice before a patient's treatment which may significantly compromise patient recruitment. A cheaper alternative is to ask another clinician to prepare the drug out of sight of the investigator. Provided the person preparing the drug is clear as to what is required and has detailed written instructions, then adequately blinded design can be achieved at reduced cost.

Sham treatments

While sham surgery is unlikely to be relevant to most clinical circumstances, it has a role and was recently used to demonstrate that knee washout was of no benefit to patients with osteoarthritis [6]. Sham treatments may be applied in other situations such as radiotherapy or hyperbaric treatment in which the patient can be placed in the clinical apparatus and exposed to all aspects of the treatment except the actual intervention (radiation or increased barometric pressure, respectively).

Some therapies may be directly detectable by the patient. For example, electroacupuncture and iontophoresis produce physical sensations inside the skin and are difficult to fully blind.

Certain drugs may appear physically similar but require special arrangements for blinding because of their different clinical characteristics. For example, remifentanil is typically given by small volume bolus injections and a continuous infusion whereas fentanyl is given as a single or small number of bolus doses and, if infused, must be stopped well in advance of the end of anaesthesia if the patient is to recover consciousness in a reasonable period. Designing a study to compare fentanyl and remifentanil required complex double-blind, double-dummy and despite this, the 'standard' regimen of application for each drug was to some extent compromised [7,8].

Personnel

Consideration should be given as to who will execute this project. Will a research nurse or the help of other members of staff be required? Research staff are expected to have appropriate training for their roles

within the study and, as a minimum, the principal investigator and other key personnel should be thoroughly familiar with the protocol and have received training in good clinical practice (GCP). Typically, this would be locally organized by institution research and development officers, but expect that ethical committees and potential funders will want to know about your competence to undertake the work you propose. Charitable bodies and other funders are interested in supporting successful projects; to this end, they are interested not only in whether your research question is meaningful, but also your competence to execute the study, write it up afterwards and then disseminate the results properly. Research groupings that are collaborative, involve a mixture of experienced — as well as less experienced — researchers and bring together complementary abilities in the delivery of the project are more likely to be funded than single-handed inexperienced researchers with no track record of research completion or publication.

Funding

There are essentially four options: drug companies, grants, 'soft' money and minimal cost projects.

Drug companies

The pharmaceutical industry usually has plenty of money but is, of course, very focused on the relevance of research to its individual products. Preference is most likely to be given to projects that will help them to obtain a product licence or develop the 'profile' of their drug.

Grant applications

The art of writing grant applications is beyond the scope of this review. However, it is clear that a plausible hypothesis, a feasible project design, a capable researcher and a reputable research institution are prerequisites to success.

'Soft' money

No research is devoid of cost and institutions are increasingly interested in identifying how their staff spend their time. Expect to be questioned about the precise impact of your research activities on the institution's clinical work load, drug costs, office and other expenses and, in particular, staff time.

Low or no cost projects

A number of projects can be pursued for minimal costs. However, institutions are increasingly aware of the 'hidden' costs of research so be prepared for questioning as to whether your project is really as inexpensive as you maintain. In addition, there is a (minority) view that cheap research is no good.

Equipment

It is essential to consider what equipment is needed and to assess whether it is available on the occasions when you need it. There may also be access charges for specialized equipment which need to be fully costed.

Statistics

The time to involve a statistician is at the planning stage of any project, in order to assess how many patients are required to test the hypothesis and how data will be managed and analysed. Resources for performing power calculations may be found on the Internet [9] but this cannot replace statistical advice.

Good will

Consider the impact of your activities on members of staff, including the surgeon, the operating room nurses, the recovery and ward staff. Extra work for them may lead to difficulties and may hinder your progress unless you convince them that it is interesting and important, and reinforce this with courtesy and regular information.

Ethical approval

Ethical committee approval will be required for most studies involving patients. Sometimes the divide between audit, which does not require approval, and research, which does, is not too clear. Therefore, always submit an ethics application if there is any doubt. In addition, if you plan to study a drug outside its licensed indications, then you require regulatory approval to do so. In the UK, applications are submitted online using the website for the Central Office for Research Ethics Committees (COREC) at www. corec.org.uk. Applications are made through COREC regardless of location in the UK, then allocated to a local research ethics committee (LREC). Multicentre studies should be submitted to a regional multicentre ethics committee for your region (MREC) also through the COREC website. LRECs also require evidence of good science — usually in the form of peer review of the proposed project.

Indemnity

If you are simply comparing two existing treatments, and if both are in current use, you may be able to argue that no indemnity is required. When testing a new drug or experimental equipment, indemnity must be provided. This may be provided by a private company, the university or additional insurance. Your LREC will require evidence of indemnity provision.

Preparing to start the study

A pilot study is often useful, which may require LREC approval even though it is a pilot study.

Pilot study

Pilot data may allow a critical decision whether to proceed with a larger study. In addition, unexpected difficulties in implementing the protocol can be resolved before committing to a much larger investigation. In addition, a pilot study will enable procurement of data required to undertake a power calculation.

Patient pack

Anaesthetists often recruit patients at a preoperative visit. Prepare yourself a small pack for each patient containing the information sheet, two copies of the consent form and the data recording form, and have these readily available so that you never miss an opportunity to recruit a patient.

Study box

Most research requires special documentation, drug

preparation or equipment. Consider a special box or bag containing all the items you need to study a patient. Prepare a comprehensive checklist including even the most mundane things that you need. If you run through this before you start, then you will not find yourself about to take a blood sample and then suddenly realizing that you do not have the necessary tubes, etc.

Case record form

You need a document (usually paper but possibly electronic in the future) into which you enter the data as you collect it. This needs to be very simple and clear, especially if it is to be used by others. Make sure that you record everything that you need for your analysis, otherwise you may find yourself going through a hundred sets of notes many months after you have completed the study in order to record the patient's weight or height!

Executing the study

In addition to the practical work of a study, you need to monitor the rate of patient recruitment and the impact of your activities on other professional groups (see above). Keep everybody happy and you should not have any problems.

Managing the paperwork

Where are you going to store the case record forms, the consent forms, etc? What are you going to write in the patients' notes? What are your arrangements for confidentiality? How are you going to enter the data on to the computer and what are the implications of this? Remember, data protection legislation requires you to notify the Data Protection Officer and they will require details of whether identifiable patient information is to be entered on the computer (usually it should not be) and who will have access. There are also restrictions on transferring data outside your institution (e.g. to a collaborator at another centre). These issues will also be considered by the ethics committee.

Analysis and report

When you have completed the study, analyse the data as agreed with your statistician and prepare a study report. This should be a comprehensive listing of all the data that you have recorded together with an appropriate analysis. In a commercial study, this can be hundreds of pages long and will represent many months of work in a data processing department. For a smaller study, it is obviously a lesser task but do look at all of your data and sort it out properly. When this is complete, you can identify which components of your results are interesting and important and submit them for publication.

Publicizing your results

Abstract

Take the relevant parts of your data (identified above) and present them as an abstract to a meeting. This is an excellent opportunity to obtain feedback on your efforts and will help you to write a better paper.

Writing the paper

This is the final stage of the process and one that if omitted, renders the research pointless. Several reviews give advice on how to do this [10,11].

References

1 Sneyd JR. Recent advances in intravenous anaesthesia. *Br J Anaesth* 2004; **93**: 725–36.
2 Scott RP, Saunders DA, Norman J. Propofol: clinical strategies for preventing the pain of injection. *Anaesthesia* 1988; **43**: 492–4.
3 Greenhalgh T. How to read a paper. The Medline database. *Br Med J* 1997; **315**: 180–3.
4 Fisher DM. Surrogate outcomes: meaningful not! *Anesthesiology* 1999; **90**: 355–6.
5 Committee MRCSiTT. Streptomycin treatment of pulmonary tuberculosis. *Br Med J* 1948; **ii**: 769–83.
6 Moseley JB, O'Malley K, Petersen NJ, *et al*. A controlled trial of arthroscopic surgery for osteoarthritis of the knee. *N Engl J Med* 2002; **347**: 81–8.
7 Coles JP, Leary TS, Monteiro JN, *et al*. Propofol anesthesia for craniotomy: a double-blind comparison of remifentanil, alfentanil, and fentanyl. *J Neurosurg Anesthesiol* 2000; **12**: 15–20.
8 Guy J, Hindman BJ, Baker KZ, *et al*. Comparison of remifentanil and fentanyl in patients undergoing

craniotomy for supratentorial space-occupying lesions. *Anesthesiology* 1997; **86**: 514–24.

9 Schoenfeld DA. Statistical considerations for clinical trials and scientific experiments. http://hedwig.mgh.harvard.edu/size.html

10 Chambers DW. How to write a research paper. *J Am Coll Dentists* 1997; **64**: 53–6.

11 Bender AE. How to write a scientific paper. *J R Soc Health* 1997; **117**: 17–9.

Index